PROTECTING CHILDREN AND YOUNG PEOPLE
Trauma Informed Care in the Perinatal Period

Protecting Children and Young People series

Sharon Vincent, *Learning from Child Deaths and Serious Abuse in Scotland* (2010)

Anne Stafford, Sharon Vincent and Nigel Parton (eds) *Child Protection Reform across the United Kingdom* (2010)

Kate Alexander and Anne Stafford, *Children and Organised Sport* (2011)

Sharon Vincent, *Preventing Child Deaths: Learning from Review* (2013)

Julie Taylor and Anne Lazenbatt, *Child Maltreatment and High Risk Families* (2014)

Caroline Bradbury-Jones, *Children as Co-researchers: The Need for Protection* (2014)

Sharon Vincent (ed.), *Early Intervention: Supporting and Strengthening Families* (2015)

Jane Appleton and Sue Peckover (eds) *Child Protection, Public Health and Nursing* (2015)

Julia Seng and Julie Taylor (eds) *Trauma Informed Care in the Perinatal Period* (2015)

See www.dunedinacademicpress.co.uk for details of all our publications

Editorial Advisory Board

PROTECTING CHILDREN AND YOUNG PEOPLE
SERIES EDITORS
JOHN DEVANEY
School of Sociology, Social Policy and Social Work,
Queen's University Belfast
and JULIE TAYLOR
School of Health and Population Sciences, University of Birmingham
and SHARON VINCENT
Social Work and Communities, Northumbria University, Newcastle

Trauma Informed Care in the Perinatal Period

Edited by

Julia Seng

*Professor of Nursing, Obstetrics and Women's Studies at the
University of Michigan, USA*

and Julie Taylor

*NSPCC Professor of Child Protection, School of Health and
Population Sciences, University of Birmingham, UK*

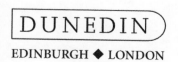

EDINBURGH ◆ LONDON

Published by Dunedin Academic Press Limited

Head Office:
Hudson House, 8 Albany Street, Edinburgh EH1 3QB

London Office:
352 Cromwell Tower, Barbican, London EC2Y 8NB

bitlit

A **free** eBook edition is available
with the purchase of this print book.

CLEARLY PRINT YOUR NAME ABOVE IN UPPER CASE
Instructions to claim your free eBook edition:
1. Download the BitLit app for Android or iOS
2. Write your name in **UPPER CASE** on the line
3. Use the BitLit app to submit a photo
4. Download your eBook to any device

ISBNs:
978-1-78046-053-6 (Paperback)
978-1-78046-545-6 (ePub)
978-1-78046-546-3 (Kindle edition)

ISSN: 1756-0691

© Dunedin Academic Press 2015
The right of Julia Seng, Julie Taylor and the contributors to be identified as the authors of their parts of this work has been asserted by them in accordance with sections 77 and 78 of the Copyright, Designs and Patents Act 1988

British Library Cataloguing in Publication data
A catalogue record for this book is available at the British Library

Typeset by Makar Publishing Production, Edinburgh, Scotland
Printed and bound by CPI Group (UK) Ltd, Croydon, CR0 4YY

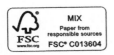

MIX
Paper from
responsible sources
FSC® C013604

CONTENTS

THE CONTRIBUTORS

Seng, Sperlich, Fisher, Rowe, Cuthbert and Taylor have been collaborating across countries for a number of years on child abuse, stress and the early years (CASEY). For this book the CASEY collaboration was joined by graduate students Acton and Choi.

Australia
Jane Fisher, BSc (Hons), PhD MAPS, is Jean Hailes Professor of Women's Health and Director of the Jean Hailes Research Unit in the School of Public Health and Preventive Medicine at Monash University. She has been Consultant Clinical Psychologist to Masada Private Hospital Mother Baby Unit, which is a twenty-bed, residential, early parenting service in Melbourne, since 1996.

Heather Rowe, BSc (Hons), PhD, is a health scientist with a background in the biological and psychological sciences and health promotion. She is Senior Research Fellow in the Jean Hailes Research Unit School of Public Health and Preventive Medicine at Monash University. Her research interests are in mental health during the perinatal life phase, including the impact of trauma on women and their health caregivers.

Catherine Acton, BSc, GDipEdPsych, MPsych (Clinical), MAPS, is a clinical psychologist working in a perinatal emotional health team at a large public maternity hospital in Melbourne, Australia. She has recently completed a PhD that investigated the impact of traumatic life events on mental health in pregnancy and adjustment following childbirth. She has a particular interest in the impact of early abuse and neglect experiences upon the transition to parenthood.

United States of America

Julia S. Seng, PhD, CNM, RN, FAAN, one of the volume editors, is a nurse-midwife and Professor of Nursing, Obstetrics, and Women's Studies at the University of Michigan in the United States. Her research focuses on the effects of post-traumatic stress disorder (PTSD) on women's health and childbearing outcomes, biological mechanisms, and interventions.

Mickey Sperlich, PhD, MSW, CPM, is an experienced midwife and Assistant Professor of Social Work at the State University of New York at Buffalo. She researches the effects of trauma and mental health challenges on childbearing and parenting and develops trauma informed perinatal interventions.

Kristen R. Choi, BSN, RN, is a nurse and PhD student at the University of Michigan School of Nursing. Her research examines trauma-related psychopathology, self-dysregulation, and health service delivery for children who have been abused and exploited.

United Kingdom

Chris Cuthbert is the Head of Strategy and Development for Children Under One at the UK's National Society for the Prevention of Cruelty to Children (NSPCC). He is in charge of fostering prevention initiatives for the zero-to-ones, including developing an evidence base for programmes that are showing the greatest promise.

Julie Taylor, PhD, RN, MSc, BSc (Hons), FRCN, is an editor in this Dunedin Academic Press series on Protecting Children and Young People. She is Professor of Child Protection in the School of Health and Population Sciences at the University of Birmingham. Her research is centred around families with complex needs.

GLOSSARY OF ABBREVIATIONS

AAP	American Academy of Pediatrics
ACE	Adverse Childhood Experiences
ACNM	American College of Nurse-Midwives
ACOG	American College of Obstetricians and Gynecologists
APA	American Psychiatric Association
CASEY	Child Abuse, Stress and the Early Years
CBT	Cognitive Behavioural Therapy
CFT	Compassion Focused Therapy
DSM	Diagnostic and Statistical Manual of Mental Disorders
EMDR	Eye Movement Desensitization and Reprocessing
FNP	Family Nurse Partnership
HPA	Hypothalamic-pituitary-adrenal
LHT	Life History Theory
NCTIC	National Center for Trauma-Informed Care
NICE	The National Institute for Health and Clinical Excellence
NSPCC	National Society for the Prevention of Cruelty to Children
OECD	Organization for Economic Cooperation and Development
PIP	Parent–Infant Psychotherapy
PTSD	Post-Traumatic Stress Disorder
PUP	Parents Under Pressure
SAMHSA	Substance Abuse and Mental Health Services Administration
STACY	Stress, Trauma, Anxiety and the Childbearing Year
WHO	World Health Organization

CHAPTER 1

Why trauma informed care in the perinatal period?

Julia Seng, University of Michigan

Introduction

Traumatic stress, a component of both toxic stress and intergenerational patterns, adversely affects population health. Traumatic stress caused by child maltreatment is often unresolved for women prior to pregnancy, with implications for her obstetric experience and subsequent relationship with her child. In order to improve perinatal outcomes and long-term health for individuals and at the population level, an emphasis on psychosocial care that is informed by a knowledge about trauma is crucial.

Professionals who work toward optimising child welfare, development and health know that preventing maltreatment is crucial both for individual outcomes and for society. Professionals who care for childbearing women in perinatal settings also realise that it is important to get the mother–infant dyad off to the best possible start. In the past, service delivery to pregnant women has been weighted towards a medical model, giving highest priority to surveillance and treatment for high-risk obstetric conditions and providing maternal support services as a secondary level of care added to address needs of vulnerable women. Currently, this prioritisation is shifting to put medical and psychosocial care on a more even footing because it is becoming clearer to all that some of the intransigent perinatal, lifespan health, developmental and social problems have intergenerational patterns that start in pregnancy.

Research across numerous academic disciplines is now demonstrating that childhood maltreatment trauma is a very important factor in patterns of deprivation, psychiatric vulnerability, ill health and violence. These problems warrant primary prevention for the infant to begin *in utero*. This presents an opportunity for child welfare professionals and maternity professionals to collaborate in creating new service delivery models that provide trauma informed care across the perinatal period – across pregnancy, birth and the 'fourth trimester' that includes the early weeks of parenting.

This book takes a broad definition of child maltreatment, in accordance with the World Health Organization policy:

Child maltreatment, sometimes referred to as child abuse and neglect, includes all forms of physical and emotional ill-treatment, sexual abuse, neglect, and

1

exploitation that results in actual or potential harm to the child's health, development or dignity. Within this broad definition, five subtypes can be distinguished – physical abuse; sexual abuse; neglect and negligent treatment; emotional abuse; and exploitation (WHO 2014).

The purpose of this book is to provide an overview of information that child welfare and perinatal professionals can use to move towards providing trauma informed care and developing trauma-specific interventions to improve intergenerational trajectories.

In this first chapter we sketch what this new knowledge includes and provide an overview of what follows. More detail about the explanatory concepts prefaced here are dealt with in subsequent chapters.

A convergence of knowledge

Psychosocial care in the perinatal period is the next frontier in advancing maternal and infant outcomes – and indeed the well-being of society at large (Shonkoff *et al.*, 2012; Renfrew *et al.*, 2014). That is a rather sweeping statement. But by the time we lay out the information that supports the statement, we think you will agree. Likely you also will allow that we have 'known' most of this information for a long time (Herman, 1992). What is true at this moment, as we write in mid-2015, is that there now is a critical mass of research findings to provide a strong impetus to strengthen psychosocial perinatal care. These come from studies conducted in numerous populations and by asking questions from biological, psychological and social standpoints. Synthesis of results provides an impetus to act on what we have surmised for a long time.

Medical advances are not enough to improve the health of the population

Medical approaches to preventing and treating obstetric complications continue to make advances, but in smaller increments than in the past. Nations with advanced healthcare systems are seeing a plateau in improving rates of sentinel public health indicators of population problems, such as prematurity and low birth weight (Martin *et al.*, 2010). Costly technological interventions that disrupt physiological processes are increasing (Childbirth Connection, 2013). While there likely are benefits for individuals from medical advances, the overall cost–benefit profile at the population level is not changing substantially. Addressing many of the remaining sources of morbidity and mortality requires that we look from the pregnant woman's position outward, to her socio-ecological context, as well as inwards, to her individual health status and biology.

Our current division of labour along bio-psychosocial lines may need revising so that the perinatal care team is acting synergistically to redress the most widespread threats to well-being at the individual and population levels. As Shamian stated in the 2014 series on midwifery in *The Lancet*:

> Interprofessional collaboration is essential to provide quality healthcare in today's complex world, and to mitigate many of the challenges faced by health systems worldwide. Patients need the range of knowledge and skills that can only be found in a wide array of health professions. Additionally, collaborative practice must include the patient as the key player in the healthcare team (Shamian, 2014, p. e41).

Emerging new conceptualisations

The emerging focus on toxic stress as a concept being applied at the forefront in child well-being may help shift attention from focusing primarily on the individual woman's health and mothering behaviour to concentrating attention on her context – which likely is shared with a whole community or population of women (Shonkoff *et al.*, 2012). Environmental justice and reproductive justice movements may be contributing ideas that will have an impact on the perinatal arena. Both movements call into view the reality that the social gradient in contexts parallels the social gradient in outcomes. But perhaps the most important shift this toxic stress conceptualisation produces is its orientation towards the form of action required, from individual efforts to more systemic ones. In a major position paper, toxic stress is defined and elevated to a significant risk factor warranting healthcare attention:

> Toxic stress can result from strong, frequent, or prolonged activation of the body's stress response systems in the absence of the buffering protection of a supportive, adult relationship ... The potential role of toxic stress and early life adversity in the pathogenesis of health disparities underscores the importance of effective surveillance

for significant risk factors in the primary healthcare setting (Shonkoff *et al.*, 2012, p. e236).

Historically, we have expected individuals to manage their own stress. But we do not count on individuals to 'manage' toxins. We seek public policy and programmatic means to control, treat or eradicate them. This opens avenues to bridge the focus on individual behaviours and the focus on environments.

When it comes to toxic stress, a single intervention is not likely to make all that much difference. So concepts of 'stepped' or 'tiered' intervention are being articulated. These pair well with the stress-biology concept of allostatic load and the notion that allostatic load can be countered by allostatic support. Allostatic load relates to the notion that repeated or unrelenting stressors do not permit a return to baseline via homeostasis, explained this way:

> When early experiences prepare a developing child for conditions involving a high level of stress or instability, the body's systems retain that initial programming and put the stress response system on a short-fuse and high-alert status. Under such circumstances, the benefits of short-term survival may come at a significant cost to longer-term health (Shonkoff *et al.*, 2009, p. 2,257).

Instead, repeated or unrelenting stressors result in a shift in baseline towards a more activated level that is evident in allostatic load: up-regulating of cardiac, respiratory, metabolic, immune and neuroendocrine functions used to counter threat. By this theory, no one stressor and no one incremental physiological change is fatal, but each single alteration entails others until the cumulative load results in morbidity. By the same token, no one intervention is likely to fix the stressors of the human condition. So every element of support that decreases one stressor or mitigates one physiologic alteration should be useful in a cumulative series of such support efforts. This body-based concept is important in framing perinatal psychosocial care because it is a mechanism, or link, that makes it logical that the provision of social care (i.e. addressing stressors and stress) can result in better outcomes not only in the social and psychological realms but also in the medical or health domains (i.e. lower rates of prematurity, fewer stress-related diseases in later life).

Maternal stress has long been implicated in adverse perinatal outcomes. Stress is one of five key pathways to prematurity articulated by the foremost US foundation that supports prevention research – the March of Dimes – and it is a priority area of research where multipronged strategies are expected to be needed:

> The March of Dimes Scientific Advisory Committee created this prioritised research agenda, which is aimed at garnering serious attention and expanding resources to make major inroads into the prevention of preterm birth, targeting six major, overlapping categories: epidemiology, genetics, disparities, inflammation, biologic stress and clinical trials. Analogous to other common, complex disorders, progress in prevention will require incorporating multipronged risk reduction strategies that are based on sound scientific discovery, as well as on effective translation into clinical care (Green *et al.*, 2005, p. 626).

Much of the funded research on maternal stress involves examining the maternal, placental and fetal contributions and pathways at the biological level, focusing on hormones in the primary stress response systems. But more macro concepts are relevant as well. Evolutionary biology theories such as life history or life course theories are being applied to understand how survival and reproduction are traded off against each other in stressful circumstances and across generations. Developmental (or fetal) origins of disease theory frame examination of how the symbiotic relationship between mother and infant results in programming *in utero* so the infant is prepared to live in the mother's world. Epigenetics extends these concepts to focus on how a person's genetic make-up is not entirely deterministic because parenting behaviour and other environmental factors can also change gene expression and affect the infant – for better or for worse:

> Early life stress has a strong impact on DNA methylation and histone modifications with subsequent alterations of gene expression and behaviour. Genome-wide approaches will very likely reveal interesting patterns of

gene classes or transcription factor binding sites that are preferentially altered by early life stress, leading to the complex behavioral and medical consequences of early life stress ... These inherited differences in the susceptibility to epigenetic changes after trauma exposure may thus serve to integrate genetic vulnerability and environmental exposure to define behavioral phenotypes (Heim and Binder, 2012, p. 108).

These macro theories draw our attention to how the mother's stress causes adaptations that may aid immediate survival yet compromise health across the lifespan. The notion of pregnancy as a stress test for life is also gaining ground, so the outcomes of stress being examined are not only those of the infant but also those of the mother (Williams, 2003). For example, we see that insulin resistance or hypertension that appears under the stress of childbearing is likely to appear again for the woman, and much earlier in the lifespan for her than for others who tolerated the 'stress test' with no adverse effects. These macro stress theories are embedded in the body, but are attentive to the larger social context. Thus the need to involve social care professionals to address stress and achieve better macro-level outcomes for the childbearing year is not a new notion, but the impetus to do so is becoming stronger.

Psychological and relational health

The psychological level within these ecological theories is also important. The middle ground of the psychological context of the woman in pregnancy and of the mother–infant dyad postnatally also has a burgeoning scientific literature. Although much of this science focuses on normative processes, to a great extent it is moving ahead rapidly now by looking at how the exception explains the rule (Schore, 2003a). From a normative perspective, the human infant learns to regulate its body, emotions and interactions in a symbiotic relationship with its primary caregiver. If all goes well, its physiology, feelings and contacts with others function well in response to daily life and to extraordinary stressors, consistent with the notion of resilience. But if all does not go well, dysregulated physiology, overwhelming affect and disruptions to developing interpersonal relationships (i.e. disorganised attachments) make the stress of life more than the child can manage from within a state of health, thereby conveying 'risk'. The obvious question to answer is 'What is going wrong?'

One answer to that question is unresolved maternal trauma, which has been referred to metaphorically as 'ghosts in the nursery' (Fraiberg et al., 1975). This metaphor comes from the psycho-analytic literature, but it captures the point that past generations are haunting the present. The metaphor may have been applied originally to describe a psychological phenomenon, but in this historic moment it can resonate with other intergenerational patterns and other broad conceptualisations. By keeping a broad lens and by considering macro-level factors as well as individual temperaments, behaviours, histories and psychopathologies pave the way for more concerted efforts to banish the ghosts.

Traumatic stress and unresolved history of childhood maltreatment

We cannot overlook the fact that traumatic stress is a part of toxic stress, and we focus on the implications of this for perinatal care in Chapter 4 and Chapter 7. One risk of using the vocabulary of toxicity is that it can obscure the role of violence and abuse in total stress. When it comes to women's health, childbearing and parenting outcomes, it is particularly important not to overlook violence, abuse and traumatic stress. One in five women has a history of childhood maltreatment (WHO, 2014). One in five has been sexually assaulted as an adult (Elliott et al., 2004). One in five has experienced severe physical violence in a dating relationship or intimate partnership (CDC, 2014). Male children are abused as well, with one in thirteen being sexually abused as a child (WHO, 2014). We are learning that those who perpetrate violence are likely to have been exposed to violence in childhood – and to have not been resilient (Gil-González et al., 2008). So, traumatic stress also fits with the concept of intergenerational patterns, which is the focus of Chapter 3. Of course, this is not really a new idea. We have had the notions of a cycle of abuse and a cycle of psychiatric vulnerability for a long time. What is shifting is how interdisciplinary science is showing clearly that:

- these cycles of abuse and psychiatric vulnerability intersect;
- there are biological, psychological, social and structural factors involved;
- the childbearing year is a crucial point in this intersection, including the early months of parenting or 'fourth trimester' as it is becoming known;
- the weight of intergenerational patterns is significant;
- these patterns can be shifted for the better: intervention matters.

There has been a coalescing of attachment theory, trauma theory and neurobiological theories pointing towards the vital importance of well-being within the mother–infant dyad for lifespan mental, physical and relational health. Including traumatic stress within the macro theories of toxic stress opens up new avenues to define a high-impact problem and to intervene with trauma informed perinatal services. Putting interventions into place to help women towards resolving childhood trauma exposures is becoming a priority arena for improving population health. This involves primary prevention for the infant and secondary or tertiary approaches for the woman. It requires that child welfare professionals and perinatal professionals share knowledge and work together for prevention to be most effective.

Child maltreatment trauma occurs across the entire social gradient. But the cumulative burden of exposures to traumatic life events is higher for populations we name as vulnerable, disadvantaged, marginalised or disenfranchised, depending on which nation's vocabulary we are using (Taylor and Lazenbatt, 2015). Among vulnerable populations the effects of childhood maltreatment can be obscured by the effects of ongoing exposures. These can be related to geographic context (e.g. crime) or to having a vulnerable social network (e.g. caregiving for ill relations, family member in prison). For women and girls, gender-based trauma exposures occur at more equal rates across socioeconomic strata (e.g. being sexually harassed, assaulted or living with domestic abuse).

The question of when to address maltreatment as a root cause of toxic stress and intergenerational patterns and when to mitigate ongoing trauma exposures likely requires a 'both-and' answer rather than an 'either-or' one. This is when having the concept of allostatic load and allostatic support is helpful, since it suggests that all beneficial actions could add up to have a positive effect.

Attention to traumatic stress with childbearing women will most often involve working with post-traumatic stress. Sometimes, safety planning to prevent ongoing violence is the priority. But in a larger proportion of cases, it is the unresolved trauma rather than an ongoing one that can be the focus of care across the perinatal period. The post-traumatic sequelae of childhood maltreatment take many forms. The developmental timing, nature of the trauma and familial genetic and relational factors all affect the constellation of adverse outcomes (Koenen *et al.*, 2008). Early trauma exposure is a risk for subsequent exposure (Messman-Moore and Long, 2003). The peak age for violence exposures reported by females in the US is in the 16- to 20-year range (Breslau, 2009). For some, this will be close to the time of first pregnancy. There will not have been much time for psychological sequelae to remit – with or without treatment. And most youth will not have had resources to focus on mental health needs at this point in the lifespan when young adult developmental requirements are so compelling. Thus, it seems highly likely that a significant proportion of childbearing women will, indeed, have psychological sequelae reflecting unresolved trauma as they enter perinatal services.

As we will see, traumatic stress includes post-traumatic stress disorder (PTSD) itself, and also depression, anxiety, substance use including smoking, dissociation, interpersonal reactivity, somatic pain and suicidality. Depression and anxiety have gained increasing attention in perinatal services, but these have been thought of largely as endogenous conditions. Screening and referral for psychotherapy or medication treatments are widespread approaches in the nations where specialty mental health services are available. Care for depression and anxiety in low-resource settings and in countries where mental health services are particularly stigmatised is still being developed. As our awareness of traumatic stress increases, we are going to see that the depression and anxiety we have been noticing is often part of the constellation of post-traumatic stress. So we are going to need to update our schema of perinatal mental health and shift how we provide services, which we will discuss in Chapter 4.

A main purpose of this book is to facilitate this updating of schemas and services. Seeing traumatic stress as a concept that links to much of what we already know provides very exciting opportunities to create psychosocial perinatal care that improves outcomes across bio-psychosocial domains and across the lifespan and across generations. No single intervention is likely to suffice fully; so having the notions of allostatic support, working at multiple eco-social levels and making progress across generations may help move us to action.

There are contributions that can be made across all roles in the child welfare and perinatal care teams when they focus together on the four trimesters of the childbearing year as a high-priority period for action. We will discuss major concepts to guide care provision that takes trauma into account looking across the pregnancy, birth and postnatal periods in Chapters 5 and 6. The time is ripe, and there are more ideas about how to do this than we have had in the past. No single professional group can accomplish what needs to be done alone, so we will be using the cross-cutting vocabulary of trauma informed care and trauma-specific interventions (www.samhsa.gov/nctic/; accessed 11 February 2015), introduced in Chapter 2, to build on momentum developing in the mental health and addiction treatment arenas where applying some of these conceptualisations is further along in influencing service delivery. As we will see in Chapters 7 and 8, individual client care provided by individual professionals is not likely to work in isolation from changes to the service delivery models. Research to develop and test interventions and their implementation is going to be needed, as well as continuing education updates for those in practice and revised curricula for those in training, as we will discuss in Chapter 9.

What the book does not cover
Despite being able to include a fairly wide range of topics, four important gaps are going to be evident. We will not be doing justice to the need for attention to partners and fathers; to women with traumatic stress from exposures other than maltreatment; to new-onset traumatic stress from a traumatic birth; or to instances where depression is the primary concern. These are topics that have their

own emerging literatures and warrant more in-depth treatment than we can provide.

Trauma history, PTSD, depression, anxiety and challenges in parenting are quite overlapping phenomena. Approaches to addressing perinatal depression and anxiety are well advanced, although not always trauma informed. So our focus here will be on instances where traumatic stress is a key factor in conceptualising the client's situation. This may include responding to low mood and anxious arousal since those are components of PTSD. Sometimes, however, even when a trauma history is part of the picture, depression is the better conceptualisation or the woman's priority to address. In those cases, the evidence-based approaches for perinatal depression or anxiety should come into play. In reality, as we will see with review of the definition of trauma informed care, key behaviours are giving control to clients and providing hope that their history can be surmounted. This means that the extent to which they want the help they receive to be trauma-specific should be up to them. They should not have to choose to address either their mental health or the parenting concerns rooted in their trauma history. We would advocate for trauma-specific help to be an option and for these services to unfold in tandem with maternity care. In most places, that will require the status quo to change.

What the book contains
The chapters that follow are in three sections. The first (chapters 1–4) defines trauma informed care, explains why a paradigm shift is warranted and provides background on the basis for changing the status quo in perinatal care. We hope those who want to adapt their way of working will be able to pull support from these chapters as rationales and frameworks. The second section (chapters 5–6) hones in on how childhood maltreatment trauma and its sequelae, especially PTSD, affect the antenatal, intrapartum and postnatal periods as well as early parenting and then focuses on implications for service models. The third section (chapters 7–9) provides resources to undergird efforts to provide trauma informed care. We draw upon technical assistance resources, look at examples of emerging trauma-specific interventions that can be part of a stepped- or tiered-care system that is trauma informed, and end with an overview of what

next steps are needed to keep this shift towards trauma informed care moving forward.

Our hope is that this book becomes dated as fast as we can write it. The influential macro-, multilevel, population health theories and their growing empirical support affirm what members of our professions have known from clinical experience at the individual client level. Coherent theory and empirical evidence crystallise a mandate for addressing the psychosocial aspects of care in the perinatal period – including addressing women's maltreatment-related traumatic stress – with the goal of preventing trauma in the next generation.

Conclusion

Here are the key points as to why attention to psychosocial care in the perinatal period is increasing and attention to traumatic stress matters:

❏ In recent years, advances in interdisciplinary science have shown that toxic stress and intergenerational patterns are affecting population health.

❏ If we are to improve perinatal outcomes and lifespan health for the majority, we are going to need to emphasise psychosocial care for the many alongside medical care for the minority who experience obstetric complications.

❏ Traumatic stress is a component of both toxic stress and intergenerational patterns adversely affecting individual and population health.

❏ Among women, traumatic stress from childhood maltreatment often has not been resolved prior to pregnancy, and this has implications for intergenerational transmission via biological, psychological and relational pathways.

❏ The childbearing year is a crucial point of intervention as primary prevention for the infant and to address unmet needs of pregnant women with a maltreatment history.

❏ Child welfare and abuse prevention professionals can play a strong part in developing and implementing perinatal services to break cycles of abuse, psychiatric vulnerability and deprivation.

❏ The purpose of this book is to assemble current theories, empirical support and ideas about how these can inform our work, so that professionals who care for childbearing women can update habits of mind and change practice to be trauma informed.

CHAPTER 2

What is trauma informed care and why is it important?

Chris Cuthbert, NSPCC (UK)
Julia Seng, University of Michigan

Introduction

If we think of the term 'trauma informed care' as meaning care that takes past trauma into account, the meaning seems straightforward enough. But if we as individual practitioners imagine trying to implement it in practice, it quickly also becomes clear that it would be very hard to do so without support at the organisational and system level. In this chapter, we will draw upon technical assistance from the US National Center for Trauma Informed Care (NCTIC) to define and describe both trauma informed care or approaches and trauma-specific interventions. Material included in the boxes in this chapter is technical assistance from their website and is used with permission (www.samhsa.gov/nctic/; accessed 11 February 2015). We will also provide an overview of the reasons why investing in trauma informed models of care and trauma-specific interventions could have major benefits for society. By the end of this chapter, it will make sense why leading-edge public sector mental health, addiction, criminal justice, child welfare, residential treatment, homelessness, HIV-related and domestic violence services are shifting their delivery models and cultures to use trauma informed approaches. This background information will provide a basis from which to advocate applying a trauma informed approach to care in the perinatal period.

Trauma informed care changes the main question from 'What's *wrong* with you?' to 'What *happened* to you?'

What is the definition of trauma informed care?

The brief and broad definition seems to be: 'Trauma informed care is an approach to engaging people with histories of trauma that recognizes the presence of trauma symptoms and acknowledges the role that trauma has played in their lives' (www.samhsa.gov/nctic/; accessed 11 February 2015). What is not immediately apparent from this definition is that trauma informed care is not (only) about what happens within a clinician–client or worker–consumer relationship. It also includes the service delivery context as an actor in providing trauma informed care.

According to SAMHSA's concept of a trauma informed approach, 'A program, organization, or system that is trauma informed:
- *realises* the widespread impact of trauma and understands potential paths for recovery;
- *recognizes* the signs and symptoms of trauma in clients, families, staff, and others involved with the system;
- *responds* by fully integrating knowledge about trauma into policies, procedures, and practices; and
- seeks to actively resist *re-traumatization*.'

A trauma informed approach can be implemented in any type of service setting or organisation and is distinct from trauma-specific interventions or treatments that are designed specifically to address the consequences of trauma and to facilitate healing.

What is the National Center for Trauma Informed Care?

The NCTIC is a part of the Substance Abuse and Mental Health Services Administration (SAMHSA), which is the US government agency that administers funding and oversees mandates for public sector mental health and addiction programming. The NCTIC's mandate is to offer consultation and technical assistance towards 'building the knowledge base on the implementation of trauma informed approaches in programs, services, and systems' (www.samhsa.gov/nctic/; accessed 11 February 2015). NCTIC defines these services broadly, but so far maternity care and medical care settings have not been a focal arena. This is not surprising given that the experiential knowledge base from which the trauma informed care implementation expertise has grown has been in behavioural health rather than physical health domains.

The NCTIC was formed in 2005, and its scope and vocabulary have grown as more implications of trauma informed care emerge. For example, in 2014 the title was expanded to be 'Trauma Informed

Care and Alternatives to Seclusion and Restraint'. This highlights the point that use of such practices in residential or in-patient settings is highly likely to be traumatising or re-traumatising and is not well-aligned with care that is trauma informed. As the trauma informed concept spreads to more sectors, word choice has also shifted from trauma informed care to trauma informed approach. Many organisations that are adopting the framework do not provide care as such, including criminal justice settings. The NCTIC mandate resonates across sectors.

'With a better collective understanding of trauma, more consumers and survivors will find their path to healing and wellness. And with a greater public commitment to trauma-informed programs and systems for survivors, NCTIC lessens and prevents a wide range of health, behavioral health, and social problems *for generations to come*' (emphasis added) (www. samhsa.gov/nctic/; accessed 11 February 2015).

The potential impact on future generations of attending to the adverse, long-term effects of trauma on people using social and health services also comes through in NCTIC's aspirations. In the next sections, we will use information from the NCTIC website to define and explain what it means to provide trauma informed care and trauma-specific interventions.

How are trauma-specific interventions defined?
The NCTIC definition of trauma-specific interventions is that these are 'interventions or treatments designed specifically to address the consequences of trauma and to facilitate healing' (www.samhsa.gov/ nctic/; accessed 11 February 2015). In specialist mental health settings, these interventions could be evidence-based treatments for formal diagnoses such as PTSD, depression, dissociation or substance misuse, including combinations of these co-morbidities.

From perinatal settings, it is sometimes possible to refer for these treatments. More often the needs for trauma-specific interventions that arise in the course of our work with childbearing woman and their families are related to both their mental health and their childbearing and parenting situation. However, trauma-specific interventions that address the consequences of trauma as it is manifesting during the childbearing year and that would facilitate healing via interventions within our scopes of practice and areas of expertise have yet to be articulated, let alone tested for efficacy. In the absence of an empirical evidence base, we resort to individual care planning based on the best information available and with informed consent (Rice, 2011). The NCTIC technical assistance provides some principles to guide this process.

Trauma-specific intervention programmes generally recognise the following:
*   the survivor's need to be respected, informed, connected, and hopeful regarding their own recovery;
*   the interrelation between trauma and symptoms of trauma such as substance misuse, eating disorders, depression and anxiety;
*   the need to work in a collaborative way with survivors, family and friends of the survivor, and other human services agencies in a manner that will empower survivors and consumers.

How can we distinguish trauma informed care from trauma-specific interventions?

It may be useful to augment the NCTIC's definitions by pointing out two distinguishing features:
*   attention to the model-level versus client level;
*   action based on general awareness versus individual assessment.

One way to distinguish trauma informed care and trauma-specific interventions are by the levels at which they can be applied. Trauma informed care is an organisation-wide framing of service delivery that attends to the context of care and the nature of all staff members' interactions with all clients and each other. By contrast, trauma-specific interventions are tailored to the needs of a particular trauma survivor client.

A second way to distinguish trauma informed care from trauma-specific interventions is what ground they rest on. Trauma informed care is based on knowing that a significant proportion of clients are trauma survivors, so all staff develop a habit of mind or basic assumption that anyone with whom they are interacting could be affected by past trauma. Trauma-specific interventions are client-specific.

We can further distinguish 'interventions' and 'treatment'. We think of trauma-specific interventions as being for clients who self-identify as having a trauma history, and which may benefit them even if they are relatively resilient (e.g. psycho-education). We think of trauma-specific treatments as being based on individual assessment of trauma history and current manifestations. In health system settings, these treatments (and the resources to implement them) will often flow from a formal diagnosis. Although there is this distinction, we will generally use 'interventions' to mean both, except in Chapter 8 where we will be more specific.

Figure 2.1 Comparative model between usual and optimal care.

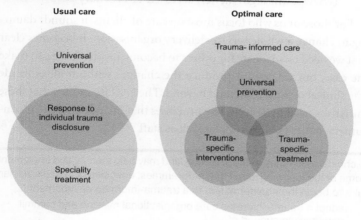

Trauma-specific interventions and trauma informed care go better together. In the context of trauma informed care, it would be routine to assess for survivor status and extent of resilience, recovery or symptomatology and use a diagnosis (if there is one that fits) or another form of naming the problem. In a trauma informed context, care planning would depend on making explicit links between trauma history and current concerns. We would hold out hope for a positive (not re-traumatising) experience of care and for post-traumatic growth – and act accordingly because doing so is part of the culture of the organisation. We would collaborate with the client so the relationship dynamics do not add to their symptomatology. In an agency using a trauma informed care approach, we would be able to expect that every member of staff would support the trauma-specific plan, uphold hopeful outcome expectations and pay attention to relationship dynamics.

This does not sound all that easy to achieve

The NCTIC describes sweeping change and expects that technical assistance will be needed for organisations to achieve that result. As it states:

> When a human services programme takes the step to become trauma informed, its entire organisation, management, and service delivery system is assessed and potentially modified to include a basic understanding of how trauma affects the life of an individual seeking services (www.samhsa.gov/nctic/; accessed 11 February 2015).

For those of us who focus most on care of clients, it sounds daunting to change a whole service delivery organisation. It becomes clear that we need to advocate for others to become involved. We can make the case, but we cannot produce the changes without allies inside our clinical organisations and beyond. The NCTIC stresses that these initiatives need to be collective processes that include clients (or consumers, patients, survivors) as well as staff.

Technical assistance of the following kind may help identify and implement some of the following steps that programmes, agencies or institutions can take to begin the transformation to a trauma-informed environment:

- adopt a trauma informed care organisational mission and commit resources to support it;
- update policies and procedures to reflect new mission;
- conduct universal trauma screening for all consumers and survivors;
- incorporate values and approaches focused on safety and prevention for consumers, survivors and staff;
- create strengths-based environments and practices that invite consumer and survivor empowerment;
- provide ongoing staff training and education in trauma informed care;
- improve and target staff hiring practices.

An approach is a process. What guides how a trauma informed approach unfolds?

SAMHSA has articulated six key principles. It is not hard to imagine how using these principles would be necessary if we are going to open our work with clients and with each other to include working attention to trauma-related issues.

A trauma-informed approach reflects adherence to six key principles rather than a prescribed set of practices or procedures. These principles may be generalizable across multiple types of settings, although terminology and application may be setting- or sector-specific:

- safety;
- trustworthiness and transparency;
- peer support;
- collaboration and mutuality;
- empowerment, voice and choice;
- cultural and historical issues and gender awareness.

From SAMHSA's perspective, it is critical to promote the linkage to recovery and resilience for those individuals and families impacted by trauma. Consistent with SAMHSA's definition of recovery, services and supports that are trauma-informed build on the best evidence available and on consumer and family engagement, empowerment and collaboration.

Does it make sense to translate these definitions for care of childbearing women?

The notion of implementing a trauma informed approach in perinatal care settings (especially in public sector maternal-infant health services) does not require much of a stretch from implementing them in mental health and child welfare settings. First, the proportion of childbearing women needing trauma-specific interventions may be lower than in public mental health services, but this is only a matter of degree. Second, intrusive and painful aspects of maternity and birth procedures have very high traumatising and re-traumatising potential that could be mitigated. Third, the intersection of cycles of abuse and psychiatric vulnerability during the childbearing year increases the likely impact of changing our paradigm because trauma informed care and trauma-specific interventions for the mother act as primary prevention for the next generation.

Of course, many individual professionals make trauma-specific care plans with their clients. Many maternal support services are aware that many of their clients have a trauma history and try to be responsive. Roles such as the specialist midwife in the UK and many certified doulas are well suited to working with clients who are trauma survivors (NSPCC, 2013; Simkin, 2011). Structures such as nurse home visiting programmes (e.g. the Family Nurse Partnership; Chapter 8) have trauma informed elements. Even practice guidelines such as those published by the UK's National Institute for Health and Care Excellence (NICE) in 2014 include attention to the needs of 'pregnant women with complex social factors' (NICE, 2014). As is evident from these definitions, however, these incremental advances are just steps on the way. More sweeping change is required to attain the goals of trauma informed care.

Is it likely to be worth it?

Collaborating to integrate psychosocial and obstetric care for child-bearing women seems warranted given what we now know about social determinants of health. But is it likely to be worthwhile to go all the way to making this integrated care trauma informed? The evidence suggesting that it is not only worth it but also essential is mounting.

The long shadow

Professor Sir Michael Rutter famously proclaimed that 'early adversity casts a long shadow' (Rutter *et al.*, 1998). In the US, the Adverse Childhood Experiences (ACE) study has demonstrated how experiences in early childhood can have a profound effect on the course of health and development over a lifetime (Felitti *et al.*, 1998). Child abuse or neglect and trauma, including witnessing violence, can alter normal child development and can have lifelong consequences. The WHO estimates that child maltreatment is responsible for almost a quarter of the burden of mental disorders. Its economic and social costs are on a par with those for all non-communicable diseases (including cancer, obesity, diabetes, heart and respiratory diseases) (Sethi *et al.*, 2013).

In addition to high chronic disease burden, US studies show that individuals who were abused or neglected have more involvement with child welfare services and the juvenile justice system; and, when adults, higher rates of sexual assault and domestic violence victimisation (Hetzel and McCanne, 2005), homelessness (Stein *et al.*, 2002) and criminality (Widom, 1989). Considering the lifelong impact of chronic illness treatment and service utilisation, the cost of abuse and neglect to US society across service sectors is estimated to be $80 to $100 billion per year (Wang and Holton, 2007; Gelles and Perlman, 2012). Based on both US and Australian studies, adjusted for population, the UK annual cost of child maltreatment is estimated at £15 billion (Access Economics Pty Ltd, Australian Childhood Foundation and Child Abuse Prevention Research Australia, 2008).

Child maltreatment is clearly a major public health concern across developed nations. The scale of the challenge is formidable. But it is increasingly clear that the costs of not acting are too great and that it is time for a decisive shift to early intervention and to break the intergenerational cycle of abuse and psychiatric vulnerability.

'We know too that not intervening now will affect not just this generation of children and young people but also the next. Those who suffer multiple adverse childhood events achieve less educationally, earn less, and are less healthy, making it more likely that the cycle of harm is perpetuated, in the following generation' (Professor Dame Sally Davies, Chief Medical Officer for England).

The first 1,001 critical days

Over recent years, there has been an explosion of research and understanding about the particular significance of pregnancy and infancy in laying the foundations for children's development (Cuthbert *et al.*, 2011). Advances in the fields of neurobiology, epigenetics and developmental psychology provide the scientific case for what until relatively recently was a matter of common sense or intuition. This new knowledge underpins a growing political consensus around the importance of 'early years intervention' and a call to increase investment in 'the first 1,001 critical days' to help children get the best possible start in life.

Pregnancy and babyhood are increasingly recognised as a unique window of opportunity to work preventatively with families. As we shall see in Chapter 8, there is much cause for optimism about the potential to achieve positive outcomes through intervention during this life stage, even among some of the most troubled and traumatised families.

A time of vulnerability

This life stage is also critically important because it is a time of exceptional vulnerability for babies, who are almost entirely dependent on their immediate caregivers. A baby's world *is* the relationship with their caregiver. A parent's capacity to respond appropriately to the emotions and needs of their baby can have a profound impact, and this early experience provides the essential foundations for all future physical, social and emotional development. However:

- Across the thirty-four Organisation for Economic Cooperation and Development (OECD) countries, risk of death by maltreatment is highest for babies under one (UNICEF, 2003).
- Babies in England and Wales are eight times more likely to be killed than older children (Smith, 2011).
- Some 39% of serious case reviews in England relate to babies under the age of one year (Brandon *et al.*, 2009).
- Just under half (42%) of children in England with a Child Protection Plan are under four years of age (Department for Education, 2012).
- Around 80% of children who are abused have a 'disorganised' attachment (Carlson *et al.*, 1989).

An additional, very important but often overlooked point is that interventions that improve child outcomes should also aim to strengthen the well-being of the mother. Addressing her unresolved trauma history and her current mental health needs would go a long way to increasing her capacity to bond with her infant and apply new skills in parenting such as reflectivity and sensitivity that will enhance outcomes for the child. Thinking of the mother–infant relationship as dyadic is crucial. Providing interventions that meet the woman's needs should be a focal part of the overall plan.

Conclusion

Here are the key points and definitions about trauma informed care and why we need it:

- ❑ Trauma informed care is an approach to engaging people with histories of trauma that recognises the presence of trauma symptoms and acknowledges the role that trauma has played in their lives.

❏ Trauma-specific interventions are interventions or treatments designed specifically to address the consequences of trauma and to facilitate recovery.

❏ While waiting for evidence-based perinatal interventions to emerge, the principles of evidence-based practice and the principles of trauma-specific interventions can be used synergistically to create care plans with individual clients.

❏ The economic and social costs of childhood maltreatment are on a par with those for all non-communicable diseases (including cancer, obesity, diabetes, heart and respiratory diseases).

❏ Prevention is a strong focus across nations, with an emphasis on early years' interventions and the first 1,001 critical days so that the outcomes for zero-to-ones are better. Whatever term is used, the aim is to intervene as early as possible.

❏ Addressing this problem in the childbearing year is a doubly important strategy because it is an opportunity to respond to unmet needs of the woman and is a chance for primary prevention for the next generation.

CHAPTER 3

What theories explain intergenerational patterns?

Julia Seng, University of Michigan,
Julie Taylor, University of Birmingham (UK)

Introduction

Given the costs to society of maltreatment, it seems very worthwhile to intervene with childbearing women to help them resolve trauma sequelae, prepare for parenting and strengthen capacity to prevent abuse and trauma exposures for their infants. But one reason why maltreatment seems such an intransigent problem is that it is a part of so many intergenerational patterns (i.e. of violence, poverty, population health). In this chapter, we will give a very brief overview of some currently influential intergenerational theories, with a little more detail provided about research on the notion of a cycle of maltreatment in particular. Our emphasis will be on how these shed light on ways to think about intervention – and to strengthen the case for intervening. To that end, we will introduce an integrating 'cycles-breaking' framework that might serve as a useful tool for trauma informed, integrated perinatal service delivery, interprofessional practice and transdisciplinary research.

What are current theories of intergenerational patterns?

Historically, the notion of intergenerational cycle (e.g. of deprivation or disadvantage) has drawn criticism as well as acceptance. It seems common sense that phenomena such as poverty or violence run in families. However, there has been scientific and political controversy about the way empirical evidence has been produced. In one well-examined instance in the UK in the 1980s (Welshman, 2009), the debate over whether the focus should be on individual behaviour or on structural factors seemed obviously political. This debate about which level to interrogate seems quite dated now. Social-ecological frameworks and multilevel statistical modelling techniques now see these as additive and interacting levels that all have to be taken into account together. Complexity studies and newer computing strategies will further change our schemas as syndemic models (resembling overlapping circles with no clear predictor-to-outcome relationship) take the place of traditional models that seek reductionist causal pathways or predictive mechanisms. Perhaps the most important problems with past research on intergenerational cycles were that interpretations of findings were focused on risk factors and evidence of continuity of problems, and seemed deterministic. Interpretative practice currently is more apt to look for resilience and risk, discontinuity as well as continuity, self-regulation as well as dysregulation, and adaptation as well as impairment. We include a focus on biological theories as well. Working across disciplinary boundaries calls for seeing the childbearing year across bio-psychosocial levels, as an embodied experienced susceptible to toxic stress.

Toxic stress

The concept of toxic stress is being used as a unifying one to explain how social determinants of health and other contextual factors contribute to ill health, i.e. premature morbidity and mortality across the lifespan. The idea is that humans can mount a response to occasional stress and return via homeostatic processes to a state of optimal health. But if the stressors are too intense or chronic they become toxic, and we pay a price as health is compromised. The American Academy of Pediatrics (AAP) has adopted toxic stress as a unifying concept to help shift the biomedical focus of paediatricians towards one that is broader and that considers larger contextual influences as not only germane to children's health but also on a par with medical issues. As it states in a major position paper:

> AAP is committed to leveraging science to inform the development of innovative strategies to reduce the precipitants of toxic stress in young children and to mitigate their negative effects on the course of development and health across the lifespan (Shonkoff *et al.*, 2012, p. e224).

Within this conceptualisation of toxic stress, there are two biological theories to explain how toxic stress in the lives of children can result in early morbidity and mortality. The first is the fetal or developmental origins of disease which focuses the toxic stress concept on the period when the mother's body is the environment for the child. The second is the stress-biology theory of allostatic load.

Fetal or developmental origins of disease

The theory of fetal origins of disease also is a general one, explaining how the stress of the mother's world 'programmes' the fetus to survive in her context. Research on this theory came to the fore as the life course health status of English children was studied in relation to maternal nutrition, infant birth weight and later cardiometabolic morbidity and mortality (Barker, 1995). Subsequent work has linked maternal psychosocial stress and hypothalamic-pituitary-adrenal (HPA) axis hormones during pregnancy to changes resulting in 'permanent changes in physiology, structure and metabolism' in the child (Reynolds, 2013, p. 1).

It is clear that prenatal maternal anxiety in particular is associated with child mental health adaptations that would be suitable for living in a dangerous world, including anxiety, aggression and attention deficit hyperactive disorder (Glover, 2011). It seems that the fetus enacts an 'adaptive predictive response' (Gluckman and Hanson, 2004) to the *in utero* stress of its mother and is born smaller and ready to survive, but with physiological adaptations that are less suitable for long-term survival. Evolutionarily, it is trading off longevity for survival long enough to reproduce. This is good for preservation of our species, but bad for individual and population health.

Allostatic load

Classic stress theories were grounded in the notion of homeostasis, which is the idea that an external stressor requires a body to mount a response and then, when the stressor is past, to return to its baseline physiologic state. The theory of allostasis accounts for what happens when the stressors are severe and prolonged. A return to homeostasis is not feasible, so a new baseline state emerges as an adaptation. Multiple body systems work together in response to stressors to optimise survival. Neuroendocrine, cardiovascular, respiratory, metabolic and immune systems all operate in concert. When they cannot return to baseline, their levels remain in a heightened state, and this takes a toll on the body.

Cascade of adaptations

The theory of allostatic load is a general one describing how a new baseline is set when homeostatic processes are not adequate due to stress that is too extreme or too chronic; it also covers how physiological adaptations occur to promote survival, but at the cost of longevity. Martin Teicher and his biological developmental psychiatry research group at Harvard University and the McLean Hospital have explained how this resetting of the baseline may happen within the neuroendocrine systems of a maltreated child (Teicher *et al.*, 2002). Teicher *et al.* explain that the HPA axis, noradrenergic/adrenaline and vasopressin-oxytocin systems are interactive, mutually regulating systems – they are 'three pillars of adaptation to childhood maltreatment'. If one system has to change, so will the others. So hormone levels in the 'fight or flight' system, such as cortisol and adrenaline (or epinephrine) become altered. That in turn causes concomitant modifications in the 'freeze' system, including oxytocin. Oxytocin is also part of a recovery system. So change in the systems that make surviving stress possible also leads to alterations in the system that makes recovering from stress possible. Changes in these hormones correspond to changes in brain anatomy and function in the areas that react to stressors and develop coping strategies (Compas, 2006). Since these hormones circulate in the body as well, health is broadly adversely affected over time. This cascade of adaptations to childhood maltreatment is one pathway through which allostatic load accrues, allostatic supports within the body erode, and toxic stressors take more of a toll than they might in the life of a person whose childhood left them with a set of healthy stress response systems.

One key implication of having changes in these 'three pillars of adaptation to childhood maltreatment' goes beyond the physical costs. These systems function under stress for the rest of the lifespan in the adapted way – unless there is concerted effort to profit from plasticity and change the systems. This goes a long way towards explaining why a person whose brain and body underwent these adaptations can have a hard time parenting. Such adaptations are useful for self-preservation under threat. But if your body reacts to stress as though it were threat, then the stress of a crying infant or the stress from deep weariness in the early months of parenting can feel much bigger to a dysregulated parent than to a healthy one (see for example Petzoldt *et al.*, 2014; Reijman *et al.*, 2014). Adrenaline can flood the parent's body. Oxytocin that would help with feeling bonded and tolerating physical closeness can be lacking (see for example Schechter *et al.*, 2008; Schore, 2003b; Teicher *et al.*, 2002). It is easy to see how irritable or angry arousal mixed with detachment or numbness is a bad combination. A trauma informed approach would take into account the differences in embodied experience and responses of parents with a maltreatment history.

Life history theory
The notion of adaptation to our environment leads to thinking about evolution and ecology systems theories. Life history theory (also referred to as a life course perspective) takes a long-term, multigenerational view of how environmental conditions including danger from abuse forces trade-offs for survival of the species. It is a population-level theory which explains that reproducing and longevity are competing interests. Life history theory (LHT) posits that a species' life history is its evolved trajectory of four aspects: growth; development; reproduction; and senescence. It models life cycles and traits in an ecological context (Chisholm, 1999), integrating evolutionary, ecological and socio-developmental perspectives (Geary, 2002). LHT illustrates how organisms must make trade-offs in the allocation of resources – including physiological ones – to these four aspects of life and how these allocations are shaped by environmental conditions (Roff, 1992).

LHT predicts that maternal physical investment in gestating offspring will be contingent upon local environmental conditions reflecting the offspring's prospects for survival. Several factors are related to the prospects of offspring survival and eventual reproduction, including the availability of food and threats from predators and members of its own species. In contemporary society, these would be akin to financial insecurity and presence of violence or abuse (Nesse and Stearns, 2008). In good-quality environments, mothers will have more resources to invest, and outcomes will tend towards the theoretical optimum for offspring fitness and thus longevity. In contexts of disadvantage or threat at the population level, we would expect to see adaptations in reproduction (Smith and Fretwell, 1973) including younger first pregnancy, more pregnancies, more vulnerability to complications, shorter gestation, lower birth weight, less breastfeeding, less bonding and worse health resulting in earlier mortality.

Epigenetics

Through the lens of LHT, genetics play a long-term role through inheritance. Genetics are also important in the short term. Epigenetics focuses on how the environment affects gene expression. Some very influential animal model studies have made us aware that the genes we inherit are only part of the story and that gene expression can be changed by behaviour and environment. Leaving aside the technical information about the gene methylation that is the mechanism, we can see how this worked from the behavioural part of the experiment conducted by Michael Meaney's team at McGill University (Meaney, 2001). Rat dams (pregnant or mother rats) have been bred to have the genetically inherited trait of being high licker-groomers or low licker-groomers. Pups of high licker-groomer dams tend to be less anxious than those of low licker-groomer dams, which exhibit less social and exploring behaviour. But if pups born to low licker-groomers are fostered by dams who are high licker-groomers, their social and exploring behaviour is not anxious. And – more surprising – their offspring in turn are more likely to be born with the genes for being high licker-groomers. That is to say, the fostering positively affected not only the pup's anxiety behaviour but also the genes for licking and grooming behaviour in the next generation.

The ways in which epigenetics undermine a deterministic view is important. Gene-by-environment interactions are common. Family patterns that may have consolidated into genetic risk over several generations can be influenced by parenting behaviours. From fetal origins of disease research, we also know that there are critical developmental windows. The pregnancy, newborn and infancy periods, known as the first 1,001 days, are critical for development. It makes sense that they are periods when trauma informed and trauma-specific care for the mother-to-be could have an impact on her capacity to disrupt the multigenerational cycles with behaviours that foster resilience and healthy development in her child. But this is no easy task. If we consider the cumulative factors of abusive family of origin, disadvantage and psychological and physical adaptations she used to survive, it stands to reason that she might need some help from professionals to achieve such a goal.

This way of understanding the impact of toxic stress in the forms of maltreatment and traumatic stress adaptations makes sense at the population health level and theoretically. Going now to a more individual level, we can review the evidence about intergenerational patterns of maltreatment, look at two concepts about how transmission of trauma could occur within the mother–infant dyad, and consider whether there is a theory we could use as a common working model for the child welfare and perinatal professional working with women in the childbearing year.

What does the research say about the intergenerational pattern of maltreatment?

The evidence

The evidence in earlier research was far from robust and revealed a range of weaknesses. A 'good deal of criticism' was levelled at these studies, according to Newcomb and Locke (2001); they found a moderately strong effect from a US community sample of 383 parents. Ertem et al. (2000), in a systematic review of studies from 1965 to 2000, point to the need to improve methodological standards, leading to a mixed evidence base. Dixon et al. (2009) found a 'moderate general relationship' in their UK study of using health visitors to assess 4,351 families. In research based on the US Rochester Youth Development Study, Thornberry and Henry (2013) found that a history of maltreatment 'significantly increases the odds' of being a perpetrator of maltreatment. Nonetheless, Thornberry et al. (2012) in their systematic review still contend that the cycle of maltreatment hypothesis has not been definitively tested and still requires empirical verification. By way of contrast, Conger *et al.* (2013) argue that the methodological limitations have been overcome in well-designed studies undertaken prospectively across time and across genders. These studies, plus their own one based on the US Family Transitions Project, a cohort of more than 500 early adolescents, have revealed 'intergenerational continuity in harsh, hostile and abusive parenting' (Conger *et al.*, 2013). A Dutch study found higher child abuse potential and lower levels of self-control among physically and sexually abused mothers (Henschel *et al.*, 2014). Jaffee *et al.* (2013) examined data from a prospective longitudinal study of mothers and children from the UK Environmental Risk Longitudinal Twin Study: this found continuity across two generations, with odds of a child experiencing physical maltreatment between three and five times greater among mothers with a history of abuse or neglect. This study also finds echoes in US research with mothers involved in child protection services, including pregnant women with older children (Schechter *et al.*, 2008; Kim *et al.*, 2014).

On the other hand, there is also evidence of discontinuity and the breaking of cycles of abuse. As Dixon *et al.* (2009) note, the majority of victimised parents do not appear to follow this pattern. A 'substantial degree of discontinuity' (77% of the study participants) was noted by Thornberry and Henry (2013). 'Cycle breakers' have been highlighted in the studies by Thornberry *et al.* (2012) and Jaffee *et al.* (2013). Both sets of researchers detected evidence that the cycle of abuse in families can be broken by safe, stable, nurturing relationships. This was demonstrated by approximately half of families in the UK-based study undertaken by Jaffee *et al.* (2013).

Recommendations

Many studies in the literature mention implications for intervention and prevention approaches, though these could be spelled out in more depth. They include universal preventive programmes to assist all parents, such as positive parenting programmes. Attention should be paid to the promotion of safe, stable, nurturing relationships (Thornberry *et al.*, 2012; Jaffee *et al.*, 2013). As well as supporting parents in engaging in warm and sensitive parenting, there should be encouragement of open communication and trust between mothers and partners (Jaffee *et al.*, 2013). Some authors refer to a need to target women with histories of abuse or neglect (Robboy and Anderson, 2011; Jaffee *et al.*, 2013). Targeted interventions for the perinatal year have yet to be developed and tested, but core concepts to include emerge from the literature. Henschel *et al.* (2014) recommend training in self-control for abused individuals (children and parents), which finds echoes in literature on reflective parenting (Slade, 2006), mindful parenting (Duncan *et al.*, 2009) and the concept of self-regulation as an overarching need of people abused in childhood who did not receive the input all infants need from parents who could self-regulate (Ford, 2013). Universal prevention and targeted interventions may not suffice for everyone. Assessment of high risk should lead to indicated treatment, whether for parental mental illness or for parenting behaviours that require one-to-one interventive or protective services.

Possible lines of future research

Why maltreatment is not perpetrated is as interesting a research question as that of the continuity of abuse and neglect across generations – perhaps more so. There should be more research interest in the 'cycle breakers' and in the notion of intergenerational resilience (Thornberry and Henry, 2013) or post-traumatic growth manifesting as protective parenting (Sperlich and Seng, 2008). This is an important concept which deserves to be followed up, as it will provide invaluable pointers for more effective prevention approaches and programmes. Moreover, this interest should be reflected in greater sensitivity in theoretical models, where simplistic and deterministic assumptions concerning the developmental trajectories of maltreated children and adults are avoided. This, in turn, should give enhanced scope to the role and function of human agency and to individual and social forms of resilience.

How does maltreatment lead to psychiatric vulnerability?

The contributions of both nature and nurture are taken for granted in the mental health fields. Family history of psychiatric illness is part of admission to mental health treatment for good reason. There is inherited genetic propensity, and also the potential for children to have worse developmental, health, educational and welfare outcomes because of impaired parenting behaviours (Champagne and Curley, 2009). PTSD is a psychiatric condition with a strong transmission pattern studied most extensively with families descended from survivors of the Nazi Holocaust (Yehuda *et al.*, 1995). In some of these families where elders have PTSD, members of the next generation (or two now) sometimes have traumatic stress even though they themselves have never been exposed to traumatic events. Not only physiology, but also world view (Foa *et al.*, 1989) and attachments (Freyd, 1998) are shaken and have to adapt in the aftermath of human-inflicted trauma exposure in particular. The literature on PTSD generally suggests that one-third of risk for having a PTSD diagnosis is from the trauma exposure, one-third from genetics and one-third from family psychiatric history (Koenen *et al.*, 2008). Research studies are now being done (mostly with mothers) and these indicate how crucial the mother's interactions with the infant are and how her mental health can adversely affect her mothering (Schechter *et al.*, 2008). It makes sense to go from the studies of holocaust survivors' families, where the trauma was 'outside the range of normal human experience' to research into maltreatment survivors where physiology, world view and attachment also have been affected (Schore, 2003a). This helps us consider more universal concepts that are important for child development and that may apply to our thinking about the childbearing woman's needs as well.

This choice of major concepts to focus on emerged from our collaboration as we focused on the question 'What are the most important things to help a new mother with maltreatment-related PTSD to understand about parenting?' It occurred to us that these ideas could also very usefully apply to our care of the woman as she looks to professionals to help her through the huge challenges of pregnancy, birth and becoming a mother. In essence, they can help us think about how we are mothering the mother.

Attachment

Since the early work in the 1950s and 1960s of John Bowlby and Mary Ainsworth (Ainsworth and Bowlby, 1991), attachment theory has a long developmental history. In a nutshell, attachment theory describes the dynamics of long-term interpersonal relationships where the pattern is created in infancy, in the ability to develop basic trust in the caregiver. (There is a very useful resource on attachment by Suzanne Zeedyk for those who want to understand the concept more: http://suzannezeedyk.com/#/resources/4579047977.)

It is generally considered that childhood maltreatment is an injury to the attachment system within the family, particularly in the relationship between primary caregiver and infant (Liotti, 2004). Women with a maltreatment history thus may enter childbearing with insecure adult attachment styles that were established in childhood in relationships with primary carers. The challenges of pregnancy, birth, breastfeeding and the early days of parenting give all of us dependency needs. Professionals across disciplines may find it useful to consider how their clients are doing in terms of navigating these needs in relationships with professionals where power dynamics and desires to be cared for and helped may reactivate old dynamics (Josephs, 1996). It may be helpful for professionals to use the lens of attachment theory to understand any problems in their relationship with the woman.

Dyadic regulation

Regulation is another important concept in parenting that may also translate up to the relationship between perinatal professionals and their clients. Women with a maltreatment history may not have experienced beneficial dyadic regulation when they were infants. That is, their mother may not have been well able to use her body, breath, voice and touch to sensitively stimulate and calm her infant (Schore, 2003b). So the woman who is our client and who is under the stress of pregnancy may require our assistance to learn to regulate her own states of attention and arousal, and she might need to develop skills in self-care, such as sleep hygiene, good nutrition and appropriate physical activity, and keeping herself safe (Bandura, 2005). Risk behaviours we recognise as critical to address in pregnancy including substance use and smoking, risky sexual behaviour and exposure to partner violence can be seen as maladaptive efforts at self-regulation (Seng et al., 2008; Lopez et al., 2011). Making self-regulation for the woman a focus of attention can improve her well-being and lay groundwork for building her capacity to provide dyadic regulation for her infant (Schore, 2003b).

Holding environment

Another important parenting concept that may usefully apply to our professional caregiving relationship with the adult woman who is our client is the notion of the caregiving relationship as a holding environment. In the child development literature (Modell, 1978), the notion goes that parents set limits and provide a predictable frame so that the child can explore within safe limits and return to a comfort zone for reassurance if the exterior challenge is too great. The challenge of pregnancy and all that follows is a big one, and maternity care services may act as a holding environment to help the mother face the challenges with a sense that she will not get lost and she is not alone.

Standard maternity services may suffice for most women, but one in five mothers with a maltreatment history may require expanded services to provide holding adequate for the number and intensity of the mother's challenges and so that no one care-providing professional becomes burdened by the potentially large extent of the mother's needs. A team to support coping with pregnancy, fears about labour, progressing through labour, starting breastfeeding, meeting her baby, managing her unique infant's temperament and difficult behaviours, and taking care of herself may suggest that an expanded holding environment includes midwife, health visitor or nurse, labour doula or designated support person, lactation consultant, paediatrician and parenting educator – and possibly a social worker if there are child safety concerns or a need to coordinate this team.

The notion of role modelling via parallel relationships

Although it may not seem like an intervention as such, caregivers attending to these three issues of attachment, dyadic regulation and the holding environment in their work with childbearing women who have a maltreatment history is likely to be a therapeutic modality in and of itself. If we respond to our clients from within our profession's role while asking ourselves how attachment theory, self-regulation and holding environment apply, we may be more likely to meet this client groups' needs. They may have more positive experiences of our care. We also role model for these mothers-to-be how to enact these considerations for their infant and child.

We will return to the three concepts of attachment, dyadic regulation and the holding environment in Chapter 6.

Is there any theory specific to the entire childbearing year – from preconception on?

Many professions, from gynaecology and sexual health in the preconception period to health visiting and paediatrics once the infant is born, intersect with the course of the childbearing year in a different, sometimes quite circumscribed location. The whole childbearing year – from conception through the fourth trimester of the postnatal period – can be seen more broadly. It is a location in the life course where cycles of abuse and psychiatric vulnerability intersect because maternal history and maternal psychological difficulties from unresolved trauma affect the maltreatment risk and psychological status of the new generation. The possibilities of diverse professions looking together at interrupting these cycles have been limited for reasons that make sense: for example, time, resources, lack of connection and collaboration. The time may have arrived to transcend these limits. A unifying theory might help.

The research on the two cycles of abuse and psychiatric vulnerability has been done mostly separately, in the fields that study violence, abuse and neglect, often led by social workers and social scientists on one hand, and in the fields that study mental disorders, often led by psychiatrists and health scientists on the other. These lines of research about cycles were somewhat siloed until fairly recently. There is now mounting evidence from research integrating attention to both maternal abuse history and maternal mental health status that intergenerational transmission of either maltreatment or psychiatric vulnerability or both is more likely when both problems are interacting in the same family (Chemtob *et al.*, 2014).

Thus, a knowledge base from population-level and individual-level theories and research tell us intervening is worthwhile and should be feasible. And the childbearing year is a crucial time because it is a point of primary prevention for the infant. Yet child welfare and psychiatric professionals have had a hard time coordinating their theories and research in the past. How much more difficult will it be for these professions to tie in their efforts with the obstetric, midwifery and nursing professions to reach across the mind–body divide that splits psychosocial and biomedical care?

A framework simple enough to be common sense to all professionals would be helpful for organising care and future research. In recent analyses from a prospective study of maltreatment-related PTSD across the childbearing year, a straightforward framework emerged from review of the literature and from the study's statistical analyses (Seng *et al.*, 2013).

Figure 3.1 Cycles-breaking framework.

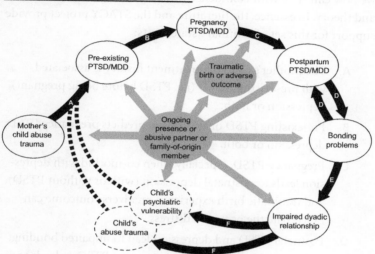

Each point in the childbearing year is an opportunity to disrupt the cycle

The Stress, Trauma, Anxiety and the Childbearing Year (STACY) project research team, including this book's contributors Seng and Sperlich, collected data in early pregnancy, late pregnancy, and at six weeks postpartum (NIH R01 NR008767, PI Seng). In the early pregnancy interview, they assessed lifetime trauma history and pre-existing PTSD and depression, and these were measured repeatedly across the series of interviews. Quality of the partner relationship and family of origin functioning were measured. The perception of care during labour and whether the experience was traumatic was also measured. Breastfeeding, postnatal mental health and mother's report of how bonded to the infant she felt were outcomes. After this study ended at six postnatal weeks, the mothers who were maltreatment survivors and their infants were recruited to continue into longer-term follow-up with another research team (NIH K23MH080147, PI Muzik). Taken together, the data augments the evidence for inter-generational patterns and also suggests points of intervention. The literature review for the latter study and the hypothesis testing and statistical modelling were reported in relationship to a cycles-breaking framework (see Figure 3.1). This practical diagram depicts what we now can state with confidence from a growing body of research and theory. In essence, the literature and the STACY project provide support for this set of summary statements:

A. The mother's child maltreatment history is associated with pre-existing PTSD (i.e. PTSD before being pregnant), depression or both.

B. Pre-existing PTSD or depression predicts pregnancy PTSD, depression or both.

C. Pregnancy PTSD, especially when co-morbid with depression leads to postnatal depression (with or without PTSD), and traumatic birth experience or adverse outcome can exacerbate the postnatal distress.

D. Postnatal PTSD and depression lead to impaired bonding; or impaired bonding triggers postnatal PTSD or leads to depression.

E. Impaired bonding leads to ongoing impairments in the mother–infant dyadic relationship.

F. Impairments in the dyadic relationship increase risk for the infant to be abused and exposed to more traumatic experiences and increase risk for psychiatric vulnerability across the lifespan:

   • the whole childbearing year chain of events can also be helped or made worse by the quality and safety of the partner relationship;
   • the safety and functioning of the family of origin can also affect the situation.

Of course, this way of explaining the linkages is all phrased in a deterministic way. This is a habit of mind and habitual language of researchers testing hypotheses about risks in studies looking for adverse outcomes. But each of those links is also a place where resilience could be noted or a locus for intervention. Actions that are support or treatment for the mother (or absence of re-traumatisation) are also primary prevention for her infant. Perhaps, a better way to depict this framework is to flatten it into a line and imagine how a small push in the right direction at any one of those points could change the trajectory for the better (see Figure 3.1). Small nudges in the appropriate direction at each of those points could add up. Changing the trajectory for this mother and infant alters the path for the next generation as well (we will say more about STACY in Chapter 5).

Interprofessional collaboration in a trauma informed context could have additive effects

Recognising that the childbearing year is a crucial time to intervene is one step towards providing trauma informed care. But multiple concerted coordinated efforts are going to be more powerful. Interprofessional collaboration is important. For example, no amount of planning with a doula to try to have a birth that does not trigger intrusive memories, feelings or dissociative episodes is going to work if the midwife, obstetrician or labour nurse will not adapt their routines or interpersonal practice. And there's only so much a healthcare provider can do for a client who screens positive for abuse-related PTSD if perinatal mental health professionals are skilled at treating only depression and anxiety. It will become clear that breaking cycles requires: integration of mental and physical healthcare professionals in interprofessional collaborations; seamless linking of the prenatal, birth and postnatal periods; and provision of both trauma informed services and trauma-specific interventions so that women who are resilient, recovered or experiencing sequelae can have the right level of response.

Transdisciplinary intervention research is needed

Similarly, no one scientific discipline can conduct the research needed to determine what perinatal interventions are beneficial for whom – especially because the interventions need to bridge medical, obstetric and psychosocial arenas. The shared conceptualisations and integrated studies that are warranted will require teams able to transcend the borders of each member's particular academic discipline. It will need to be very creative work to develop cycle-breaking interventions. Research will have to be innovative to include a focus on prevention and on resilience. Looking for positive outcomes of trauma informed care and trauma-specific interventions implemented by numerous professions at multiple time points across the perinatal period will require a level of collaboration not routinely applied to perinatal problem.

A. The woman had a warm trusting relationship when she was a girl with someone who encouraged, supported and validated her, perhaps a teacher. She did not develop full PTSD.

B. Her prenatal clinic diagnosed partial PTSD, provided a psycho-education course about PTSD, and were allies to reduce triggers.

C. A labour doula along with her partner, nurse and midwife used strategies to reduce sexual abuse flashbacks. Memories still intruded, but she felt supported.

D. A postnatal nurse visited to teach strategies to manage the baby's crying. She used brief exposure therapy to decrease intrusive memories of and sadness about the birth experience.

E. The mother feels herself rest after the therapy session while her baby rests. She notices the baby curl up against her and senses he is happy to be with her.

F. These early periods of noticing contentment and comfort with her baby help the mother to find calm and patience when the baby cries a lot. On tough days, she messages her partner that she's going to need a break when he gets home from work. He takes the baby on a walk and makes supper.

Conclusion

This chapter has focused on contemporary theories about intergenerational patterns as they apply to health and human development and pertain to the childbearing year.

❏ In the past, these theories have caused debates about whether individual or structural levels were more important and about whether the notion of cycles was deterministic.

❏ Recent research on maltreatment patterns shows a degree of intergenerational continuity. Intersecting cycles of maltreatment and psychiatric vulnerability are providing better explanations. Evidence of substantial discontinuity reminds us that these patterns are not deterministic and that resilience and intervention are often left out of the equation.

❏ This body of research makes recommendations on the need to identify and better support parents with history of abuse and neglect and to prevent continuity.

❏ The intergenerational pattern theories tend to explain transmission at either the interpersonal or biological levels, but integrative theories are needed to foster interventions that take the embodied experience of trauma, PTSD and parenting into account.

❏ A theory is needed that combines attention to the dual cycles of maltreatment and psychiatric vulnerability to underpin interprofessional care and transdisciplinary research across the perinatal period.

❏ Replacing the metaphor of 'cycle' with the metaphor of 'trajectory' may usefully undermine simplistic and deterministic assumptions concerning the life course of maltreated children and adults.

CHAPTER 4

How does focusing on post-traumatic stress disorder shift perinatal mental health paradigms?

Mickey Sperlich, State University of New York at Buffalo

Introduction

This chapter tracks the developing history of trauma informed thinking about the perinatal period. It provides a rationale for making a paradigm shift in perinatal mental health to be more trauma informed through focusing on post-traumatic sequelae. It also addresses the logical question of whether assessing for PTSD alone will be able to facilitate this paradigm shift properly.

Why is trauma informed perinatal care not very DEVELOPED?

Trauma informed care is an idea whose time has come for maternity services – but only just recently. By the early 1990s, public sector mental health and addiction fields became very aware that trauma history affected a majority of their clients (see Table 4.1).

In maternity care settings, the proportion is not as high, and the effects have taken longer to see. In the same early-1990s period, when the movement for trauma informed care gained momentum in mental health and substance abuse settings, a few maternity care professionals also called for the provision of care in pregnancy, birth and gynaecologic settings that would take women's trauma-related needs into account. Midwives, nurses and obstetrician-gynaecologists gave voice to this concept in clinical case reports and literature reviews that sought to translate information from the fields studying violence

Table 4.1 Timeline of key (mainly US) events: The evolution of incorporating attention to maltreatment sequelae and PTSD into care of adult women.

1977	Review of case studies estimates that one in a million girls in the English-speaking world are the victims of incest (Weinberg, 1955; 1976)
1983	Diane Russell's landmark study shows a much higher incidence of childhood sexual abuse — 38% of girls by age eighteen (Russell, 1983)
1985	Mary Koss reports about the 'hidden rape victim' by showing that only 10–50% of women disclose when they have been raped (Koss, 1985). Gail Elizabeth Wyatt reveals high rates of child sexual abuse in both white and black girls in California (Wyatt, 1985)
1990	In their national study, Finkelhor et al. affirm high incidence of childhood sexual assault of girls (Finkelhor et al., 1990)
1991	Call for changing standard (DSM) trauma definition from 'outside the range of usual human experience' to include maltreatment, rape and battering, which are all too common (Brown, 1991)
1992	Judith Herman publishes Trauma and Recovery — arguing for including complex PTSD, a sequela of maltreatment (i.e. domestic captivity) in the DSM-IV (Herman, 1992)
1992	WHO's ICD adds a complex PTSD diagnosis using the term 'Disorders of Extreme Stress Not Otherwise Classified; DESNOC (WHO, 1992)
1993 on	Epidemiology shows that PTSD occurs at twice the rate among women than men (Resnick et al., 1993; Kessler et al., 1995; Breslau et al., 1998)
1994	DSM-IV PTSD diagnostic criteria includes abuse/rape as potential traumas but does not make complex PTSD a diagnosis (APA, 1994)
2013	DSM-BV narrows trauma criteria so that some forms of childhood maltreatment again may not be a 'qualifying trauma' other than for sexual abuse and physical violence (APA, 2013) [despite the evidence of impact of emotional abuse — authors]

against women, child abuse and neglect, and trauma psychology into the field of women's health (see Table 4.2).

By the late 1990s, research on childhood sexual abuse began to appear in the main journals read by perinatal clinicians, and in 2001 the American College of Obstetricians and Gynecologists (ACOG) published an education bulletin calling for screening women for history of childhood sexual abuse because adverse effects on women's health across the lifespan were becoming clear. Yet this recommendation seemed to languish in implementation, likely because these health professionals did not know what to provide in response.

Now trauma and traumatic stress are moving to a more central focus in women's health. In the decade of the 2000s, research on PTSD in pregnancy and on birth as a traumatic event brought these concerns to the forefront. Since 2010, there have been several large studies showing that pregnancy PTSD is associated with adverse outcomes

Table 4.2 Timeline with examples from several nations of papers typical of the state of the science about trauma, PTSD and childbearing outcomes.

1992–1994	A survivor of childhood sexual abuse speaks out about the triggering effect of birth, and nurses and a childbirth educator responds (Rose, 1992; Courtois and Riley, 1992; Simkin, 1992). Nurse-midwives report a higher prevalence of abuse among those choosing midwifery care (Sampselle et al., 1992). Recommendations for midwifery care of survivors of childhood sexual abuse appear in publications for survivors (Sperlich, 1993–1994). First qualitative studies are published (e.g. Rhodes and Hutchinson, 1994)
1995–1998	Nurse-midwives and obstetricians call for routine screening for childhood sexual abuse (Bohn and Holz, 1996; Horan et al., 1998)
2001	First exploratory, population-focused report of PTSD associated with pregnancy complications in large service-use data set (Seng et al., 2001)
2001	American College of Obstetricians and Gynecologists' education bulletin recommends screening for childhood sexual abuse (ACOG, 2001)
2004 – 2009	Numerous papers are written on prevalence of PTSD in pregnancy among diverse populations and links with risk behaviours (Loveland Cook et al., 2004; Kim et al., 2014; Morland et al., 2007; Rodriguez et al., 2008; Seng et al., 2009)
Across this entire period	Key papers are published on birth as a new trauma that can cause PTSD and a re-traumatizing event that can cause recurrence (Czarnocka and Slade, 2000; Beck and Watson, 2008; Kitzinger and Kitzinger, 2007; Söderquist et al., 2004)
2011–2014	Large, well-designed studies show PTSD is associated with a range of adverse outcomes, including lower birth weight and shorter gestation and breastfeeding problems, and show intergenerational transmission pattern across the childbearing year (Seng et al., 2011b; 2013; Shaw et al., 2014; Yonkers et al., 2014)
2011 +	Beginning of reporting on interventions for maltreatment history and PTSD for childbearing women (Sperlich et al., 2011; Seng et al., 2011c; Rowe et al., 2014)

(Seng *et al.*, 2011; Shaw *et al.*, 2014; Yonkers *et al.*, 2014), and that birth is also a 're-traumatizing' event for women who have previous trauma history (Seng *et al.*, 2013). Thus, we are now in a period when trauma informed care in the perinatal period is beginning to make sense for reasons that are important to healthcare providers.

It probably also could go without saying that one other likely reason why maternity care is not yet trauma informed is that healthcare in general has not moved in this direction except in isolated arenas. Although the ACE study in the 1990s demonstrated a pattern of risk for several poor health outcomes due to childhood adversity (Felitti *et al.*, 1998), it has taken over fifteen years for this information to start to make it into mainstream consciousness. There has been positive movement, certainly. For example, the traumatising effects of cancer or traumatic injury are making oncology and emergency medicine more trauma informed, especially where children and their parents are involved. Care of veterans with PTSD is also making trauma informed primary care more widespread in settings that care for this population. The tipping point has yet to be reached. However, collaborations between psychosocial care professionals and obstetric healthcare providers that are being forged now to reduce perinatal health disparities and improve population health provide an opportunity not to be missed.

What justifies shifting our perinatal mental health paradigm?

Considerable attention (rightfully so) has been paid to the detection and treatment of postnatal depression and more recently antenatal depression. But far less attention has been brought to addressing trauma sequelae, including PTSD. And yet we now know that PTSD is quite common among women (Breslau *et al.*, 1991; Kessler *et al.*, 1995), and that depression and post-traumatic stress are highly comorbid with one another in general (Pietrzak *et al.*, 2011) and among pregnant women specifically (Seng *et al.*, 2009). A recent review of the research on child sexual abuse and PTSD among pregnant and postnatal women concludes that there are positive associations between child sexual abuse and clinical PTSD or PTSD symptomatology (Wosu *et al.*, 2015).

Just as mental healthcare for all women with maltreatment sequelae has evolved, so too must our understanding of the trauma-related needs of women during the childbearing year. A lack of attention to trauma sequelae is highly problematic because women experience PTSD symptoms during healthcare encounters and during birth. Doctors, midwives, and nurses are often in the position of witnessing post-traumatic reactions that are triggered either by pregnancy or the birth process itself, or else by the way that women are treated. During the birth process, there is no possibility to refer women to mental health services for current post-traumatic symptoms. Therefore, it is incumbent upon those who provide maternity care services to increase their understanding of trauma and how it affects women during the childbearing year, and to develop strategies for helping minimise the potential for healthcare routines in maternity care and birth to re-traumatise. They have to be able to respond in the moment, at the bedside.

We must make a collective shift in our perinatal mental health paradigm to include attention to:

- trauma exposure past and current;
- PTSD as an organising framework for understanding risk;
- preventing and responding to 'triggers';
- the challenge of co-morbidity and health risks;
- intergenerational transmission of risk;
- the opportunity presented by trauma informed maternity care.

Past and current trauma exposure
The effects of having been sexually abused as a child are so far-reaching that it has been suggested that such exposure should be considered a non-specific risk factor for a range of psychological disturbance (Maniglio, 2009). Both women and men are at the peak age of exposure to violence trauma during the ages of sixteen to twenty (Breslau *et al.*, 1998). Young women, in particular, are exposed to sexual abuse at high rates during childhood or adolescence, with one study showing that more than 26% of young women have had such experiences (Finkelhor *et al.*, 2014), and other research stated that one in five women experience either physical or sexual violence in their dating relationships (Vagi *et al.*, 2015). Given the age of exposure, there may be little time for treatment and recovery before beginning a pregnancy.

Some of these women will have contracted sexually transmitted infections or become pregnant as a result of rape, and may have psychological sequelae related not only to the rape trauma but also to any stigma or insensitive treatment they may have subsequently experienced in accessing medical care related to these conditions.

Trauma is also happening in the here and now for many women. Intimate partner relationships that involve violence place women at high risk during pregnancy for a range of problems. These include prematurity and low birth weight of infants (Alhusen *et al.*, 2015), and, importantly, women in such situations are at risk of being killed by their intimate partner, or of committing suicide (Palladino *et al.*, 2011). Although clinicians in healthcare systems across the globe have been asking routinely about current domestic abuse/intimate partner violence for some time, opinions are divided about whether or not this is advisable (Feder *et al.*, 2013; Moyer, 2013), since there is at this time insufficient evidence to demonstrate that screening alone results in benefits to women (Taft *et al.*, 2013; Hegarty *et al.*, 2015).

It is clear from close examination of the research on intimate partner violence and on eliciting disclosure of abuse trauma in general that what is lacking in particular is clinician training on the effects of trauma during the childbearing year, and effective screening coupled with capacity to respond appropriately to disclosure of past trauma and intimate partner violence (Feder *et al.*, 2006; Seng *et al.*, 2008). Thus screening for current violence that occurs within a system of trauma informed care may enhance responses to screening and improve benefits to women.

PTSD as an organising framework for understanding risk
A trauma informed approach to perinatal mental healthcare involves abandoning the question of 'What is wrong with you?' and instead asking 'What happened to you?' That is a first step, however. We also need a way of identifying those who are not resilient and who may be at risk. Using the concept of PTSD may be the best tool we have to do this. Those with PTSD will have symptoms that cause significant distress and impair functioning in a variety of settings (work, school, home/relationships). Understanding the features of PTSD not only allows us to gain a better comprehension of trauma sequelae, but also compels us to ask 'How is this affecting you now?' Understanding the answer to that question helps identify specific ways that we must tailor our mental health and maternity care to facilitate optimal treatment and to identify priority needs for resource facilitation and allocation. Subsequent chapters in this book will explore in more detail the connections between PTSD and trauma informed care both for pregnancy and the postnatal period. The current American Psychiatric Association (APA, 2013) and International Classification of Diseases (WHO, 1992) diagnostic criteria for PTSD are presented in very brief form in Table 4.3.

Table 4.3 Comparison of PTSD diagnostic criteria.

American Psychiatric Association (DSM-V) 2013	ICD-10 World Health Organization International Classification of Diseases (ICD-10) 1992
A. Exposure to actual or threatened death, serious injury or sexual violence: direct exposure, witnessing, in person, indirectly (relative or friend exposed to trauma), indirect exposure to trauma in the course of professional duties	A. Exposure to a stressful event or situation of exceptionally threatening or catastrophic nature
B. Persistent re-experiencing of the traumatic event: recurrent, involuntary and intrusive memories, traumatic nightmares, dissociative reactions, marked physiologic reactivity after exposure	B. Persistent remembering or reliving the stressor by intrusive flashbacks, vivid memories, recurring dreams, distress
C. Persistent avoidance of distressing trauma-related stimuli (thoughts or feeling, external reminders)	C. Actual or preferred avoidance of circumstances resembling or associated with the stressor
D. Negative alterations in cognitions and mood after the traumatic event: inability to recall key features, negative beliefs and expectations about oneself or the world, distorted blame of self or others, negative trauma-related emotions, diminished interest in significant activities, feeling alienated from others, constricted affect	D. Either: (a) inability to recall, partially or completely, some aspects of the period of exposure to the stressor, or (b) persistent symptoms of increased psychological sensitivity and arousal: sleep difficulty, irritability or anger, difficulty concentrating, hypervigilance, exaggerated startle response
E. Trauma-related alterations in arousal and reactivity after the traumatic event: irritable or aggressive behaviour, self-destructive or reckless behavior, hypervigilance, exaggerated startle response, problems in concentration, sleep disturbance **Specify if:** (1) with dissociative symptoms: in reaction to trauma, high levels of either: (a) depersonalization — experience of being an outside observer or detached from oneself; or (b) derealisation — experience of unreality, distance or distortion (2) with delayed expression: onset related to new reminder of old trauma	E. For some purposes, onset delayed more than six months may be included

Preventing and responding to triggers

One out of three women experience birth as traumatic, with 1–3% of women at risk of developing new-onset PTSD and another 4–5% of women experiencing it as a recurrent trigger for PTSD symptoms related to a previous trauma exposure (Seng *et al.*, 2013). We may not be able to save women from experiencing their birth as traumatic. So what can we do?

First, do no further harm. Women who have experienced maltreatment trauma report that post-traumatic stress symptoms including re-experiencing, avoidance and numbing, and arousal are features of their pregnancy and birth experiences (Seng *et al.*, 2004; Sperlich and Seng, 2008). These may manifest in response to any number of maternity care procedures that may serve as triggers, including: undressing and having one's genitalia exposed to relative strangers; being confined to bed and/or restrained by tubes, monitors, belts, etc.; being drugged; undergoing invasive procedures including epidural placement and internal pelvic examinations; operative deliveries; being ignored despite calls for assistance; enduring pain; and feeling out of control of one's own body (Hobbins, 2004; Sperlich and Seng, 2008). Given that these potential triggers are regular aspects of maternity care, 'doing no further harm' means that we must develop expertise in modifying and adapting such procedures in order to lessen their traumagenic influence.

Second, we must respond to symptoms triggered by aspects of the pregnancy, labour and birth experience with compassion. This includes developing an understanding of what being triggered looks like. Anticipating that there will be the potential for triggering in labour and birth, some women will choose a non-interventionist and unmedicated approach to childbirth in the belief that this will afford them more control over the process; other women will express a desire for analgesia/anaesthesia in order to numb potential triggers due to pain and discomfort (Seng *et al.*, 2004).

There is no single way that a woman with maltreatment history might respond to triggers in labour and birth. She may fight what is happening or dissociate from the experience altogether (Rhodes and Hutchinson, 1994). Efforts on the part of caregivers to calm her may be counterproductive: for example, telling a woman with a history of sexual abuse to 'calm down' and 'relax' may replicate the original abusive scenario. Ideally, understanding how an individual woman may react to triggering events would be done throughout pregnancy in the context of the developing relationship between care provider and client. However, conditions are not always ideal, and often women do not have the benefit of having developed a relationship with the care provider who attends them during labour and birth. Thus, we need to have strategies for helping in the moment.

At the minimum, we must adequately explain what we are doing in terms of procedures, and why we are doing it, and must be patient and give the mother a moment to react to what is happening. If this is not possible, then we need to acknowledge that what we are doing is causing distress, and that we are sorry for that. To the fullest extent possible, we need to develop a model of shared power and control, which honours both individualistic needs, and what is happening in the moment (i.e. addressing an emergency). It is important also to note that meeting the individual requirements of the client may outstrip available resources and time. Because of this, we need to identify support resources: for example, engaging the services of a doula; or additional labour support person who is known and trusted by the mother.

Shifting paradigms to focusing on preventing and responding to triggers during labour and birth suggests opportunity for interprofessional exchanges involving case histories and simulations. This would allow for improvements in skill in addressing mental health on the part of maternity care professionals and also could help therapists, social carers and educators who support women understand the perspective and unique challenges of working with women during the childbearing year. The extract from the UK social media website for mothers (Netmums) gives a good example of what support could look like – in this case, engaging with a doula for support where the trauma history is a previous traumatic birth.

Extract from Netmums (2012) concerning how a doula can help

After a very distressing back-to-back first labour (followed by PND/PTSD) I have been left with an absolute fear of childbirth and being in the hands of midwives. My current midwife is very understanding and has recommended I have a c-section to reduce my anxiety and related problems (anxiety attacks/nightmares/insomnia/tearfulness etc.) which has been agreed by my consultant. I'm not keen on a c-section but the thought of having to face labour is causing significant mental health problems. As it stands I've no idea what to do!

I'm considering hiring a doula as I'd feel more comfortable knowing I have an advocate to get my point across to the midwives if I went through labour … I would hope that as an independent birth partner a doula would be taken a bit more seriously as she would be objective whilst ensuring my wishes were taken into account. I'd also want someone there to reassure my partner as I don't cope well with pain and completely went to pieces in my last labour when they let the pain relief run out suddenly – it upset both my ex and mum to see me terrified and distressed when they could do nothing to help and I don't want to put him through that without someone to say 'it's ok, this is all part of labour and she can get through it'.

My only hesitation is that I don't want a doula who has an emphasis on natural birth and this seems to be the big focus on websites. I want a doula who'll support me and argue for me to get an epidural when I feel I need one rather than when the midwives think I'm in enough pain. I also only had contact with a midwife for about five minutes every four hours over a twenty-hour period (up to the point I had an epidural) in my last labour which left me feeling very scared and isolated so having someone to support me if the midwives don't would be a massive help to me.

I guess I think the most important quality for a doula is to listen to the mother's wishes about the birth whether they be natural or medical and to support her as much as possible to get the birth she wants even if it means marching straight down to the hospital at the first sign of pain and ensuring that pain relief is offered (www.netmums.com/coffeehouse/pregnancy-64/birth-labour-256/734413-has-anyone-out-there-used-doula-all.html/; accessed 6 July 2015).

The challenge of co-morbidity and health risks

Perinatal depression puts mothers and babies and their families at great risk, and is likely on the radar for most clinicians. Researchers and clinicians alike have also been recognising the co-morbidity that exists among mood disorders and anxiety disorders for some time, and have in fact shifted nomenclature from looking exclusively at postnatal depression and instead prefer 'perinatal mood and anxiety disorders' (e.g. Bradley and Hill, 2011). However, a similar move has not occurred in relation to bringing attention to the co-morbidity between mood disorders and post-traumatic stress. This is problematic because emerging studies show that not only does PTSD itself matter in terms of poor outcomes but also the co-morbidity between the two, evidenced by a gradient pattern of risk for prematurity, low birth weight, pregnancy substance using and postnatal bonding with infants (Seng et al., 2011; Shaw et al., 2014; Yonkers et al., 2014). Yet, many of these affected women are not coming to our clinical attention because we are not asking about trauma, and are not assessing for PTSD.

A closer examination of this co-morbidity suggests interplay of PTSD and depression in perhaps unexpected ways. When looking at those who meet major depression diagnosis in one perinatal study, we find that the majority of those with depression have had a significant

Figure 4.1 Sperlich's (2015) sample of pregnant women.

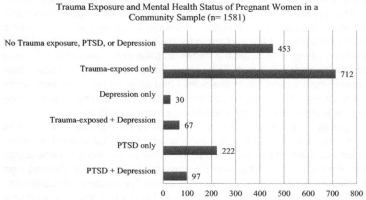

Trauma Exposure and Mental Health Status of Pregnant Women in a Community Sample (n= 1581)

traumatic exposure, and either have a subclinical level of PTSD or meet the full diagnosis for PTSD (Sperlich, 2015). In fact, of 194 women with depression only thirty (15.5%) did not report having had a major trauma consistent with the type that may lead to PTSD (see Figure 4.1).

Furthermore, it appears that PTSD symptoms in pregnancy, either by themselves or co-morbid with depression, are a more accurate predictor of meeting criteria for postnatal depression than is antenatal depression by itself (Sperlich, 2015). This suggests that there is an interplay between PTSD and depression (Ruscio *et al.*, 2002), and is respondent to accumulating trauma and allostatic pressure. It also indicates that the co-morbidity between PTSD and depression might be an entity in itself and that there may be such a thing as post-traumatic mood disorder (Sher, 2005) in itself. Yet another way to conceptualise co-morbidity is to assume that it is responsive to accumulation of trauma. For example, the ACE study (Felitti *et al.*, 1998) found dose-response relationships not only between the number and severity of ACE (toxic stress) and a wide number of health problems, but also for the co-morbid conditions of substance using, depression and suicide (PTSD was not assessed in the ACE study).

The opportunity presented by trauma informed maternity care
The frequent schedule of antenatal/postnatal visits represents a unique opportunity for treatment engagement. Trauma informed

maternity care would thereby present multiple opportunities for clinical contact to facilitate case-finding, non-triggering care, referral and treatment engagement, if care providers are aware of these issues and if there is true coordination between physical and behavioural health services. A shift in paradigm entails making sure there is a team that can be pulled together to facilitate meeting the needs of women who experience maltreatment-related sequelae. This team would include maternity care professionals and mental health professionals at the core, but would ideally reach out as needed to include local domestic violence agency personnel, suicide prevention counselling, labour support providers including doulas, childbirth educators and lactation consultants sensitive to trauma history. While such teams often exist in principle, there may be a lack of coordination and their care may not be trauma informed.

What are the implications for specialty service delivery?
Shifting our paradigm means that we must develop safety and evidence-based treatments for PTSD in pregnancy and the postnatal period. During the initial period where trauma informed perinatal care needs to be invented, we would need coordinated liaisons between those providing maternity care professionals (including obstetricians, midwives, nurses, health visitors, childbirth educators, doulas) and those providing specialty care (including social workers, therapists and other psychiatric care professionals), in order to develop ways to manage the ongoing presence of triggers that maternity care presents. Liaisons should also be extended to those who provide care for women during the fourth semester, including infant mental health specialists and parenting support professionals.

Why can't we just add PTSD to the list of conditions to address by screening and referring?

What are the implications for the rest of the perinatal care system and staff? Many of the one in five women with a maltreatment history have been resilient or have recovered from mental health conditions rooted in the trauma they experienced. Yet others begin their pregnancy having not yet recovered. Currently, such women are not routinely being screened and referred for specialty mental healthcare services to address traumatic sequelae. So it is logical to wonder whether it would be advisable and expedient simply to add PTSD to the list of conditions for which maternity care personnel routinely screen and refer. Unfortunately, this is likely to be problematic for a number of reasons, including:

- issues related to disclosure;
- competing priorities during the childbearing year;
- unique features of post-traumatic stress;
- paucity of trauma informed and pregnancy-specific treatment options.

All of these reasons must be taken into account, and have implications for those who provide perinatal care and for the entire perinatal care system.

Issues related to disclosure

Women by and large are not disclosing their history of traumatic exposure to maternity care providers at the same rates that they disclose in research contexts (Seng *et al.*, 2008). Many barriers to divulging trauma have been identified, and include both woman-centric barriers (e.g. concerns about safety; confidentiality; feeling it is not relevant to their care; stigma; and previous negative responses to previous disclosures) and provider-centric barriers (e.g. the belief that there are no existing strategies to help women; lack of confidence or comfort with asking; and lack of education). There are also system-centric reasons (e.g. language and cultural barriers; and inadequacy of privacy and time). Adding to this, many women who present to care for pregnancy have not yet sought treatment for PTSD because of the short intervening time between the traumatic exposure and the pregnancy.

These barricades suggest that simply adding PTSD to the checklists at intake will not be sufficient. Systemic change is needed in order to address the identified barriers, including enhancement to maternity provider education, further integration of behavioural health services into maternity care settings, and development of trauma informed and pregnancy-specific treatments. In the meantime, it has been demonstrated recently that primary care physicians who adopt a positive attitude towards outpatient mental healthcare are able to increase positive attitudes in their patients towards the uptake of such mental healthcare (Hornik-Lurie *et al.*, 2014).

Competing priorities during the childbearing year

The childbearing year brings many challenges for women and there are often many competing demands such as obtaining adequate housing, income and negotiating the increased physical demands of pregnancy. What this means in practical terms is that, even if we identify women with PTSD, a mental health referral might not fit with their priority needs. It is therefore incumbent for maternity care professionals to anticipate the ways in which PTSD may present an additional challenge during the childbearing year: for example, by managing potential triggers inherent to maternity care; meeting the needs for parenting support; and guiding a woman to make decisions about the future safety for her child, including determining who in her family or social sphere are safe to have contact with her child or to act as childcare providers.

Unique features of post-traumatic stress

One of the central features of PTSD that may inhibit disclosure is the avoidance of reminders of the trauma and anything that might trigger such memories. For a subset of women with PTSD, there will also be a dissociative element, meaning that they experience depersonalisation or derealisation, as well. Women who are trying to avoid memories of trauma or who feel disconnected from themselves or their surroundings may therefore be less likely to discuss their trauma or traumatic sequelae with maternity care providers.

The implications of these unique features of PTSD are that maternity care providers will often have to 'listen for unspoken messages' of the abuse survivors under their care (Montgomery *et al.*, 2015). In the absence of disclosure, care providers will be left with making a presumptive diagnosis. The subtlety required to do this, however, is dependent on adequacy of clinician education to facilitate sensitive care.

Paucity of trauma informed and pregnancy-specific treatment options

Maternity care providers are not mental health experts, nor should they be expected to be. They therefore need ready access to liaisons with mental health professionals and new primary care approaches to working with trauma survivors in the context of the maternity care setting. It makes sense that a midwife or doctor is reticent to ask about past trauma or PTSD if they perceive that there are no trauma informed and pregnancy-specific treatments available.

The good news is that there are trauma informed and pregnancy-specific interventions under development. Chapter 8 will describe these and their current state of development.

Conclusion

This chapter has focused on demonstrating the need for a shift in the collective perinatal mental health paradigm to become more trauma informed and to include attention to understanding how post-traumatic stress is experienced by women during the childbearing year:

❑   In the past, we have focused on perinatal mood and anxiety disorders; a focus on trauma and maltreatment and PTSD are more recent developments.

❑   There is considerable co-morbidity between depression and PTSD, making it clear that focusing on depression alone is not adequate.

❑   Clinical and research evidence for the deleterious effects of maltreatment and PTSD during the childbearing year has been accruing and suggests the need for a paradigm shift in the way we think about perinatal care.

❑   PTSD brings unique challenges. We cannot just refer women with maltreatment history to mental healthcare providers, since women experience triggering events in the context of maternity care. Therefore, we must do a better job of educating and supporting maternity care specialists towards optimal care of maltreatment survivors.

❑   Shifting paradigms suggests that we must develop trauma informed and pregnancy-specific interventions that serve the needs of pregnant women and their families.

CHAPTER 5

How does traumatic stress affect pregnancy and birth?

Julia Seng, University of Michigan

Introduction

In this chapter we will review the trajectory of research on traumatic stress and pregnancy – from a qualitative focus on women's experiences to quantitative work on outcomes, and back again. This body of work has significant gaps to fill, but the accumulating knowledge indicates that trauma informed care and trauma-specific interventions are warranted, especially in settings where vulnerable populations are served. In this chapter we also point out that providing trauma informed care is not only about risk; it also is about supporting resilient women and promoting post-traumatic growth. In addition, we give some space to discussing the challenges to providers who work closely with traumatised clients. The information in this chapter is largely told from the maternity care provider's perspective, which will give child welfare and mental health professionals a glimpse of what things look like from the bedside. At the end of the chapter we will turn to the obvious point that our work at the bedside and our well-being as practitioners of interpersonal practice professions can be enhanced by interprofessional collaboration.

Coming full circle?

When we look back on the progress of research on post-traumatic stress effects on pregnancy, it would seem that the first quantitative papers examining PTSD effects on pregnancy were published around the year 2000 (Neuberg *et al.*, 1998; Chang *et al.*, 2002; Seng *et al.*, 2001; Yehuda *et al.*, 2005). There was relevant scholarship starting ten or so years earlier, beginning around 1990, but the focus had been on child sexual abuse history: for example, looking at women's experiences of childbearing qualitatively (e.g. Rhodes and Hutchinson, 1994). It made sense that this was the focus of early studies because the maternity care providers writing the early case study, literature review and qualitative research papers likely would not have put the PTSD vocabulary front and centre, though it may have been mentioned in discussion. The whole issue likely came to their attention because they were observing flashbacks, dissociation and interpersonal reactions that are part and parcel of the sequelae of child sexual abuse.

Moreover, the prevalence of abuse history and of PTSD among women was just beginning to be known in the mental health and child welfare professions in the 1980s, including the extent to which all forms of maltreatment were overlapping. This information was only beginning to leak into the knowledge base of women's health-care providers.

Early publications and the focus on experiences of care
As perinatal professionals started out studying traumatic stress and pregnancy, they focused on the experience of women with child-hood sexual abuse in their history, often using the language of survivorship rather than the language of diagnosis. This literature focused on how each woman's history seemed to affect her experi-ence of care adversely. An influential series of papers was published under the leadership of Penny Simkin, a physiotherapist and child-birth educator, in the international multidisciplinary journal *Birth* in 1992; the series included a survivor's perspective (Rose, 1992). An article written in 1993 for abuse survivors about giving birth was by one of this book's co-authors, Mickey Sperlich, in a publication for survivors called *Above a Whisper* (Sperlich, 1993). The earliest case report we have found was written by a clinical psychologist, Laura Josephs, in 1996 for a psychology and psychiatry journal urging interprofessional work between maternity care and mental health professionals – and with clients, to improve relationship dynam-ics (Josephs, 1996). Literature reviews integrating knowledge from mental health disciplines appeared in perinatal professional jour-nals across disciplines (Bohn and Holz, 1996; Horan *et al.*, 1998; 2000) including an education bulletin by ACOG calling for routine screening for history of childhood sexual abuse, which appeared in 2001 (ACOG, 2001).

Qualitative reports contributing information from both women's and clinicians' perspectives have been appearing steadily for the past two decades. Although based on studies conducted in many nations, the themes and concerns engendered a sense of familiarity among clinicians and researchers in the field that suggests the phenomenon has commonalities across cultures. Early survey research, also from the 1990s, focused mostly on the experiences of gynaecologic care of women with a history of childhood sexual abuse, likely because the common procedure of pelvic examination was a trigger for many women and a clinical challenge for healthcare providers who wanted to do a better job of meeting their needs. It seems in hindsight that distress in response to this intrusive contact and its power dynamics was the tip of an iceberg or a sentinel sign of a problem we did not yet have the lens to see.

Shifting the focus to maltreatment survivors' risk exposures

Awareness of childhood sexual abuse survivors' presence among gynaecology and maternity clients intersected with the emerging body of social work and psychology literature that was raising the profile of abuse survivors' behavioural risk exposures. From these reports, gynaecology and perinatal studies followed, showing that known risks for adverse perinatal outcomes including smoking, substance abuse, disordered eating, high-risk sexual activity and adult re-victimisation were concentrated among maltreatment survivors (Seng *et al.*, 2008; Morland *et al.*, 2007). Yet in these studies samples were generally cross-sectional and did not have sample sizes large enough to examine birth outcomes.

Moving towards studying psychosocial stress and outcomes

Also during this period psychosocial stress in the forms of violence, depression and socio-demographic disadvantage (including disparities for minority groups) was being studied as a pathway to preterm birth and low birth weight (Reagan and Salsberry, 2005). It was often a vulnerable subset of the sample that experienced the most risk for adverse outcomes. These studies had not taken lifetime trauma exposures into account, including the maltreatment trauma that can be a basis for vulnerability. Trauma was not the concept of interest, since the focus was still on stress.

These studies also occurred prior to publication of the *Diagnostic and Statistical Manual of Mental Disorders, Fourth Edition* (APA, 1994) where the definition of trauma changed from experiences 'outside the range of usual human experience' to include abuse and sexual assault and prior to publication of epidemiological studies reported in 1993 and 1995 (Resnick *et al.*, 1993; Kessler *et al.*, 1995) showing that PTSD was twice as prevalent among women as among men.

Focusing on PTSD's effect on outcomes

The first PTSD studies that reported on perinatal outcomes were conducted in the aftermath of disasters (e.g. Yehuda *et al.*, 2005; Neuberg *et al.*, 1998; Chang *et al.*, 2002). Knowledge about PTSD in civilian populations has often been advanced by post-disaster studies, where the exposure to trauma is a natural experiment, measurable and not subject to recall bias. These studies of perinatal outcomes among women exposed to earthquake, hurricane and terrorism trauma compared those who did and did not develop disaster-related PTSD, and they had inconsistent results. A limitation of these projects was that they did not assess lifetime trauma exposure including maltreatment or pre-existing PTSD.

Another influential study (and one to which we have referred many times) in the 1990s, the ACE study, reported that among 17,000 adults the more adverse childhood experiences (ACEs) reported, the greater the correlation with early morbidity and mortality from the leading causes of death – independently of other risk exposures (Felitti *et al.*, 1998). This raised the question of what could connect the relationship of maltreatment to disease across decades. Numerous health research studies conducted around this time consistently showed PTSD to be a mediator between trauma exposure (of many types, including child and adult abuse) and health problems (Schnurr and Green, 2004). It seemed logical to extend this work to determine if PTSD also mediated the relationship between trauma exposure and adverse perinatal outcomes.

As summarised in Table 5.1, three large (non-disaster) studies now show association of PTSD with shorter gestation and lower birth weight (Seng *et al.*, 2011; Shaw *et al.*, 2014; Yonkers *et al.*, 2014). The three studies used different methods, different samples and had

Table 5.1 Results of three recent PTSD and perinatal outcome studies in relation to the public health outcomes of gestational age and birth weight.

Study	Design and sample	PTSD and adverse birth outcomes
Seng et al., 2011b	Prospective cohort study, 839 women	PTSD was associated with shorter gestation and lower birth weight (283 grams less than for trauma-exposed, resilient women)
Shaw et al., 2014	Analysis of service use data, 16,334 deliveries	Mothers with PTSD were significantly more likely to suffer preterm birth; two out of a hundred preterm births were attributable to PTSD
Yonkers et al., 2014	Prospective cohort study, 2,654 women	Women with PTSD and depression were at a fourfold increased risk of preterm birth

slightly different focal questions, but all three found PTSD was associated with adverse outcomes. Replication is important, adding credence to findings and building a case for taking action.

One of these, our study known as the STACY project, focused on the question of whether the type of antecedent trauma mattered by assessing trauma history in detail and analysing the predictive relationships of five categories of trauma exposure (Seng et al., 2009). The answer was yes; trauma type matters. Women with a maltreatment history had the highest (twelvefold) risk of PTSD in pregnancy and worse outcomes across every outcome examined. Although maltreatment trauma in childhood was not a focal predictor in the two subsequent studies (Shaw et al., 2014; Yonkers et al., 2014), these investigators showed that experiencing military sexual trauma, meeting PTSD diagnostic criteria in pregnancy and having PTSD that is co-morbid with depression are strong risk factors for prematurity. These predictors parallel the re-victimisation, active PTSD in pregnancy and depression co-morbidity seen in the group with maltreatment-related PTSD in the STACY study. Together, these results indicate that further research on biological mechanisms and on perinatal interventions should concentrate particularly on the women with a history of maltreatment – both resilient women and those affected by PTSD and associated morbidity.

PTSD and its greater adverse impact in low-resource populations

One key finding of the STACY study that is important to take into account when creating trauma informed care and trauma-specific interventions is that PTSD in pregnancy seems to have a strong social gradient. STACY was a US study where African American women are disadvantaged and experience disparities in health and in perinatal outcomes. In this study, a very key finding was that European American and African American women did not have differences in risk for maltreatment, sexual trauma or lifetime PTSD. They did reveal a strong variation in rates of PTSD in pregnancy, with the minority women having nearly five times the rate (14% versus 3%) of meeting PTSD diagnostic criteria in early pregnancy (Seng *et al.*, 2011a). This is likely a function of at least four factors:

- younger age at first pregnancy, which would leave less time for recovery;
- greater total number of types of trauma exposure, which likely means more recent exposure;
- more chronic life stressors including racism that likely interact with traumatic stress and foster depression;
- fewer of the resources that enhance resilience and recovery such as education, safety, belonging to the dominant culture, and treatment.

This constellation of factors that seems to increase risk for pregnancy PTSD probably generalises beyond the US to many low-resource settings. Trauma informed care likely should be prioritised for public sector maternity clinics and maternal support services and should articulate with and look for synergies by linking with existing models of care that address the needs of vulnerable populations.

The STACY study has been able to examine many research questions. The study was designed to answer questions about health, mental health and relational outcomes. But it has been possible to address many other questions along the way. Table 5.2 summarises findings across papers that have been published to date.

Table 5.2 Main findings from STACY project reports.

Reference	Main findings
King *et al.*, 2008	• The impacts (i.e. effect sizes) of socio-economic stress, smoking and PTSD on the stress hormone cortisol were similar among women in the first half of pregnancy
Seng *et al.*, 2008	• The risk behaviours and exposures that adversely affect pregnancy outcomes were concentrated among childhood maltreatment survivors • Women disclosed maltreatment and sexual trauma more in research interviews than in new patient interviews in maternity care. The ratio was 11:1, 33% versus 3%
Seng *et al.*, 2009	• The prevalence of lifetime PTSD was 20.2% and of PTSD in pregnancy was 7.9% in this US community sample of women in the first half of pregnancy • Rates differed by socioeconomic context, with women in an affluent town having a pregnancy PTSD rate of 2.7% versus 13.9% for women in an impoverished urban area • Maltreatment history conveyed twelvefold risk for meeting PTSD diagnostic criteria in pregnancy • Depression diagnosis rates were: 3.4% among the group with no trauma exposure; 4.7% in the trauma-exposed, resilient women; 27% among those with lifetime PTSD (recovered); and 35% among those meeting PTSD criteria in pregnancy
Seng *et al.*, 2010	• Comparing this pregnant sample with a national sample studied with the same standardised interview, PTSD rates were higher in the pregnant sample • Younger age and lower socio-economic status in the pregnancy sample accounted for only a small proportion of the increased prevalence, suggesting pregnancy triggers symptoms • PTSD symptom profile among pregnant women indicated the most frequently reported symptoms in pregnancy were detachment, loss of interest, anger and irritability
Seng *et al.*, 2011a	• Minority (African American) women and majority (European American) women had no difference in their rates of exposure to maltreatment and sexual trauma • There were no differences in rates of lifetime PTSD • But minority women had higher rates of PTSD during pregnancy. In this study this likely was because they were younger and so closer to the 16–21 peak age of trauma exposure, had fewer resources for treatment or recovery, and had more total non-abuse trauma exposures including more recent exposures
Seng *et al.*, 2011b	• PTSD was associated with shorter gestation and lower birth weight compared with trauma-exposed but resilient women and compared to non-exposed women • This relationship was strongest in the sample where the antecedent trauma exposure was maltreatment (as opposed to the sample where the index trauma was something else such as accidents, illness, robbery or natural disaster) • Prenatal care was not protective among the women with maltreatment history • When PTSD was taken into account, minority (African American) race was no longer independently predictive of prematurity
Lopez *et al.*, 2011	• Women who were not able to quit smoking in pregnancy had higher rates of PTSD and were more likely to report abuse as their worst trauma exposure • PTSD arousal symptoms were predictive of not quitting • This has implications for smoking cessation treatment among pregnant women. Dual-diagnosis approaches may be more effective

Reference	Main findings
Kruse *et al.*, 2013	• The quality of the partner relationship was a better predictor of outcomes than partnered status alone • Since women with a maltreatment history were more likely to be in abusive partner relationships, including an indicator of their satisfaction and safety would improve outcomes research
Bell *et al.*, 2012	• Childhood maltreatment history and pre-pregnancy use of mental health treatment were associated with using adequate prenatal care • PTSD, interpersonal reactivity, low scores on alliance with the maternity care providers, substance use and public insurance were associated with not using adequate prenatal care
Seng *et al.*, 2013	• The rate of postnatal PTSD in this study was 6%, consistent with other studies. 75% of postnatal PTSD cases were among women who had PTSD prior to birth • Lifetime PTSD was a better predictor of postnatal depression than pregnancy depression • PTSD mediated the relationship between maltreatment history and postnatal depression and bonding impairment • Bonding impairment was associated with postnatal depression, but only when it was co-morbid with PTSD • The multivariable, stepwise, regression models of postnatal outcomes confirmed the literature from multiple disciplines showing intergenerational patterns of abuse and psychiatric vulnerability intersecting in the childbearing year
Seng *et al.*, 2014	• There were almost no cases of PTSD that were not co-morbid with depression or complicated by interpersonal reactivity, dissociation or somatisation (eight cases out of 319 women in the PTSD cohort)
Lopez *et al.*, 2014	• Smoking and PTSD interacted in their impact on stress hormone (cortisol) levels, causing the highest levels • PTSD and smoking both exert toxic effects on pregnancyes
Kruse *et al.*, 2014	• Structural equation modelling suggested that bonding impairment was a cause of postnatal depression as well as a result of depression • Bonding impairment was predictable antenatally by the PTSD symptom of detachment and by parenting sense of competence assessed antenatally • This suggested that attention to attachment concerns antenatally may help prevent cases of postnatal depression
Choi and Seng (date to be confirmed)	• Dissociation in labour was predicted by childhood maltreatment history, pre-pregnancy PTSD, depression and dissociation, by appraisals of the labour experience and care received in labour as poor • Dissociation in labour was a strong predictor of postnatal PTSD, postnatal depression and impaired bonding
Seng *et al.*, under review	• In a subset of 395 of the STACY participants, PTSD was associated with higher stress hormone (cortisol) levels across the day • The highest levels were among those with the dissociative subtype of PTSD • In a subset of 111 STACY participants who gave saliva sample twelve times from early pregnancy to six weeks postpartum, the PTSD group had consistently higher levels across a curve that peaked just before birth • The dissociative subtype group was highest to begin with — so high that it did not have any peak

Looking also at the opposite causal direction – PTSD as the outcome, not the predictor

At the same time as research was taking off on PTSD as a cause of adverse childbearing outcomes, there was also progress in a large body of research internationally looking at traumatic childbearing as a reason for PTSD. Studies have demonstrated that PTSD results from childbirth in approximately 6% of cases, with a higher proportion experiencing significant symptomatology that does not reach the diagnostic level (Ayers *et al.*, 2015). [Note, however, Seng *et al.*'s (2013) further breakdown of this in Chapter 4: of those 6%, the majority are women who had PTSD previously and for them the birth was a re-triggering event (4–5%), whereas only 1–3% of women experienced their birth as a new-onset trauma (meaning they did not previously have PTSD.] Predictors of postnatal, birth-related PTSD include both predisposing and precipitating factors (Slade, 2006).

It became clear early in this trajectory of studies that interpersonal components of the birth experience, i.e. care by providers perceived to be insensitive or incompetent, were consistent precipitating factors for post-birth PTSD (Slade, 2006). Previous trauma including abuse emerged as a predisposing factor (Slade, 2006). This postnatal PTSD research then linked to the research on fear of childbirth, and leading researchers in psychosomatic obstetrics suggested that women with a maltreatment history might be suffering in pregnancy from what could be called pre-traumatic stress (Söderquist *et al.*, 2004; 2009). Thus, in relation to postnatal birth-related PTSD also, future research and interventions should attend to lifetime trauma history. We would expect a proportion of women with post-birth PTSD to have birth as a first traumatic life event and new-onset PTSD. It seems, however, that a majority will be women for whom postnatal PTSD is recurrent or chronic, exacerbated by birth as a re-traumatisation.

Coming back to the beginning about women's experiences

These outcomes studies, taken together, suggest that post-traumatic stress that has childhood maltreatment as its antecedent is a particularly important risk factor for adverse childbearing experiences and adverse outcomes. New research about the experiences of women in childbirth holds promise to inform care, including intrapartum services (see Table 5.3). The finding that it is women with a maltreatment history who have the worst outcomes has spurred a return to qualitative work to improve understanding of the phenomenon for this one in five subgroup.

A recent meta-synthesis of eight qualitative studies undertaken with women with a history of childhood sexual abuse distilled and themes led to a clear conclusion that building trusting relationships, facilitating a sense of control and avoiding actions and dynamics that remind women of the past trauma are key areas for professionals to attend to (Montgomery, 2013).

Another recent study used surveys to learn what women who experienced traumatic or difficult births identified as 'hotspots', defined as moments in memory that can become the content of PTSD-intrusive, re-experiencing symptoms. In this study, dissociation in labour and fear and lack of control predicted re-experiencing the worst hotspots. Dissociation, fear and lack of control and obstetric events predicted postnatal PTSD, while hotspots of interpersonal difficulties were the most predictive factor (Harris and Ayers, 2012).

These research findings align well with psychoanalytic and maternal development literature from the mid-twentieth century. These writers observed that pregnancy is an embodied psychosexual experience and a sensitive period when a woman's development as a mother involves harkening back in memory, dreams and subconsciously to how she was mothered (Deutsch, 1945; Bibring, 1959). For women maltreated by family members (including emotional, physical or sexual maltreatment), this developmental process would likely include activation or re-activation of trauma-related psychological distress. This, in turn, coincided logically with the finding of twelvefold risk for PTSD in pregnancy conveyed by maltreatment history (Seng *et al.*, 2009) and the clinical awareness that internal examinations, the inescapable major physical and emotional challenge of birth, and dependence on caregivers and the power dynamics in healthcare relationships were triggers (Montgomery, 2013; Harris and Ayers, 2012).

Taken together, a focus on the needs of maltreatment survivors in pregnancy, birth and in the immediate aftermath is warranted in

Table 5.3 Recent reports of studies about intrapartum risk factors for adverse experiences and post-traumatic stress that highlight the relational aspects of risk

Study	Design and sample	Findings
Montgomery, 2013	Meta-synthesis of eight qualitative reports focused on the needs of childbearing women with a childhood sexual abuse history	**Needs during childbirth:** • sense of control; • feeling safe; • disclosure opportunities; • healing opportunities. • Unmet needs lead to: • remembering (triggers, flashbacks); • dissociation (loss of control); • feelings of vulnerability. **Overall synthesis:** • women could feel safe and experience healing if they could retain control and forge positive, trusting relationships with healthcare professionals; • re-enactments of abuse occur with reminders of abusive situations, absence of control and absence of a trusting relationship.
Harris and Ayers, 2012	Survey of 675 women with traumatic birth experiences to characterise intrapartum hotspots that increase risk for post-birth PTSD	**Intrapartum hotspots fall into three categories.** *Interpersonal events:* • being ignored; • lack of support; • poor communication; • being abandoned; • being put under pressure. *Events concerning the baby:* • problems with the baby; • being separated from the baby. *Obstetric events and pain:* • non-painful obstetric events; • pain. *Overall findings:* • re-experiencing symptoms (flashbacks, nightmares, unwanted recollections) of the worst hotspot were more likely if there was also dissociation and fear and lack of control; • PTSD was predicted by those and obstetric complications, but the interpersonal difficulties factor was the largest predictor.

research, clinical care and policy to shape what is feasible in terms of service delivery in health and social care. The boundaries of this work are hard to delineate because the needs of trauma survivors do not stop with birth. And the requirements of trauma survivors also are going to affect their caregivers.

Expanding attention to trauma

As maternity care providers have become more aware of the impact of trauma and PTSD on women's childbearing experiences and outcomes, they also are becoming more cognisant of vicarious trauma. 'Listening to women' is a major theme of the US midwifery profession (www.midwife.org/Our-Mission-Vision-Values/; accessed 6 July 2015). As maternity professionals open themselves to seeing traumatic stress reactions and hearing trauma narratives in their practice, they begin to encounter the same risk for vicarious trauma as psychotherapists (Pearlman and Saakvitne, 2013). There are perhaps some added layers for maternity professionals (Beck, 2011; Leinweber and Rowe, 2010). First, pregnancy and birth can have catastrophic outcomes in some cases or professionals can make mistakes, so exposure to real-time trauma occurs in the workplace. Second, not all healthcare team members have equal power or control over how care is delivered, so less powerful members often feel helpless or victimised themselves or are placed in situations where they feel as though they are perpetrating or accomplices to someone else enacting violence. Finally, most healthcare professionals do not have sophisticated training about counter-transference reactions where they empathise with or react to their clients' intense emotions – consciously or not – in ways that warrant awareness, reflection, self-monitoring and potentially self-care to remain effective and healthy over the long-term. Similarly, the central goal of midwifery is that of being with the woman, but this connection in itself may increase exposure to traumatic memories.

So far we also have focused on maltreatment trauma (and birth re-traumatisation) as the index trauma for PTSD. But as we become more trauma informed, other types of traumatic experience will garner more attention. Among these are other potential triggers to pregnancy PTSD. These include sexual trauma in adulthood.

Sexual assault of adult women occurs at high rates in civilian and military settings (Elliott *et al.*, 2004; Skinner *et al.*, 2000). Although pregnancy that results from rape seems to occur at low rates (Holmes *et al.*, 1996), these mothers may have needs for trauma informed care and trauma-specific interventions for pregnancy, birth and bonding with the infant. Previous medical trauma – whether from the condition or the treatment procedures – may also trigger PTSD in pregnancy, which is a highly medicalised situation in Western contexts (Hamama *et al.*, 2010).

Previous perinatal loss, previous traumatic birth or loss of a child also can result in PTSD that may be ongoing or recurrent in subsequent pregnancies (Engelhard *et al.*, 2001; Hamama *et al.*, 2010). Parents whose infant's life is at risk also may experience PTSD and need postnatal trauma informed and trauma-specific help (Feeley *et al.*, 2011).

Finally, women from non-Western groups may have culturally specific situations that are potentially salient as traumatic stressors around the time of birth. Examples include women with genital cutting or infibulation that could complicate birth (ACNM, 2000) or women of indigenous cultures required to give birth in Western medical settings (Linehan, 1992).

As we become more organised and proficient about applying trauma informed care, tailored responses for more types of salient trauma exposures and for particular populations can be advanced.

Not to forget resilience and post-traumatic growth

By focusing on all the reasons why women with a maltreatment history are at risk for adverse experiences and outcomes and warrant trauma informed care, there is a real risk of ignoring resilience. And we could easily overlook the potential power we have to foster post-traumatic growth as well as address or prevent post-traumatic disorders.

Resilience is the flip side of the PTSD coin that is easily ignored. A significant proportion of women with a maltreatment history do not develop PTSD, depression, dissociation, substance misuse or relationship problems. They used engaged or creative coping strategies, connected to other adults who give them love and support, or managed life-affirming escape paths into adulthood (Agaibi and Wilson, 2005). Others may have experienced some sequelae but managed to recover, on their own or with help, by the time they have a child. Thus, while some pregnant women may have diagnosable mental health sequelae and need or want specialist treatment, others may require only some acknowledgement of concerns and trauma informed supports such as care planning to avoid triggers or opportunities to talk about protective parenting strategies and resources to use if they become overwhelmed.

Quantitative research affirms that resilient women are different from women who have not been exposed to maltreatment or other major traumas. In the STACY project, sometimes the maltreated but resilient women do seem a little bit worse off than non-exposed women. For example, they have slightly more depression symptoms, smoke more and worry more about how competent they will be as parents compared with women who have never been maltreated. But sometimes the resilient women seem to do better. They show strengths in forming alliance with caregivers, and intend to breastfeed at higher rates than others. Qualitative studies by different research teams have shown repeatedly that women with a maltreatment history often hope – and manage – to do better for their children than their parents did for them. There are themes and narratives, too, from qualitative studies of survivors' birth experiences indicating that a positive birth was not only uplifting but also a special challenge that changed their perceptions of themselves for the better and gave them a needed opportunity to take pride in their strength and to experience an intense instance of being well cared for by someone in a position of power (Sperlich and Seng, 2008). These phenomena point to the potential for the challenges of pregnancy, birth and breastfeeding to be opportunities for positive emotions, nurturing relationships and post-traumatic growth that could not come at a better time if they strengthen the woman as she starts her development as a mother.

As we will see more in the next chapter, one of the most powerful strategies professionals may be able to use in the perinatal period is to role model in relationship with the woman the same types of relational strategies she will ideally enact with her infant – fostering a secure attachment, providing a holding environment where it is safe to respond to a major challenge, and expecting to need to work with the woman to regulate fear, anxiety, PTSD and other intense emotions provoked by pregnancy, birth and parenting.

Perhaps another important reason to try to keep a focus on resilience and post-traumatic growth is actually for the sake of the caregivers. Listening to women about their trauma-related needs and providing trauma informed care can extract a cost (Leinweber and Rowe, 2010). This may be especially true in the early days of doing so, when there is a steep learning curve or resistance in the organisation or even backlash from colleagues. Supporting a resilient woman or fostering post-traumatic growth is also important work. Noticing, documenting and feeling satisfaction from successes will make trauma informed care's value evident and increase likelihood of sustainability.

Collaborating across the mental versus physical health divide early on

Maternity care providers have likely been observing traumatic stress reactions in some (or many) clients since the beginnings of their professional lives. But care of women experiencing maltreatment sequelae in the form of traumatic stress is not yet a core element of nursing, midwifery or obstetric training. Therefore, many perinatal clinicians who are expert in other domains feel ill-prepared to address PTSD with their pregnant or labouring clients. Social care, child welfare and mental health professionals have more training and experience in this domain and could help.

Removing system-level logistic barriers to integrated care may yet take some time, but in the immediate future individuals could begin to collaborate informally or formally – one phone call, cup of coffee or case consultation at a time. Maternity care professionals who have taken an interest in working with trauma-affected clients tell stories of how helpful it was to debrief with a social work colleague after a difficult case – and of how they consulted proactively the next time they wanted ideas.

Nurses could create in-service meetings where they invite a mental health professional, share case stories and start listing best practices and supporting each other to modify unit routines. Mental health professionals who find themselves treating a pregnant woman with maltreatment-related needs could ask the client for formal permission to communicate with the maternity care provider and offer suggestions for integrated care.

Such one-to-one opportunities to share expertise can ease the learning curve and build momentum for larger changes. We can also share with each other what we learn in our work with clients who disclose and are good collaborators in planning their own care.

Conclusion

Current research findings about how PTSD affects pregnancy and birth have built from case studies and qualitative research begun in the 1990s. Now that we know more from large quantitative studies, we understand that there is justification for interventions, especially in low-resource settings. Here is key information about how PTSD affects childbearing:

❑ Early clinical literature and qualitative studies suggested that pregnancy, antenatal care procedures and birth were triggers for PTSD morbidity in pregnancy for women with maltreatment history.

❑ Quantitative research now confirms that maltreatment history conveys higher risk for having PTSD in pregnancy.

❑ PTSD in pregnancy, maltreatment history, sexual trauma and depression co-morbidity have been found to contribute to the important public health problems of shorter gestation and lower birth weight in three large studies to date.

❑ The experience of birth – regardless of outcome – can be traumatic and trigger new-onset of PTSD or be re-traumatising and exacerbate existing PTSD.

❑ Other types of trauma exposure may also be salient to subgroups of women and could also be addressed with trauma informed care tailored to special populations.

❑ Disadvantaged women bear a greater burden of traumatic stress sequelae during pregnancy, so trauma informed care should be a priority in low-resource settings where trauma informed care and trauma-specific interventions should articulate and synergise with existing models of care for vulnerable women.

❑ Trauma informed care can meet the needs of resilient women as well as those with mental health sequelae of maltreatment. Supporting resilient women and promoting post-traumatic growth would also probably improve population outcomes.

❑ Providing bedside care may place maternity care professionals at risk for vicarious trauma that is similar to that which psychotherapists can experience.

❑ Starting to collaborate across the health versus mental health divide in the earliest phases of implementing trauma informed care may increase comfort-level and sophistication more quickly and lead to evidence of success on which to build.

CHAPTER 6

The postnatal period – opportunities for creating change

Catherine Acton Jane Fisher, and Heather Rowe, Monash University, Australia, Julie Taylor, University of Birmingham (UK)

Introduction

Postnatal care has in the past been focused primarily on physical recovery from birth and on infant feeding, health and development. However, there is growing systematic attention to maternal postnatal mental health in high income countries and a recognition that the term 'postnatal depression' includes other psychological states including anxiety and trauma reactions. Mental health professionals have theoretical frameworks and skills to address perinatal psychological needs, and they will be able to apply a trauma informed approach. But many perinatal healthcare and child welfare workers may not feel they have adequate theory or skills training to take an active role in this domain.

This chapter describes how past maltreatment experiences might affect a woman's adjustment in the postnatal period. It then focuses on three theory-based concepts that can provide a common language for interprofessional care that is consistent with a trauma informed approach and that also is pertinent to all new mothers: 'attachment', 'dyadic regulation' and the 'holding environment'. The chapter also outlines some clinical skills useful for front-line care providers, especially those who do home visiting, to support healthcare professionals to be more confident to assess for and respond to women with mental health problems including PTSD.

Understanding the psychological needs of women who have recently given birth

The birth of a baby is a major adaptive challenge for any woman. In having a baby, a woman has to relinquish, at least temporarily, her personal autonomy and liberty, occupational identity, capacity to generate an income and social and leisure activities in service of infant care. The adaptation to new required roles, major responsibilities, multiplication of the unpaid workload and, for some, harm to bodily integrity through unexpected adverse reproductive events places great demands on individual psychological resources and existing relationships. Psychological disequilibrium, characterised by uncertainty, ambivalence, confusion and a sense of being underequipped or ill-prepared for new expectations, is normal during life transitions and in adaptation to change. However, there is now general agreement that mental health can be compromised among women who have recently given birth (Fisher *et al.*, 2009). There are debates about whether mental health problems are most accurately conceptualised as positions on a spectrum of distress or as discrete specific conditions, but the most widely used framework is that psychotic illnesses are rare and that non-psychotic problems which are associated with reduced functioning are more prevalent.

Postnatal depression is a clinical and research construct used to describe experiences of major or minor depression occurring among women who have recently given birth. Postnatal depression is characterised by the persistent presence for at least two weeks of cognitive and affective symptoms including low mood, guilt, despondency, self-criticism, lack of pleasure, impaired concentration, irritability, elevated anxiety, rumination and social withdrawal. The somatic symptoms of sleep and appetite disturbance are also present, but are not uncommon in normal postnatal adjustment. Brockington (2004) in a review of postnatal psychiatric disorders concludes, however, that women identified through screening using self-report questionnaires as 'depressed' actually have heterogeneous conditions including panic, phobic and generalised anxiety disorders and adjustment disorders as well as depression. These are situation focused, disabling and often reflect adversity (Brockington *et al.*, 2006).

PTSD occurring among women after childbirth has more recently been investigated. Most of the focus has been on determining the potential of childbirth to meet the trauma exposure criterion for PTSD (APA, 1994) in that a woman can perceive birth as involving threatened death or serious injury or harm to physical integrity and respond to it with intense fear, helpless or horror. In a recent systematic review and meta-analysis of studies which had investigated PTSD among women occurring between one and eighteen months after they had given birth, Grekin and O'Hara (2014) distinguish between PTSD caused by childbirth and PTSD caused by 'other events'. There is a lack of specificity in what has been assessed as a 'history of trauma' or 'past traumatic event'. However, postnatal PTSD was overall more common among women with a past history of exposure to trauma and psychiatric illness (Grekin and O'Hara, 2014). There is increasing recognition that we need to distinguish new-onset postnatal PTSD that is related to a traumatic birth experience from chronic or recurrent PTSD from maltreatment history that is triggered by a birth experience that was re-traumatising.

Perinatal distress and mental health problems can be complex. Non-psychotic postnatal mental health problems often co-occur (for example Grekin and O'Hara found a correlation between PTSD and depression), and there is substantial overlap of symptoms among them. So in practice it is more relevant to recognise indicators of poor psychological functioning which warrant more detailed assessment. Mental health problems also always reflect both lifetime experiences and current circumstances (Fisher *et al.*, 2014). These can include in the past:

- childhood neglect and maltreatment;
- having had a parent with a personality disorder or a severe mental illness;
- foster care, special schooling or poverty, marginalisation and social exclusion;

and in the present:

- unintended or unwanted pregnancy;
- being un-partnered or in a relationship with a partner who is physically or emotionally abusive or who misuses alcohol or drugs;
- unstable housing;
- geographic separation from family of origin;
- low literacy;
- insufficient income or having a child with special needs.

For professionals who are not specialists in mental health assessment and treatment, this complexity can be daunting.

Using theory-based, relationship-oriented concepts as common ground

Theory that cuts across the boundaries between disciplines can facilitate interprofessional work. We propose that there are a few relationship-focused concepts that can provide a common vocabulary and serve as concepts to organise and communicate about care. Relationship functioning is a crucial focus for the woman and infant in the postnatal period. It is also a domain where maltreatment trauma history can leave particular deficits or impairments that make sense if the woman was deprived of a solid relationship with a trustworthy caregiver in her own infancy and childhood.

Women whose own experiences of being cared for have been suboptimal or abusive can have more difficulty learning to care well for their baby than those who have experienced sensitive, responsive and consistent care. It is commonly understood in mental health settings that the therapist–client relationship is a crucial element for healing. Women with a maltreatment history in qualitative research also have been articulate in expressing the importance of their health and social care relationships to their well-being (Sperlich and Seng, 2008; Harris and Ayers, 2012; Montgomery, 2013).

A working knowledge of relevant psychological theories pertinent to relationships can help with making explicit links between how past relationships can affect present relationships, including the early parenting relationship. We have already briefly described these concepts in relation to providing perinatal care to the woman. Here we present more information about them and link them to maternal development and well-being.

Attachment

Attachment pertains to the nature of an individual's patterns of relating to others, which are first experienced as the emotional tie that develops during the interaction between an infant and the primary caregiver, typically the mother. The theory was first articulated by John Bowlby (Bowlby, 1983) to explain patterns of behaviour in infants who had been separated from their mothers. The emotional attachment that arises from the infant's need for proximity to the caregiver for survival is promoted by behaviours such as crying, smiling and vocalising, which function to keep the mother nearby. Proximity to the primary caregiver enables access to food, social interaction and protection from harm. 'Attachment theory' should be distinguished from 'attachment parenting' – a descriptor for a style of parenting that advocates continuous close physical contact between parent and infant, including bed sharing (Sears and Sears, 2003).

A 'secure' attachment arises in an infant and child when the caregiver is physically and psychologically available to them. The caregiver recognises the infant's cues, interprets them accurately, responds in a timely way, cooperates rather than interferes with the infant's behaviour and accepts rather than rejects the infant's needs. Secure attachment in turn facilitates the development of trust, emotional regulation, empathy and resilience in the child and later the adult.

In contrast, experiences of neglectful or abusive care during infancy and childhood may result in an 'insecure' attachment style. Attachment theory recognises several distinct categories of insecure attachment, but in general if caregiving has been insensitive, inconsistent or intrusive, the infant and child may learn to doubt that caregivers can be depended on, to mistrust others and to be unconcerned about others' concerns. Dismissing and rejecting parenting behaviours may lead the child to learn that their distress is not easily tolerated by others, is unreasonable, unwarranted or annoying, that the child is not worthy of care and is unlovable. The child is likely to become apprehensive, fearing that the caregiver is missing or unhelpful, and thus reluctant to develop independence.

A parent with poor emotional regulation may respond to their infant's distress in an emotive, exaggerated or chaotic way. In this case, the infant can experience the caregiver as unpredictable, helpless or overwhelmed and is likely to internalise an exaggerated sense of their own distress. Caregivers with severe impairment can alternate between unresponsiveness or neglect and intrusive frightening interactions or abuse including hitting or shaking the infant. In this case, the mother is the source of the infant's fear as well as safety; the child becomes chronically afraid and may experience difficulty maintaining emotional and behavioural control. A parent with their own experiences of child maltreatment, attachment difficulties and impaired emotional regulation may have problems relating to their infant contingently, sensitively and appropriately and thus perpetuate the cycle of maltreatment.

The nature of a parent's own attachment relationships, established with their primary caregiver, is of central importance to the quality of relationships that they develop with their own children and the parenting that they provide. However, caregiving abilities are able to be modified by emotional support and specific skills in reflective parenting, and there is debate as to what extent attachment patterns are repeated through subsequent generations (Shah *et al.*, 2010). A woman's developing attachment to her baby begins during pregnancy (Condon, 1993), so prenatal assessment of her attachment patterns, her thoughts about parenting and her emerging ideas about her developing baby (Zeanah *et al.*, 2011) could lead to education and treatment that prepares her for mothering.

'Having once been helped to recognize and recapture the feelings which she herself had as a child and to find that they are accepted tolerantly and understandingly, a mother will become increasingly sympathetic and tolerant toward the same things in her child' (Bowlby, 1940, p. 23).

Mothers who are doing well recognise that not every interaction can be perfect, but they provide a consistently nurturing environment and are able to reflect on the infant's signals of distress as real, legitimate, meaningful and manageable and to respond appropriately. This enables the child to turn to this parent with confidence in times of need. Through repeated experiences with a sensitive caregiver, the child learns to interpret accurately, validate and respond effectively to their own internal states.

As we will see in Chapter 8, there are numerous examples of universal and trauma-specific programmes that teach about and promote attachment and provide attachment-focused interventions for mothers experiencing impaired bonding in the postnatal period.

Dyadic regulation
The close physicality of the mother–baby relationship continues long after the separation of birth. Biological explanations of this

connection contribute to understanding intergenerational patterns of child maltreatment and provide clues about how to intervene.

In a well-known pair of books, Allan Schore (2003a; 2003b) synthesises attachment theory, trauma theory and neurobiology to describe how disorders of the self and their repair have a basis in close physical relationships. The overarching concept is that of self-regulation. As Schore explains it, self-regulation develops within the physical and emotional exchanges between the mother–infant dyad.

'If ... an infant ... does not have adequate experiences of being part of an open dynamic system with an emotionally responsive adult human, its corticolimbic organization will be poorly capable of coping with the stressful chaotic dynamics that are inherent in all human relationships. Such a system tends to become static and closed, and invested in defensive structures to guard against anticipated interactive assaults that potentially trigger disorganizing and emotionally painful psychobiological states. Due to its avoidance of novel situations and diminished capacity to cope with challenging situations, it does not expose itself to new socioemotional learning experiences that are required for the continuing experience-dependent growth of the right brain. This structural limitation, in turn, negatively impacts the future trajectory of self-organization' (Schore, 1997).

During early development, an infant has limited independent capacity to maintain an optimal level of arousal. The role of the caregiver is to act as a 'neurobiological regulator' while the infant's own regulatory processes are developing. The role involves helping the infant to calm her or himself during stress, as well as providing enough stimulation for growth and development. Many of these actions involve the mother's body: holding, feeding, using touch, conveying her own pace of breathing and heart rate, using the sound of her voice. Insufficient nurturing as well as over-protection can hinder development of the infant's own optimal self-regulation. Extremes of this kind include neglect and intrusive overstimulation. Consistent with attachment theory, poor emotion regulation on the part of the mother is likely to impair her ability to regulate her infant.

The mother's own emotional state is central to this embodied experience of nurturing. But the relationship between a mother and infant is dynamic and interactive. The infant also contributes to the dyadic process. Mothers are gratified by an infant who responds to their attempts to soothe, who quietens to sleep and who develops along a normal trajectory. This contributes to the mother's sense of competence and confidence. Conversely, an infant who cries inconsolably, wakes up after short sleeps and does not respond to a mother's efforts to soothe can be experienced as critical and unappreciative and can contribute to the mother's hyperarousal, anxiety and demoralisation.

Practical help can be vital as an intervention to promote dyadic regulation. Women with a maltreatment history may not have experienced effective regulation through parental care and may be unable to imagine how it would feel. They may have no strategies to use. When the baby is unsettled, the woman may become extremely distressed herself and be unable to recognise her infant's needs or meet them successfully. If a professional observes a woman who is distressed to a point of needing help to 'regulate', taking actions that make use of this concept can be helpful to the woman in the moment, can give her the real-time, embodied experience of being understood and helped, and can serve as a basis for talking about how the caregiver fulfilled the 'external regulator' role.

Ideas for responding to a woman who is highly dysregulated:
- remain calm yourself;
- create a containing and supporting environment in the moment;
- describe her baby's sleep needs and developmental capacities;
- help her to focus on keeping the baby's internal state in mind;
- encourage her to establish a predictable pattern of daily care;
- show her how to settle her baby to sleep;
- remind her that her baby is not deliberately trying to annoy her;
- provide her with consistent validation and encouragement.

Unsettled infant behaviour including prolonged crying and waking after short sleeps is difficult for any parent to manage, but especially for those with impaired emotional regulation. Caring for an infant is a highly skilled activity that needs to be learnt. It involves understanding the baby's individual temperament and behaviour and knowing how to respond appropriately. Establishing a predictable pattern of daily care is a first step to regulating the baby's and thereby the mother's emotions.

Parenting education can include teaching caregiving skills in the early weeks of an infant's life. This helps to prevent unsettled behaviour including prolonged crying and waking after short sleeps (Rowe and Fisher, 2010b). The aim is to establish a sustainable, three- to four-hour pattern of daytime care. Parents are educated about infant sleep needs, states of sleep, sleep associations, sleep cycles and how to recognise cues that the infant is tired. Parents are advised to avoid sleep associations that are not sustainable such as rocking, walking, carrying and suckling to sleep, and to use a wrap, sleeping bag or transitional object such as a small soft toy, instead.

Parents learn to recognise their baby's signs of tiredness, including eye rubbing, ear pulling and grizzling, after the baby has been awake for one and a half to two hours, and how to settle the baby to sleep. The baby is put into bed while still awake, and comforted using a slow rhythmic 'heart beat' pat and gentle body rocking without making eye contact until the baby is quiet. Being put to bed in a quiet dark room, with a cot with minimal distractions or toys in or over it, helps the infant to associate this safe space with sleep rather than play. Infants who wake after one sleep cycle (40–50 minutes) are resettled to sleep using the same strategies without being picked up out of bed.

Parents are encouraged to separate feeding from sleeping with a play period, during which the parents interact with the baby in an age-appropriate way. This helps parents to understand their baby's developmental capacities and needs, to be empathic to their baby's internal state and to interpret the infant's cues accurately. When the infant shows signs of tiredness, the 'feed-play-sleep' cycle is begun again and the baby is settled to sleep in bed. Infants cared for in this way are likely to have their sleep needs met and to learn that life is predictable and safe. Parental fatigue is reduced and their sense of competence and confidence grows (Fisher *et al.*, 2010).

There are examples of postnatal programmes that focus on dyadic regulation. At a universal level, parenting education and support programmes can teach parents about infant temperament, capacities and needs and how to settle the baby to sleep (Rowe and Fisher, 2010b). Programmes such as 'What were we thinking', developed by authors Rowe and Fisher, teach and practise the above skills and also focus on the couple relationship and negotiating of parenting work to enhance parental well-being by reflective recognition of needs and problem-solving.

At a secondary level, Australia's residential early parenting services provide brief admissions for parents who are experiencing difficulties with caregiving. Residential early parenting services offer structured 4–5 night admissions where parents learn to manage unsettled infant behaviour in a supported environment. There is good evidence that helping the baby to regulate by building specific caregiving skills has sustained benefits for the woman's emotional state and well-being (Fisher *et al.*, 2011). Almost a quarter of women admitted to one service reported having been physically abused during childhood and nearly as many reported having been sexually abused; 10% stated that they had had childhood experiences of both physical and sexual abuse (Rowe and Fisher, 2010a). These rates are somewhat higher than those for Australia generally (https://aifs.gov.au/cfca/publications/prevalence-child-abuse-and-neglect/; accessed 28 May 2015), suggesting that help to regulate the infant may be needed particularly by women with a maltreatment history.

The holding environment

All women who have recently given birth benefit from appropriate emotional and practical support, but women with maltreatment experiences, especially those with impaired relationships, may not have the support they need. They are less likely to have partners and more often have partners who are abusive. It is probable that their relationships with their families of origin – the grandparents, aunts and uncles of the infant – are troubled or broken. Pregnancy is sometimes the impetus for women to sever relationships with parents or partners as a means to keep the child safe from abuse (Sperlich and Seng, 2008).

In order to undertake the physically and emotionally demanding work of mothering a newborn, a woman requires a supportive 'holding environment'. Psychotherapists Winnicott (1965) and Stern (1995) note that, in order for a new mother to protect her child effectively, she requires a containing psychological environment in which she feels protected, validated, encouraged and supported.

- A positive holding environment helps the mother to manage the exhaustion and overwork that result from caring for a newborn.
- The company of an experienced mother promotes competence and confidence in the new mother.
- A central figure in the holding environment is usually a woman's own mother.
- Creation of the holding environment commences during pregnancy; a woman's reflection on her own mother as a mother is often the beginning of this process.

The relationship with her own mother is centrally important to a woman who is mothering a newborn. A woman whose relationship with her mother is impaired because of abuse or neglect, death or geographical separation may have deficits in her sense of herself as a mother and in relationship with others. Among a cohort of women admitted to an Australian residential early parenting service, women who recalled emotionally cold and unresponsive maternal relationships during childhood were more likely to be experiencing clinically significant symptoms of depression at admission than others (Fisher *et al.*, 2002). Skilled professional care can assist women in these circumstances.

Professional care providers form an important part of the holding environment for all women who have recently given birth, but may be especially significant for women whose social networks are limited, abusive or undermining. Home visiting nursing programmes, extended family support, outreach programmes and other services for vulnerable populations may fill a crucial gap.

Skills for providing psychological care, including trauma informed care

Part of providing a holding environment for new mothers is paying close attention to their mental health status and parenting capacity. Collaborating with other professionals is likely to be important. But cooperating with the woman is also essential, and in the postnatal period, especially with women whose mental health and parenting are adversely affected by trauma-related problems, this may require particular skills. We will focus on assessment conversations, transference and counter-transference reactions, safety issues and vicarious traumatic stress.

Using an observation-enquiry assessment process

Assisting women and their infants when things are not going well involves communicating across divides of language, literacy and disability. This is difficult even when focused on practical matters, but is especially challenging when discussing emotional experiences and needs. Emotional vocabulary varies and can be quite limited, so women might not have the words to describe their mood, frustrations, needs, aspirations and daily experiences. Making connections between past trauma and current feelings and functioning can also be useful but sensitivity is required. A routine use of observation and enquiry is a useful skill.

Woman

Observations
A woman might:

- be agitated and restless, or, less commonly, slowed in her movements and speech;
- avoid eye contact;
- appear to be distracted.

Enquiry
A woman might disclose spontaneously or in response to questions that she is:

- feeling sad or in low mood;
- not experiencing pleasure in things that she would usually enjoy;
- being irritable, especially with the people near her;
- feeling despondent or hopeless about the future;
- not wanting to see her friends;
- being excessively self-critical;
- crying easily;
- waking at night apart from caring for the baby;
- finding that worries are going over and over in her mind;
- finding it difficult to concentrate or to think clearly;
- find it difficult to describe her situation or needs in a coherent narrative;
- experience intrusive disturbing images or thoughts;
- feel 'nothing' or be 'numb'.

Observation and enquiry are iterative processes of monitoring, forming a mental question about what any problems might be, testing them through enquiry and then beginning the process again. It is always important to observe the interactions between a woman and her baby. Optimally, these are characterised by sensitivity to the baby's cues, and contingent timely responses, which lead to mutually gratifying exchanges. However, if a woman is experiencing a mental health problem and is living in difficult circumstances, these interactions can be problematic.

Breastfeeding is one area where the observation and enquiry process may be particularly useful. There are reasons to think that breastfeeding is more problematic for women with a maltreatment history (Coles, 2009) because they intend to breastfeed at high rates but are less likely to be doing so after initial attempts. A successful breastfeeding relationship can be a source of healing for the woman. Choosing not to breastfeed or ceasing breastfeeding may be a relief from an unwelcome or uncomfortable experience for others. However, women can experience extreme distress and internal conflict if breastfeeding is much desired but unable to be continued (Coles and Jones, 2009).

Observation of feeding and sensitive exploration of feelings associated with how things are going may be helpful in the early days and weeks after birth as part of the holding environment. Lactation consultants may be more accustomed to providing practical help and problem-solving and not know how to bring trauma-related issues into their conversations with women struggling to breastfeed. Those who work from a trauma informed perspective will understand that, for some, breastfeeding may be difficult because it evokes memories of past abuse. They can use this assessment process to enquire about the women's experience, to ask if trauma-specific help might be useful to her, and to help the mother to make the right decision for her, balancing her own and her infant's needs.

Interactions between a woman and her baby

Observations
The mother might:
- attribute hostile motives or intentions to the baby;
- fail to respond when the baby 'signals' to her with vocalisations or gestures;

- be physically intrusive or speak too loudly to the baby;
- handle the baby roughly;
- become agitated or panicky when the baby cries or is irritable;
- be disparaging about her baby's needs or experiences;
- not be affectionate in her interactions with her baby.

The baby might:
- avoid eye contact;
- not be distressed when separated from or unable to see her/his mother;
- explore without reference to her/his mother.

Enquiry
A mother might disclose spontaneously or in response to questions that she:
- dislikes or resents the baby;
- thinks the baby harmed her body;
- doesn't like touching the baby or having the baby touch her;
- experiences breastfeeding as 'disgusting'.

Paying attention to relationship dynamics: transference and counter-transference
When providing care for women with these difficulties, it is important to understand the notions of transference, which is the emotional reactions that people receiving care have to the care provider, and counter-transference, which is the feelings and thoughts that develop in providers about their clients. It is almost inevitable that people in these extremely difficult circumstances will have experienced repeated disappointments in their relationships and will find it challenging to trust new caregivers. They can be acutely attuned to the slightest indications of disapproval or rejection. Providers have the dual task of being sensitive to their client's needs while managing their own reactions to situations that can be confronting and seem overwhelming or insoluble. It requires particular self-awareness to be thoughtful not only about how questions are asked and what is suggested but also about what is conveyed non-verbally.

Trauma informed care recognises that women with experiences of early maltreatment are sensitised to perceive rejection from caregivers, that they are not liked or that other clients are preferred.

Frequent changes of healthcare providers, or when practitioners depart without warning, can be perceived by the woman as abandonment. Women may behave in ways that can be challenging for the care provider: they may be mistrustful, complain about their care or miss appointments. These behaviours are more likely to be manifestations of abuse experiences than deliberate attempts by the woman to be difficult.

The professional may also have reactions and feelings that seem uncharacteristic or uncomfortable. Counter-transference reactions can include having a desire to rescue the client or feeling infuriated at demanding or needy interactions. It is helpful for the professional to be able to reflect on both the client's responses and their own, and to apply a curious enquiring attitude rather than a judgemental or punitive one. The feelings being provoked are usually informative and can be used to navigate the relationship. This type of reflection about what behaviours and emotions mean role-models mindfulness and self-regulation. It contributes to a holding environment by building a sense of safety because problems in the relationship can be thought about and repaired.

The presence of a skilled professional in the holding environment can be a means to 'mother the mother', assist her to regulate her emotions and model sensitive caregiving. The most valuable approach to take, including with people who are vulnerable and multiply disadvantaged, is a solution-focused or problem-solving one. People can be helped to feel less overwhelmed if the practitioner can, with them, frame solutions as a series of small problems, which can be addressed one-by-one on the way to realising a larger, long-term goal. It is useful to make a list together and then to work out which problems are the most pressing and what assistance would be required or wanted to address them.

Approaches that foster autonomy rather than promote dependence are important. Achievement of small goals can be reviewed and celebrated at subsequent meetings. Affirmation and recognition of progress are always psychologically beneficial. One topic for problem-solving collaboration can be how to expand the mother's support system so that demands on professional care providers remain within workable limits.

It is more difficult to attend to transference and counter-transference while visiting someone at home rather than having the meeting in an office where there are parameters about privacy, placement of furniture, the keeping of notes and records, times for appointments to begin and end, and other colleagues in the building. Reflection on relationship dynamics may occur after the fact rather than in the moment. Case discussions with colleagues may be an additional way to get input and grow in expertise at focusing on the dynamics that can arise at more intense levels when working with survivors of maltreatment.

Not assuming safety

Nurses and health visitors receive training about personal safety when entering clients' homes. Staying focused on the issue of personal safety is salient when working with families where maltreatment may have taken violent forms in the past and where a member of the family or partner or poorly trained animals may present some danger.

Assessing the woman's social support network for safety also is important. Women are often encouraged to enlist the assistance of their own mothers and their partners to share the work of infant care and household tasks. Caregivers may make unwarranted assumptions that others who might be available will be able to provide unconditional and affirming practical and emotional support. Trauma informed care challenges these assumptions by recognising that a family of origin may not be a safe source of positive support. Care providers must assess a woman's close relationships and assist the woman to prioritise the needs of herself and her baby. The care provider can assist her to acquire the skills to recognise her own needs and set limits on the involvement of others without attributing blame.

Care providers must also remain alert to the quality of a woman's relationship with her intimate partner. Mothers and fathers with maltreatment experiences may lack role models for 'firm but fair' parenting and may need explicit help to regulate their own frustration and anger and to develop a shared understanding about what are safe limits and how these can be set. A trauma informed model of care suggests that parenting education be available throughout the child's development as new parenting challenges emerge. It is important to remember that conflict and abuse can be exacerbated by the demands of the perinatal period, and safety of mother and baby should be routinely assessed.

Questions you can ask to assess the nature of supportive relationships:

- How are things at home?
- Does someone share the household work with you?
- Is there someone you can leave your baby with when you need to go out or take a brief break?

Home visiting programmes seek to assist women and their children, and this raises questions from time to time not only about the safety of the woman but also of young children. For the professional, this involves the most delicate challenge of maintaining a positive alliance while having to raise unwelcome topics and keeping legal obligations about the rights of all parties in mind. Women with a maltreatment history may have been involved in child protection services in their own childhoods. They may see themselves as being at risk for harming or failing to protect their child and resist having professionals involved in their parenting because they fear losing custody of their child. Being clear and direct about both the preventive supportive goals of the services being offered and the duty for safeguarding may strengthen alliance with women who fear the worst; it may also build trust that the mother will not be betrayed by the professional with whom she is collaborating to achieve good outcomes.

Working successfully with a woman who has attachment difficulties means establishing a trustworthy relationship at the outset. Ways to demonstrate trustworthiness include communicating promptly and sensitively when appointment times are unable to be kept. Model firm but fair interactions; a woman who is anxious or mistrustful can then learn to interact in a trustworthy way herself. Set clear but considerate boundaries so that the woman knows the limits of your assistance but is not in doubt about your understanding. It is important to avoid personalising a woman's apparent hostility; this involves recognising that this is not about you the practitioner personally, but about the woman's general mistrust and fear of others.

Vicarious trauma

The challenges of working with traumatised people can take a toll. Despair can be infectious, and there is inevitably potential for compassion fatigue, secondary traumatisation and burnout in this work. By definition, providing trauma informed care requires making explicit the role of past trauma in present difficulties. It also entails holding out hope that the trauma-related difficulties can be surmounted.

In order to maintain this optimism, professionals and the organisations where they work need to foster their own resilience. Strategies include practising in a team; using regular scheduled opportunities to review professional experiences in supportive, peer-to-peer supervision or with a mentor; and consulting others about potential approaches and solutions to unfamiliar situations or problems that appear intractable. Organisations working in trauma informed ways need to keep the work environment non-traumagenic for staff and provide opportunities to deal with crises, vicarious trauma and the chronic stressors of providing services to vulnerable people. Finally, self-care strategies such as regular holidays and nurturing a sense of humour are essential to maintaining the psychological well-being that is fundamental to the capacity to be professionally helpful to others.

Care of women in the postnatal period provides rich opportunities to support well-being and enhance both maternal and infant development. When the woman is suffering psychological distress or mental health problems, care can be complex. It can involve co-occurring conditions, with roots in past and present circumstances, and where mental health and parenting issues are entangled. When maltreatment in the past is affecting the present, trauma informed care can make a difference.

Conclusion

Here are key points that may help in managing the complexities of postnatal care when the woman's trauma-related mental health and parenting needs require interprofessional approaches:

❏ Postnatal care has traditionally focused on physical health needs more than psychological ones. Recent advances in perinatal mental health services are helping to shift this balance. Making postnatal care trauma informed can be a powerful way to improve women's well-being and child outcomes.

❏ The concepts of attachment, dyadic regulation and the holding environment can provide a common framework for postnatal care and facilitate interprofessional collaboration.

❏ As health visitors and perinatal professionals begin to focus more on trauma-related needs, they may have to hone skills that are particularly salient to working with women with a maltreatment history. These include:

  ❏ using assessment skills of observation and enquiry;

  ❏ attending to relationship dynamics, including reflecting on transference and counter-transference reactions;

  ❏ making safety issues an area of focus, including providing safety for the woman in the caregiving relationship by being clear about roles and goals of the professional care or programmes offered;

  ❏ retaining optimism in the face of constant attention to the effects of trauma by preventing or redressing vicarious trauma with organisational, collegial and personal strategies that nurture well-being.

CHAPTER 7

What does trauma informed perinatal care look like?

Mickey Sperlich, State University of New York at Buffalo
Julia Seng, University of Michigan

Introduction

So far we have looked at how childhood maltreatment trauma and post-traumatic stress can adversely affect pregnancy and the postnatal period. We have generated some thematic ideas of how professionals who specialise in each of those domains can begin to frame their thinking about the needs of women with maltreatment history in terms of attachment, dyadic regulation and a holding environment. In this chapter, we take a step back and look at the big picture again. We use the cycles-breaking conceptual framework that points to opportunities to intervene – the action points – and provide some examples of trauma informed practices and trauma-specific interventions at each action point. We start off making recommendations for advocacy and policy action as well, because changing perinatal care to break cycles of maltreatment and psychiatric vulnerability brings up the need for service delivery systems that are seamless and integrated, as well as trauma informed.

Service model evolution to seamless maternity and postnatal care

Although we have perpetuated the antenatal versus postnatal divide in our presentation of pregnancy and postnatal concerns in separate chapters, trauma informed care probably would be better delivered via a seamless perinatal care model. By seamless, we mean perinatal care that the woman experiences as a continuous relationship with one team from planning for pregnancy through her child's first 1,001 critical days. Different nations have diverse systems. Some already approach this seamless ideal. Others have a distinct break between maternity care that ends with the birth and paediatric care that focuses on the child. Many systems are evolving to make better articulation, especially via home visiting programmes where nurses bridge these domains. For women with a maltreatment history, this seamlessness may be particularly invaluable. Congruent with the themes from the previous chapters, it is straightforward to see how a continuous relationship with the perinatal care team would attend to attachment, regulation and holding environment needs.

Attachment in the caregiving relationship

Continuity of care acknowledges that caregiver–client relationships are important. For women with a maltreatment history, attachment trauma may have left long-term difficulties navigating caregiving relationships. Capacity of both client and caregiver to achieve optimal outcomes of perinatal care likely would be increased if they could work from a base of secure attachment, in the sense that the system would foster their staying connected across the long-term. Both parties would be able to invest in the relationship as a significant one that fostered intimacy, trust and accountability.

From the client's perspective having one main person to turn to (e.g. a nurse or midwife) who would facilitate disclosure of trauma-related needs and care planning among a small group of others who worked together routinely (e.g. an obstetrician, lactation consultant, paediatrician, parenting educator) could improve outcomes. It also could decrease stress and maximise the psychological benefits of positive experiences of care.

From the caregivers' perspectives, long-term relationships would allow more accurate responses to particular needs that come from truly knowing the client, leading to better outcomes. It also could shift the caregiving experience from one marked by frustration at dealing with a 'difficult patient' to satisfaction at having been able to make a difference by sticking with the woman across a deeply challenging period in her life. Of course, not all providers would be interested either in continuity models or in working with this client population. Creative solutions may be required, potentially including use of continuity in prenatal care and a designated labour support person or doula for the hospital component. Midwives who specialise in care of trauma survivors using a continuity model with a smaller but more intensive caseload might be another model to try. Innovative and local solutions are a place to start.

Dyadic regulation as a skills-building process that takes time

Seamless service models may also prove useful for enhancing parenting outcomes because they support learning over a sustained period, which is required to build skill. Continuity across maternity and paediatric domains would provide for frequent repeated opportunities to support the woman's self-care initially and her care of the infant over time. Sensitive reflective parenting is an embodied process of perceiving and responding to needs. Using the overarching concept of dyadic regulation, the woman is using her embodied self – voice, warmth, heartbeat and respiration, gaze, holding and movement – to soothe or stimulate her infant according to the infant's cues.

Starting to teach this complex skill after the birth may be too late for this population. Women with a maltreatment history are more likely to be physically and emotionally dysregulated themselves and may have poor self-care capacity. Seamless attention to developing her self- and infant-care ability from early pregnancy could get better results. The woman also may experience longer-term continuity of attention to her self-care and to her growth in mothering as role modelling of patience, consistency and firm expectations that will serve her well. Continuity of support could be a vital improvement over current episodic care, too, because early warning signs could lead to appropriate proactive help and surveillance for high-risk dyads, and a team would be more powerful in taking concerted action.

Seamlessness to enhance the holding environment

Scope of practice for midwives and obstetricians and for paediatricians and parenting specialists has been loosely delimited by the moment of cutting the cord. The handover of the baby from birth attendant to the infant caregivers marks the beginning of the end of the nine-month relationship of the pregnant woman with those who got her through the birth. Many women experience this structural reality as abandonment. In cases where the birth experience was traumatic or the infant experienced complications, the woman can feel alone and/or angry (and sometimes relieved if the caregiver's behaviour was the source of the trauma) in managing the aftermath. Systems that would permit staying connected to antenatal caregivers during this transition might enhance the holding environment for the woman, including chances to work through negative experiences, but this would involve major change to current practice.

Enhanced holding would decrease the mother's stress by allowing the continuous caregiver to play an active role in the early weeks of postnatal care. This nurse or midwife could talk with her about her birth experience, move from the abstract planning for breastfeeding to its reality, help the partner engage well, and observe the mother–infant dyad in the earliest days through eyes that know the woman's vulnerabilities enough to spot difficulties and to reinforce successes. Having been able to work with the woman antenatally to face concerns and worries related to her trauma history, this caregiver would be positioned to notice and point out strengths and post-traumatic growth in a way that an entirely new team could not.

Giving birth is a rite of passage that takes place in a liminal state – a place of psychological, spiritual and physical openness that facilitates changing to a new identity (Davis-Floyd, 2004). In a system without seamless care across this period, the new mother is required to leave behind those who have been her professional support system to make the rest of this deep adjustment while needing to form new caregiver relationships. In systems with scant postnatal care, she is making the rest of this adjustment without any established trusted relationship.

Seamless perinatal care is not a new idea. Calls for continuity models for vulnerable populations with complex needs are long-standing and are being implemented in some primary care areas (e.g. in 'medical homes' in the US); but often the emphasis is on a one-stop-shopping experience to provide multiple services efficiently under a single roof. Health visiting in the UK is another approach that incorporates continuity and has a long track record – more than 150 years. Health visitors provide a universal and public health preventive service to all preschool children and their families. There are calls to return to continuity of care across the perinatal year as well. Most recently, the emphasis has been on providing continuity in order to give better attention to psychosocial needs including maternal mental health (NICE, 2014; NSPCC, 2013; Renfrew et al., 2014).

Perinatal home visiting programmes such as the Nurse Family Partnership (Family Nurse Partnership in the UK) (Olds *et al.*, 2014; Roman *et al.*, 2014) go a long way towards offering seamless support to first-time mothers because the nurse–client relationship extends from early pregnancy to the infant's second year. Further progress toward seamless care would occur if the other professionals including mental health and child welfare professionals joined in the process of smoothing the transition from maternity to paediatric care relationships and of focusing on continuity of relationships as a means to meet trauma informed care ideals. Interprofessional case notes and case conferences for clients with complex issues or challenging behaviours could enhance consistency, increase the sophistication of all team members for addressing trauma-related needs and promote *esprit de corps* for teams engaging over the long-term trajectory of these dyads and families.

Service model evolution towards integration of physical and mental healthcare

As pointed out in Chapter 4, focusing on maternal trauma history and post-traumatic stress calls for a paradigm shift in the structure of perinatal services towards integration. Current structures tend towards a screen-and-refer routine. This remains appropriate in many instances where women need immediate involvement of psychiatric specialists familiar with the woman's mental health morbidity and experienced in treating during pregnancy and breastfeeding. Some women with maltreatment history and PTSD will want referral to specialist mental health services, so being able to refer to trauma-specific treatment is a necessary component of trauma informed service models. Yet trauma informed perinatal care delivered to a high standard would mean that referral alone is no longer sufficient for at least two reasons.

First, to help women with a maltreatment history to break cycles of maltreatment and psychiatric vulnerability, we need to address needs that go beyond treating diagnosable PTSD, depression, anxiety or other features of complex traumatic stress including dissociation and substance misuse. Many appropriate responses sit at the level of targeted intervention – between universal prevention and indicated treatment. And the interventions likely need to be specific to the salient concerns of the perinatal period: pregnancy self-care, fear of labour, deciding about breastfeeding, worries about parenting, keeping the infant safe from perpetrators of abuse in the family system. Since these issues may concern as many as one in five pregnant women, or more in settings serving disadvantaged populations, equipping perinatal professionals to deliver these targeted interventions within antenatal, postnatal and paediatric settings is warranted.

Second, we know from meta-synthesis of qualitative research (Montgomery, 2013) that medical procedures that impinge on body integrity (e.g. vaginal examinations, delivery procedures, breastfeeding support, infant vaccination) are triggers to PTSD reactions for some women. Thus, the healthcare providers who implement these procedures need to be able to respond therapeutically in the moment. Integration of mental and physical healthcare for this population would mean not only co-locating practitioners but also having them influence each other's practice. True integration would mean that perinatal and infant mental health professionals have expertise about pregnancy and postnatal periods, which they already have, and also that obstetricians, midwives, perinatal nurses, health visitors and paediatric specialists have expertise about trauma, PTSD, abuse prevention and therapeutic relationships that attend with some sophistication to mental health needs that they must address in the moment. These include issues that can fall into the categories of attachment, dyadic regulation and holding environment. System change is needed so that perinatal mental health providers can be part of the team rather than only an outside resource to which women can be referred. Interprofessional collaboration may also protect against providers feeling isolated and might decrease vicarious trauma (Saakvitne, 2002).

In the meantime
Advocating for system change to create service delivery models that are trauma informed will take time. Until then, professionals caring for women with a maltreatment history must continue to provide the best care they can in their circumstances. This is challenging at the current moment when the evidence base is scant for trauma

informed perinatal care and trauma-specific interventions for the childbearing year. Nevertheless, the evidence-based practice paradigm can still guide us because it supports use of individual care plans developed in collaboration with clients and entered into with informed consent – including sharing the information that there is, as yet, no evidence to go on (Rice, 2011). Although it surely would be easier to be supported by a trauma informed system of care, we need not wait for system change to begin to create trauma informed care – one client at a time, if need be – with all the allies we can assemble.

Using the cycles-breaking framework to imagine and coordinate interventions

In Chapter 3 we presented the cycles-breaking conceptual framework that is based on the literature from numerous professions and academic disciplines. The links connect one profession's domain and the next (see Figures 3.1 and 7.1), while the framework shows action points where we could positively disrupt the cycles.

Figure 7.1 Cycles breaking conceptual framework.

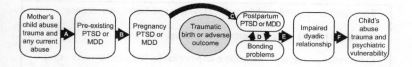

It is helpful to think of actions we could take as being part of a tiered or stepped system of care, so we can provide the right level of response. These levels go from actions that are universal prevention, to targeted interventions based on having the history, to indicated treatment based on assessment and diagnosis. The AAP describes them as part of the 'social-emotional safety nets' within a public health approach to toxic stress (AAP, n.d.)

Universal primary preventions include:

- programmes such as 'Bright futures', 'Reach out and read', 'Connected kids' and 'Circle of security' and seeing relationships as a 'vital sign';
- evidence-based child development competencies.

Targeted interventions include:

- screening for risks (e.g. substance dependency or domestic abuse) and referring to and advocating evidence-based interventions as well as collaborating to develop them to meet specific needs;
- mid-level competencies.

Indicated treatments include:

- assessing for diagnosis and referring to and advocating for evidence-based treatments as well as collaborating to develop them to meet specific needs;
- advanced competencies.

The childbearing year is a crucial time for taking action. Using the cycles-breaking framework we can see schematically the points of intervention between the last generation's parenting and the next. Action could take the form of universal prevention, targeted interventions that are trauma informed or indicated treatment that is trauma-specific. Development of evidence-based approaches are strongly needed for the perinatal-specific points in the cycle. Here are the action points and priority tasks aiming at helping the woman break the cycles:

A: prevent or respond to child maltreatment in childhood/adolescence;

B: resolve trauma sequelae prior to pregnancy;

C: intervene prenatally – including with planning for birth and breastfeeding – and watch for parenting concerns; signs of high-risk parenting; and emerging 'internal working models' of the child;

D: intervene postnatally – including providing parenting support, remembering that bonding problems may lead to mental health morbidity as well as vice versa;

E: plan to help regulate the dyad, because the infant learns self-regulation in relation to the mother, and the mother's capacity to regulate is affected by the infant's temperament and behaviours;

F: consider persistently dysregulated dyads high risk and collaborate with child welfare professionals for intensive support and surveillance:

- remember that the partner/father may also be impaired;
- bear in mind that family of origin may not be a safe source of social support or babysitting.

We provide two case illustrations written in alignment with the above framework. The A and B action points may have passed before perinatal professionals begin their relationship with the client. Action point F stretches beyond the perinatal period, but in a seamless system groundwork for targeted interventions or indicated treatment in this period would have been laid and some perinatal care relationships might provide continuity in cases where women's involvement is intense and long-term. In the following scenarios, we mark elements that could be seen as universal prevention, targeted intervention and indicated treatment so that what we mean by these terms starts to become clear. We define these in relation to trauma informed and trauma-specific services after the cases.

Amanda's case is an example of a resilient woman in trauma informed care using a targeted intervention, while that of Susan is an example of a PTSD-affected woman in trauma informed care using a targeted intervention and also indicated treatment. Although Susan's case is a US-based example, note the key ingredients that are applicable in any country.

AMANDA	
A: Prevent or respond to child maltreatment in childhood/ adolescence	Amanda's childhood neighbour was aware that her mother was often enraged, verbally and physically abusive. She gave Amanda a safe haven and helped her succeed in apprenticeship helped her choose an apprenticeship in another town as a means to leave home
B: Resolve trauma sequelae prior to pregnancy	Amanda saw a counsellor at a youth centre and decided not to go back home anymore to live. She sees her mother some holidays
C: Intervene prenatally – including with birth and breastfeeding – and watch for parenting concerns and signs of high risk parenting	Amanda answered 'yes' to maltreatment history screening questions and had a few PTSD and depression symptoms, especially arousal and irritability [Prevention]. She declined offers to discuss programmes or referral information [Intervention], saying her midwives were very kind and supportive, and she felt comfortable
D: Intervene postnatally – including providing parenting support, remembering that bonding problems may lead to mental health morbidity as well as vice versa	Amanda's concerns about breastfeeding were well addressed by the nurse and she felt pleased that they were off to a good start. After a few days at home, Amanda called her midwives because she was overwhelmed by the baby's crying. She felt a lot of 'adrenaline' and anger when the baby would not stop. She feared she would be like her mother. The midwives offered a postnatal parenting programme for women with a maltreatment history that would help Amanda understand and manage these reactions that resembled the irritability/anger of PTSD and keep the baby safe [Intervention]. Amanda felt very relieved and found the programme suited her needs, was helpful for learning about PTSD reactions and gave her a sense of being a strong protective mother

AMANDA

E: Plan to help regulate the dyad, because the infant learns self-regulation in relation to the mother, and she may be impaired	The nurse who taught the programme followed up to verify that the strategies Amanda learnt to calm her own irritability and angry edge and to soothe the baby were working [Intervention]. Amanda used the contacts with the nurse to decide to go back to work part-time, using childcare, because that amount of relief from parenting seemed right to keep her from feeling overwhelmed
F: Consider persistently dysregulated dyads high risk and collaborate with child welfare professionals for intensive support and surveillance	Amanda and her infant did well after the first rough month. The baby's development was on track, and mother and baby were relaxed and enjoying each other when the nurse continued to visit [Intervention]
• Remember that the partner/ father may also be impaired	Amanda's partner collaborated in making sure she and the baby got enough rest and had a routine that prevented exhaustion for Amanda. He used strategies the nurse had taught to de-escalate situations and provide calm and comfort for his partner and daughter [Intervention]. As a couple, they attended a parenting education programme together [Prevention]. At a subsequent nurse visit, Amanda said she and her partner did not agree about physical punishment. She was afraid his approach was harsh and would resemble to her the physical abuse Amanda endured as a child. The nurse got them access to a parenting class for people with maltreatment histories and/or PTSD [Intervention]
• Remember that family of origin may not be a safe source of social support or babysitting	Amanda used that trauma-specific parenting programme to make decisions about her own mother's relationship with the baby [Intervention]. She decided it would be okay to take the baby to visit on holidays, but she supervised these visits between grandmother and granddaughter. She declined her mother's offers to babysit

SUSAN

A: Prevent or respond to child maltreatment in childhood/ adolescence	Susan's childhood was chaotic and characterised by several moves to new houses and schools. She does not remember much of her early years, but she was a good student and buried herself in hard work to make it through a prestigious university and into a high-powered job
B: Resolve trauma sequelae prior to pregnancy	None of her romantic relationships worked out, so at thirty-five she opted to become pregnant and raise a child on her own. In her preconception visits, she answered 'no' to the questions about childhood abuse and sexual trauma but disclosed some symptoms of PTSD, depression and dissociation, and she was still smoking [Intervention]. She declined referrals to address these issues prior to conceiving [Intervention or Treatment] saying 'I just get that way when I work too hard.' The gynaecologist noted dissociation during the insemination [Intervention] and made a point at the end of the visit to say that Susan could reconnect any time if she wanted a referral 'for stress or anything that might come up' [Intervention]

SUSAN	
C: Intervene prenatally – including with birth and breastfeeding – and watch for parenting concerns and signs of high risk parenting	Susan became pregnant from the first insemination and booked in with a community midwife but kept cancelling her appointment because she was panicking at the thought of being examined. Finally, with the midwife becoming rather insistent on the phone, Susan explained her panicky feelings. The midwife suggested two things: obtaining the gynaecologist's record so the initial pregnancy examinations need not be repeated [Intervention], and switching Susan to a specialist midwife who had additional education to work with psychological issues in pregnancy [Intervention]. Susan agreed. The specialist midwife obtained the record with the notes about screening results and the observed dissociation. At her first visit with Susan, she undertook a more in-depth assessment in conversation about the 'out of body' experiences, Susan's amnesia for early childhood and her panic about antenatal examinations [Intervention]. She offered Susan enrolment in a group antenatal care programme for women with depression, anxiety, PTSD and maltreatment histories that Susan could join because of her panic and dissociation, whether she had a maltreatment history or not [Intervention]. Susan was glad for that opportunity to be with other pregnant women who had in common that they were not feeling 'all perfect and glowing' as she put it, especially since she did not have a partner and it was a way not to be alone in healthcare visits. Susan liked the group and appreciated the information they received about coping with mental health symptoms, even though she did not think she had been abused. But at the 34-week visit when the midwife was doing the swabs of her vagina and anus for group B strep cultures, she started sobbing and felt like a little girl and like something terrible was happening, even though her friend from the antenatal care group was with her, and she knew she was safe. The midwife gently suggested that this might be a 'flashback' where Susan was re-experiencing emotions from a traumatic event when she was a little girl [Intervention]. She strongly encouraged Susan to allow her to facilitate a visit with the perinatal therapist who works with trauma survivors as soon as possible so she could work through the feelings and not be alone with them [Intervention]. Susan saw the therapist that afternoon and agreed to use an evidence-based PTSD treatment approach to reduce the intensity of the trigger and to make plans for managing PTSD reactions during the birth [Treatment]. Since the birth was likely less than six weeks away, she set up twice-weekly sessions. The midwife also referred her to a doula who was experienced working with women with sexual trauma history and PTSD who would help her implement her strategies in labour [Intervention]
D: Intervene postnatally –including providing parenting support, remembering that bonding problems may lead to mental health morbidity as well as vice versa	Susan worked well with her therapist, midwife and doula, but it was an emotionally intense and draining time. She chose to see a psychiatrist to use medication for help sleeping and to line up trying an antidepressant after the birth if she was not doing well with PTSD and low mood [Treatment]. She did not go into labour until 41 weeks and chose to use an epidural because she was surprised at the level of pain and felt her planned strategies for managing PTSD reactions would work only if she could concentrate [Intervention]. She felt surrounded by good care and support to use her strategies [Intervention], she did not get overwhelmed, and she felt proud of herself, grateful to her team and very happy to have her baby in her arms. She was content with her decision to bottle feed the baby, and she felt supported by the other mothers in her antenatal care group who came to visit her [Intervention]. She saw her therapist a week after the birth to tell her the story and check in about her emotional health [Treatment]. She felt relieved and proud of herself, but she also felt depleted and worried that her 'baby blues' would deepen into the low mood of PTSD or depression, so she started on the selective serotonin re-uptake inhibitor and set an appointment to pick up with therapy in a month, once she was on her feet with mothering [Treatment]

SUSAN

E: Plan to help regulate the dyad, because the infant learns self-regulation in relation to the mother, and she may be impaired	Susan enrolled in a parenting class for women with a maltreatment history with another woman from the antenatal care group [Intervention]. She found it helpful. She did not use any sleeping medication now that the baby was born because she feared she would not hear the baby wake up in the night. But she used a routine she had developed in the class, including a warm bath, infant massage and warm milk for herself while the baby had her warm bottle so they both would get a solid 4–5 hours of sleep before the next feed. Susan took her full twelve weeks of maternity leave, but she talked with her closest peer in the antenatal care group [Intervention] about the possibility of using childcare on a limited basis when she started up her therapy again, so she could have some time to herself on those days
F: Consider persistently dysregulated dyads high risk and collaborate with child welfare professionals for intensive support and surveillance	Through her therapy [Treatment], Susan came to understand that the intense drive for academic success as an adolescent had been her 'escape plan' to get away from her family of origin where sexual abuse and her parents' substance misuse kept them in chaos. Her intense drive to succeed at work also was a sort of 'escape' because it kept her too busy to focus on her inner life, which helped keep the trauma out of her awareness. But the triggers of antenatal care made it so she now 'knew' and the rigours of single parenting meant that she needed to work at a more normal pace to take care of herself and her baby. Even though she was not a low-income woman, she asked for nurse home-visiting [Intervention] so that she would have someone checking on her and motivating her to try to keep a good routine and slow down enough to enjoy her daughter's infancy. She felt that she was using this chance to give herself the sweetness of a good childhood as she gave that to her daughter
• Remember that the partner/father may also be impaired.	Susan could see that her difficulties in romantic relationships in the past were related to the past sexual abuse trauma. She was hopeful that she might work through her issues and find a partner in the future. But she felt 'complete' on her own, at least for now
• Remember that family of origin may not be a safe source of social support or babysitting.	Susan latched on to the notion of 'family of choice' that some of the women in her antenatal care group had talked about developing when they decided not to stay connected to their family of origin [Intervention], and she set about connecting to people in her life who were good and loving, but with whom she had lost touch during her years of over-working. She chose to become actively involved in the community of parents at her daughter's daycare centre

Trauma- or PTSD-specific interventions and treatments for pregnancy and the postnatal period have yet to be developed and carried to the point of having an evidence base. Using the action points on the cycles-breaking framework, it is clear that there are numerous types of interventions or treatments that could be created.

Universal prevention programmes are likely to provide benefit to women with a maltreatment history. Numerous programmes that are not intended solely for maltreatment survivors are probably quite beneficial because they are based on attachment theory (e.g. 'Circle of security', 'Mom power') (Powell *et al.*, 2014; LePlatte *et al.*, 2012); they help with self-regulation or dyadic regulation (e.g. some types of yoga or mindfulness training, infant massage) (Muzik *et al.*, 2012; Diego *et al.*, 2014); or they amplify the holding environment (e.g. nurse home visiting programmes) (Olds *et al.*, 2014; Roman *et al.*, 2014).

Home visiting programmes that bridge the antenatal and postnatal period could be especially helpful platforms for supporting women to use multiple interventions and to engage in treatment as appropriate. Articulating with ongoing universal services or programmes is efficient. This sort of stepped or tiered approach allows targeted interventions to be more focused because they can build on general information. Women whose maltreatment history or mental health symptoms were missed during intake screening may be identified by prevention programmes providers. This can minimise missed opportunities to guide women towards targeted interventions.

These can take several forms – they could be actions we do not think of as interventive, including screening and assessment, since tools and conversations in these processes can include consciousness raising, information giving and stigma reduction. Interventions also could include care-planning routines or protocols to empower survivors and provide tailored responses to their needs. Front-line programmes could be broadly provided (e.g. psychoeducation, birth planning tools, recommended readings, websites or videos). Tailored services provided by a range of professionals who want to work with trauma survivor clients could be developed at a protocol level, with evaluation or outcomes research efforts to demonstrate their usefulness (e.g. group antenatal care that provides peer support, doulas specialised in labour support for women with PTSD, midwives, obstetricians, labour nurses and lactation consultants who specialise in care of this population). None of these interventions aims to 'cure' the mental health condition, but each addresses trauma-related needs in ways that lead to better outcomes in other domains – often by strong efforts not to trigger or exacerbate distress.

Indicated treatment is the level of trauma-specific care that aims to improve or cure the mental health sequelae. A research base has emerged for treatments specific to perinatal depression. A similar situation can be created in the near term as evidence-based treatments for PTSD also are applied in the perinatal context. Adult perinatal mental health and infant mental health professionals have strong contributions to make in developing therapies so that woman-centred, family and dyadic therapy modalities become available.

Collaborations across the healthcare and mental health professional divide are as important as referral capacity in the near term. Interprofessional case consultations are an immediate step to use in order to start building both integrated service delivery models and more sophisticated knowledge and skills for providing trauma informed care in maternity and paediatric settings.

As providers become more comfortable with breaking the taboo of talking about maltreatment-related needs across the childbearing year, women will have greater opportunities to express their needs and accept input and targeted support at this crucial time. Individual women will be helped to experience post-traumatic growth and to break the cycles. The perinatal care system will also be moved forward towards better addressing the psychosocial risk and toxic and traumatic stress that takes such a toll on the population.

Conclusion

This chapter has focused on what trauma informed care in the perinatal period might look like in the future. We have offered some ideas to organise this envisioning and creating:

❑ Bearing in mind the themes of attachment, dyadic regulation and the holding environment may be useful. These overarching concepts can help organise trauma informed approaches to meeting the needs of the new mother and her infant.

❑ Trauma informed care can fit into a stepped or tiered system of care. Levels in this system can be described as universal prevention, targeted intervention and indicated treatment. Trauma-specific interventions and treatments ideally will articulate with and build upon universal prevention strategies.

❑ Interprofessional relationships will be needed. These can start out as consulting and case-conferencing exchanges to improve the shared knowledge base and grow into collaborative service models.

❑ Ideal service delivery structures probably should integrate mental and physical healthcare and seamlessly connect care across the antenatal, postnatal and early childhood periods.

❑ Advocating for system change may be a long-term process. Developing and testing interventions and treatments will take time too. In the meantime, we can practice within an evidence-based framework by planning care in collaboration with individual clients within a process that includes informed consent about the limits of current knowledge.

CHAPTER 8

Where are we on the journey towards trauma-specific interventions and treatments for the perinatal period?

Chris Cuthbert, NSPCC (UK)

Introduction

With the growth in awareness of maltreatment-related traumatic stress and adverse effects on pregnancy and the transition to motherhood, we would expect to see the emergence of a range of health and social care system responses that address the trauma-related needs of childbearing women. Some will be more focused on the mother's needs, and some on nurturing the mother–infant bond and addressing relational trauma in the dyad. Using a stepped or tiered approach, there could be targeted interventions and indicated treatments offered within a system that is trauma informed and seeks to identify the one in five women with a maltreatment history who may want or need trauma-specific help. This chapter describes a range of emerging efforts to reduce the harms of past maltreatment and post-traumatic mental health and relational sequelae into the future, beginning with prevention programmes.

Characteristics of trauma-specific interventions and treatments

The hope of the contributors to *Trauma Informed Care* is that this chapter will become outdated almost as fast as it can be published.. In it, the focus is on trauma-specific targeted interventions and indicated treatments for women who are pregnant and postnatal and who have a maltreatment history or trauma-related mental health conditions.

By trauma-specific targeted intervention, we mean that it is for maltreatment survivors, to an extent that it would not be a fit for anyone else (i.e. who did not have a maltreatment history). Interventions could be taken up by resilient women because they want the information, support and strategies provided.

By indicated treatment, we mean an individualised psychotherapy or medication provided to address significant distress or impairment, where the clinical problem is framed by attention to the role maltreatment trauma history is playing, whether the agreed-upon goal of the therapy is resolving the trauma or another higher priority clinical problem.

Treatments are a step up from interventions in that a clinical indication or diagnosis based on individual assessment will usually be needed. Such targeted interventions and indicated treatments are trauma-specific when the link between past trauma and current needs and focus is explicit.

A key starting point is finding ways to get trauma-specific interventions and treatments to the women who need then. Prevention programmes within a trauma-informed system have a key role to play, because they can articulate with trauma-specific interventions and treatment options. Also, their content often addresses needs women with a maltreatment history may have and may well satisfy the desires of women who do not want trauma-specific help.

Limitations on the scope of this chapter

We searched the literature for trauma-specific interventions and treatments by using keywords including trauma, abuse, maltreatment and post-traumatic stress. It is very important to point out that there probably are hundreds more interventions and treatments that could become trauma-specific with very small adaptations. Numerous perinatal interventions have garnered evidence for their efficacy in relation to depression, anxiety or parenting outcomes.

Many women with depression, anxiety and parenting challenges in the perinatal period will, in fact, be those who also have a maltreatment history and PTSD (see Table 5.2). Maltreatment history and PTSD would not have been taken into account when these interventions were developed. Yet modifying or tailoring these to be trauma-specific might increase their benefits for the maltreatment survivor subset of users. So, for example, a mindfulness yoga intervention for pregnant women that has published data about depression and attachment outcomes (Muzik *et al.*, 2012) would likely also be useful for PTSD because mindfulness and yoga have some evidence of efficacy with PTSD (not in pregnancy) (King *et al.*, 2013; Spinazzola *et al.*, 2011). Another example would be interpersonal psychotherapy designed to treat perinatal depression by improving the women's key relationships (O'Hara *et al.*, 2000). Making this therapy trauma-specific by adding a focus on family violence and perpetrators and measuring PTSD outcomes as well as depression outcomes would probably be feasible. That focus may already occur in specific cases, but this adaptation or tailoring information has not yet been added to the published outcomes literature.

As we will see next, there has been very limited research to test the safety and efficacy of evidence-based PTSD treatments when used with pregnant women. Thus, adapting existing evidence-based pregnancy interventions for mental health and parenting to create trauma-specific versions may be efficient.

We will not go into medication therapy for PTSD in pregnancy except to say that the front-line drugs for PTSD are largely the same drugs as those for depression, so some safety data is available, but data on their efficacy for treating PTSD in pregnancy is limited (Yonkers *et al.*, 2011). As with management of depression in pregnancy and during lactation, decision-making would need to be individualised and based in an informed consent dialogue (Einarson *et al.*, 2001) that includes the most up-to-date analyses of short- and long-term risk for the child.

Tiered or stepped framework within a trauma informed system of care

Universal perinatal programmes such as maternity care and parent education have a goal to improve physical perinatal outcomes, enhance maternal development and mental health status, ease the transition to parenting, promote sensitive and reflective parenting, and enhance the likelihood of secure attachment for the infant. The natural corollary or flip side of the coin for these goals is case-finding to identify high-risk pregnancies and struggling or high-risk parents and move them up the stepped or tiered levels to intervention and possibly treatment. In a trauma informed system of care, staff would recognise that a key source of the struggle and risk in some cases is likely to be trauma history and post-traumatic sequelae. Prevention programmes can play a key role.

Prevention examples

Family Nurse Partnership

The original US programme was the Nurse Family Partnership, which has a lengthy history of rigorous development and several decades of research providing evidence of its effectiveness with young and poor women in improving maternal health and child development outcomes, including reduced child maltreatment (Olds, 2006). The UK's version of this is the Family Nurse Partnership (FNP), which is an example of a home visiting programme that is being broadly implemented across the UK context. The FNP model is underpinned by a clear theoretical framework, drawing on attachment, human ecology and self-efficacy theories. FNP in the UK uses experienced and qualified health visitors who undergo significant preparation for and supervision within the role.

Compassionate Minds

Home visiting programmes are well suited to augmentation and the development of additional modules. One such augmentation programme – Compassionate Minds – is being tried within the UK's FNP and is a module that family nurses can use to enable individuals to understand compassion, appreciate the importance of self-compassion and learn skills and techniques to use in their daily lives, which in turn helps manage emotional dysregulation or distress. It was introduced to FNP in England in 2010 as an optional and experimental approach to help clients, particularly those with mental health problems, to get the most from the FNP programme. It is based on Compassion Focused Therapy (CFT), which was developed from other forms of mindfulness and was originally created for people with personality disorders rooted in shame or self-critique. The theory of change of CFT is that practising compassion activates the 'soothing' system in the body, balancing the 'drive' and 'threat' systems.

A formative evaluation of Compassionate Minds suggests it is valued by family nurses, who report benefits to themselves and their clients (Renshaw and Wrigley, 2015). The evaluators recommend further work to embed the module and there is a need for further outcomes-based research.

Baby Steps

Structured education packages are another example of prevention within the English Healthy Child programme. Baby Steps is a nine-session perinatal intervention that supports expectant mothers and their partners during the transition to parenthood, and is implemented with support from the major UK charity, the National Society for the Prevention of Cruelty to Children (NSPCC; www. nspcc.org.uk/; accessed 6 July 2015). It combines home visiting and group classes and spans the antenatal and postnatal periods. The programme is designed to be engaging and responsive for families that health and children's services might traditionally consider 'hard to reach'. Baby Steps covers the health and care topics that parents expect from traditional antenatal education – birth, breastfeeding, physical changes in pregnancy and the practicalities of parenting. However, the programme also recognises that this life stage is a time of major psychological and relational reorganisation. Key themes therefore include: supporting parents' emotional well-being; encouraging communication and the couple relationship; building social capital and social networks; enhancing the relationship with the child and capacity for reflective functioning; and understanding child development.

A formative evaluation of the Baby Steps programme, using a pre-post measures design among a sample of more than 200 parents, has shown a range of positive impacts including reductions in symptoms of anxiety, improvements in self-esteem, positive birth outcomes and better-quality relationships with their babies (Coster *et al.*, 2015).

Minding the Baby

This is a programme that combines nurse home visiting and elements of parent–infant psychotherapy and is directed at vulnerable mothers and their babies from pregnancy until the baby reaches age two. It targets the relationship disruptions that stem from mothers' early trauma and derailed attachment history (Slade, 2005). Minding the Baby aims to promote 'reflective functioning', helping mothers develop the capacity to envision mental states (thoughts, feelings, needs, desires) in their babies. Reflective functioning refers not only to the capacity to recognise mental states, but also to link mental states to behaviour in meaningful and accurate ways. A reflective individual has a sophisticated internal working model of emotion and intentions, which facilitates affect regulation (the ability to maintain positive feelings and regulate stress levels) and productive social relationships.

A randomised controlled trial of Minding the Baby in the US found no significant impact on maternal mental health, but at twelve months significantly more babies in the intervention group were securely attached to their mothers compared with the control group (Sadler *et al.*, 2013). Also, the control group was significantly more likely to have disorganised attachment. The programme has been replicated in three settings in the UK by the NSPCC, with a randomised controlled trial currently underway led by University College London (Fearon *et al.*, 2014).

The extent to which these prevention programmes aim explicitly to prevent maltreatment varies, but in all of them the focus on trauma is explicit enough that they appeared in our search using abuse and neglect and trauma as key words. Each focuses on maternal (and some also paternal) mental health, parent–infant relationship, and each is aware of potential for distress and problems from past abuse and

Table 8.1 Trauma informed programmes.

Universal prevention	Focus on mother	Focus on parent–infant relationship
Family Nurse Partnership	✔✔	✔✔
Compassionate Minds	✔✔	✔✔
Baby Steps	✔✔	✔✔
Minding the Baby	✔✔	✔✔✔

neglect in the lives of the parents that could impinge on positive outcomes. These programmes include relationships with professionals via which referral up the tiers to interventions and treatment could easily take place as trauma-specific interventions and treatments become available.

Trauma-specific interventions

Using our definition, trauma-specific interventions are designed for women (or families) based on history; that is, they address trauma-related needs and could be useful to a woman with a maltreatment history whether she is affected by post-traumatic mental health conditions or is resilient. Here are two examples of trauma-specific interventions that address maternal needs via manualised programmes that do not require diagnosis and could benefit resilient women.

Mom Power

This is a ten-week group intervention created in the US for young mothers (15–21 years) with young children (0–6 years) that aims to build secure attachment bonds between the mother and her child (LePlatte *et al.*, 2012). It includes strengthening mother–child interactions, improving parenting skills, teaching self-care practices and strengthening or establishing connections with social support systems and healthcare systems. Mothers are taught to cope with stressful life circumstances and mental health symptoms while being responsive and sensitive parents. They learn to regulate their emotions, think clearly under stress and recover from problems with mental health (e.g. anxiety, depression, addiction, anger, social isolation, dissociation) to feel safe and adequate as parents. Each of the ten programme sessions specifically addresses these topics in a group setting.

In 2012, Mom Power was found to be feasible and effective in a small study of twenty-four teenage mothers (LePlatte *et al.*, 2012). On programme completion, participants demonstrated significant decreases in depression, PTSD symptoms and self-rated guilt and shame regarding parenting. An additional pilot study published in 2015 by Muzik *et al.* used a sample of sixty-eight mother–child dyads to examine Mom Power for feasibility, acceptability and pilot outcomes. The study found significant reductions in depression, PTSD and caregiving helplessness, a dose-response relationship for the intervention, and favourable perception of the intervention by participants. These results suggest that further testing of Mom Power is warranted in randomised controlled trials (Muzik *et al.*, 2015).

Survivor Moms' Companion

The Survivor Moms' Companion is a ten-module, self-study psychoeducation programme developed to address the pregnancy-specific needs of abuse survivors affected by traumatic stress to improve affect regulation, reduce interpersonal reactivity and support PTSD symptom management despite the presence of triggers (Seng *et al.*, 2011a). The programme was developed by by collaborators connected via the University of Michigan and followed their pioneering investigation into women's experiences of pregnancy, birth, mothering and healing after sexual abuse (Sperlich and Seng, 2008).

The Survivor Moms' Companion is provided to participants in hard copy workbook format and comprises ten self-study modules, which are accompanied by structured telephone or face-to-face tutoring sessions with social workers or perinatal nurses. The modules each include learning objectives and written information on the topic, followed by vignettes that are used to support simulated problem-solving and skills practice (Sperlich *et al.*, 2011).

Results from a pilot study of the Survivor Moms' Companion showed improvements in anger expression, interpersonal reactivity and PTSD symptom management, affirming the theory of change (Seng *et al.*, 2011a). Outcomes analyses show improvements in birth experience, postnatal mental health status and maternal to infant bonding, suggesting that participation in the programme is beneficial to mothers (Rowe *et al.*, 2014). These results suggest that the

Table 8.2 Trauma-specific interventions.

Universal prevention	Focus on mother	Focus on parent-infant relationship
Mom Power	✔✔	✔✔✔
Survivor Moms' Companion	✔✔✔	✔✔

programme merits larger-scale evaluation including measurement of outcomes for the child.

Trauma-specific treatments

In this section, we describe examples of treatments for women who probably would meet diagnostic criteria for a trauma-related disorder such as PTSD, depression, dissociation or personality disorder. These therapies have in common a purpose to redress sequelae of childhood maltreatment trauma at the level of psychopathology in stress response, relationships, self-esteem or self-regulation. They are primarily for individual expectant or new mothers, sometimes including the infant, and they are sometimes delivered in groups. These interventions are examples chosen to span a range of theoretical perspectives and differ in their relative emphasis between a focus on the mother and on the mother–infant relationship.

Cognitive behavioural therapy for PTSD

Trauma-focused cognitive behavioural therapy (CBT) for PTSD focuses on the trauma and aims to help people develop strategies to reduce their sense of current threat and thereby reduce PTSD symptoms. The treatment involves supporting mothers to relive traumatic memories and modify unhelpful appraisals of their experiences. This process of elaboration and contextualisation of the trauma memory is intended to decrease fear of the memory and facilitate discrimination between the past and the present. The therapist works with the client to identify the 'hotspots' in these memories and the different emotions that they trigger, with the aim of ultimately reducing the intensity of emotions by changing their meaning. Prolonged Exposure and Eye Movement Desensitisation and Reprocessing are additional individual psychotherapies with CBT underpinnings that have an evidence base for treatment of PTSD (Bisson and Andrew, 2007).

Meta-analyses (cf. Roberts *et al.*, 2009) and systematic reviews (Bisson *et al.*, 2007) have shown that treatments focusing on memories and the meaning of trauma are consistently more effective than non-trauma focused ones. There is not yet an evidence base for CBT's efficacy or safety for use with pregnant women, but the clinical trials literature shows decrease in symptom levels across treatment. This suggests that the treatment may be less stressful than persistent untreated PTSD in women experiencing high levels of intrusions and arousals. For now, as with medication use, individualised decision-making with careful informed consent will be needed (Rice, 2011). Direct investigation of risks and benefits for the maternal–fetal dyad are very much needed for these psychotherapies as well as for medication use.

Compassion Focused Therapy

Therapies with their basis in a mindfulness and compassion approach have also been developed to address personality disorders rooted in trauma. CFT recognises the sense of constant threat that hangs over the lives of those who have experienced trauma and abuse (Lee, 2012). But it places particular emphasis on shame and self-criticism as products of such experiences. CFT offers a way to work with these socially constructed emotions, which may be difficult to access or influence using self-focused CBT techniques. CFT is based on the premise that we cannot think our way out of shame, but we need to feel our way out by accessing emotional memories of safeness and being able to calm ourselves. Thus, CFT targets activation of the soothing system so that it can be used to help regulate threat-based emotions of anger, fear, disgust and shame.

There is a modest amount of empirical evidence that CFT, when provided alongside concurrent support from mental health services, may impact stress, depression, anxiety, self-criticism and self-compassion for adults with severe mental health difficulties (Renshaw and Wrigley, 2015). However, while this approach might seem well suited to the circumstances of women in the perinatal period who have histories of trauma, to date there is no research evidence on its effectiveness specifically with adolescents, or with pregnant or postnatal women.

Parent–Infant Psychotherapy

Parent–Infant Psychotherapy (PIP) Is a dyadic therapy that involves working simultaneously with the parent and the infant. The aim of PIP is to help mothers to address their own past trauma and to recognise the 'ghosts in the nursery' (Fraiberg, 1980). Parents tend to raise children as they themselves were raised. Yet it is not the quality of childhood experiences that predicts this intergenerational transmission, but how parents talk and think (intrapsychic representation) about their experiences in the present (Stern, 1995). Through empathy, respect, concern and unfailing positive regard, therapists foster healthy relationships between mother and baby (Baradon, 2010). These therapies fall most closely into the psychodynamic orientation where the focus is on how internal representation of experiences is organised around interpersonal relations, and where the relationship between the therapist and client is a key factor in the modality (Shedler, 2010).

A recent systematic review examined the evidence on the effectiveness of parent–infant/toddler psychotherapy (Barlow *et al.*, 2015). Meta-analyses indicate that parents who received PIP were more likely to have an infant who was securely attached to the parent after intervention than those in a no-treatment control group; however, there were no significant differences between groups in studies comparing outcomes of PIP with other kinds of treatment (such as video-interaction guidance, counselling or CBT). Barlow *et al.* (2015) conclude that PIP is a promising model in terms of improving infant attachment in high-risk families but that further research is needed into its impact on potentially important mediating factors, such as mental health, reflective functioning and parent–infant interaction.

Parents Under Pressure

This is a treatment programme that combines elements of mindfulness, attachment theory and attention to self-regulation. It is an intensive, twenty-week home visiting treatment, originally designed in Australia to support methadone-maintained mothers and their children aged 2–8 years. More recently, Parents Under Pressure (PUP) has been developed to work with parents of newborn babies and infants aged up to two-and-a-half-years and the programme eligibility criteria have been broadened to include drug and alcohol misuse. PUP is underpinned by an ecological model of child development, reflecting the importance of social contextual factors such as social isolation, poverty and poor housing on family functioning.

The model recognises the high proportions of substance-misusing parents who have histories of abuse and trauma. PUP therapists aim to build a therapeutic alliance with their clients and use mindfulness as a means to help parents regulate their emotions. The programme draws on behaviourist and attachment-based parenting approaches to improve the quality and sensitivity of parent–child interaction.

A small-scale, randomised, controlled trial in Australia demonstrated reductions in parenting stress, child abuse potential inventory scores and improvements in child behaviour (Dawe and Harnett, 2007). The NSPCC is working with the programme developers to test the effectiveness of the adapted PUP programme in a multicentre controlled trial in the UK. This independent evaluation will measure the impacts of the programme, its cost-effectiveness and fit with UK delivery systems (Barlow *et al.*, 2013).

Table 8.3 Trauma-specific treatment.

Universal prevention	Focus on mother	Focus on parent-infant relationship
Parents Under Pressure	✔✔	✔✔
CBT for PTSD	✔✔✔	(not specific to pregnancy)
Compassion Focused Therapy	✔✔✔	(not specific to pregnancy)
Parent-Infant Psychotherapy	✔✔	✔✔✔

Looking towards the future

This chapter has described a range of innovative and promising approaches to helping women with histories of maltreatment trauma and PTSD during the transition to parenthood. Yet, despite the clear and urgent need for such interventions, trauma-specific and trauma informed approaches remain exotic features in the current landscape of perinatal healthcare. Those that do exist are fairly specialised, requiring staff training and resources – features not available in many jurisdictions. Indeed, while there has been an upsurge in understanding about the importance of early years' intervention, much practice in the early years' field remains blind to the corrosive impacts of parents' histories of trauma and overlooks the crucial importance of intervening in pregnancy.

It would be easy to become fatalistic in the face of so much suffering, such limited awareness and such a low base in routine practice. Yet, the pioneering examples in this chapter suggest that there is cause for optimism, indeed that much can be done to help women heal the wounds of their trauma and successfully navigate the transition to parenthood. Perhaps in the future we will see increased integration between trauma-specific models of intervention for expectant mothers and the equally exciting set of interventions that focus on building the mother–child relationship. In the future, this integration between maternal and infant mental health could unlock improved outcomes for both mother and baby.

Conclusion

Here are the main points from this chapter about the state of the science in trauma-specific interventions and treatments:

❏ Awareness of the impact of maltreatment history and PTSD on childbearing and early parenting is new compared to knowledge about perinatal depression, but trauma-specific interventions and treatments are emerging.

❏ Prevention programmes usually also include case-finding to refer high-risk people to intervention. Attending to maltreatment history and post-traumatic sequelae as risk factors would take universal prevention programmes a step towards becoming trauma informed.

❏ Tiered or stepped perinatal care systems can include trauma-specific interventions for any woman with a maltreatment history – resilient or not – and trauma-specific treatment for women meeting diagnostic criteria or other threshold understood by the service delivery context.

❏ Some existing, evidence-based programmes for pregnant women who have depression or anxiety could perhaps be adapted or tailored to become trauma-specific.

❏ Current treatments for PTSD that have an evidence base for use with the general population need to be studied for safety and efficacy in pregnancy.

❏ Medications for PTSD include many already used for depression in pregnancy, so focus could be on study of efficacy in pregnancy for PTSD symptoms.

❏ While waiting for the perinatal PTSD treatment evidence base to be built, we can use the processes of mutual decision-making and informed-consent dialogues to create individual plans with our clients.

CHAPTER 9

What are the next steps for trauma informed care in education and research?

Kristen R. Choi, University of Michigan
Julie Taylor, University of Birmingham (UK)

Introduction

So far, this book has focused on what we need to do in practice to provide trauma informed care and to try to influence service delivery models from within our professional roles and leadership positions. However, to advance this agenda, we also need to provide education for professionals and create empirical evidence on which to base our work and with which to lay claim to resources. In this chapter, we focus on the education and research domains and outline ideas for next steps.

Education needs

The body of literature on the prevalence of maltreatment and traumatic stress and their toxic effects on lifespan health is building quickly and solidly. The literature on their adverse effects on perinatal outcomes is more recent. Perinatal healthcare professionals currently in practice received limited or no training on how to address maltreatment trauma and PTSD in their pre-qualifying education. Pre-qualifying programmes in nursing, midwifery and medicine are beginning to include more content about post-traumatic stress (White, 2014), but postgraduate opportunities to fill this training gap will be needed into the future. Addressing this hole in both pre-qualifying and postgraduate education is essential to creating service delivery systems that are trauma informed.

As mentioned in earlier chapters, child welfare and mental health professionals have more background in this arena. Interprofessional opportunities to train and move collaboratively from novice to expert hold promise as a means not only to bring the healthcare providers on the team up to speed, but also to advance the linkages and relationships needed to provide integrated seamless models of care. Technical assistance from organisations such as the NCTIC in the USA can be extremely useful, but these materials are not yet tailored for healthcare or perinatal professionals. Local education offerings that can be studied and published for broader use will be needed.

Continuing education on trauma informed care is required to address gaps in pre-qualifying curricula. Our qualitative research suggests that perinatal care providers wish to provide high-quality care to clients with histories of trauma, accommodate their trauma-related needs and preferences and learn best practices for trauma informed care (Choi and Seng, 2014). Topics they wanted to have addressed in continuing education programmes include: the neurobiology of trauma and pathophysiology of PTSD; how to recognise signs of post-traumatic stress; on-the-spot interventions to address symptoms of post-traumatic stress or PTSD reactions that may arise in perinatal care settings; therapeutic communication strategies including how to invite disclosure; and pertinent screening to consider for closely related issues (e.g. anxiety, depression, domestic violence). Communication strategies, in particular, such as the observation and enquiry process described in Chapter 6, are an important skill to address because post-traumatic stress is often triggered within the provider–client interpersonal context. A large UK survey on the topic of postgraduate education needs found that most midwives did not feel prepared to respond to or address disclosures of past sexual abuse. This study suggested that provider education is needed on how to discuss sexuality and trauma in general (Jackson and Fraser, 2009).

Educational programmes should be available in a variety of formats and for different levels of knowledge. In a small study of knowledge, attitudes and skills developed via a one-hour, 'all hands', in-service meeting for perinatal service agencies (Choi and Seng, date TBC), it became clear that different offerings had to have different goals. For example, administrative, medical and nursing professionals may need information that is really too basic for the child welfare and mental health staff, but team-building could be an objective of this mixed-level programme where common language and shared understandings are an outcome. Social workers and therapists may require more advanced sessions about dilemmas in practice or advanced information on treatment.

One-size-fits-all offerings are unlikely to satisfy as some clinicians will be very interested in working with this client group or will liaise with populations where trauma is more prevalent and will want in-depth learning opportunities. Here, however, we have distilled three particular topics that warrant inclusion in even basic educational offerings.

Avoiding triggering and re-traumatisation
Re-traumatisation of clients often happens at the hands of healthcare providers, and provider–client relationships and service delivery structures are laden with power dynamics that put clients in subordinate positions for managing their own care. Re-traumatisation can occur when providers use non-therapeutic words, attitudes and actions, but it can also transpire when care appears to be courteous and professional, but is not trauma informed. These interactions can activate PTSD reactions. Intrusive healthcare procedures and birth and breastfeeding also can be triggers. Providers need consciousness-raising, strategising and skill-building opportunities to learn to provide sensitive care and repair ruptures in relationship caused by triggering. Training for healthcare providers may need to include a focus on how empowering clients or patients to make their own choices about care can prevent the construction of non-therapeutic, oppressive power dynamics and about how this contributes to trauma informed care.

Vicarious trauma
Many professionals including emergency first-responders and psychotherapists are quite familiar with the concept of vicarious trauma. However, healthcare professionals are less likely to know about this or to have strategies in place by which to protect themselves. We use this definition from the psychotherapy professional literature:

Vicarious traumatization refers to a transformation in the therapist's (or other trauma worker's) inner experience resulting from empathetic engagement with clients' trauma material. That is, through exposure to clients' graphic accounts of sexual abuse experience and to the realities of people's intentional cruelty to one another, and through the inevitable participation in traumatic re-enactments in the therapy relationship, the therapist is vulnerable through his or her empathetic openness to the emotional and spiritual effects of vicarious traumatization. These effects are cumulative and permanent, and evident in both a therapist's professional and personal life (Pearlman and Saakvitne, 2013, p. 151).

Healthcare providers may also witness traumatic memories and PTSD reactions happening *in vivo* from their position at the side of the examination table or birthing bed. Because of the highly empathetic nature of provider–woman relationships during the perinatal period, healthcare providers might find their own mental health and capacity to provide care at risk (Leinweber and Rowe, 2010).

Perinatal professionals who work with populations with high rates of trauma exposure should be cognisant of the signs of vicarious traumatisation and self-care practices for managing vicarious trauma. The key sign of vicarious trauma is disruption of the professional's frame of reference including sense of identity, worldview and spirituality (Pearlman and Saakvitne, 2013). The person may begin to question their identity as a helping professional. Those with a maltreatment history of their own may be more susceptible than others. If vicarious trauma becomes severe, professionals may also question their worldviews, values and spirituality. They may experience changes in interpersonal relations (e.g. social withdrawal, feeling alienated from intimate relationships and sexual partners, unable to enjoy leisure activities) and behaviours (e.g. self-deprecation, avoidance). Education programmes that address vicarious traumatisation in maternity care can focus on the same three domains for attention that experts in the psychotherapy profession recommend: personal, professional and organisational (Pearlman and Saakvitne, 2013).

To identify signs of vicarious traumatisation early and promote self-care, it is important for professionals to take time to reflect on their own practice. Self-regulatory learning theories suggest that both cognitive (critical thinking) and metacognitive (reflective thinking) reflection on one's practice facilitate professional growth (Kuiper and Pesut, 2004). Establishing habits of regular reflection will allow professionals who work with traumatised clients to identify their own feelings and seek input about what they might need to continue in order to provide sensitive care and safeguard their own well-being.

Diagnostic frameworks

Healthcare professionals will be most effective securing resources for care and producing credible care plans if they can call upon a diagnostic framework instead of documenting only a history of maltreatment. Education programmes should include information about assessment tools, the range of trauma-related diagnoses in national or international taxonomies and a range of treatment options. PTSD is perhaps the 'root' diagnosis, but others including

Table 9.1 Suggestions for training content and format.

Content
• neurobiology of trauma and PTSD;
• recognising signs of post-traumatic stress;
• interventions to address post-traumatic stress;
• therapeutic communication strategies for use with triggered client;
• language for communicating with the woman and other healthcare professionals;
• how to invite disclosure;
• screening for related mental health and social issues;
• discussing sexual trauma effects on sexual health:
• avoiding triggering and re-traumatisation;
• vicarious trauma;
• diagnostic frameworks.

Format	
Pre-qualifying programmes:	Postgraduate and continuing professional development:
• problem-focused learning scenarios; • gynaecologic teaching assistants leading scenarios and role playing; • content modules or lectures; • webinars or web-blended format.	• case conferences; • journal club; • focused issues of professional journals; • in-service programmes; • training workshops or conference sessions; • certification courses; • webinars.

depression, substance misuse, dissociation, somatisation and personality pathologies can come into play. Understanding the complexity of maltreatment effects and how these appear in antenatal, intrapartum and postnatal care should be solidly addressed in healthcare professional trainings.

Next steps for research

Throughout this book, it has been pointed out where research is needed because the evidence base does not yet exist, or where interventions have not yet been tried in different population groups. This last section draws those points together to suggest a research agenda for trauma informed care in the perinatal period. We know from a wealth of evidence that the effects of childhood maltreatment and PTSD during the childbearing year are severe, long-lasting and extend to following generations. There is a need for a paradigm shift in the way we think about perinatal care in practice and in research.

New service delivery models

There is now an opportunity for child welfare professionals and maternity professionals to collaborate in creating new service delivery models that provide trauma informed care across the perinatal year – across pregnancy, birth and the fourth trimester, which includes the early weeks of parenting. We have suggested that a continuity model offers most promise, but this has not been tested in research. It would be a challenging endeavour, but if coupled with economic analysis could provide some useful alternatives to current models. Continuity models could be developed in a number of ways: for example, specialist trauma midwives with smaller, more intensive caseloads. Furthermore, interprofessional collaboration and integration are espoused as the gold standard and certainly make sense. It is perhaps time to observe what such teams contribute during the perinatal year, to look at best composition, process and outcome.

Revise divisions of labour

While there are benefits for individuals from medical advances, addressing many of the remaining sources of morbidity and mortality requires a bifocal lens from the pregnant woman's position:

outward, to her socioecological context; and inward, to her individual health status and biology. Our current division of research endeavour along biological, psychological and social lines needs revision and bringing together to address perinatal threat at the individual and population levels. For example, much of the funded research on maternal stress examines the maternal, placental and fetal contributions and pathways at the biological level, focusing on hormones in the primary stress response systems. Yet evolutionary biology theories such as life history or life course theories are being applied to understand how survival and reproduction are traded off against each other in stressful circumstances and across generations. Relevant research into biomedics, epigenetics, trauma, child protection, maternity care etc. could be usefully integrated in unique ways that are currently missing.

Pregnancy as a stress test for life
The idea that pregnancy is a stress test for life is also gaining ground, so the outcomes of stress being examined are not only those of the infant but also of the mother. For example, insulin resistance or hypertension that appears under the stress of childbearing is likely to reappear later for the woman, and much earlier in the lifespan for her than for others who tolerated the 'stress test' with no adverse effects. Such macro stress theories are embedded in the body, but are attentive to the larger social context.

Partners and fathers
We have not covered the roles of partners and fathers in this book, and there is research to be done in this area. What might be the protective elements in these relationships? And what might be the components that increase the risk? We know little about the effects of childbirth and the early weeks on fathers who were maltreated in childhood, and next to nothing about this group of men who also have PTSD symptomatology.

Trauma-specific interventions
Trauma- or PTSD-specific interventions and treatments for pregnancy and the postnatal period have yet to be developed and carried

to the point of having an evidence base. Using the action points on the cycles-breaking framework (Chapters 3 and 7), it is clear that there are numerous types of interventions or treatments that could be created at multiple action points across the perinatal period.

Targeted interventions for the perinatal year have yet to be developed and tested, but core concepts might include training in self-control for abused individuals (children and parents) and the concept of self-regulation as an overarching need of people abused in childhood who did not receive the input all infants need from parents.

Lifetime trauma history
In relation to postnatal birth-related PTSD, future research and interventions should attend to lifetime trauma history. Although for some women giving birth will be a first traumatic life event and lead to new-onset PTSD, it seems that a majority will be women for whom postnatal PTSD is recurrent or chronic, exacerbated by birth as a re-traumatisation. Tailoring post-birth interventions for women with new-onset versus recurrent PTSD is an area for further research.

Child and maternal outcomes in tandem
Interventions that improve child outcomes should also aim to improve maternal well-being. By addressing the mother's unresolved trauma history and current mental health needs, we might also strengthen her capacity to bond with her infant and apply new skills in parenting such as reflectivity and sensitivity that will enhance outcomes for the child. Thinking of the mother–infant relationship as dyadic is crucial. Providing interventions that meet the woman's needs can also be measured in terms of short- and long-term outcomes for the child.

Intergenerational resilience
Why maltreatment is not perpetrated is as interesting a research question as that of the continuity of abuse and neglect across generations. There is a need for more research into those who are 'cycle breakers', who did well despite trauma or whose post-traumatic growth results in more protective parenting. Research into intergenerational resilience should be reflected in greater sensitivity in

theoretical models, where simplistic and deterministic assumptions concerning the developmental trajectories of maltreated children and adults are avoided.

Replication and testing tailored adaptations
Replication is important where studies are few or underpowered, adding credence to findings and building a case for taking action in a variety of settings. Duplication of studies in different settings, cultures, populations and countries is critical. Other types of trauma exposure may also be significant to subgroups of women and could also be addressed with trauma informed care tailored to special populations.

There are likely to be many interventions and treatments that could become trauma-specific with little adaptation: for example, diverse evidence-based perinatal interventions in relation to depression, anxiety and parenting outcomes. When they were developed, it is unlikely that maltreatment history and PTSD would have been taken into account. Modifying or tailoring these to be trauma-specific might increase their benefits for maltreatment survivors.

There has been no research to test the safety and efficacy of evidence-based PTSD treatments when used with pregnant women. Adapting and testing existing evidence- based PTSD treatments for pregnant and postnatal women may be efficient.

While there are a range of adaptations that could be made, the models we have articulated have largely been interventions in well-resourced, English-speaking health systems. Feasibility and acceptability studies in other cultures and settings are also needed. In many areas, a baseline mapping of current provision and understanding would be an essential first research step.

Methodologies and theories
A research agenda sensitive to trauma informed care in the perinatal period would need to think carefully about a range of approaches, both qualitative and quantitative. The burgeoning field of implementation science (cf. Fixsen *et al.*, 2009; Curran *et al.*, 2012) might be applied well within this field. New conceptualisations or revising of current models are required. Methodological advances in

informatics and big data analytics may permit analyses of data collected across health, education and social care systems to answer questions about trajectories over time, with and without interventions.

Educational research

It could go without saying, but those who develop pre-qualifying curricula or postgraduate workshops would do a great service by conducting evaluation and learning outcome research and publishing the findings, as well as considering sharing the curriculum itself. Local solutions are important, but much of what we need to know has commonalities across healthcare roles and could be designed for interprofessional use.

Impact on professionals and systems

There is potential for trauma informed care and trauma-specific interventions not only to improve outcomes for women with a maltreatment history and their infants but also to advance the well-being of the professionals who work with them. Research is warranted to learn how changing structures, processes and outcomes to be trauma informed could enhance our professional relationships and career longevity. Greater self-efficacy and sense of effectiveness could lead to higher satisfaction, less job-related stress and greater retention in our challenging professions.

Conclusion

Here are the main points from this chapter about the next steps for education and research:

- ❏ Pre-qualifying and postgraduate programmes in nursing, midwifery and medicine need to include maltreatment trauma and PTSD in their curricula.
- ❏ Although one size does not fit all, the three topics that are needed in all educational offerings are:
  - ❏ avoiding triggering and re-traumatisation;
  - ❏ vicarious trauma;
  - ❏ diagnostic frameworks.
- ❏ There is a need for a paradigm shift in the way we think about perinatal care research.

❑ Research is needed:

  ❑ to test new service delivery models and develop new trauma-specific interventions for women with childhood maltreatment histories;

  ❑ across disciplines and sciences;

  ❑ with different client groups and settings;

  ❑ in modifying and revising existing interventions;

  ❑ accounting for lifetime trauma history.

❑ New methodologies and conceptualisations may need to be applied to this field of work.

REFERENCES

AAP (n.d.) 'Social emotional safety net diagram' (online). Available from URL: www.aap.org/en-us/advocacy-and-policy/aap-health-initiatives/EBCD/Documents/SE_Safety_Nets.pdf (accessed 17 April 2015)

Access Economics Pty Ltd, Australian Childhood Foundation and Child Abuse Prevention Research Australia (2008) 'The cost of child abuse in Australia', Monash University. Available from URL: www.childhood.org.au/~/media/Files/Research/Research%20Cost%20of%20Child%20Abuse%20in%20Australia%202009.ashx (accessed 20 April 2015)

ACNM (2000) 'Position statement: Female circumcision' (online). Available from URL: www.midwife.org/ACNM/files/ACNMLibraryData/UPLOAD-FILENAME/000000000068/Female%20Circumcision%20Sept%202012.pdf (accessed 21 April 2015)

ACOG (2001) 'Adult manifestation of childhood sexual abuse, number 259, July 2000', ACOG educational bulletin: Clinical management guidelines for obstetrician-gynecologists, *International Journal of Gynaecology and Obstetrics: The Official Organ of the International Federation of Gynaecology and Obstetrics*, Vol. 74, No. 3, p. 311

Agaibi, C. E. and Wilson, J. P. (2005) 'Trauma, PTSD, and resilience: A review of the literature', *Trauma, Violence, & Abuse*, Vol. 6, No. 3, pp. 195–216; doi:10.1177/1524838005277438

Ainsworth, M. D. S. and Bowlby, J. (1991) 'An ethological approach to personality development', *American Psychologist*, Vol. 46, pp. 331–41

Alhusen, J. L., Ray, E., Sharps, P. and Bullock, L. (2015) 'Intimate partner violence during pregnancy: Maternal and neonatal outcomes', *Journal of Women's Health*, Vol. 24, pp. 100–106; doi:10.1089/jwh.2014.4872

APA (1994) *Diagnostic and Statistical Manual of Mental Disorders, Fourth Edition (DSM-IV)*, Washington, DC: American Psychiatric Association

APA (2013) *Diagnostic and Statistical Manual of Mental Disorders, Fifth Edition (DSM-V)*, Arlington, VA: American Psychiatric Publishing

Ayers, S., McKenzie-McHarg, K. and Slade, P. (2015). 'Post-traumatic stress disorder after birth', *Journal of Reproductive and Infant Psychology*, pp. 1–4; doi/full/10.1080/02646838.2015.1030250

Bandura, A. (2005) 'The primacy of self-regulation in health promotion', *Applied Psychology*, Vol. 52, No. 2, pp. 245–54; doi:10.1111/j.1464-0597.2005.00208.x

Baradon, T. (ed.) (2010) *Relational Trauma in Infancy: Psychoanalytic, Attachment and Neuropsychological Contributions to Parent–Infant Psychotherapy*, New York, NY: Routledge

Barker, D. J. P. (1995) 'Fetal origins of coronary heart disease', *BMJ*, Vol. 311, pp. 171–4; doi:10.1136/bmj.311.6998.171

Barlow, J., Bennett, C., Midgley, N., Larkin, S. and Yinghui, W. (2015) 'Parent–infant psychotherapy for improving parental and infant mental health', *Cochrane Database of Systematic Reviews*; doi:10.1002/14651858. CD010534.pub2

Barlow, J., Sembi, S., Gardner, F., Macdonald, G., Petrou, S., Parsons, H., Harnett, P. and Dawe, S. (2013) 'An evaluation of the parents under pressure programme: A study protocol for a randomised controlled trial into its clinical and cost effectiveness', *Trials*, Vol. 14, p. 210; doi:10.1186/1745–6215–14–210

Beck, C. T. (2011) 'Secondary traumatic stress in nurses: A systematic review', *Archives of Psychiatric Nursing*, Vol. 25, No. 1, pp. 1–10; doi:10.1016/j. apnu.2010.05.005

Beck, C. T. and Watson, S. (2008) 'Impact of birth trauma on breast-feeding: A tale of two pathways', *Nursing Research*, Vol. 57, No. 4, pp. 228–36; doi:10.1097/01.NNR.0000313494.87282.90

Bell, S. A. and Seng, J. (2013) 'Childhood maltreatment history, post-traumatic relational sequelae, and prenatal care utilization', *Journal of Obstetric, Gynecologic, & Neonatal Nursing*, Vol. 42, No. 4, pp. 404–15; doi:10.1111/1552–6909.12223

Bibring, G. L. (1959) 'Some considerations of the psychological processes in pregnancy', *The Psychoanalytic Study of the Child*, Vol. 14, pp. 113–21

Bisson, J. and Andrew, M. (2007) 'Psychological treatment of post-traumatic stress disorder (PTSD)', *Cochrane Database of Systematic Reviews*, Vol. 3, No. CD003388; doi:10.1002/14651858.CD003388.pub3

Bohn, D. K. and Holz, K. A. (1996) 'Sequelae of abuse: Health effects of childhood sexual abuse, domestic battering, and rape', *Journal of Nurse-Midwifery*, Vol. 41, No. 6, pp. 442–56; doi:10.1016/S0091–2182(96)80012–7

Bowlby, J. (1940) 'The influence of early environment in the development of neurosis and neurotic character', *International Journal of Psycho-Analysis*, Vol. XXI, pp. 1–25

Bowlby, J. (1983) [1969] *'Attachment: Attachment and Loss'*, Vol. 1, No. 2, New York, NY: Basic Books

Bradley, P. and Hill, L. (2011) 'Perinatal mood and anxiety disorders screening program: It's more than depression', *Journal of Obstetric, Gynecologic, & Neonatal Nursing*, Vol. 40, No. 1, pp. S4–S5; doi:10.1111/j.1552–6909.2011.01242_3.x

Brandon, M, Bailey, S. and Belderson, P. (2009) *Building on the Learning from Serious Case Reviews: A Two Year Analysis*, London: Department for Education

Breslau, N. (2009) 'The epidemiology of trauma, PTSD, and other post-trauma disorders', *Trauma, Violence, & Abuse*, Vol. 10, No. 3, pp. 198–210; doi:10.1177/1524838009334448

Breslau, N., Davis, G. C., Andreski, P. and Peterson, E. (1991) 'Traumatic events and post-traumatic stress disorder in an urban population of young adults', *Archives of General Psychiatry*, Vol. 48, No. 3, pp. 216–22;

doi:10.1001/archpsyc.1991.01810270028003

Breslau, N., Kessler, R. C., Chilcoat, H. D., Schultz, L. R., Davis, G. C. and Andreski, P. (1998) 'Trauma and post-traumatic stress disorder in the community: The 1996 Detroit Area Survey of Trauma', *Archives of General Psychiatry*, Vol. 55, No. 7, pp. 626–32; doi:10.1001/archpsyc.55.7.626

Brockington, I. (2004) 'Postpartum psychiatric disorders', *The Lancet*, Vol. 363, p. 8

Brockington, I., Macdonald, E. and Wainscott, G. (2006) 'Anxiety, obsessions and morbid preoccupations in pregnancy and the puerperium', *Archives of Women's Mental Health*, Vol. 9, No. 5, pp. 253–63

Brown, L. S. (1991) 'Not outside the range: One feminist perspective on psychic trauma', *American Imago*, Vol. 48, pp. 119–33

Carlson, V., Cicchetti, D., Barnett, D. and Braunwald, K. (1989) 'Disorganised/disoriented attachment relationships in maltreated infants', *Developmental Psychology*, Vol. 25, pp. 25–31; doi:10.1037/0012-1649.25.4.525

Centers for Disease Control and Prevention (2014) 'Prevalence and characteristics of sexual violence, stalking, and intimate partner violence victimization – National Intimate Partner and Sexual Violence Survey, United States, 2011', *Morbidity and Mortality Weekly Report*, Vol. 63, No. SS08, pp. 1–18; doi:10.2105/AJPH.2015.302634. Available from URL: www.cdc.gov/mmwr/preview/mmwrhtml/ss6308a1.htm?s_cid=ss6308a1_e (accessed 16 April 2015)

Champagne, F. A. and Curley, J. P. (2009) 'Epigenetic mechanisms mediating the long-term effects of maternal care on development', *Neuroscience and Biobehavioral Reviews*, Vol. 33, No. 4, pp. 593–600; doi:10.1016/j.neubiorev.2007.10.009

Chang, H. L., Chang, T. C., Lin, T. Y. and Kuo, S. S. (2002) 'Psychiatric morbidity and pregnancy outcome in a disaster area of Taiwan 921 earthquake', *Psychiatry & Clinical Neurosciences*, Vol. 56, No. 2, pp. 139–44; doi:10.1046/j.1440-1819.2002.00948.x

Chemtob, C. M., Gudino, O. G. and Laraque, D. (2014) 'Maternal post-traumatic stress disorder and depression in pediatric primary care: Association with child maltreatment and frequency of child exposure to traumatic events', *JAMA Pediatrics*, Vol. 167, No. 11, pp. 1011–18; doi:10.1001/jamapediatrics.2013.2218

Childbirth Connection (2013) 'The cost of having a baby in the United States: Executive summary' (online). Available from URL: http://transform.childbirthconnection.org/wp-content/uploads/2013/01/Cost-of-Having-a-Baby-Executive-Summary.pdf (accessed 16 April 2015)

Chisholm, J. S. (1999) *Death, Hope and Sex: Steps to an Evolutionary Ecology of Mind and Morality*, Cambridge: Cambridge University Press

Choi, K. R. and Seng, J. S. (2014) 'Trauma-informed care with childhood maltreatment survivors: What do maternity professionals want to learn?' *International Journal of Childbirth*, Vol. 4, No. 3, pp. 191–201

Choi, K. R. and Seng, J. S. (under review). 'Dissociation in labor: Identifying "trait" and "state" dissociation and creating prevention, intervention, and follow-up strategies'.

Coles, J. (2009) 'Qualitative study of breastfeeding after childhood sexual assault', *Journal of Human Lactation*, Vol. 25, pp. 317–24

Coles, J. and Jones, K. (2009) 'Universal precautions': Perinatal touch and examination after childhood sexual abuse', *Birth*, Vol. 26, pp. 230–6

Compas, B. E. (2006) 'Psychobiological processes of stress and coping: Implications for resilience in childhood and adolescence', *Annals of the New York Academy of Sciences*, Vol. 1,094, pp. 226–34; doi:10.1196/annals.1376.024

Condon, J. (1993) 'The assessment of antenatal emotional attachment: Development of a questionnaire instrument', *British Journal of Medical Psychology*, Vol. 66, pp. 167–83

Conger, R. D., Schofield, T. J., Neppl, T. K. and Merrick, M. T. (2013) 'Disrupting intergenerational continuity in harsh and abusive parenting: The importance of a nurturing relationship with a romantic partner', *Journal of Adolescent Health*, Vol. 53, No. 4, Supplement, pp. S11–S17; doi:10.1016/j.jadohealth.2013.03.014

Coster, D., Brookes, H. and Sanger, C. (2015) *Evaluation of the Baby Steps Programme: Pre- and Post-Measures Study*, London: NSPCC. Available from URL: http://www.nspcc.org.uk/globalassets/documents/research-reports/baby-steps-evaluation-pre-post-measures-study.pdf (accessed 11 June 2015)

Courtois, C. A. and Riley, C. C. (1992) 'Pregnancy and childbirth as triggers for abuse memories: Implications for care', *Birth*, Vol. 19, No. 4, pp. 222–3; doi:10.1111/j.1523–536X.1992.tb00408.x

Curran, G. M., Bauer, M., Mittman, B., Pyne, J. M. and Stetler, C. (2012) 'Effectiveness-implementation hybrid designs', *Annals of Health Service Research*, Vol. 50, No. 3, pp. 217–26

Cuthbert, C., Rayns, G. and Stanley, K. (2011) *All Babies Count: Prevention and Protection for Vulnerable Babies*, London: NSPCC. Available from URL: http://cslp.psu-tests.co.uk/userfiles/documents/resources/fellows/Kate_Stanley/NSPCC-All-babies-count-research.pdf (accessed 20 April 2015)

Czarnocka, J. and Slade, P. (2000) 'Prevalence and predictors of post-traumatic stress symptoms following childbirth', *British Journal of Clinical Psychology*, Vol. 29, No. 1, pp. 31–51; doi:10.1348/014466500163095

Davies, Professor Dame Sally (2013) *Chief Medical Officer's Annual Report*, London: Department of Health. Available from URL: www.gov.uk/government/uploads/system/uploads/attachment_data/file/413196/CMO_web_doc.pdf (accessed 20 April 2015)

Davis-Floyd, R. (2004) *Birth as an American Rite of Passage*, Oakland, CA: University of California Press

Dawe, S. and Harnett, P. H. (2007) 'Improving family functioning in methadone maintained families: Results from a randomised controlled trial', *Journal of Substance Abuse Treatment*, Vol. 32, pp. 381–90

Department for Education (2012) 'Table D6 in main table: Characteristics of children in need in England', 2011–12 (Excel), London: Department for Education

Deutsch, H. (1945) *The Psychology of Women: A Psychoanalytic Interpretation*, New York: Grune & Stratton

Diego, M.A., Field, T. and Hernandez-Reif, M. (2014) 'Pre-term infant weight gain is increased by massage therapy and exercise by different underlying mechanisms', *Early Human Development*, Vol. 90, No. 3, pp. 137–41; doi:10.1016/j.earlhumdev.2014.01.009

Dixon, L., Browne, K. and Hamilton-Giachritsis, C. (2009) 'Patterns of risk and protective factors in the intergenerational cycle of maltreatment', *Journal of Family Violence*, Vol. 24, No. 2, pp. 111–22; doi:10.1007/s10896-008-9215-2

Duncan, L. G., Coatsworth, D. and Greenberg, M. T. (2009) 'A model of mindful parenting: Implications for parent-child relationships and prevention research', *Clinical Child and Family Psychology Review*, Vol. 12, No. 3, pp. 255–70; doi:10.1007/s10567-009-0046-3

Einarson, A., Selby, P. and Koren, G. (2001) 'Abrupt discontinuation of psychotropic drugs during pregnancy: Fear of teratogenic risk and impact of counselling', *Journal of Psychiatry and Neuroscience*, Vol. 6, No. 1, pp. 44–9; PMCID: PMC1408034

Elliott, D. M., Mok, D. S. and Briere, J. (2004) 'Adult sexual assault: Prevalence, symptomatology, and sex differences in the general population', *Journal of Traumatic Stress*, Vol. 17, No. 3, pp. 203–11; doi:10.1023/B:JOTS.0000029263.11104.23

Engelhard, I. M., van den Hout, M. A. and Arntz, A. (2001) 'Post-traumatic stress disorder after pregnancy loss', *General Hospital Psychiatry*, Vol. 23, No. 2, pp. 62–6; doi:10.1016/S0163-8343(01)00124-4

Ertem, I. O., Leventhal, J. M. and Dobbs, S. (2000) 'Intergenerational continuity of child physical abuse: How good is the evidence?', *The Lancet*, Vol. 356, No. 9232, pp. 814–19; doi:10.1016/S0140-6736(00)02656-8

Fearon, P., Murray, L., Fonagy, P., Longhi, E. and MacKenzie, K. (2014) 'Minding the baby' (online). Available from URL: http://annafreud.org/training-research/research/understanding-mental-health-and-resilience/minding-the-baby (accessed 17 April 2015)

Feder, G. S., Hutson, M., Ramsay, J. and Taket, A. R. (2006) 'Women exposed to intimate partner violence: Expectations and experiences when they encounter health care professionals: A meta-analysis of qualitative studies', *Archives of Internal Medicine*, Vol. 166, No. 1, pp. 22–37; doi:10.1001/archinte.166.1.22

Feder, G., Wathen, C. N. and MacMillan, H. L. (2013) 'An evidence-based response to intimate partner violence: WHO guidelines', *JAMA*, Vol. 310, No. 5, pp. 479–80; doi:10.1001/jama.2013.167453

Feeley, N., Zelkowitz, P., Cormier, C., Charbonneau, L., Lacroix, A. and Papageorgiou, A. (2011) 'Post-traumatic stress among mothers of very low birthweight infants at 6 months after discharge from the neonatal intensive care unit', *Applied Nursing Research*, Vol. 24, No. 2, pp. 114–17; doi:10.1016/j.apnr.2009.04.004

Felitti, V. J., Anda, R. F., Nordenberg, D., Williamson, D. F., Spitz, A. M., Edwards, V., Koss, M. and Marks, J. S. (1998) 'Relationship of childhood abuse and household dysfunction to many of the leading causes of death in adults: The Adverse Childhood Experiences (ACE) Study', *American*

Journal of Preventive Medicine, Vol. 14, No. 4, pp. 245–58; doi:10.1016/S0749-3797(98)00017-8

Finkelhor, D., Hotaling, G., Lewis, I. and Smith, C. (1990) 'Sexual abuse in a national survey of adult men and women: Prevalence, characteristics, and risk factors', *Child Abuse & Neglect*, Vol. 14, No. 1, pp. 19–28; doi:10.1016/0145-2134(90)90077-7

Finkelhor, D., Shattuck, A., Turner, H. A. and Hamby, S. L. (2014) 'The lifetime prevalence of child sexual abuse and sexual assault assessed in late adolescence', *Journal of Adolescent Health*, Vol. 55, No. 3, pp. 329–33; doi:10.1016/j.jadohealth.2013.12.026

Fisher, J. R., Wynter, K. H. and Rowe, H. J. (2010) 'Innovative psycho-educational program to prevent common postpartum mental disorders in primiparous women: A before and after controlled study', *BMC Public Health*, Vol. 10, p. 432

Fisher, J. R. W., Feekery, C. J. and Rowe-Murray, H. J. (2002) 'Nature, severity and correlates of psychological distress in women admitted to a private mother-baby unit', *Journal of Paediatrics and Child Health*, Vol. 38, pp. 140–5

Fisher, J., Feekery, C. and Rowe, H. (2011) 'Psychoeducational early parenting interventions to promote infant mental health', in Fitzgerald, H., Puura, K., Tomlinson, M. and Paul, C. (eds), *International Perspectives on Children and Mental Health: Prevention and Treatment,* Santa Barbara, CA: ABC-CLIO, Vol. 2, pp. 205–36

Fisher, J. R. W., Herrman, H., Cabral de Mello, M. and Chandra, P. (2014) 'Women's mental health', in Patel, V., Prince, M., Cohen, A. and Minas, H. (eds), *Global Mental Health: Principles and Practice*, New York, NY: Oxford University Press, pp. 354–84

Fisher, J. R. W., Cabral de Mello, M, and Isutzu, T. (2009) *Pregnancy, Childbirth and the Postpartum Year: Mental Health Aspects of Women's Reproductive Health: A Global Review of the Literature*, Geneva: World Health Organization and United Nations Population Fund, pp. 8–43

Fixsen, D. L., Blase, K. A., Naoom, S. F. and Wallace, F. (2009) 'Core implementation components', *Research on Social Work Practice*, Vol. 19, pp. 531–40; doi:10.1177/1049731509335549

Foa, E. B., Steketee, G. and Rothbaum, B. O. (1989) 'Behavioral/cognitive conceptualizations of post-traumatic stress disorder', *Behavior Therapy*, Vol. 20, No. 2, pp. 155–76; doi:10.1016/S0005-7894(89)80067-X

Ford, J. D. (2013) 'How can self-regulation enhance our understanding of trauma and dissociation?', *Journal of Trauma & Dissociation*, Vol. 14, pp. 237–50; doi:10.1080/15299732.2013.769398

Fraiberg, S. (1980) *The Motherhood Constellation*, London: Karnac Books

Fraiberg, S., Adelson, E. and Shapiro, V. (1975) 'Ghosts in the nursery: A psychoanalytic approach to the problems of impaired infant-mother relationships', *Journal of American Academy of Child Psychiatry*, Vol. 14, No. 3, pp. 387–421; doi:10.1016/S0002-7138(09)61442-4

Freyd, J. (1998) *Betrayal Trauma: Logic of Forgetting Childhood Abuse*, Cambridge, MA: Harvard University Press

Geary, D. C. (2002) 'Sexual selection and human life history', *Advances in Child Development and Behavior*, Vol. 30, pp. 41–101

Gelles, R. J. and Perlman, S. (2012) *Estimated Annual Cost of Child Abuse and Neglect*, Chicago: Prevent Abuse America. Available from URL: www.preventchildabusenc.org/assets/preventchildabusenc/files/cms/100/1299. pdf (accessed 16 April 2015)

Gil-González, D., Vives-Cases, C., Ruiz, M. T., Carrasco-Portiño, M. and Álvarez-Dardet, C. (2008) 'Childhood experiences of violence in perpetrators as a risk factor of intimate partner violence: A systematic review', *Journal of Public Health*, Vol. 30, No. 1, pp. 14–22; doi:10.1093/pubmed/fdm071

Glover, V. (2011) 'Annual research review: Prenatal stress and the origins of psychopathology: An evolutionary perspective', *Journal of Child Psychology and Psychiatry*, Vol. 52, pp. 356–67; doi:10.1111/j.1469-7610.2011.02371.x

Gluckman, P. D. and Hanson, M. A. (2004) 'The developmental origins of the metabolic syndrome', *Trends in Endocrinology & Metabolism*, Vol. 15, No. 4, pp. 183–7; doi:10.1016/j.tem.2004.03.002

Green, N. S., Damus, K., Simpson, J. L., Iams, J., Reece, E. A., Hobel, C. J., Merkatz, I. R., Greene, M. F., Schwarz, R. H. and the March of Dimes Scientific Advisory Committee on Prematurity (2005) 'Research agenda for preterm birth: Recommendations from the March of Dimes', *American Journal of Obstetrics and Gynecology*, Vol. 193, pp. 626–35; doi:10.1016/j.ajog.2005.02.106

Grekin, R. and O'Hara, M. W. (2014) 'Prevalence and risk factors of postpartum post-traumatic stress disorder: A meta-analysis', *Clinical Psychology Review*, Vol. 34, No. 5, pp. 389–401; doi:10.1016/j.cpr.2014.05.003

Hamama, L., Rauch, S. A., Sperlich, M., Defever, E. and Seng, J. S. (2010) 'Previous experience of spontaneous or elective abortion and risk for post-traumatic stress and depression during subsequent pregnancy', *Depression and Anxiety*, Vol. 27, No. 8, pp. 699–707; doi:10.1002/da.20714

Harris, R. and Ayers, S. (2012) 'What makes labour and birth traumatic? A survey of intrapartum "hotspots" ', *Psychology & Health*, Vol. 27, No. 10, pp. 1166–77; doi:10.1080/08870446.2011.649755

Hegarty, K., O'Docherty, L., Taft, A., Chondros, P., Brown, S., Valpied, J., Astbury, J., Taket, A., Gold, L., Feder, G. and Gunn, J. (2015) 'Screening and counselling in the primary care setting for women who have experienced intimate partner violence (WEAVE): A cluster randomised controlled trial', *The Lancet*, Vol. 382, No. 9888, pp. 249–58

Heim, C. and Binder, E. B. (2012) 'Current research trends in early life stress and depression: Review of human studies on sensitive periods, gene-environment interactions, and epigenetics', *Experimental Neurology*, Vol. 233, No. 1, pp. 102–11; doi:10.1016/j.expneurol.2011.10.032

Henschel, S., de Bruin, M. and Möhler, E. (2014) 'Self-control and child abuse potential in mothers with an abuse history and their preschool children', *Journal of Child and Family Studies*, Vol. 23, No. 5, pp. 824–36; doi:10.1007/s10826-013-9735-0

Herman, J. (1992) *Trauma and Recovery: The Aftermath of Violence-from*

Domestic Abuse to Political Terror, New York, NY: Basic Books

Hetzel, M. D. and McCanne, T. R. (2005) 'The roles of peritraumatic dissociation, child physical abuse, and child sexual abuse in the development
of post-traumatic stress disorder and adult victimization', *Child Abuse &
Neglect*, Vol. 29, No. 8, pp. 915–30; doi:10.1016/j.chiabu.2004.11.008

Hobbins, D. (2004) 'Survivors of childhood sexual abuse: Implications for
perinatal nursing care', *Journal of Obstetric, Gynecologic, & Neonatal Nursing*, Vol. 33, No. 4, pp. 485–97; doi:10.1177/0884217504266908

Holmes, M. M., Resnick, H. S., Kilpatrick, D. G. and Best, C. L. (1996)
'Rape-related pregnancy: Estimates and descriptive characteristics from a
national sample of women', *American Journal of Obstetrics and Gynecology*, Vol. 175, No. 2, pp. 320–5; doi:10.1016/S0002–9378(96)70141–2

Horan, D. L., Hill, L. D. and Schulkin, J. (2000) 'Childhood sexual abuse and
preterm labor in adulthood: An endocrinological hypothesis', *Women's
Health Issues: Official Publication of the Jacobs Institute of Women's Health*,
Vol. 10, No. 1, pp. 27–33; doi:10.1016/S1049–3867(99)00038–9

Horan, D. L., Klein, L., Schimdt, L. A. and Schulkin, J. (1998) 'Domestic
violence screening practices of obstetrician-gynecologists', *Obstetrics &
Gynecology*, Vol. 92, No. 5, pp. 785–9

Hornik-Lurie, T., Lerner, Y., Zilber, N., Feinson, M. C. and Cwikel, J. G.
(2014) 'Physicians' influence on primary care patients' reluctance to use
mental health treatment', *Psychiatric Services*, Vol. 65, No. 4, pp. 541–5;
doi:10.1176/appi.ps.201300064

Jackson, K. B. and Fraser, D. (2009) 'A study exploring UK midwives' knowledge and attitudes towards caring for women who have been sexually
abused', *Midwifery*, Vol. 25, No. 3, pp. 253–63

Jaffee, S. R., Bowes, L., Ouellet-Morin, I., Fisher, H. L., Moffitt, T. E., Merrick, M. T. and Arseneault, L. (2013) 'Safe, stable, nurturing relationships
break the intergenerational cycle of abuse: A prospective nationally
representative cohort of children in the United Kingdom', *Journal of
Adolescent Health*, Vol. 53, No. 4, Supplement, pp. S4–S10; doi:10.1016/j.
jadohealth.2013.04.007

Josephs, L. (1996) 'Women and trauma: A contemporary psychodynamic
approach to traumatization for patients in the OB/GYN psychological consultation clinic', *Bulletin of The Menninger Clinic*, Vol. 60, No. 1, pp. 22–38;
PMID:8742670

Kessler, R. C., Sonnega, A., Bromet, E., Hughes, M. and Nelson, C. B. (1995)
'Post-traumatic stress disorder in the National Comorbidity Survey',
Archives of General Psychiatry, Vol. 52, No. 12, pp. 1048–60; doi:10.1001/
archpsyc.1995.03950240066012

Kim, H. G., Harrison, P. A., Godecker, A. L. and Muzyka, C. N. (2014) 'Post-
traumatic stress disorder among women receiving prenatal care at three
Federally Qualified Health Care centers', *Maternal and Child Health Journal*, Vol. 18, No. 5, pp. 1056–65; doi:10.1007/s10995–013–1333–7

King, A. P., Erickson, T. M., Giardino, N. D., Favorite, T., Rauch, S. A. M.,
Robinson, E., Kulkarni, M. and Liberzon, I. (2013), 'A pilot study of group
mindfulness-based cognitive therapy (MBCT) for combat veterans with

posttraumatic stress disorder (PTSD)', *Depress Anxiety*, Vol. 30, No. 7, pp. 638–45; doi:10.1002/da.22104

King, A. P., Leichtman, J. N., Abelson, J. L., Liberzon, I. and Seng, J. S. (2008) 'Ecological salivary cortisol analysis – Part 2: Relative impact of trauma history, posttraumatic stress, comorbidity, chronic stress, and known confounds on hormone levels', *Journal of the American Psychiatric Nurses Association*, Vol. 14, No. 4, pp. 285–96; doi:10.1177/1078390308321939

Kitzinger, C. and Kitzinger, S. (2007) 'Birth trauma: Talking with women and the value of conversation analysis', *British Journal of Midwifery*, Vol. 15, No. 5, pp. 256–64; doi:10.12968/bjom.2007.15.5.23397

Koenen, K. C., Nugent, N. R. and Arnstadter, A. B. (2008) 'Gene-environment interaction in post-traumatic stress disorder', *European Archives of Psychiatry and Clinical Neuroscience*, Vol. 258, No. 2, pp. 82–96; doi:10.1007/s00406–007–0787–2

Koss, M. P. (1985) 'The hidden rape victim: Personality, attitudinal, and situational characteristics', *Psychology of Women Quarterly*, Vol. 9, No. 2, pp. 193–212; doi:10.1111/j.1471–6402.1985.tb00872.x

Kruse, J. A., Low, L. K. and Seng, J. S. (2013) 'Validation of alternative indicators of social support in perinatal outcomes research using quality of the partner relationship', *Journal of Advanced Nursing*, Vol. 69, No. 7, pp. 1562–73; doi:10.1111/jan.12015

Kruse, J. A., Williams, R. A. and Seng, J. S. (2014) 'Considering a relational model for depression in women with postpartum depression', *International Journal of Childbirth*, Vol. 4, No. 3, pp. 151–68; doi:10.1891/2156–5287.4.3.151

Kuiper, R. A. and Pesut, D. J. (2004) 'Promoting cognitive and metacognitive reflective reasoning skills in nursing practice: Self-regulated learning theory', *Journal of Advanced Nursing*, Vol. 45, No. 4, pp. 381–91; PMID: 14756832

Lee, D. (2012) *The Compassionate Mind Approach to Recovering from Trauma Using Compassion Focused Therapy*, London: Constable & Robinson

Leinweber, J. and Rowe, H. J. (2010) 'The costs of "being with the woman": Secondary traumatic stress in midwifery', *Midwifery*, Vol. 26, No. 1, pp. 76–87; doi:10.1016/j.midw.2008.04.003

LePlatte, D., Rosenblum, K. L., Stanton, E., Miller, N. and Muzik, M. (2012) 'Mental health in primary care for adolescent parents', *Mental Health in Family Medicine*, Vol. 9, No. 1, pp. 39–45; PMCID: PMC3487608

Linehan, S. (1992) 'Giving birth the "White Man's Way" ', *Health Sharing*, Vol. 13, pp. 11–15

Liotti, G. (2004) 'Trauma, dissociation, and disorganized attachment: Three strands of a single braid', *Psychotherapy: Theory, Research, Practice, and Training*, Vol. 41, No. 4, pp. 472–86; doi:10.1037/0033–3204.41.4.472

Lopez, W. D., Konrath, S. H. and Seng, J. S. (2011) 'Abuse-related posttraumatic stress, coping, and tobacco use in pregnancy', *Journal of Obstetric, Gynecologic, & Neonatal Nursing*, Vol. 40, No. 4, pp. 422–31; doi:10.1111/j.1552–6909.2011.01261.x

Lopez, W. D. and Seng, J. S. (2014) 'Post-traumatic stress disorder, smoking, and cortisol in a community sample of pregnant women', *Addictive Behaviors*, Vol. 39, No. 10, pp. 1408–13; doi:10.1016/j.addbeh.2014.04.027

Loveland Cook, C. A., Flick, L. H., Homan, S. M., Campbell, C., McSweeney, M. and Gallagher, M. E. (2004) 'Post-traumatic stress disorder in pregnancy: Prevalence, risk factors, and treatment', *Obstetrics & Gynecology*, Vol. 103, No. 4, pp. 710–17; doi:10.1097/01. AOG.0000119222.40241.fb

Maniglio, R. (2009) 'The impact of child sexual abuse on health: A systematic review of reviews', *Clinical Psychology Review*, Vol. 29, pp. 647–57; doi:10.1016/j.cpr.2009.08.003

Martin, J. A., Osterman, M. J. K. and Sutton, P. D. (2010) 'Are preterm births on the decline in the United States? Recent data from the National Vital Statistics system', *NCHS Data Brief No. 39*. Available from URL: www.cdc. gov/nchs/data/databriefs/db39.pdf (accessed 16 April 2015)

Meaney, M. J. (2001) 'Maternal care, gene expression, and the transmission of individual differences in stress reactivity across generations', *Annual Review of Neuroscience*, Vol. 24, pp. 1161–92; doi:10.1146/annurev. neuro.24.1.1161

Messman-Moore, T. L. and Long, P. J. (2003) 'The role of childhood sexual abuse sequelae in the sexual revictimization of women: An empirical review and theoretical reformulation', *Clinical Psychology Review*, Vol. 23, No. 4, pp. 537–71; doi:10.1016/S0272-7358(02)00203-9

Modell, A. H. (1978) 'The conceptualization of the therapeutic action of psychoanalysis: The action of the hold environment', *Bulletin of the Menninger Clinic*, Vol. 42, No. 6, pp. 493–504

Montgomery, E. (2013) 'Feeling safe: A metasynthesis of the maternity care needs of women who were sexually abused in childhood', *Birth*, Vol. 40, No. 2, pp. 88–95; doi:10.1111/birt.12043

Montgomery, E., Pope, C. and Rogers, J. (2015) 'A feminist narrative study of the maternity care experiences of women who were sexually abused in childhood', *Midwifery*, Vol. 31, No. 1, pp. 54–60; doi:10.1016/j. midw.2014.05.010

Morland, L., Goebert, D., Onoye, J., Frattarelli, L., Derauf, C., Herbst, M., Matsu, C. and Friedman, M. (2007) 'Post-traumatic stress disorder and pregnancy health: Preliminary update and implications', *Psychosomatics*, Vol. 48, No. 4, pp. 304–8; doi:10.1176/appi.psy.48.4.304

Moyer, V. A. (2013) 'Screening for intimate partner violence and abuse of elderly and vulnerable adults: US Preventive Services Task Force recommendation statement', *Annals of Internal Medicine*, Vol. 158, No. 6, pp. 478–86; doi:10.7326/0003-4819-158-6-201303190-00588

Muzik, M., Hamilton, S., Rosenblum, K. L., Waxler, E. and Hadi, Z. (2012) 'Mindfulness yoga during pregnancy for psychiatrically at-risk women: Preliminary results from a pilot feasibility study', *Complementary Therapies in Clinical Practice*, Vol. 18, No. 4, pp. 235–40; doi:10.1016/j. ctcp.2012.06.006

Muzik, M., Rosenblum, K. L., Alfafara, E. A., Schuster, M. M., Miller, N. M., Waddell, R. M. and Kohler, E. S. (2015) 'Mom Power: Preliminary outcomes of a group intervention to improve mental health and parenting among high risk mothers', *Archives of Women's Mental Health*, epub ahead-of-print; doi:10.1007/s00737–014–0490-z

Nesse, R. M. and Stearns, S. C. (2008) 'The great opportunity: Evolutionary applications to medicine and public health', *Evolutionary Applications*, Vol. 1, pp. 28–48; doi:10.1111/j.1752–4571.2007.00006.x

Neuberg, M., Pawlosek, W., Lopuszanski, M. and Neuberg, K. (1998) 'The analysis of the course of pregnancy, delivery and postpartum among women touched by flood disaster in Kotlin Klodzki in July 1997', *Ginekologia Polska*, Vol. 69, No. 12, pp. 866–70; PMID:10224743

Newcomb, M. D. and Locke, T. F. (2001) 'Intergenerational cycle of maltreatment: A popular concept obscured by methodological limitations', *Child Abuse & Neglect*, Vol. 25, No. 9, pp. 1219–40; doi:10.1016/S0145–2134(01)00267–8

NICE (2014) 'Pregnancy and complex social factors overview' (online). Available from URL: http://pathways.nice.org.uk/pathways/pregnancy-and-complex-social-factors (accessed 16 April 2015)

NSPCC (2013). 'Specialist mental health midwives: What they do and why they matter' (online). Available from URL: www.baspcan.org.uk/files/MMHA%20SMHMs%20Report.pdf (accessed 16 June 2015)

O'Hara, M. W., Stuart, S., Gorman, L. L. and Wenzel, A. (2000). 'Efficacy of interpersonal psychotherapy for postpartum depression', *Archives of General Psychiatry*, Vol. 57, No. 11, pp. 1039–45; doi:10.1001/archpsyc.57.11.1039

Olds, D. L. (2006) 'The Nurse-Family Partnership: An evidence-based preventive intervention', *Infant Mental Health Journal*, Vol. 27, No. 2, pp. 5–25; doi:10.1002/imhj.20077

Olds, D. L., Kitzman, H. K., Knudtson, M. D., Anson, R., Smith, J. A. and Cole, R. (2014) 'Effect of a home visiting program on maternal and child mortality: Results of a 2-decade follow-up of a randomized clinical trial', *JAMA Pediatrics*, Vol. 168, No. 9, pp. 800–6; doi:10.1001/jamapediatrics.2014.472

Palladino, C. L., Singh, V., Campbell, J., Flynn, H. and Gold, K. (2011) 'Homicide and suicide during the perinatal period: Findings from the national violent death reporting system', *Obstetrics and Gynecology*, Vol. 118, No. 5, p. 1056; doi:10.1097/AOG.0b013e31823294da

Pearlman, L. A. and Saakvitne, K. W. (2013) 'Treating therapists with vicarious traumatization and secondary traumatic stress disorders', in Figley, C. R. (ed.) *Compassion Fatigue: Coping with Traumatic Stress Disorder in Those Who Treat the Traumatized*, London: Routledge, pp. 150–5

Petzoldt, J., Wittchen, H-U., Wittich, J., Einsle, F., Höfler, M. and Martini, J. (2014). Maternal anxiety disorders predict excessive infant crying: A prospective longitudinal study, *Archives of Disease in Childhood*, Vol. 99, pp. 800–6; doi:10.1136/archdischild-2013–305562

Pietrzak, R. H., Goldstein, R. B., Southwick, S. M. and Grant, B. F. (2011) 'Prevalence and Axis I comorbidity of full and partial post-traumatic stress disorder in the United States: Results from wave 2 of the National

Epidemiologic Survey on alcohol and related conditions', *Journal of Anxiety Disorders*, Vol. 25, pp. 456–65; doi:10.1016/j.janxdis.2010.11.010

Powell, B., Cooper, G., Hoffman, K. and Marvin, B. (2014) *The Circle of Security Intervention: Enhancing Attachment in Early Parent–Child Relationships*, New York, NY: Guilford Press

Reagan, P. B. and Salsberry, P. J. (2005) 'Race and ethnic differences in determinants of preterm birth in the USA: Broadening the social context', *Social Science & Medicine*, Vol. 60, No. 10, pp. 2217–2228; doi:10.1016/j.socscimed.2004.10.010

Reijman, S., Alink, L. R. A., Compier-de Block, L. H. C. G., Werner, C. D., Maras, A., Rijnberk, C., van IJzendoorn, M. H. and Bakermans-Kranenburg, M. J. (2014). 'Autonomic reactivity to infant crying in maltreating mothers', *Child Maltreatment*, Vol. 19, No. 2, pp. 101–12; doi:10.1177/1077559514391115

Renfrew, M. J., Homer, C. S. E., Downe, S., McFadden, A., Muir, N., Prentice, T. and Hoope-Bender, P. (2014) 'Midwifery: An executive summary for *The Lancet*'s series', *The Lancet*. Available from URL: http://www.thelancet.com/pb/assets/raw/Lancet/stories/series/midwifery/midwifery_exec_summ.pdf (accessed 16 April 2015)

Renshaw, J. and Wrigley, Z. (2015) 'Service evaluation of the Compassionate Minds module of the Family Nurse Partnership programme' (online), Darlington Social Research. Available from URL: http://dartington.org.uk/wp-content/uploads/2015/02/Compassionate-minds-service-evaluation-final-report-2015.pdf (accessed 11 June 2015)

Resnick, H. S., Kilpatrick, D. G., Dansky, B. S., Saunders, B. E. and Best, C. L. (1993) 'Prevalence of civilian trauma and post-traumatic stress disorder in a representative national sample of women', *Journal of Consulting and Clinical Psychology*, Vol. 61, No. 6, pp. 984–91; doi:10.1037/0022–006X.61.6.984

Reynolds, R. M. (2013) 'Glucocorticoid excess and the developmental origins of disease: Two decades of testing the hypothesis', *Psychoneuroendocrinology*, Vol. 38, No. 1, pp. 1–11; doi:10.1016/j.psyneuen.2012.08.012

Rhodes, N. and Hutchinson, S. (1994) 'Labor experiences of childhood sexual abuse survivors', *Birth*, Vol. 21, No. 4, pp. 213–20; doi:10.1111/j.1523–536X.1994.tb00532.x

Rice, M. (2011) 'Evidence-based practice principles: Using the highest evidence when evidence is limited', *Journal of the American Psychiatric Nurses Association*, Vol. 17, No. 6, pp. 445–8; doi:10.1177/1078390311426289

Robboy, J. and Anderson, K. G. (2011) 'Intergenerational child abuse and coping', *Journal of Interpersonal Violence*, Vol. 26, No. 17, pp. 3526–41; doi:10.1177/0886260511403758

Roberts, N. P., Kitchiner, N. J., Kenardy, J. and Bisson, J. I. (2009) 'Systematic review and meta-analysis of multiple-session early interventions following traumatic events', *American Journal of Psychiatry*, Vol. 166, No. 3, pp. 293–301. Available from URL: http://dx.doi.org/10.1176/appi.ajp.2008.08040590

Rodriguez, M. A., Heilemann, M. V., Fielder, E., Ang, A., Nevarez, F. and Mangione, C. M. (2008) 'Intimate partner violence, depression, and PTSD among pregnant Latina women', *Annals of Family Medicine*, Vol. 6, No. 1, pp. 44–52; doi:10.1370/afm.743

Roff, D. A. (1992) *The Evolution of Life Histories: Theory and Analysis*, New York, NY: Springer

Roman, L., Raffo, J. E. and Meghea, C. I. (2014) 'A statewide Medicaid enhanced prenatal care program: Impact on birth outcomes', *JAMA Pediatrics*, Vol. 168, No. 3, pp. 220–7; doi:10.1001/jamapediatrics.2013.4347

Rose, A. (1992) 'Effects of childhood sexual abuse on childbirth: One woman's story', *Birth*, Vol. 19, pp. 214–18; doi:10.1111/j.1523–536X.1992. tb00405.x

Rowe, H. and Fisher, J. (2010a) 'The contribution of Australian residential early parenting centres to comprehensive mental health care for mothers of infants: Evidence from a prospective study', *International Journal of Mental Health Systems*, Vol. 11, No. 4, p. 6; doi:10.1186/1752–4458–4–6

Rowe, H. and Fisher, J. (2010b) 'Development of a universal psycho-educational intervention to prevent common postpartum mental disorders in primiparous women: A multiple method approach', *BMC Public Health*, Vol. 18, No. 10, p. 499; doi:10.1186/1471–2458–10–499

Rowe, H., Sperlich, M., Cameron, H. and Seng, J. (2014) 'A quasi-experimental outcomes analysis of a psychoeducation intervention for pregnant women with abuse-related post-traumatic stress', *Journal of Obstetric, Gynecologic, & Neonatal Nursing*, Vol. 43, No. 2, pp. 282–93; doi:10.1111/1552–6909.12312

Ruscio, A. M., Ruscio, J. and Keane, T. M. (2002) 'The latent structure of post-traumatic stress disorder: A taxometric investigation of reactions to extreme stress', *Journal of Abnormal Psychology*, Vol. 111, pp. 290–301; doi:10.1037/0021–843X.111.2.290

Russell, D. E. (1983) 'The incidence and prevalence of intrafamilial and extrafamilial sexual abuse of female children', *Child Abuse & Neglect*, Vol. 7, No. 2, pp. 133–46; doi:10.1016/0145–2134(83)90065–0

Rutter, M., Giller, H. and Hagell, A. (1998) *Antisocial Behaviour by Young People*, New York, NY: Cambridge University Press

Saakvitne, K. W. (2002) 'Shared trauma: The therapist's increased vulnerability', *Psychoanalytic Dialogues: The International Journal of Relational Perspectives*, Vol. 12, No. 3, pp. 443–9; doi:10.1080/10481881209348678

Sadler, L. S., Slade, A., Close, N., Webb, D. L., Simpson, T., Fennie, K. and Mayes, L. C. (2013) 'Minding the baby: Enhancing reflectiveness to improve early health and relationship outcomes in an interdisciplinary home visiting program', *Infant Mental Health Journal*, Vol. 34, No. 5, pp. 391–405; doi:10.1002/imhj.21406

Sadler, L. S., Slade, A. and Mayes, L. C. (2006) 'Minding the baby: A mentalization-based parenting program', in Allen, J. G. and Fonagy, P. (eds), *Handbook of Mentalization-Based Treatment*, Wiley Online Library; doi:10.1002/9780470712986

Sampselle, C., Petersen, B. A., Murtland, T. C. and Oakley, D. J. (1992) 'Prevalence of abuse among pregnant women choosing certified midwives or physician providers', *Journal of Nurse Midwifery*, Vol. 37, pp. 425–8;

doi:10.1016/0091–2182(92)90131

Schechter, D. S., Coates, S. W., Kaminer, T. *et al.* (2008) 'Distorted maternal mental representations and atypical behavior in a clinical sample of violence-exposed mothers and their toddlers', *Journal of Trauma & Dissociation,* Vol. 9, N°o. 2, pp. 123–47; doi:10.1080/15299730802045666

Schnurr, P. P. and Green, B. L. (2004) *Trauma and Health: Physical Health Consequences of Exposure to Extreme Stress,* Washington, DC: American Psychological Association

Schore. A. H. (1997) 'Early organization of the nonlinear right brain and development of a predisposition to psychiatric disorders', *Development and Psychopathology,* Vol. 9, No. 4, pp. 595–631

Schore, A. H. (2003a) *Affect Dysregulation and Disorders of the Self,* New York, NY: Norton

Schore, A. H. (2003b) *Affect Regulation and Repair of the Self,* New York, NY: Norton

Sears, W. and Sears, M. (2003) *The Baby Book: Everything You Need to Know About Your Baby From Birth to Age Two,* New York: NY: Little, Brown, pp. 4–10

Seng, J. S., D'Andrea, W. and Ford, J. D. (2014) 'Complex mental health sequelae of psychological trauma among women in prenatal care', *Psychological Trauma,* Vol. 6, No. 1, pp. 41–9

Seng, J. S., King, A. P., Li. Y. X., Lee, H., Rowe, H., Sperlich, M., Muzik, M., Ronis, D., Ford, J.D. and Liberzon, I. (under review) 'Posttraumatic stress and dissociation effects on cortisol levels across pregnancy and postpartum'

Seng, J. S., Kohn-Wood, L. P., McPherson, M. D. and Sperlich, M. (2011a) 'Disparity in post-traumatic stress disorder diagnosis among African American pregnant women', *Archives of Women's Mental Health,* Vol. 14, No. 4, pp. 295–306; doi:10.1007/s00737–011–0218–2

Seng, J. S., Low, L. K., Sparbel, K. J. H. and Killion, C. (2004) 'Abuse-related post-traumatic stress during the childbearing year', *Journal of Advanced Nursing,* Vol. 46, No. 6, pp. 604–13; doi:10.1111/j.1365-2648.2004.03051.x

Seng, J. S., Low, L. K., Sperlich, M., Ronis, D. and Liberzon, I. (2009) 'Prevalence, trauma history, and risk for post-traumatic stress disorder among nulliparous women in maternity care', *Obstetrics and Gynecology,* Vol. 114, No. 4, pp. 839–47; doi:10.1097/AOG.0b013e3181b8f8a2

Seng, J. S., Low, L. K., Sperlich, M., Ronis, D. and Liberzon, I. (2011b) 'Posttraumatic stress disorder, child abuse history, birthweight and gestational age: A prospective cohort study', *British Journal of Obstetrics and Gynecology,* Vol. 118, No. 11, pp. 1329–39; doi:10.1111/j.1471–0528.2011.03071.x

Seng, J. S., Oakley, D. J., Sampselle, C. M., Killion, C., Graham-Bermann, S. and Liberzon, I. (2001) 'Association of post-traumatic stress disorder with pregnancy complications', *Obstetrics & Gynecology,* Vol. 97, pp. 17–22; doi:10.1016/S0029–7844(00)01097–8

Seng, J. S., Rauch, S. A., Resnick, H., Reed, C. D., King, A., Low, L. K. and Liberzon, I. (2010) 'Exploring posttraumatic stress disorder symptom profile among pregnant women', *Journal of Psychosomatic Obstetrics & Gynecology,* Vol. 31, No. 3, pp. 176–87; doi:10.3109/0167482X.2010.486453

Seng, J. S., Sperlich, M. and Low, L. K. (2008) 'Mental health, demographic, and risk behavior profiles of pregnant survivors of childhood and adult abuse', *Journal of Midwifery and Women's Health*, Vol. 53, No. 6, pp. 511–21; doi:10.1016/j.jmwh.2008.04.013

Seng, J., Sperlich, M., Low, L. K., Ronis, D., Muzik, M. and Liberzon, I. (2013) 'Childhood abuse history, post-traumatic stress disorder, post-partum mental health, and bonding: A prospective cohort study', *Journal of Midwifery and Women's Health*, Vol. 58, No. 1, pp. 57–68; doi:10.1111/j.1542-2011.2012.00237.x

Seng, J. S., Sperlich, M., Rowe, H., Cameron, H., Harris, A., Rauch, S. A. M. and Bell, S. A. (2011c) 'The survivor moms' companion: Open pilot of a post-traumatic stress specific psychoeducation program for pregnant survivors of childhood maltreatment and sexual trauma', *International Journal of Childbirth*, Vol. 1, pp. 111–21; doi:10.1891/2156-5287.1.2.111

Sethi, D., Bellis, M. A., Hughes, K., Gilbert, R., Mitis, F. and Galea, G. (2013) *European Report on Preventing Child Maltreatment*, Copenhagen: World Health Organization Regional Office for Europe

Shah, P. E., Fonagy, P. and Strathearn, L. (2010) 'Is attachment transmitted across generations? The plot thickens', *Clinical Child Psychology and Psychiatry*, Vol. 15, No. 3, pp. 329–45; doi:10.1177/1359104510365449

Shamian, J. (2014) 'Interprofessional collaboration, the only way to save every woman and every child', *The Lancet*, Vol. 384, No. 9948, pp. e41–2; doi:10.1016/S0140–6736(14)60858–8

Shaw, J. G., Asch, S. M., Kimerling, R., Frayne, S. M., Shaw, K. A. and Phibbs, C. S. (2014) 'Post-traumatic stress disorder and risk of spontaneous preterm birth', *Obstetrics & Gynecology*, Vol. 124, No. 6, pp. 1111–19; doi:10.1097/AOG.0000000000000542

Shedler, J. (2010) 'The efficacy of psychodynamic psychotherapy', *American Psychologist*, Vol. 65, No. 2, pp. 98–109; doi:10.1037/a0018378

Sher, L. (2005) 'The concept of post-traumatic mood disorder', *Medical Hypotheses*, Vol. 65, No. 2, pp. 205–10; doi:10.1016/j.mehy.2005.03.014

Shonkoff, J. P., Boyce, T. and McEwen, B. S. (2009) 'Neuroscience, molecular biology, and the childhood roots of health disparities: Building a new framework for health promotion and disease prevention', *JAMA*, Vol. 301, No. 21, pp. 2252–9; doi:10.1001/jama.2009.754

Shonkoff, J. P., Garner, A. S., Committee on Psychosocial Aspects of Child and Family Health, Committee on Early Childhood, Adoption, and Dependent care, and Section on Development and Behavioral Pediatrics (2012) 'The lifelong effects of early childhood adversity and toxic stress', *Pediatrics*, Vol. 129, No. 1, pp. e232–46; doi:10.1542/peds.2011-2663

Simkin, P. (1992) 'Overcoming the legacy of childhood sexual abuse: The role of caregivers and childbirth educators', *Birth*, Vol. 19, pp. 224–5; doi:10.1111/j.1523–536X.1992.tb00409.x

Simkin, P. (2011) 'Pain, suffering, and trauma in labor and prevention of subsequent posttraumatic stress disorder', *The Journal of Perinatal Education*, Vol. 20, No. 3, pp. 166–76; doi:10.1891/1058-1243.20.3.166

Skinner, K. M., Kressin, N., Frayne, S., Tripp, T. J., Hankin, C. S., Miller, D. R.

and Sullivan, L. M. (2000) 'The prevalence of military sexual assault among female Veterans' Administration outpatients', *Journal of Interpersonal Violence*, Vol. 15, No. 3, pp. 291–310; doi:10.1177/088626000015003005

Slade, A. (2005) 'Minding the baby: A reflective parenting programme', *The Psychoanalytic Study of the Child*, Vol. 60, pp. 74–100

Slade, A. (2006) 'Reflective parenting programs: Theory and development' (online). Available from URL: http://reflectiveparenting.org/wp-content/uploads/2011/06/Reflective_Parenting_Programs.pdf (accessed 16 April 2015)

Slade, P. (2006) 'Towards a conceptual framework for understanding post-traumatic stress symptoms following childbirth and implications for further research', *Journal of Psychosomatic Obstetrics and Gynaecology*, Vol. 27, No. 2, pp. 99–105; doi:10.1080/01674820600714582

Smith, C. C., and Fretwell, I. A. (1973) 'The optimal balance between size and number of offspring', *American Naturalist*, Vol. 108, pp. 499–508

Smith, K. (ed). (2011) *Homicides, Firearms Offences and Intimate Violence 2009/2010*, Vol. 2 (supplementary), Crime in England and Wales 2009/10, London: Home Office

Söderquist, J., Wijma, B., Thorbert, G. and Wijma, K. (2009) 'Risk factors in pregnancy for post-traumatic stress and depression after childbirth', *BJOG: An International Journal of Obstetrics & Gynaecology*, Vol. 116, No. 5, pp. 672–80; doi:10.1111/j.1471–0528.2008.02083.x

Söderquist, J., Wijma, K. and Wijma, B. (2004) 'Traumatic stress in late pregnancy', *Journal of Anxiety Disorders*, Vol. 18, No. 2, pp. 127–42; doi:10.1016/S0887–6185(02)00242–6

Sperlich, M. (1993–1994) 'Boundary waters: A series of articles on caring for sexually abused midwifery clients', *Michigan Midwives Association Newsletter*, reprinted in the *Above a Whisper Newsletter* in 1994

Sperlich, M. (2015) 'Trauma exposure, post-traumatic stress, and depression in a community sample of first-time mothers', Unpublished dissertation

Sperlich, M. and Seng, J. S. (2008) *Survivor Moms: Women's Stories of Birthing, Mothering and Healing After Sexual Abuse*, Eugene, OR: Motherbaby Press

Sperlich, M., Seng, J. S., Rowe, H., Cameron, H., Harris, A., McCracken, A., Rauch, S. A. M. and Bell, S. A. (2011) 'The survivor moms' companion: Feasibility, safety, and acceptability of a post-traumatic stress specific psychoeducation program for pregnant survivors of childhood maltreatment and sexual trauma', *International Journal of Childbirth*, Vol. 1, pp. 122–35; doi:10.1891/2156–5287.1.2.122

Spinazzola, J., Rhodes, A. M., Emerson, D., Earle, E. and Monroe, K. (2011) 'Application of yoga in residential treatment of traumatized youth', *Journal of the American Psychiatric Nurses Association*, Vol. 17, No. 6, pp. 431–44; doi:10.1177/1078390311418359

Stein, J. A., Leslie, M. B. and Nyamathi, A. (2002) 'Relative contributions of parent substance use and childhood maltreatment to chronic homelessness, depression, and substance abuse problems among homeless women: Mediating roles of self-esteem and abuse in adulthood', *Child Abuse &*

Neglect, Vol. 26, No. 10, pp. 1011–27; doi:10.1016/S0145–2134(02)00382–4

Stern, D. N. (1995) *The Motherhood Constellation: A Unified View of Parent–infant Psychotherapy*, London: Karnac Books

Taft, A., O'Doherty, L., Hegarty, K., Ramsay, J., Davidson, L. and Feder, G. (2013) 'Screening women for intimate partner violence in healthcare settings' (online), Cochrane Library. doi:10.1002/14651858.CD007007.pub2

Taylor, J. and Lazenbatt, A. (2015). *Child Maltreatment and High Risk Families*, Edinburgh: Dunedin Academic Press

Teicher, M. H., Andersen, S. L., Polcari, A., Anderson, C. M. and Navalta, C. P. (2002) 'Developmental neurobiology of childhood stress and trauma', *Psychiatric Clinics of North America*, Vol. 22, No. 2, pp. 397–426; PMID:12136507

Thornberry, T. P. and Henry, K. L. (2013) 'Intergenerational continuity in maltreatment', *Journal of Abnormal Child Psychology*, Vol. 41, No. 4, pp. 555–69; doi:10.1007/s10802-012-9697-5

Thornberry, T. P., Knight, K. E. and Lovegrove, P. J. (2012) 'Does maltreatment beget maltreatment? A systematic review of the intergenerational literature', *Trauma, Violence, & Abuse*, Vol. 13, No. 2, pp. 135–52; doi:10.1177/1524838012447697

UNICEF (2003) 'A league table of child maltreatment deaths in rich nations' (online). Available from URL: www.unicef-irc.org/publications/353 (accessed 20 April 2015)

Vagi, K. J., O'Malley Olsen, E., Basile, K. C. and Vivolo-Kantor, A. M. (2015) 'Teen dating violence (physical and sexual) among US high school students: Findings from the 2013 National Youth Risk Behavior Survey', *JAMA Pediatrics*, Vol. 169, No. 5, pp. 474–82; doi:10.1001/jamapediatrics.2014.3577

Wang, C. and Holton, J. (2007) *Total Estimated Cost of Child Abuse and Neglect in the United States*, Chicago: Prevent Abuse America; doi:10.1.1.192.2911

Weinberg, S. K. (1955) *Incest Behavior*, New York, NY: Citadel Press

Weinberg, S. K. (1976) *Incest Behavior 'Revised Edition'*, Secaucus, NJ: Citadel Press

Welshman, J. (2009) 'Where less angels might have feared to tread: The social science research council and transmitted deprivation', *Contemporary British History*, Vol. 23, No. 2, pp. 199–219; doi:10.1080/13619460802636425

White, A. (2014) 'Responding to prenatal disclosure of past sexual abuse', *Obstetrics and Gynecology*, Vol. 123, No. 6, pp. 1344–7; doi:10.1097/AOG.0000000000000266

WHO (1992) *The ICD-10 Classification of Mental and Behavioral Disorders: Clinical Descriptions and Guidelines*, Geneva: World Health Organization

WHO (2014) 'Child maltreatment' (online). Available from URL: www.who.int/mediacentre/factsheets/fs150/en (accessed 16 April 2015)

Widom, C. S. (1989) 'Child abuse, neglect, and adult behavior: Research design and findings on criminality, violence, and child abuse', *American Journal of Orthopsychiatry*, Vol. 59, No. 3, pp. 355–67; doi:10.1111/j.1939–0025.1989.tb01671.x

Williams, D. (2003) 'Pregnancy: A stress test for life', *Current Opinion in Obstetrics and Gynecology*, Vol. 15, No. 6, pp. 465–71

Winnicott, D. (1965) *The Maturational Process and the Facilitating Environment*, New York: International Universities Press

Wosu, A. C., Gelaye, B. and Williams, M. A. (2015) 'Child sexual abuse and post-traumatic stress disorder among pregnant and postpartum women: Review of the literature', *Archives of Women's Mental Health*, Vol. 18, No. 1, pp. 61–72

Wyatt, G. E. (1985) 'The sexual abuse of Afro-American and white-American women in childhood', *Child Abuse & Neglect*, Vol. 9, No. 4, pp. 507–19; doi:10.1016/0145–2134(85)90060–2

Yehuda, R., Engel, S. M., Brand, S. R., Seckl, J., Marcus, S. M. and Berkowitz, G. S. (2005) 'Transgenerational effects of post-traumatic stress disorder in babies of mothers exposed to the World Trade Center attacks during pregnancy', *Journal of Clinical Endocrinology & Metabolism*, Vol. 90, No. 7, pp. 4115–18; doi:10.1210/jc.2005–0550

Yehuda, R., Kahana, B., Schmeidler, J., Southwick, S. M., Wilson, S. and Giller, E. L. (1995) 'Impact of cumulative lifetime trauma and recent stress on current post-traumatic stress disorder symptoms in holocaust survivors', *American Journal of Psychiatry*, Vol. 152, No. 12, pp. 1815–18

Yonkers, K. A., Gotman, N., Smith, M. V., Forray, A., Belanger, K., Brunetto, W. L., Lin, H., Burkman, R. T., Zelop, C. M. and Lockwood, C. J. (2011) 'Does antidepressant use attenuate the risk of a major depressive episode in pregnancy?' *Epidemiology*, Vol. 22, No. 6, pp. 848–54; doi:10.1097/EDE.0b013e3182306847

Yonkers, K. A., Smith, M. V., Forray, A., Epperson, C. N., Costello, D., Lin, H. and Belanger, K. (2014) 'Pregnant women with post-traumatic stress disorder and risk of preterm birth', *JAMA Psychiatry*, Vol. 71, No. 8, pp. 897–904; doi:10.1001/jamapsychiatry.2014.558

Zeanah, C. H., Berlin, L. J. and Boris, N. W. (2011) 'Practitioner review: Clinical applications of attachment theory and research for infants and young children', *Journal of Child Psychology and Psychiatry*, Vol, 52, No. 8, pp. 819–33; doi:10.1111/j.1469–7610.2011.02399.x

INDEX

Note: page numbers in *italics* refer to figures or tables

16/04/2025

14658578-0001

BIOLOGICAL SLUDGE MINIMIZATION AND BIOMATERIALS/BIOENERGY RECOVERY TECHNOLOGIES

Edited by

ETIENNE PAUL
YU LIU

WILEY

A JOHN WILEY & SONS, INC., PUBLICATION

Published by John Wiley & Sons, Inc., Hoboken, New Jersey.
Published simultaneously in Canada.

For general information on our other products and services or for technical support, please contact
our Customer Care Department within the United States at (800) 762-2974, outside the United States
at (317) 572-3993 or fax (317) 572-4002.

Wiley also publishes its books in a variety of electronic formats. Some content that appears in print
may not be available in electronic formats. For more information about Wiley products, visit our
web site at www.wiley.com.

Library of Congress Cataloging-in-Publication Data:

Biological sludge minimization and biomaterials/bioenergy recovery technologies / edited by
Etienne Paul and Yu Liu.
    p. cm.
  Includes index.
  ISBN 978-0-470-76882-2 (cloth)
  1. Water treatment plant residuals—Purification. 2.   Waste products as fuel. 3.   Water—
Purification. 4.   Biochemical engineering. I. Paul, Etienne, 1964- II. Liu, Yu, 1964-
  TD899.W3B56 2012
  628.3—dc23

                                                                                    2011045240
Printed in the United States of America

10 9 8 7 6 5 4 3 2 1

CONTENTS

PREFACE

Activated sludge systems have been employed to treat a wide variety of wastewaters, and most municipal wastewater treatment plants use it as the core of the treatment process. The basic function of a biological treatment process is to convert organics to carbon dioxide, water, and bacterial cells. The cells can then be separated from the purified water and disposed of in a concentrated form called *excess sludge*. Assuming that activated sludge has a conversion growth yield efficiency of 0.3 to 0.5 mg dry weight per milligram of chemical oxygen demand (COD), 1 kg of COD removed will generate 0.3 to 0.5 kg of dry excess sludge. As a result, a large amount of sewage sludge is currently generated annually: around 10 million tons of dry solids in the European Union, and 8 million tons of dry solids in the United States in 2010. In China, due to improvements in wastewater treatment systems, sludge production is expected to increase radically and should have reached more than 11 million tons of dry solids in 2010. With the expansion of population and industry, the increased excess sludge production is generating a real global challenge. It should be realized that the excess sludge generated from the biological treatment process is a secondary solid waste that must be disposed of in a safe and cost-effective way. The ultimate disposal of excess sludge has been and continues to be one of the most expensive problems faced by wastewater utilities; for example, the treatment of the excess sludge may account for 25 to 65% of the total plant operation cost. So far, sludge production and disposal are entering a period of dramatic change, driven mainly by stringent environmental legislation. Sludge disposal to all the established outlets could become increasingly difficult or, in the case of sea disposal, will become illegal. Environmental pressures on sludge recycling to land may lead to restrictions on applications in terms of nitrogen content and more stringent limits for metals in soils.

At least four technical approaches have been seriously considered with respect to excess sludge handling: (1) conversion of excess sludge to value-added materials (e.g, construction materials and activated carbon); (2) recovery of useful resources from sludge (e.g., production of fuel by-products through sludge melting or sludge pyrolysis and extraction of useful chemicals from sludge (e.g. poly(hydroxyalkanoate)]; (3) reduction of sludge production from the wastewater treatment process rather than the post-treatment or disposal of the sludge generated; and (4) sludge incineration. In the past, sewage sludge was considered as a waste, today, it is treated as a misplaced resource. Reducing sludge production can be done through a variety of technologies targeting microbial growth yield or the biodegradability of the matter accumulated. In most cases, mechanisms behind these technologies have not been well understood, leading to limited full-scale applications. The waste-to-energy or waste-to-useful materials strategies have received extensive attention. Energy recovery from sewage sludge can be realized through anaerobic digestion for biogas production (e.g., methane or hydrogen), pyrolysis and gasification for generating syngas, and potentially, biochar or incineration with optimal drying for direct production of electricity. Production of bioplastics from sewage sludge using a mixed culture has attracted intensive research effort and indeed represents a new option for sludge-to-high value material. Therefore, in this book we provide up-to-date and comprehensive coverage of sludge reduction and valorization technologies which are important for sustainable development of the global wastewater industry.

The book is organized into 15 chapters. Chapter 1 provides a comprehensive review of the fundamentals of biological processes for wastewater treatment, covering wastewater microbiology, microbial metabolism, and biological processes that are the basis for better understanding of how excess sludge is produced. Chapter 2 is more focused on sludge production mechanisms and prediction. Prediction of primary sludge and waste activated sludge production is one of the major tasks and challenges in the design and operation of a wastewater treatment plant. Such prediction is based on detailed characterization of influent organic and inorganic components. Therefore, in Chapter 3, detailed characterization methods of wastewater and sludge are presented.

Technologies for sludge reduction are discussed in Chapters 4 to 8, with the primary focus on strategies to reduce microbial growth yield as well as to enhance sludge disintegration in various biological processes, such as the oxic-settling-anaerobic process for enhanced microbial decay (Chapter 4), the energy uncoupling-assisted activated sludge process (Chapter 5), the reduction of excess sludge production through ozonation and chlorination (Chapter 6), the high-dissolved-oxygen biological process for sludge reduction (Chapter 7), and membrane bioreactors as an alternative for minimizing excess sludge production (Chapter 8).

Microbial fuel cells for sustainable treatment of organic wastes and electrical energy recovery are discussed in Chapter 9. For decades, in-plant anaerobic digestion of sewage sludge has been employed for biogas recovery. Anaerobic digestion in terms of process fundamentals, design, and operation is discussed in detail in Chapter 10. During anaerobic digestion of sewage sludge, cell hydrolysis has been identified as a limiting step in the overall process. In Chapter 11 we look into mechanical pretreatment of sewage sludge for enhanced biological treatment, including ultrasonication, grinding, high-pressure homogenization, collision plate homogenization, and lysis centrifuging.

Thermal treatment of sludge has been used in main activated sludge treatment plants (sidestream treatment) or as a pretreatment in anaerobic sludge digestion. Chapter 12 covers the representative thermal treatment technologies that have been used successfully for the reduction of waste activated sludge as well as for enhanced conversion of sludge to biogas. Waste sludge conversion to energy can be realized through gasification, pyrolysis, and combustion of sewage sludge, as detailed in Chapter 13. In Chapter 14, aerobic granulation technology, a novel biological process for wastewater treatment, is discussed with a focus on its potential in sludge reduction. Chapter 15 offers an excellent overview and technical details regarding the production of biodegradable bioplastics from fermented sludge, wastes, and effluents.

The audience for the book includes scientists, engineers, graduate students, and everyone who has an interest in sludge reduction and valorization technologies.

We extend our gratitude to Ya-Juan Liu for her invaluable editorial assistance.

ETIENNE PAUL
YU LIU

CONTRIBUTORS

Damien J. Batstone, INRA, UR050, Advanced Water Management Centre, The University of Queensland, Brisbane St Lucia, Queensland, Australia

Yolaine Bessière, Université de Toulouse; INSA, UPS, INP; LISBP, Toulouse, France; INRA, UMR792, Ingénierie des Systèmes Biologiques et des Procédés, Toulouse, France; CNRS, UMR5504, Toulouse, France

Hélène Carrère, INRA, UR050, Laboratoire de Biotechnologie de l'Environnement, Narbonne, France

Bo Jiang, Division of Environmental and Water Resources Engineering, School of Civil and Environmental Engineering, Nanyang Technological University, Singapore

Duu-Jong Lee, Department of Chemical Engineering, National Taiwan University of Science and Technology, Taipei, Taiwan

Dominique Lefebvre, Université Paul Sabatier, Laboratoire de Biologie Appliquée à l'Agroalimentaire et à l'Environnement, Auch, France

Xavier Lefebvre, Université de Toulouse; INSA,UPS,INP; LISBP, 135 Avenue de Rangueil, F-31077 Toulouse, France; INRA, UMR792, Ingénierie des Systèmes Biologiques et des Procédés, F-31400 Toulouse, France; CNRS, UMR5504, F-31400 Toulouse, France

Qi-Shan Liu, School of Architecture and the Built Environment, Singapore Polytechnic, Singapore

Yong-Qiang Liu, Institute of Environmental Science and Engineering, Nanyang Technology University, Singapore

Yu Liu, Division of Environmental and Water Resources Engineering, School of Civil and Environmental Engineering, Nanyang Technological University, Singapore

Elisabeth Neuhauser, Université de Toulouse; INSA, UPS, INP; LISBP, 135 Avenue de Rangueil, F-31077 Toulouse, France; INRA, UMR792, Ingénierie des Systèmes Biologiques et des Procédés, F-31400 Toulouse, France; CNRS, UMR5504, F-31400 Toulouse, France

Bing-Jie Ni, Department of Chemistry, University of Science and Technology of China, Hefei, China

Etienne Paul, Université de Toulouse; INSA, UPS, INP; LISBP, 135 Avenue de Rangueil, F-31077 Toulouse, France; INRA, UMR792, Ingénierie des Systèmes Biologiques et des Procédés, F-31400 Toulouse, France; CNRS, UMR5504, F-31400, Toulouse, France

Nan-Qi Ren, State Key Laboratory of Urban Water Resource and Environment, School of Municipal and Environmental Engineering, Harbin Institute of Technology, Harbin, China

Kuan-Yeow Show, Department of Environmental Engineering, Faculty of Engineering and Green Technology, University Tunku Abdul Rahman, Jalan University, Bandar Barat, Kampar, Perak, Malaysia

Mathieu Spérandio, Université de Toulouse; INSA, UPS, INP; LISBP, 135 Avenue de Rangueil, F-31077 Toulouse, France; INRA, UMR792, Ingénierie des Systèmes Biologiques et des Procédés, F-31400 Toulouse, France; CNRS, UMR5504, F-31400 Toulouse, France

Joo-Hwa Tay, Department of Environmental Science and Engineering, Fudan University, Shanghai, China

Jianfang Wang, School of Environmental Science and Engineering, Suzhou University of Science and Technology, Suzhou, China

Jianlong Wang, Laboratory of Environmental Technology, INET, Tsinghua University, Beijing, China

Zhi-Wu Wang, Bioscience Division, Oak Ridge National Laboratory, Oak Ridge, Tennessee

Philip Chuen-Yung Wong, Division of Environmental and Water Resources Engineering, School of Civil and Environmental Engineering, Nanyang Technological University, Singapore

Shi-Jie You, State Key Laboratory of Urban Water Resource and Environment, School of Municipal and Environmental Engineering, Harbin Institute of Technology, Harbin, China

Han-Qing Yu, Department of Chemistry, University of Science and Technology of China, Hefei, China

Qing-Liang Zhao, State Key Laboratory of Urban Water Resource and Environment, School of Municipal and Environmental Engineering, Harbin Institute of Technology, Harbin, China

1

FUNDAMENTALS OF BIOLOGICAL PROCESSES FOR WASTEWATER TREATMENT

JIANLONG WANG

Laboratory of Environmental Technology, INET, Tsinghua University, Beijing, China

1.1 INTRODUCTION

In this chapter we offer an overview of the fundamentals and applications of biological processes developed for wastewater treatment, including aerobic and anaerobic processes. Beginning here, readers may learn how biosolids are eventually produced during the biological treatment of wastewater. The fundamentals of biological treatment introduced in the first six sections of this chapter include (1) an overview of biological wastewater treatment, (2) the classification of microorganisms, (3) some important microorganisms in wastewater treatment, (4) measurement of microbial biomass, (5) microbial nutrition, and (6) microbial metabolism. Following the presentation of fundamentals, the remaining four sections introduce applications of biological wastewater treatment, including the functions of wastewater treatment, the activated sludge process, the suspended and attached-growth processes, and sludge production, treatment, and disposal. The topics covered include (1) aerobic biological oxidation, (2) biological nitrification and denitrification, (3) anaerobic biological oxidation, (4) biological phosphorus removal, (5) biological removal of toxic organic compounds and heavy metals, and (6) biological removal of pathogens and parasites.

Biological Sludge Minimization and Biomaterials/Bioenergy Recovery Technologies, First Edition.
Edited by Etienne Paul and Yu Liu.
© 2012 John Wiley & Sons, Inc. Published 2012 by John Wiley & Sons, Inc.

1.2 OVERVIEW OF BIOLOGICAL WASTEWATER TREATMENT

Biological treatment processes are the most important unit operations in wastewater treatment. Methods of purification in biological treatment units are similar to the self-purification process that occurs naturally in rivers and streams, and involve many of the same microorganisms. Removal of organic matter is carried out by heterotrophic microorganisms, which are predominately bacteria but also, occasionally, fungi. The microorganisms break down the organic matter by two distinct processes, biological oxidation and biosynthesis, both of which result in the removal of organic matter from wastewater. Oxidation or respiration results in the formation of mineralized end products that remain in wastewater and are discharged in the final effluent, while biosynthesis converts the colloidal and soluble organic matter into particulate biomass (new microbial cells) which can subsequently be separated from the treated liquid by gravity sedimentation because it has a specific gravity slightly greater than that of water.

The fundamental mechanisms involved in biological treatment are the same for all processes. Microorganisms, principally bacteria, utilize the organic and inorganic matter present in wastewater to support growth. A portion of materials is oxidized, and the energy released is used to convert the remaining materials into new cell tissue. The aim in this chapter will help students and technicians in environmental science and engineering to recognize the role that environmental microbiology plays in solving environmental problems. The principal purposes of this chapter are (1) to provide fundamental information on the microorganisms used to treat wastewater and (2) to introduce the application of biological process fundamentals for the biological treatment of wastewater.

1.2.1 The Objective of Biological Wastewater Treatment

From a chemical point of view, municipal wastewater or sewage contains (1) organic compounds, such as carbohydrates, proteins, and fats; (2) nitrogen, principally in the form of ammonia; and (3) phosphorus, which is principally in the form of phosphate from human waste and detergents. In addition, municipal wastewater contains many other types of particulate and dissolved matter, such as pathogens, plastics, sand, grit, live organisms, metals, anions, and cations. All these constituents have to be dealt with at wastewater treatment plants. However, not all of these are important for the modeling and design of a wastewater treatment plant. Usually, the carbonaceous, nitrogenous, and phosphorus constituents are mainly objects to be considered because they influence biological activity and eutrophication in the receiving water.

When municipal wastewater is discharged to a water body, the organic compounds will stimulate the growth of the heterotrophic organisms, causing a reduction in the dissolved oxygen. When oxygen is present, the ammonia, which is toxic to many higher life forms, such as fish and insects, will be converted to nitrate by the nitrifying microorganisms, resulting in a further demand for oxygen. Depending on the volume of wastewater discharged and the amount of oxygen available, the water body can become anoxic. If the water body does become anoxic, nitrification of ammonia to nitrate by the autotrophic bacteria will cease. However, some of the heterotrophic bacteria will use nitrate instead of oxygen as a terminal electron acceptor and continue their metabolic reactions. Depending on the relative amount of organics and nitrate, the nitrate may become depleted. In this case, the water will become anaerobic and transfer to fermentation. When the organic compounds of the wastewater have been depleted, the water body will begin to recover, clarify, and again becomes aerobic. But most of the nutrients, nitrogen (N) and phosphorus (P), remain and stimulate aquatic plants such as algae to grow. Only when the nutrients N and P are depleted and the organic compounds sufficiently reduced can the water body became eutrophically stable again.

From these considerations, the overall objectives of the biological treatment of domestic wastewater are to (1) transform (i.e., oxidize) dissolved and particulate biodegradable constituents into acceptable end products that will no longer sustain heterotrophic growth; (2) transform or remove nutrients, such as ammonia, nitrate, and particularly phosphates; and (3) in some cases, remove specific trace organic constituents and compounds. For industrial wastewater treatment, the objective is to remove or reduce the concentration of organic and inorganic compounds. Because some of the constituents and compounds found in industrial wastewater are toxic to microorganisms, pretreatment may be required before industrial wastewater can be discharged to a municipal collection system.

1.2.2 Roles of Microorganisms in Wastewater Treatment

The biological wastewater treatment is carried out by a diversified group of microorganisms. It is the bacteria that are primarily responsible for the oxidation of organic compounds. However, fungi, algae, protozoans, and higher organisms all have important roles in the transformation of soluble and colloidal organic pollutants into carbon dioxide and water as well as biomass. The latter can be removed from the liquid by settlement prior to discharge to a natural watercourse.

Many water pollution problems and solutions deal with microorganisms. To solve water pollution problems, environmental scientists require a background in microbiology. By understanding how microbes live and grow in an environment, environmental engineers can develop the best possible solution to biological waste problems. After construction of the desired treatment facilities, environmental engineers are responsible to operate them properly to produce the desired results at the least cost.

Learning to use mixtures of microorganisms to control the major environmental systems has become a major challenge for environmental engineers. Environmental microbiology should help operators of municipal wastewater and industrial waste treatment plants gain a better understanding of how their biological treatment unit work and what should be done to obtain maximum treatment efficiency. Design engineers should gain a better understanding of how microbes provide the desired treatment and the limitations for good design. Even regulatory personnel can obtain a better understanding of the limits of their regulations and what concentration of contaminants can be allowed in the environment.

The stabilization of organic matter is accomplished biologically using a variety of microorganisms, which convert the colloidal and dissolved carbonaceous organic matter into various gases and into protoplasm. It is important to note that unless the protoplasm produced from the organic matter is removed from the solution, complete treatment will not be accomplished because the protoplasm, which itself is organic, will be measured as biological oxygen demand (BOD) in the effluent.

1.2.3   Types of Biological Wastewater Treatment Processes

Biological treatment processes are typically divided into two categories according to the existing state of the microorganisms: suspended-growth systems and attached-growth systems. *Suspended systems* are more commonly referred to as *activated sludge processes*, of which several variations and modifications exist. *Attached-growth systems* differ from suspended-growth systems in that microorganisms attached themselves to a medium, which provides an inert support. Trickling filters and rotating biological contactors are most common forms of attached-growth systems.

The major biological processes used for wastewater treatment are typically divided into four groups: aerobic processes, anoxic processes, anaerobic processes, and a combination of aerobic/anoxic or anaerobic processes. The individual processes are further subdivided into two categories: suspended-growth systems and attached-growth systems, according to the existing state of microorganisms in the wastewater treatment systems.

1.3   CLASSIFICATION OF MICROORGANISMS

Conventional taxonomic methods used to identify a bacterium rely on physical properties of the bacteria and metabolic characteristics. To apply this approach, a pure culture must first be isolated. The culture may be isolated by serial dilution and growth in selective growth media. The cells are harvested and grown as pure culture using sterilization techniques to prevent contamination. Historically, the types of tests that are used to characterize a pure culture include (1) microscopic observations, to determine morphology (size and shape); (2) Gram staining technique; (3) the type of electron acceptor used in oxidation–reduction reactions; (4) the type of carbon source used for cell growth; (5) the ability to use various nitrogen and sulfur sources; (6) nutritional needs; (7) cell wall chemistry; (8) cell characteristics, including pigments, segments, cellular inclusions, and storage products; (9) resistance to antibiotics; and (10) environmental effects of temperature and pH. An alternative to taxonomic classification is a newer method, termed *phylogeny.*

1.3.1   By the Sources of Carbon and Energy

Microorganisms may be classified by their trophic levels, that is, by their energy and carbon source and their relationship to oxygen. Energy is derived principally from two sources and carbon from two sources, and these form convenient criteria to categorize organisms, in particular the microorganisms involved in water quality control and wastewater treatment. Microbes can be grouped nutritionally on the basis of how they satisfy their requirements for carbon, energy, and electrons or hydrogen. Indeed, the specific nutritional requirements of microorganisms are used to distinguish one microbe from another for taxonomic purposes.

Microorganisms may be grouped on the basis of their energy sources. Two sources of energy are available to microorganisms. Microbes that oxidize chemical compounds (either organic or inorganic) for energy are called *chemotrophs*; those that use sunlight as their energy sources are called *phototrophs*. A combination of these terms with those employed in describing carbon utilization results in the following nutritional types:

1. *Chemoautotrophs.* microbes that use inorganic chemical substances as a source of energy and carbon dioxide as the main source of carbon.
2. *Chemoheterotrophs.* microbes that use organic chemical substances as a source of energy and organic compounds as the main source of carbon.
3. *Photoautotrophs.* microbes that use light as a source of energy and carbon dioxide as the main source of carbon.
4. *Photoheterotrophs.* microbes that use light as a source of energy and organic compounds as the main source of carbon.

Microorganisms also have two sources of hydrogen atoms or electrons. Those that use reduced inorganic substances as their electron source are called *lithotrophs*. Those microbes that obtain electrons or hydrogen atoms (each hydrogen atom has one electron) from organic compounds are called *organotrophs*.

A combination of the terms above describes four nutritional types of microorganisms:

1. *Photolithotrophic autotrophs.* also called *photoautotrophs*, they use light energy and carbon dioxide as their carbon source, but they employ water as the electron donor and release oxygen in the process, such as cyanobacteria, algae, and green plants.
2. *Photo-organotrophic heterotrophs.* also called *photoheterotrophs*, they use radiant energy and organic compounds as their electron/hydrogen and carbon donors, such as purple and green non-sulfur bacteria.
3. *Chemolithotrophic autotrophs.* also called *chemoautotrophs*, they use reduced inorganic compounds, such as nitrogen, iron, or sulfur molecules, to derive both energy and electrons/hydrogen. They use carbon dioxide as their carbon source, such as the nitrifying, hydrogen, iron, and sulfur bacteria.
4. *Chemo-organotrophic heterotrophs.* also called *chemoheterotrophs*, they use organic compounds for energy, carbon, and electrons/hydrogen, such as animals, most bacteria, fungi, and protozoans.

Chemotrophs are important in the transformations of the elements, such as the conversion of ammonia to nitrate and sulfur to sulfate, which occur continually in nature. Usually, a particular species of microorganism belongs to only one of the four nutritional types. However, some microorganisms have great metabolic flexibility and can alter their nutritional type in response to environmental change. For example, many purple non-sulfur bacteria are photoheterotrophs in the absence of oxygen, and they can become chemoheterotrophs in the presence of oxygen. When oxygen is low, photosynthesis and oxidative metabolism can function simultaneously.

In the biosphere, the basic source of energy is solar radiation. The photosynthetic autotrophs (e.g., algae) are able to fix some of this solar energy into complex organic compounds (cell mass). These complex organic compounds then form the energy source for other organisms—the heterotrophs. The general process whereby the sunlight energy is trapped and then flows through the ecosystem (i.e., the process whereby life forms grow) is a sequence of reduction–oxidation ("redox" reactions).

In chemistry the acceptance of electrons by a compound (organic or inorganic) is known as *reduction* and the compound is said to be reduced, and the donation of electrons by a compound is known as *oxidation* and the compound is said to be oxidized. Because the electrons cannot remain as entities on their own, the electrons are always transferred directly from one compound to another so that the reduction–oxidation reactions, or electron donation–electron acceptance reactions, always operate as couples. These coupled reactions, known as *redox reactions*, are the principal energy transfer reactions that sustain temporal life. The link between redox reactions and energy transfer can best be illustrated by following the flow of energy and matter through an ecosystem.

1.3.2 By Temperature Range

Temperature has an important effect on the selection, survival, and growth of microorganisms. Microorganisms may also be classified by their preferred temperature regime. Each species of bacteria reproduces best within a limited range of temperatures. In general, optimal growth for a particular microorganism occurs within a fairly narrow range of temperature, although most microorganisms can survive within much broader limits. Temperatures below the optimum typically have a more significant effect on growth rate than do temperatures above the optimum. The microbial growth rates will double with approximately every 10°C increase in temperature until the optimum temperature is reached. According to the temperature range in which they function best, bacteria may be classified as psychrophilic, mesophilic, or thermophilic. Typical temperature ranges for microorganisms in each of these categories are presented in Table 1.1.

Three temperature ranges are used to classify them. Those that grow best at temperatures below 20°C are called *psychrophiles. Mesophiles* grow best at temperatures between 25 and 40°C. Between 55 and 65°C, the *thermophiles* grow best. The growth range of facultative thermophiles extends from the thermophilic into the mesophilic range. These ranges are qualitative and somewhat subjective. Bacteria will grow over a range of temperatures and will survive at a very large range of

TABLE 1.1 Temperature Classifications of Microorganisms

Type	Temperature Range (°C)	Optimum Range (°C)
Psychrophilie	10–30	12–20
Mesophilie	20–50	25–40
Thermophilie	35–75	55–65

temperatures. For example, *Escherichia coli,* classified as mesophiles, will grow at temperatures between 20 and 50°C and will reproduce, albeit very slowly, at temperatures down to 0°C. If frozen rapidly, they and many other microorganisms can be stored for years with no significant death rate.

1.3.3 Microorganism Types in Biological Wastewater Treatment

In municipal wastewater treatment incorporating biological nutrient removal, two basic categories of organisms are of specific interest: the heterotrophic organisms and the lithoautotrophic nitrifying organisms, including the ammonia and nitrite oxidizers. The former group utilizes the organic compounds of the wastewater as electron donor and either oxygen or nitrate as terminal electron acceptor, depending on whether or not the species is obligate aerobic or facultative and the conditions are aerobic or anoxic. Irrespective of whether obligate aerobic or facultative, the heterotrophic organisms obtain their catabolic (energy) and anabolic (material) requirements from the same organic compounds. In contrast, the latter group, which are lithoautotrophs, obtain their catabolic and anabolic requirements from different inorganic compounds: the catabolic (energy) from oxidizing ammonia in the wastewater to nitrite and nitrate, and the anabolic (material) from dissolved carbon dioxide in the water. Being obligate aerobic organisms, only oxygen can be used as an electron acceptor, and therefore the nitrifying organisms require aerobic conditions.

In activated sludge plants, irrespective of whether or not biological N and P removal is incorporated, the heterotrophic organisms dominate and make up more than 98% of the active organism mass in the system. If the organism retention time (sludge age) is long enough, the nitrifying bacteria may also be sustained. However, because of their low specific yield coefficient compared to the heterotrophs and relatively small amount of ammonia nitrified compared to organic material degraded, they make up a very small part of the active organism mass (less than 2%). Therefore, in terms of sludge production and oxygen or nitrate utilization, the heterotrophs have a dominating influence on the activated sludge system.

From a bioenergetic point of view, an understanding of basic heterotrophic organism behavior will form a sound foundation on which many important principles in biological wastewater treatment are based, such as (1) growth yield coefficient and its association with oxygen or nitrate utilization, and (2) energy balances and its association with wastewater strength measurement.

In contrast to the lithoautotrophs, the heterotrophs obtain the energy requirements (catabolism) and material requirement (anabolism) from the same organic compounds, irrespective of the type of external terminal electron acceptor. This difference in the metabolism of the autotrophic and heterotrophic organisms is the principal reason why the cell yield (i.e., the organism mass formed per electron donor mass utilized) is different. It is low for autotrophs [e.g., 0.10 mg volatile suspended solids (VSS) mg^{-1} NH_4^+-N nitrified for the nitrifiers] and high for heterotrophs (e.g., 0.45 mg VSS mg^{-1} COD utilized). Not only is the energy requirement in anabolism to convert carbon dioxide to cell mass far greater than that required to convert organic compounds to cell mass, but also the energy released (catabolism) in oxidizing inorganic compounds is less than that in oxidizing organic compounds.

1.4 SOME IMPORTANT MICROORGANISMS IN WASTEWATER TREATMENT

Microbiology forms one of the cornerstones of biological wastewater treatment. Bacteria have attracted the greatest attention in microbiology because they are easy to cultivate and study in pure cultures, and they have a major influence on the health of people. Fungi are also important in the treatment of some industrial wastewaters and in composting of solid wastes. Algae are photosynthetic microorganisms that have unique growth characteristics. Since algae depend on light for their source of energy, they are found primarily in water and on moist surfaces exposed to light. Algae can conserve nitrogen and phosphorus in their protoplasm, so they have a special role to play in water pollution control. Protozoans are found in almost every aquatic environment and are widely distributed. They play an important role in the treatment of wastewater. Higher animals, such as rotifers, crustaceans, and worms, live on bacteria, algae, and small protozoans. The higher animals have complex digestive systems and are much more sensitive to toxic materials than are the other microorganisms. A number of field studies have been made, using organism counts and species diversity to indicate water toxicity: for example, using *Ceridaphnia* as an indicator of wastewater effluent toxicity.

1.4.1 Bacteria

Understanding bacteria provides the basis for understanding the other microorganisms involved in environmental concerns. Learning how bacteria metabolize different organic compounds will provide the basis for designing and operating new biological wastewater treatment systems. De spite all the knowledge that we have on bacteria, it has been indicated that the majority of bacteria have yet to be found and examined in pure culture. New media and new techniques will still be required to find and study these unknown bacteria that currently inhabit our environment.

Bacteria are the most important group of microorganisms in the environment. Their basic mission is to convert dead biological matter to stable materials that can be recycled back into new biological matter. Bacteria are also the highest population of microorganisms in a wastewater treatment plant. They are single-celled organisms that use soluble food. Conditions in the treatment plant are adjusted so that chemoheterotrophs predominate.

The Shape and Size of Bacteria Bacteria are indeed the simplest form of life. Bacteria are the most numerous of living organisms on Earth in terms of number of species, number of organisms, and total mass of organisms. Their prokaryotic cell structure is significantly different from higher forms such as the single-celled algae and protozoans, invertebrates, plants, and animals. Each cell is small, typically 1 to 2 μm in diameter and length, and has a total mass of 1 to 10 pg. Under optimal conditions of temperature, pH, and nutrient availability, some bacterial species have generation times of less than 30 min. Such short generation times account for the rapid progression of infectious diseases.

Individual bacteria can be seen with the help of an optical microscope. There are three basic shapes of bacteria: spheres, rods, and spirals. The spherical bacteria are called *cocci*. The rod-shaped bacteria are called *baccillus;* and the spiral-shaped bacteria are called *spirillum*. As shown in Fig. 1.1, the *cocci* can exist as single cells, as diplos (two cells), as squares (four cells), as cubes (eight cells), as chains, or as large clumps having no specific size or shape. The *bacillus* is found as a single cell, diplo cells, and in chains. The *spirillum* exists primarily as single cells or diplos.

The Basic Cell Structure All bacteria have the same general structure. For a single bacterium, observing from the outside to the inside, we would find a slime layer, a cell wall, a cell membrane, and the cytosol within the membrane. The slime layer appears to be part of the cell wall that has lost most of its proteins. The chemical structure of the slime layer is primarily polysaccharide material of relatively low structural strength. Figure 1.2 is a schematic drawing of a typical rod-shaped bacterium.

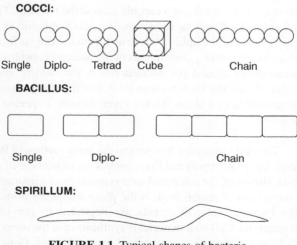

COCCI:

Single   Diplo-   Tetrad   Cube   Chain

BACILLUS:

Single   Diplo-   Chain

SPIRILLUM:

FIGURE 1.1 Typical shapes of bacteria.

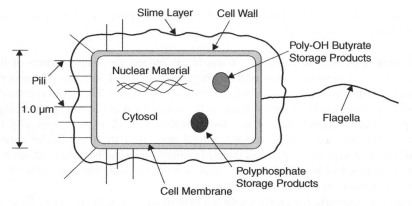

FIGURE 1.2 Schematic diagram of a bacterium cell.

Cell Wall Gram-positive bacteria have thicker cell walls than those of gram-negative bacteria. The basic cell wall materials for both types of bacteria are similar. The major component for cell walls is peptidoglycan. Cell walls are continuously synthesized from the inside surface as the cell expands to form two new cells. It appears that both proteins and lipids are integrated into the cell wall as it is synthesized. The cell wall gives the shape to the bacteria and helps control movement of materials into and out of the cell. The proteins in the cell walls are largely hydrolytic enzymes designed to break down complex proteins and polysaccharides in the liquid around the bacteria into smaller molecules that can move across the cell wall to the cell membrane and into the cell.

As bacteria age, the synthesis of new cell wall material at the cell membrane surface causes the cell wall to increase in thickness. Young bacteria move rapidly through the liquid, where hydraulic shear forces cause the outer layer of the cell wall to break off, giving a uniform cell wall. As the bacteria slow their motility, the cell wall increases its thickness, producing a capsule around the bacteria. The proteins in the cell wall tend to break off and move into the surrounding liquid as extracellular, hydrolytic enzymes. Some of the lipids are also lost from the cell surface. This leaves the polysaccharides as the primary constituents of the bacteria capsules. The capsular material that accumulates around the bacteria has a low density and is not very chemically reactive. When the bacteria lose their motility, the polysaccharide cell wall material accumulates to a much thicker layer without a specific shape and is called the *slime layer*.

Cell Membrane The cell membrane lies next to the inner surface of the cell wall. It is primarily a dense lipoprotein polymer that controls the movement of materials into and out of bacteria. However, the cell membrane is much more important than simply controlling the movement of materials. It is the place where the primary metabolic reactions for the bacteria occur. Nutrients are degraded to provide energy for synthesis of cell materials. Cell wall material is synthesized at the membrane surface, while RNA, DNA, and proteins are synthesized inside the cell. Generally, the cell membrane is a well-organized complex of enzymes that allows the most efficient transfer of energy from the substrate to be metabolized to the production of all the cell components.

Cytosol   Cytosol is the major material inside the cell membrane. It is a colloidal suspension of various materials, primarily proteins. Colloids are tiny particles that have very large surface area/mass ratios, making them highly reactive. These protein fragments are important to the success of the bacteria, providing the building blocks for all of the key enzymes that the cell needs. The large size of these colloidal fragments prevents their movement out of the cell until the cell membrane is ruptured.

Since bacteria do not have a defined nucleus, their nuclear material is dispersed throughout the cytosol. The DNA in the bacteria determines their biochemical characteristics and exists as organic strands in the cytosol. The DNA is surrounded by RNA, which is responsible for protein synthesis. The dispersed nature of bacterial nuclear material and the permeability of bacteria cells permit transfer of small nuclear fragments from one cell to another, changing the biochemical characteristics of the bacteria. If the changes in biochemical characteristics are permanent, the process is known as *mutation*. If the changes in biochemical characteristics are controlled by the environmental conditions around the bacteria, the process is known as *adaptation*. Both adaptation and mutation are important environmental processes. Adaptation occurs far more often than mutation and is reversible. It is hoped that bacteria with one set of characteristics will develop a second set of characteristics. Although artificial gene transfer is relatively new, natural gene transfer has been occurring since time began and will continue in the future. Gene transfer among bacteria is a never-ending process.

If the bacteria are in a medium that has excess nutrients, the bacteria cannot process all the nutrients into cell components as quickly as the bacteria would like. The excess nutrients that the bacteria remove, but cannot use in the synthesis of new cell mass, are converted into insoluble storage reserves for later metabolism when the available substrate decreases. Excess carbohydrates in the media can be stored as glycogen under the proper environmental conditions. Some bacteria convert excess carbohydrates into extracellular slime that cannot be further metabolized, rather than storing the excess carbohydrates inside the cell. Excess acetic acid can be stored as a poly(hydroxybutyric acid) polymer. Storage of nutrients inside the cell does not occur in a substrate-limited environment. When the nutrient substrate is limited, the bacteria use all the nutrients as fast as they can for the synthesis of new cell mass.

Flagella and Pili   Flagella are protein strands that extend from the cell membrane through the cell wall into the liquid. Energy generated at the cell membrane causes the flagella to move and propel the bacteria through the liquid environment. The flagella can be located at one end of the bacteria, at both ends of the cell, or covering the bacteria completely. Flagella are very important for rod-shaped bacteria, allowing them to move in search of nutrients when necessary. Some bacteria move by flexing their bodies rather than using flagella. A spirillum has flagella at the end of the cell that produce a corkscrew-type motion. Spherical bacteria are

TABLE 1.2 Bacteria Cell Structure and Their Functions

Cell Structure	Function
Cell wall	Provides strength to maintain the cell shape and protects the cell membrane. Some bacteria can produce a sticky polysaccharide layer outside the cell wall, called a capsule or slime layer.
Cell membrane	Controls the passage of dissolved organics and nutrients into the cell and the waste materials and metabolic by-products out of the cell.
Cytoplasm	Contains the material within the cell to carry out cell functions and includes water, nutrients, enzymes, ribosomes, and small organic molecules.
Cytoplasmic inclusions	Contains storage material that can provide carbon, nutrients, or energy. These may be carbohydrate deposits, such as poly(hydroxybutyrate) or glycogen, polyphosphates, lipids, and sulfur granules.
Deoxyribonucleic acid (DNA)	A double-stranded helix-shaped molecule that contains genetic information that determines the nature of the cell protein and enzymes that are produced.
Plasmid DNA	Small circular DNA molecules that can also provide genetic characteristics for the bacteria.
Ribosomes	Particles in the cytoplasm that are composed of RNA and protein and are the sites where proteins are produced.
Flagella	Protein hairlike structures that extend from the cytoplasm membrane several bacteria lengths out from the cell and provide mobility by rotating at high speeds.
Fimbriae and pili	Short protein hairlike structures (pili are longer) that enable bacteria to stick to surfaces. Pili also enable bacteria to attach to each other.

Source: Adapted from Metcalf & Eddy, Inc. (2003).

devoid of flagella and lack motility. As bacteria age, they appear to produce many small protein projections that look like flagella. These small protein projections, called *pili*, appear to help the bacteria attach to various surfaces, including other bacteria. The flagella and pili are best observed using an electron microscope.

The difference in basic cell structure allowed microorganisms to be placed into two major groups: *prokaryotes*, cells without a defined nucleus, and *eukaryotes*, cells with a defined nucleus. Bacteria were classified as prokaryotes, and all the other microorganisms were classified as eucaryotes. The important components of the prokaryotic cell and their functions are described in Table 1.2.

1.4.2 Fungi

Fungi are multicellular, nonphotosynthetic, heterotrophic microorganisms that metabolize organic matter in a manner similar to bacteria. Fungi are obligate aerobes, requiring dissolved oxygen and soluble organic compounds for metabolism. They are predominately filamentous and reproduce by a variety of methods, including fission, budding, and spore formation. Their cells require only half as much nitrogen as bacteria, so that in a nitrogen-deficient wastewater, they predominate over the bacteria.

Unlike bacteria, fungi have a nucleus that is self-contained within each cell. They are larger than bacteria and can produce true cell branching in their filaments. Fungi have more complex phases in their life cycle than do bacteria. The identification of fungi has been based entirely on their physical characteristics and on the different phases of their life cycle. Current emphasis on genetic structure may result in significant changes in the identification and classification of fungi. Over the years, mycologists have placed greater emphasis on identification of fungi than on their biochemistry. More than 10^5 species of fungi have been identified. Currently, fungi are classified in the Eucarya domain. Although fungi are very important in applied environmental microbiology, it is not essential to know the names of the fungi to recognize their value. Fortunately, most fungi are nonpathogenic and play an important role in the degradation of dead plant tissue and other organic residues. Anyone involved in organic waste processing needs to have a general knowledge of fungi and their metabolic characteristics.

Fungi contain 85 to 90% water. The dry matter is about 95% organic compounds with 5% inorganic compounds. Growth of fungi in a high-salt environment will have a greater inorganic fraction than that of fungi grown in normal-salt media, in the same way as for bacteria. The organic fraction of fungi contains between 40 and 50% carbon and between 2 and 7% nitrogen. Protein analyses show that the fungi cell mass contains only 20 to 25% proteins. Proteins are a major difference between fungi and bacteria. Fungi produce protoplasm with less protein than bacteria and require less nitrogen per unit cell mass synthesized. Fungi also have less phosphorus than bacteria, containing from 1.0 to 1.5% P in the fungi cell mass. Fungi do not produce significant amounts of lipids, usually less than 5.0%. The fungal protoplasm is largely polysaccharide. The fungi cell wall structure is a lipo–protein–polysaccharide complex. Lipids make up less than 8% of the fungi cell walls and proteins are less than 10%. The majority of the cell wall composition is chitin, a polysaccharide composed of N-acetylglucosamine.

Since fungi must hydrolyze complex organic solids the same as bacteria, the lipids and proteins in the cell wall are very important for metabolism. The chemical composition analysis of *Aspergillus niger* was 47.9% carbon, 5.24% nitrogen, 6.7% hydrogen, and 1.58% ash. By difference oxygen was 38.6%. The chemical analysis *of A. niger* appears to be typical for fungi as a group, yielding an empirical analysis of $C_{10.7}H_{18}O_{65}N$ for the organic solids when $N = 1.0$. Although the empirical formula for fungi protoplasm is quite different from bacterial protoplasm, the metabolic energy requirements for fungi are essentially the same as those for bacteria, $31.6\,kJ\,g^{-1}$ VSS.

Aerobic metabolism permits the fungi to obtain the maximum energy from the substrate for synthesis of new cell protoplasm. Surface enzymes allow the fungi to hydrolyze complex organic compounds to simple soluble organics prior to entering the cell, in the same way as for bacteria. Hydrophobic organic compounds enter through the lipids in the cell wall structure. Inside the cell, enzymes oxidize the organic compounds to organic acids and then to carbon dioxide and water. Since the fungi have less protein than bacteria, metabolism of protein substrates by fungi results in more ammonia nitrogen being released to the environment than during bacteria metabolism of the same quantity of proteins in the substrate. Without sufficient dissolved oxygen, fungi metabolism results in the release of organic acid intermediates into the environment and a decrease in pH. The low protein content of fungi allows them to be more tolerant than bacteria of low–pH environments. Fungi have the ability to grow at pH levels as low as 4.0 to 4.5 with an optimum pH between 5.0 and 7.0. From a temperature point of view, fungi grow between 5 and 40°C with an optimum temperature around 35°C. There are a few thermophilic fungi that grow at temperatures up to 60°C. The low oxygen solubility at high temperatures limits the growth of fungi at thermophilic temperatures.

One of the more interesting aspects of fungi metabolism is the ability of some fungi to metabolize lignin. The white rot fungi *Phanerochaete chrysosporium* have been studied in detail because of their ability to metabolize substituted aromatic compounds that accumulate from industrial wastes and to metabolize lignin. Lignin is a complex plant polymer that protects plant cellulose from attack by bacteria. Terrestrial fungi have the ability to metabolize lignin and cellulose, recycling all the dead plant tissue back into the environment. Unfortunately, there are no aquatic fungi capable of metabolizing lignin. Efforts to develop aquatic fungi capable of metabolizing lignin in the aqueous environment have all been unsuccessful. Terrestrial fungi also have the ability to degrade bacteria cell wall polysaccharides in the soil environment. The dead cell mass of fungi and the nonbiodegradable plant tissue form a complex organic mixture that has been designated as *humus*.

In the natural environment fungi compete with bacteria for nutrients to survive. Bacteria normally have the advantage over fungi in the natural environment. Bacteria simply have the ability to obtain more nutrients and can process the nutrients at a faster rate than can fungi. Since both groups of microorganisms metabolize soluble nutrients, both groups survive according to their ability to obtain and process nutrients. The greater surface area/mass ratio permits bacteria to obtain nutrients at a faster rate than fungi under normal metabolic conditions. The presence of higher animal forms in the environment favors the fungi since the higher animals can eat bacteria easier than they can consume fungi. The filamentous fungi are difficult for microscopic animals to metabolize. The environment has a number of factors that allow the fungi to be competitive with bacteria. By understanding the various factors affecting the growth of the bacteria and fungi, the environmental microbiologist can recognize how to adjust the environment of different treatment systems to favor one group of microorganisms or the other.

Moisture content is very important for the growth of fungi. Unlike bacteria, fungi can grow in environments with limited amounts of water. The lower nitrogen and phosphorus content of fungi protoplasm than bacteria protoplasm gives the fungi an advantage over bacteria when metabolizing organic compounds in low-nitrogen and low-phosphorus environments. The ability to grow at low pH levels also favors the growth of fungi over bacteria. Both bacteria and fungi grow under aerobic conditions. As the dissolved oxygen is used up, the fungi cannot continue normal metabolism, but the facultative bacteria shift from aerobic metabolism to anaerobic metabolism. Controlling the oxygen level can be an important tool for environmental microbiologists to minimize the growth of fungi.

Since fungi do not produce dispersed cells, growth cannot be measured by numbers of cells. Growth is measured by dry weight mass, in the same way as bacteria are measured.

1.4.3 Algae

Algae are photosynthetic microorganisms containing chlorophyll. They can be single cell or multicell, motile or nonmotile. Algae use light as their source of energy for cell synthesis and inorganic ions as their source of chemicals for cell protoplasm. Algae have both a positive and a negative impact on the environment. One of the positive aspects of algae is the production of oxygen in proportion to the growth of new cells. On the negative side, algae are responsible for tastes and odors in many surface water supplies. Algae also take stable inorganic ions and convert them into organic matter that ultimately must be stabilized.

Like fungi, algae are identified by their physical characteristics. The primary characteristic of algae is pigmentation. The green algae are largely grouped as Chlorophycophyta. The Chlorophycophyta grow as individual cells, motile and nonmotile, and as filaments. *Chlorella* has been the most widely studied green algae. *Chlorella* appears as small spherical nonmotile cells about 5 to 10 μm in diameter. *Chlorella* can be found as dispersed cells or as clumps of cells, depending on the growth environment. *Ochromonas* is a motile single-celled alga with two flagella. Diatoms are the most common Chrysophycophyta. The most important characteristic of diatoms is their ability to create a silica shell around a cell.

Algae use light as their source of energy for synthesizing cell protoplasm. Sunlight furnishes the light in the natural environment for algae. Since light energy is absorbed by water, growth of the algae occurs near the water surface. The photosynthetic pigments in the algae convert light energy into chemical energy by electron transfer. The rate of energy production in algae is a function of the surface area of photosynthetic pigments and the light intensity.

In addition to light, algae need a source of carbon for cell protoplasm. Carbon dioxide is the primary carbon source for algae. The air atmosphere contains about 0.03% carbon dioxide, giving very little pressure for transferring carbon dioxide into natural waters. Alkalinity forms the primary source of carbon dioxide in natural waters. Algae grow much better in waters containing high concentrations of bicarbonate alkalinity than in waters with low bicarbonate alkalinity. Water is the source of hydrogen for algae. Removal of hydrogen from water leaves the oxygen to form dissolved oxygen in the water.

Nitrogen is important to form proteins for algae protoplasm. Ammonia nitrogen is the primary source of nitrogen for algae, with nitrates as the secondary source. Nitrates must be reduced to ammonia for incorporation into protoplasm. Part of the light energy must be expended in the nitrate reduction, limiting the amount of potential synthesis.

Phosphorus is a critical element for the growth of algae. Although algae do not need a large quantity of phosphorus, it is important in energy transfer for the algae, the same as for other microorganisms. Phosphates are the primary source of phosphorus for the algae. Since phosphates are limited in the natural environment, phosphorus availability is often the limiting factor in the growth of algae. Eutrophication of lakes and reservoirs has been caused by the discharge of excess phosphates from domestic wastewater and fertilizer runoff with the subsequent algae growth.

Algae also need sulfates and trace metals. The sulfates in natural waters are adequate to supply the algae demands. The trace metal needs are quite small compared with those of the other elements; but they are essential if normal algae growth is to occur. Iron is needed for electron transfer. Magnesium is required for chlorophyll. Other important trace metals include calcium, potassium, zinc, copper, manganese, and molybdenum. The lack of sufficient trace metals will limit the magnitude of algae growth.

Algae also play a positive role in wastewater treatment for many small communities. Wastewater stabilization ponds have been widely used to treat municipal wastewater from small communities. While bacteria play the primary role in stabilization ponds, algae play an important secondary role. The algae metabolism at the pond surface provides oxygen to keep the bacteria aerobic and ties up some nitrogen and phosphorus in the dead algae cell mass that accumulates along with the dead bacteria cell mass on the bottom of the stabilization pond. The keys to using algae in wastewater treatment systems lie in understanding the basic biochemistry of the algae, the wastewater characteristics, and the practical engineering design concepts.

1.4.4 Protozoans

Protozoans are a large collection of organisms with considerable morphological and physiological diversity. Protozoans are all eukaryotic and considered to be single-celled organisms that can reproduce by binary fission (dividing in 2). The majority of them are chemoheterotrophs, and they often consume bacteria. Because certain species possess chloroplasts, they can also practice photoautotrophy. Protozoans are found in almost every aquatic environment and are widely distributed. They play an important role in all aspects of environmental microbiology, ranging from their health impacts as human pathogens through to their role in the treatment of wastewater. They are desirable in wastewater effluents because they act as polishers in consuming the bacteria.

In nature, bacteria form the major food supply for protozoans. The bacteria concentrate various nutrients into their protoplasm, making them the perfect food for the protozoans. A portion of the organic matter from the bacteria is oxidized to yield energy for the synthesis of new protoplasm from the remaining organic matter. The energy–synthesis relationships for protozoans are similar to the bacteria energy–synthesis relationships, 38% oxidation and 62% new cell mass. Large protozoans can also eat small algae. Most protozoans are aerobic, requiring dissolved oxygen as their electron acceptor. There are a few anaerobic protozoans. The problem with anaerobic protozoans is even more acute than with anaerobic bacteria.

To understand fully the contribution of protozoans to aquatic ecosystems and to exploit these same properties in engineered systems, it is essential to be able to identify and then classify them. Protozoans are classified on the basis of their morphology, in particular as regards their mode of locomotion. There are four major groups of protozoans: (1) Mastigophora: flagellated protozoans (*Euglena*); (2) Sarcodina: amoeba-like protozoans (*Amoeba*); (3) *Sporozoa*, parasitic protozoans (*Plasmodium* malaria); (4) Ciliophora: ciliated protozoans (*Paramecium*). The first three classes are the free-swimming protozoans and the last class comprises the parasitic protozoans. The full scheme is illustrated in Fig. 1.3.

Protozoans are primarily aerobic organisms, requiring dissolved oxygen as their electron acceptor. Although protozoans can be grown in concentrated, complex nutrient media, they prefer to use bacteria as their source of nutrients. The protozoans metabolize the biodegradable portion of the bacteria for energy and synthesis and excrete the nonbiodegradable fraction back into the environment. Although the majority of protozoans are aerobic organisms, there are anaerobic protozoans. Like their bacteria counterparts, the anaerobic protozoans must eat tremendous quantities of nutrients to obtain sufficient energy for cell synthesis. The low bacteria growth in anaerobic environments means that anaerobic protozoans will be found only in high-organic-concentration environments.

Protozoans undergo reproduction by fission, splitting into two cells along the longitudinal axis. It takes several hours for the two cells to split completely. Growth

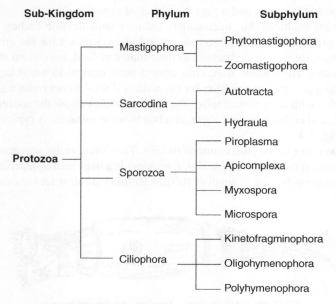

FIGURE 1.3 Classification of protozoans.

continues as long as environmental conditions are favorable. When environmental conditions begin to turn bad for continued growth of the protozoans, they form cysts. Each cyst is produced by coating the nucleus with a hard shell, allowing the nucleus to survive in adverse environments. The rest of the cell tissues become nutrients for additional bacteria growth. When the cyst finds a reasonable environment for growth, the nucleus begins to expand, creating new protozoans.

Environmental factors such as pH and temperature have the same relative effect on protozoans as on bacteria. Protozoans grow best at pH levels between 6.5 and 8.5. Strongly acidic or strongly alkaline conditions are toxic to protozoans. As far as temperature is concerned, protozoans can be either mesophilic or thermophilic, the same as bacteria. Most protozoans are mesophilic, having a maximum temperature for growth of around 40°C. Protozoans change their rate of metabolism by a factor of 2 for each 10°C temperature change, the same as the other organisms. Protozoans have difficulty surviving at temperatures below 5°C because the viscosity of the water increases, making it more difficult for the protozoans to move and obtain food.

1.4.5   Rotifers and Crustaceans

Both rotifers and crustaceans are animals: aerobic multicellular chemoheterotrophs. The rotifer derives its name from the apparent rotating motion of two sets of cilia on its head. The cilia provide mobility and a mechanism for catching food. Rotifers consume bacteria and small particles of organic matter. Crustaceans, a group that includes shrimp, lobsters, and barnacles, are characterized by their shell structure. They are a source of food for fish and are not found in wastewater treatment systems to any extent except in underloaded lagoons. Their presence is indicative of a high level of dissolved oxygen and a very low level of organic matter.

Rotifers are multicellular, microscopic animals with flexible bodies. They are larger than protozoans and have complex metabolic systems. Like the other microscopic animals, rotifers prefer bacteria as their source of food, but can eat small algae and protozoans. The rotifers have cilia around their mouths to assist in gathering food. The cilia also provide motility for the rotifers if they do not remain attached to solid particles with their forked tails. The flexible bodies allow the rotifers to bend around and feed on bacteria and algae attached to solid surfaces. A typical rotifer is shown in Fig. 1.4.

Philodina is one of the most common rotifers. The cilia give the appearance of two rotating wheels at the head of the rotifer. *Epiphanes* is a large rotifer, reaching 600 μm in length. Some rotifers are as small as 100 μm. Rotifers are all strict aerobes and must

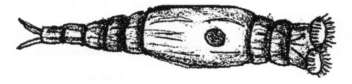

FIGURE 1.4 Schematic diagram of a typical rotifer.

have several micrograms per liter of dissolved oxygen in order to grow. They can survive for several hours in low dissolved oxygen (DO) environments, but not for long periods. In the presence of large bacteria populations and adequate DO, rotifers will quickly eat most of the bacteria, even if the bacteria are flocculated. In a suitable environment the rotifers can quickly metabolize all the bacteria and then starve to death. Excessive growth of rotifers can be controlled by reducing the dissolved oxygen to prevent them from growing so rapidly. The DO can be reduced to around $1.0 \, \text{mg} \, \text{L}^{-1}$ to favor the metabolism of aerobic bacteria and protozoans and slow the growth of rotifers. As large complex organisms, rotifers require lots of bacteria in their growth. Rotifers can remove the bacteria attached to solid surfaces and can ingest small, flocculated masses of bacteria. They are more sensitive to environmental stresses than either bacteria or protozoans. Temperature affects rotifers in the same way that temperature affects the other microorganisms. Their metabolism slows as the temperature decreases and increases as the temperature rises. There do not appear to be any thermophilic rotifers. Reproduction in rotifers occurs through egg formation rather than by binary fission. Rotifer eggs can remain dormant for a considerable period of time if environmental conditions are not satisfactory for growth. It has been difficult to study the quantitative growth characteristics of rotifers since they cannot be grown free of bacteria.

Rotifers play an important role in the overall food chain from bacteria and algae to higher organisms. They are widely found in the aquatic environment, where there is a suitable environment for growth. Rivers, lakes, and reservoirs are good sources of rotifers. The environments that favor rotifers tend to favor other higher animal forms.

Crustaceans are multicellular animals with hard shells to protect their bodies. They also have jointed appendages attached to their bodies. The appendages assist in movement and food gathering. The large size of the crustaceans, 1.5 to 2 mm, makes them visible to the naked eye if one looks very carefully. Being more complex than rotifers, they grow more slowly and are more sensitive to environmental changes. The crustaceans feed on bacteria, algae, protozoans, and solid organic materials.

Daphnia and *Cyclops* are two common crustaceans. They are easily found in freshwater lakes in the warm summer months. They require high levels of DO and a moderate level of nutrients. It has been estimated that *Daphnia* require about 80% of their body weight each day for maximum growth. Only about 20% of the food consumed ends up as cell mass. The larger mass of the *Daphnia* requires a considerable number of smaller organisms to remain alive and to grow. Since the *Daphnia* are relatively large, they become food for macroscopic organisms in the water environment.

The presence or absence of sufficient concentrations of trace metals in the bacteria or algae used as their food source also affects the magnitude of growth of the different species of crustaceans. The U.S. Environmental Protection Agency (EPA) has proposed the use of *Ceridaphnia* as the indicator organism for effluent toxicity from wastewater treatment plants. Unfortunately, *Ceridaphnia* is a very sensitive crustacean that can be difficult to maintain in the laboratory for routine use. Researchers are currently examining other *Daphnia* in an effort to find a suitable crustacean that is both sensitive to toxic substances and easy to maintain in the laboratory.

1.4.6   Viruses

Viruses belong neither to prokaryotes nor to eukaryotes. They carry out no catabolic or anabolic function. Their replication occurs inside a host cell. The infected cells may be animal or plant cells, bacteria, fungi, or algae. Viruses are very small (25 to 350 nm) and most of them can be observed only with an electron microscope.

A virus is made of a core of nucleic acid (double- or single-stranded DNA; double- or single-stranded RNA) surrounded by a protein coat called a *capsid*. Capsids are composed of arrangements of various numbers of protein subunits known as *capsomeres*. The combination of capsid and nucleic acid core is called *nucleocapsid*.

Bacterial phages have been used as models to elucidate the phases involved in virus replication. The various phases are as follows (Fig. 1.5):

1. *Adsorption and entry.* This is the first step in the replication cycle of viruses. In order to infect the host cells, the virus must adsorb to receptors located on the cell surface. Animal viruses adsorb to surface components of the host cell. The receptors may be polysaccharides, proteins, or lipoproteins. Then the virus or its nucleic acid enters the host cell. Bacteriophages "inject" their nucleic acid into the host cell. For animal viruses the entire virion penetrates the host cell by endocytosis.

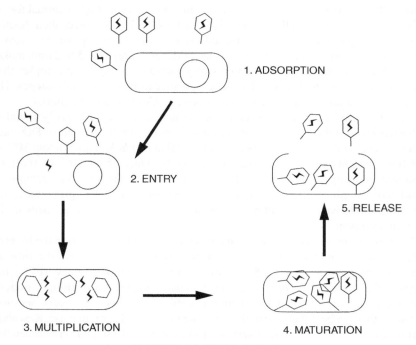

FIGURE 1.5 Viral lytic cycle.

2. *Eclipse.* During this step, the virus is "uncoated" (i.e., stripping of the capsid), and the nucleic acid is liberated.
3. *Replication.* This step involves the replication of the viral nucleic acid.
4. *Maturation and release.* The protein coat is synthesized and is assembled with the nucleic acid to form a nucleocapsid. Virus release is generally attributable to the rupture of the host cell membrane.

1.5 MEASUREMENT OF MICROBIAL BIOMASS

Various approaches are available for measuring microbial biomass in laboratory cultures or in environmental samples, as shown in Fig. 1.6.

1.5.1 Total Number of Microbial Cells

The total number of cells (live and dead cells) can be measured by using special counting chambers such as the Petroff–Hauser chamber for bacterial counts or

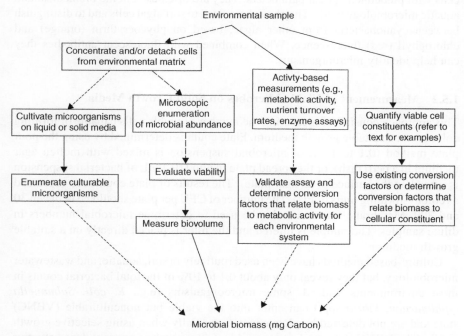

FIGURE 1.6 Experimental approaches commonly used for estimating microbial biomass. Dashed arrows indicate steps in the procedures in which current methods may introduce bias or uncertainty to the final biomass determination. The extent of bias or uncertainty is indicated by the size of the dash; finely dashed lines indicate that current methods for measurement or calculation of these parameters may be indeterminate. [From Sutton (1991).]

the Sedgewick–Rafter chamber for algal counts. The use of a phase-contrast microscope is required when nonphotosynthetic microorganisms are under consideration. Presently, the most popular method consists of retaining the cells on a membrane filter treated to suppress autofluorescence (use of polycarbonate filters treated with Irgalan black) and staining the cells with fluorochromes, such as acridine orange or 4′,6-diamidino-2-phenylindol (DAPI). The microorganisms are subsequently counted using an epifluorescence microscope. An advantage of DAPI is its stable fluorescence. A wide range of other fluorochromes are available for many applications in environmental microbiology studies, including PicoGreen, SYBR-Green 1 and 2, Hoechst 33342, YOYO-1, and SYTO dyes (green, red, and blue).

Scanning electron microscopy has also been considered for measuring total microbial numbers. Electronic particle counters are also used for determining the total number of microorganisms in a sample. These instruments do not differentiate, however, between live and dead microorganisms, and very small cells may be missed.

Flow cytometers are fluorescence-activated cell sorters and include a light source (argon laser or a mercury lamp) and a photodetector, which measures fluorescence (use correct excitation wavelength) and scattering of the cells. They sort and collect cells with predefined optical parameters. They are often used in the biomedical and aquatic microbiology fields. They have been used to sort algal cells and to distinguish between cyanobacteria from other algae, based on phycoerythrin (orange) and chlorophyll (red) fluorescence. When combined with fluorescent antibodies they can help identify microorganisms.

1.5.2 Measurement of Viable Microbes on Solid Growth Media

This approach consists of measuring the number of viable cells capable of forming colonies on a suitable growth medium. Plate count is determined by using the pour plate method (0.1 to 1 mL of microbial suspension is mixed with molten agar medium in a petri dish), or the spread plate method (0.1 mL of bacterial suspension is spread on the surface of an agar plate). The results of plate counts are expressed as colony-forming units (CFU). The number of CFU per plate should be between 30 and 300. Membrane filters can also be used to determine microbial numbers in dilute samples. The sample is filtered and the filter is placed directly on a suitable growth medium.

Culture-based methods have been used routinely in soil, aquatic, and wastewater microbiology, but they reveal only about 0.1 to 10% of the total bacterial counts in most environments. Indeed, some microorganisms (e.g., *E. coli*, *Salmonella typhimurium*, *Vibrio* spp.) can enter into the viable but nonculturable (VBNC) state and are not detected by plate counts, especially when using selective growth media. The VBNC state can be triggered by factors such as nutrient deprivation or exposure to toxic chemicals. This phenomenon is particularly important for pathogens that may remain viable in the VBNC state for longer periods of time than previously thought. The VBNC pathogens may remain virulent and cause disease in humans and animals.

1.5.3 Measurement of Active Cells in Environmental Samples

Several approaches have been considered for assessing microbial viability or activity in environmental samples as shown in Fig. 1.7 (Keer and Birch, 2003). Epifluorescence microscopy, in combination with the use of oxido-reduction dyes, is used to determine the percent of active cells in aquatic environments. The most popular oxido-reduction dyes are INT [2-(p-iodophenyl)-3-(p-nitrophenyl)-5-phenyltetrazoliumchloride] and CTC (cyanoditolyl tetrazolium chloride). A good correlation was found between the number of CTC-positive *E. coli* cells and the CFU count, regardless of the growth phase.

The direct viable count (DVC) method was pioneered by Kogure and his collaborators in Japan (Kogure et al., 1984). The sample is incubated with trace amounts of yeast extract and nalidixic acid, the latter blocks DNA replication but not RNA synthesis. This leads to cell elongation of active cells, which are counted using epifluorescence microscopy. Some methods allow detection in aquatic samples of specific bacterial pathogens, including those in the VBNC state. One such method combines fluorescent in situ hybridization with DVC, followed by cell enumeration using a laser scanning cytometer. This approach gives information on the identity of the bacteria (Baudart et al., 2002). To detect specific bacteria in aquatic environments, the cells can be labeled simultaneously with a fluorescent antibody (FA technique) in combination with viability and activity markers such as

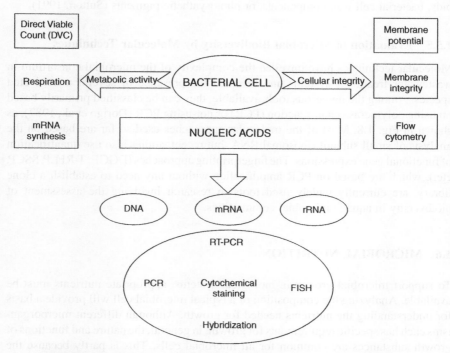

FIGURE 1.7 Approaches used for assessing microbial viability or activity.

cyanoditolyl tetrazolium chloride or propidium iodide, which is an indicator of membrane integrity.

Fluorescein diacetate (FDA) is transformed by esterase enzymes to a fluorescent compound, fluorescein, which accumulates inside the cells (FDA is a nonpolar compound and fluorescein is a polar compound). The active fluorescent cells are counted under a fluorescent microscope. This method is best suited for active fungal filaments but can be applied to bacterial cells.

1.5.4   Determination of Cellular Biochemical Compounds

Technical problems and experimental biases associated with traditional biomass measures prompted microbial ecologists to use a biochemical approach for studying microorganisms in the environment. The biochemical index molecule should be (1) common to all cells, (2) present in a constant proportion in all microbial cells regardless of physiological state, (3) present only in viable cells and be rapidly degraded on cell death, and (4) present in sufficient quantity to be readily extracted from environmental samples. The quantity of this component should be easily related to biomass. Finally methods should be readily available for quantitative extraction and sensitive detection of the specific component within environmental samples. A number of different biochemical components have been used for the estimation of microbial biomass, including adenosine triphosphate (ATP), DNA, RNA, proteins, phospholipids, bacterial cell wall components, or photosynthetic pigments (Sutton, 1991).

1.5.5   Evaluation of Microbial Biodiversity by Molecular Techniques

Molecular techniques have unveiled the complexity of the microbial consortium in wastewater treatment systems and revealed the presence of several uncultivated species. Among the numerous tools available, they can be classified primarily based on using polymerase chair reaction (PCR) or not-using PCR (Dorigo et al., 1987), as shown in Fig. 1.8. Most of the molecular approaches used so far are based on the analysis of small subunit ribosomal RNA, but recent studies also use quantification of functional gene expressions. The fingerprinting approaches (DGGE, T-RFLP, SSCP, etc.), which are based on PCR amplification without any need to establish a clone library, are currently widely used tools in research involving the assessment of biodiversity in aquatic microbial communities.

1.6   MICROBIAL NUTRITION

To support microbial growth in biological systems, appropriate nutrients must be available. Analyzing the composition of a typical microbial cell will provide a basis for understanding the nutrients needed for growth. Although different microorganisms each has specific requirements for growth, in general, the nature and functions of growth substances are common for all microbial cells. This is partly because the chemical composition of microbial cells is more or less similar. In order to grow,

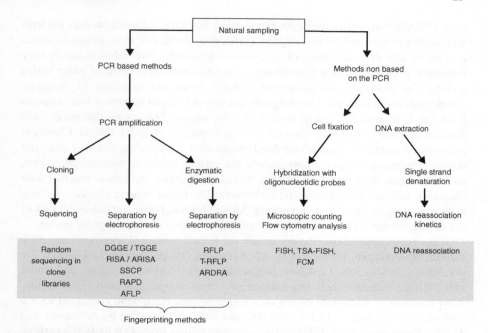

FIGURE 1.8 Various molecular approaches to assessing the genetic diversity of microbial communities: DGGE, denaturing gradient gel electrophoresis; TGGE, temperature gradient gel electrophoresis; RISA, ribosomal intergenic spacer analysis; ARISA, automated ribosomal intergenic spacer analysis; SSCP, single-stranded conformation polymorphism; RAPD, random amplified polymorphic DNA; AFLP, amplified fragment length polymorphism; (t)-RFLP, (terminal)-restriction fragment length polymorphism; ARDRA, amplified ribosomal DNA restriction analysis; (TSA)-FISH, (tyramide signal amplification)-fluorescence in situ hybridization; FCM, flow cytometry.

microorganisms must have proper essential chemical elements. The main chemical elements for cell growth include C, N, H, O, S, and P—the same elements that form the chemical composition of the cells. For example, all microbes require a carbon source because carbon is a component of protoplasm; nitrogen is a component of many major macromolecules, such as protein and nucleic acids. Over 95% of a cell's dry weight is made up of a few major elements, such as C, O, H, S, P, K, Ca, Mg, and Fe. All these substances must be put together by biosynthesis to form cellular material. However, not all growth substances are incorporated into cell material. Some are used instead as energy sources. For example, carbon compounds are frequently used as energy sources by many microorganisms.

1.6.1 Microbial Chemical Composition

Bacteria are approximately 70 to 80% water and 20 to 30% dry matter. The dry matter in bacteria is both organic and inorganic. The percentages of organic and inorganic matter depend on the chemical characteristics of the media in which the bacteria are grown. Media that contain high concentrations of inorganic salts will produce bacteria with higher concentrations of inorganic compounds in the cell mass than will media containing low concentrations of inorganic compounds. This relationship is very important in environmental microbiology since the mineral content of water varies widely. The growth media determine both the types and quantities of inorganic compounds in the bacteria. The inorganic fraction in bacteria in normal media ranges from 5 to 15%, with an average around 10% dry weight. This means that the organic fraction in bacteria will vary from 85 to 95%, averaging 90% dry weight. Chemical analyses of bacteria are made on the dried residue after centrifuging, washing, and oven drying. The major inorganic ions include the various oxides of sodium, potassium, calcium, magnesium, iron, zinc, copper, nickel, manganese, and cobalt, together with chlorides, sulfates, phosphates, and carbonates. The major organic elements include carbon, hydrogen, oxygen, and nitrogen. Although phosphorus and sulfur are part of the organic matter in bacteria, they are measured as part of the inorganic matter.

It has been reported that the dry matter for *E. coli* contained approximately 50% carbon, 20% oxygen, 14% nitrogen, 8% hydrogen, 3% phosphorus, 1% sulfur, 2% potassium, 0.05% each of calcium, magnesium, and chlorine, 0.2% iron, and a total of 0.3% trace elements, including manganese, cobalt, copper, zinc, and molybdenum. A typical aerobic bacterium grown on a single organic compound contained 45.6% carbon, 7.6% hydrogen, 12.1% nitrogen, and 3.0% ash. Oxygen by difference was 31.7%. Analyses of three different bacteria gave ranges from 43.6 to 48.0% carbon, 6.64 to 7.14% hydrogen, 26.8 to 35.4% oxygen, 9.9 to 11.8% nitrogen, and 7.5 to 11.2% ash. These data confirmed that carbon, hydrogen, oxygen, and nitrogen are the main components of the organic fraction of bacteria. The ash or inorganic fraction of the cell mass varies with the media used for growth. Some bacteria require high inorganic salt concentrations for good growth. The salt-loving bacteria *Halobacteria* will definitely have higher ash fractions than indicated for normal bacteria. Typical values for the composition of bacterial cells are listed in Table 1.3.

TABLE 1.3   Typical Bacterial Cellular Elements

Elements	Dry Weight (%)
Carbon	50.0
Oxygen	22.0
Nitrogen	12.0
Hydrogen	9.0
Phosphorus	2.0
Sulfur	1.0
Potassium	1.0
Sodium	1.0
Calcium	0.5
Magnesium	0.5
Chlorine	0.5
Iron	0.2
Other trace elements	0.3

Source: Adapted from Madigan et al. (1984).

TABLE 1.4 Typical Bacterial Cellular Materials

Constituent	Dry Weight (%)
Protein	55.0
Polysaccharide	5.0
Lipid	9.1
DNA	3.1
RNA	20.5
Other (sugars, amino acids)	6.3
Inorganic ions	1.0

Source: Adapted from Madigan et al. (1984).

The chemical analyses of bacteria showed that carbon and hydrogen percentages remain fairly constant while oxygen and nitrogen vary. As the bacteria release ammonia nitrogen, it is replaced by oxygen. The percentage of nitrogen in the cell mass decreases with time, while the percentage of oxygen in the cell mass increases.

Another way to look at bacterial protoplasm is to examine its major chemical compounds. Most of the bacteria protoplasm is protein, about 60% of the organic compounds. The nucleic acids RNA and DNA make up about 25% of the organic compounds. Lipids consist of about 10% of the organic compounds, leaving the remaining 5% as polysaccharides. The general analyses of the organic compounds in bacteria indicate that the total N could be about 14%. Typical values for the composition of bacterial cell materials are listed in Table 1.4.

1.6.2 Macronutrients

The major elements (macroelements), such as C, H, N, O, S, and P, are used in large amounts by microorganisms. The minor elements (microelements), such as K, Ca, Mg, Na, and Fe, are used in smaller quantities, while the trace elements, such as Mn, Zn, Co, Mo, Ni, and Cu, are used in relatively very much smaller amounts. The amount of an element used by a microbe does not correlate with its relative importance; even one used in a trace amount may be essential to the growth or life of a microbial cell.

Carbon to Build Cells Carbon is one of the most important chemical elements required for microbial growth. Microorganisms obtain their carbon for cell growth from either organic matter or carbon dioxide. Carbon accounts for about 50% of the dry weight of any cell; thus all organisms require carbon in some form. Carbon forms the backbone of three major classes of organic nutrients: carbohydrates, lipids, and proteins. These compounds provide energy for cell growth and serve as building blocks of cell material.

Heterotrophs use organic compounds as their major carbon source for the formation of new biomass, and they obtain such organic molecules by absorbing them as solutes from the environment. Autotrophs use carbon dioxide (the most oxidized form of carbon) as their major or even sole source of carbon, and they can live exclusively on relatively simple inorganic molecules and ions absorbed from the aqueous and gaseous environment. The conversion of carbon dioxide to cellular carbon compounds requires a reductive process, which requires a net input of energy. Autotrophic organisms must therefore spend more of their energy for synthesis than do heterotrophs, resulting in generally lower yields of cell mass and growth rates.

Nitrogen to Build Cells   All microorganisms require nitrogen in some form. It is an essential part of amino acids that comprise cell proteins. Nitrogen is needed for the synthesis of purine and pyrimidine rings that form nucleic acids, some carbohydrates and lipids, enzyme cofactors, murein, and chitin. Many prokaryotes use inorganic nitrogen compounds such as nitrates, nitrites, or ammonium salts. Unlike eukaryotic cells, some bacteria (e.g., the free-living *Azotobacter* and the symbiotic *Rhizobium* of legume plants) and some archaeons (e.g., the methanogens *Methanococcus* and *Methanobacterium*) can use atmospheric or gaseous nitrogen for cell synthesis by a nitrogen-fixation process. Some microbes require organic nitrogen compounds such as amino acids or peptides. Some microorganisms use nitrate as an alternative electron acceptor in electron transport.

Phosphorus to Synthesize ATP (Energy Carrier) and DNA   Phosphorus is essential for the synthesis of nucleic acids and ATP. It is a component of teichoic acids and teichuronic acids in the cell walls of gram-positive bacteria as well as a component of various membrane phospholipids.

Hydrogen, Oxygen, and Sulfur   Other elements essential to the nutrition of microorganisms are hydrogen, oxygen, and sulfur. Hydrogen and oxygen are components of many organic compounds. Because of this, the requirements for carbon, hydrogen, and oxygen often are satisfied together by the availability of organic compounds. Free oxygen is toxic to most strict anaerobic bacteria and some archaeons, although aerobic microorganisms use oxygen as a terminal electron acceptor in aerobic respiration. Sulfur is needed for the biosynthesis of the amino acids cysteine, cystine, homocysteine, cystathione, and methionine, as well as the vitamins biotin and thiamine. Reduced forms of sulfur may serve as sources of energy for chemotrophs or as sources of reducing power for phototrophs. Sulfate may serve as a terminal electron acceptor in electron transport.

1.6.3   Micronutrients

Many other essential elements, the microelements and trace elements, are required in smaller amounts than the macroelements by microorganisms in their nutrition. Some of their functions in supporting the growth of microorganisms are summarized in Table 1.5. For example, sodium is required by the permease that transports the sugar melibiose into the cells of the colon bacterium *E. coli*. Sodium is required by marine microorganisms for maintaining cell integrity and growth. Some "salt-loving" prokaryotes, the red extreme halophiles, cannot grow with less than 15% sodium chloride in their environment. Essential elements are often required as cofactors for

TABLE 1.5 Functions of Some Microelements and Trace Elements

Element	Major Functions in Some Microorganisms
Sodium	Enzyme activator
	Transport across membranes
	Maintenance of cell integrity
	Facilitates growth
	Salt form of some required organic acids
Potassium	Cofactor for enzymes
	Maintenance of osmotic balance
Iron	Component of cytochromes, heme-containing enzymes, electron transport compounds, and proteins
	Energy source
Magnesium	Enzyme activator, particularly for kinase reactions
	Component of chlorophyll
	Stabilizes ribosomes, cell membranes, and nucleic acids
Calcium	Enzyme activator, particularly for protein kinases
	Component of dipicolinic acid in bacterial endospores
Cobalt	Component of vitamin B_{12} and its coenzyme derivatives
Manganese	Enzyme activator, particularly for enzymes transferring phosphate groups
Molybdenum	Enzyme activator for nitrogen fixation

enzymes. Because iron is a key component of the cytochromes and electron-carrying iron–sulfur proteins, it plays a key role in cellular respiration. However, most inorganic iron salts are highly insoluble in water. Thus, to utilize this element many microbes must produce specific iron-binding agents called *siderophores*. Siderophores are chelating agents that solubilize iron salts and transport iron into the cell. Many enzymes, including some involved in protein synthesis, specifically require potassium. Magnesium functions to stabilize ribosomes, cell membranes, and nucleic acids and is needed for the activity of many enzymes.

Trace elements, needed in extremely small amounts for nutrition by microorganisms, include manganese, molybdenum, cobalt, zinc, and copper. For example, molybdenum is required by nitrogenase, the enzyme that converts atmospheric nitrogen to ammonia during the nitrogen-fixation process. Manganese aids many enzymes to catalyze the transfer of phosphate groups. Cobalt is a component of vitamin B_{12} and its coenzyme derivatives.

1.6.4 Growth Factor

Some microorganisms have good synthetic capability and thus can grow in a medium containing just a few dissolved salts. The simpler the cultural medium to support growth of a species of microbe, the more complex or advanced is the microbe's nutritional synthetic capability. Thus, the photoautotrophs are the most complex in their nutritional physiology.

Because they cannot be synthesized specifically, organic compounds required in the nutrition of microorganisms are called *growth factors*. Growth factors are needed by an organism as precursors or constituents of organic cell material which cannot be synthesized from other carbon sources. Although growth factor requirements differ from one organism to another, the major growth factors fall into the following three classes: (1) amino acids, (2) nitrogen bases (i.e., purines and pyrimidines), and (3) vitamins. Proteins are composed of about 20 amino acids. Some bacteria and archeons cannot synthesize one or more of these and require them preformed in the medium. For example, *Staphylococcus epidermidis*, the normal resident on the human skin, requires proline, arginine, valine, tryptophan, histidine, and leucine in the medium before it can grow. Requirements for purines and pyrimidines, the nucleic acid bases, are common among the lactic acid bacteria. Vitamins are small organic compounds that make up all or part of the enzyme cofactors (nonprotein catalytic portion of enzymes). Lactic acid bacteria such as species of *Streptococcus, Lactobacillus,* and *Leuconostoc* are noted for their complex requirements of vitamins, and hence many of these species are used for microbial assays of food and other substances. Vitamins most commonly required by microorganisms are thiamine (vitamin B_1), biotin, pyridoxine (vitamin B_6), and cyanocobalamin (vitamin B_{12}). The functions of some vitamins for the growth of microorganisms are summarized in Table 1.6.

TABLE 1.6   Functions of Some Vitamins in the Growth of Microorganisms

Vitamin	Function
Folic acid	One-carbon transfers
	Methyl donation
Biotin	Carboxyl transfer reactions
	Carbon dioxide fixation, β-decarboxylations
	Fatty acid biosynthesis
Cyanocobalamin (B_{12})	Carries methyl groups
	Synthesis of deoxyribose
	Molecular rearrangements
Lipoic acid	Transfer of acyl groups
Nicotinic acid (niacin)	Precursor of NAD^+ and $NADP^+$
	Electron transfer in oxidation–reduction reactions
Pantothenic acid	Precursor of coenzyme A
	Carries acyl groups
Riboflavin (B_2)	Precursor of FMN and FAD in flavoproteins involved in electron transport
	Dehydrogenations
Thiamine (B_1)	Aldehyde group transfer
	Decarboxylations
Pyridoxal–pyridoxamine group (B_6)	Amino acid metabolism (e.g., transamination and deamination)
Vitamin K group; quinones	Electron transport
	Synthesis of sphingolipids
Hydroxamates	Iron-binding compounds
	Solubilization of iron and transport into cell
Heme and related tetrapyrroles	Precursors of cytochromes

1.6.5 Microbial Empirical Formula

The C, H, O, N data provide a reasonable evaluation of the organic fraction of the bacterial protoplasm. Environmental microbiologists have tended to favor the formula using N as unity, whereas bacteriologists have favored the formula using C as unity. Overall, both formulas are identical, making the choice of the specific presentation a personal issue rather than a technical issue. The corrected values of the four primary chemical elements in cell mass are the important values to be used for comparative purposes. Another factor of importance is the use of fractional values of the different elements. There has been a tendency to round off the number of each element to the nearest whole number when using $N = 1.0$.

The most widely used empirical formula for the organic fraction of cells is $C_5H_7O_2N$. About 53% by weight of the organic fraction is carbon. The formulation $C_{60}H_{87}O_{23}N_{12}P$ can be used when phosphorus is also considered. It should be noted that both formulations are approximations and may vary with time and species, but they are used for practical purposes. Nitrogen and phosphorus are considered macronutrients because they are required in comparatively large amounts. Prokaryotes also require trace amounts of metallic ions, or micronutrients, such as zinc, manganese, copper, molybdenum, iron, and cobalt. Because all of these elements and compounds must be derived from the environment, a shortage of any of these substances would limit and, in some cases, alter growth.

For municipal wastewater treatment sufficient nutrients are generally present, but for industrial wastewaters nutrients may need to be added to the biological treatment processes. The lack of sufficient nitrogen and phosphorus is common especially in the treatment of food-processing wastewaters or wastewaters high in organic content. Using the formula $C_{60}H_{87}O_{23}N_{12}P$ for the composition of cell biomass, about 12.2 g of nitrogen and 2.3 g of phosphorus are needed per 100 g of cell biomass.

1.7 MICROBIAL METABOLISM

Metabolism is the sum of biochemical transformations that includes interrelated catabolic and anabolic reactions. Catabolic reactions are exergonic and release energy derived from organic and inorganic compounds. Anabolic reactions (i.e., biosynthetic) are endergonic: They use the energy and chemical intermediates provided by catabolic reactions for biosynthesis of new molecules, cell maintenance, and growth.

Assimilated nutrient substances need to be metabolized. *Metabolism* refers to the totality of organized biochemical activities carried out by an organism. Such activities, usually catalyzed by enzymes, are of two types: those involved in generating energy, and those involved in using energy. Some microorganisms use nutrients absorbed by the cell as the source of energy in a process called *catabolism*, which is the reverse of biosynthesis (anabolism). Catabolism includes all the biochemical processes by which a substrate is degraded to end products with the release of energy. In wastewater treatment, the substrate is oxidized (Davis and Cornwell, 1991). The oxidation process releases energy that is transferred to an

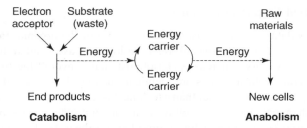

FIGURE 1.9 General scheme of microbial metabolism.

energy carrier that stores it for future use by the bacterium (Fig. 1.9). In catabolism, large molecules are degraded in sequential stepwise reactions by enzymes and a portion of the energy released is trapped in the form of chemical energy. Other microorganisms derive their energy from the trapping of light and also convert it into chemical energy. This chemical energy is then harnessed to do work for the cell. A microorganism must perform many different types of work, such as synthesis of physical parts of the cell, repair or maintenance of cell components, and growth. Some chemical compounds released by catabolism are used by the bacterial cell for its life functions. Anabolism includes all the biochemical processes by which the bacterium synthesizes new chemical compounds needed by the cells to live and reproduce. The synthesis process is driven by the energy that was stored in the energy carrier. Thus metabolism may be viewed as the coupling of energy generation and energy utilization. The types of nutrients and how they are assimilated and fed into the various metabolic pathways for energy production and utilization in microorganisms are introduced in this section.

1.7.1 Catabolic Metabolic Pathways

A catabolic metabolic pathway is a pathway by which organisms obtain energy in a useful form for carrying out biological work involved in protoplasm (organism mass) synthesis. A fraction of the organic molecules taken up by an organism is oxidized enzymatically to CO_2 and water, and a large amount of energy is released. A part of this energy is captured by the organism and is available for performing useful biological work; the part the organism is unable to "capture" is lost as heat to the surroundings.

Microorganisms use a wide variety of chemical compounds as energy sources. Sometimes these compounds are large molecules such as proteins, lipids, or polysaccharides that must first be broken down to smaller molecules before they can be dissimilated or used to supply energy. Microorganisms use enzymes to break down proteins to amino acids, fats to glycerol and fatty acids, and polysaccharides to monosaccharides.

Chemotrophic microorganisms derive energy by a series of consecutive enzyme-catalyzed chemical reactions called a *dissimilatory pathway*. Such pathways serve not only to liberate energy from nutrients but also to supply precursors or building blocks from which a cell can construct its structure.

Although highly diverse in their metabolism, microorganisms such as bacteria do not have individually specific pathways for each of the substances they dissimilate. Instead, a relatively few central pathways of metabolism that are essential to life are found in bacteria and, indeed, in all cellular forms. The ability of bacteria to oxidize a wide spectrum of compounds for energy reflects their ability to channel metabolites from unusual substances into the central metabolic pathways.

The central metabolic pathways are those pathways that provide precursor metabolites, or building blocks, for all of the biosynthetic pathways of the cell. They also generate ATP and reduced coenzymes, such as NADH, that can enter electron transport systems and generate a proton motive force. The most important central metabolic pathways are the Embden–Meyerhof–Parnas pathway (also called the glycolytic pathway), the pentose phosphate pathway, and the Entner–Doudoroff pathway. The latter pathway has been found only among the prokaryotes.

Glycolysis Glycolysis ("splitting of sugar") is the most common dissimilatory pathway, which occurs widely and is found in animal and plant cells as well as in microorganisms. The majority of microbes utilize the glycolytic pathway for the catabolism of carbohydrates such as glucose and fructose. This series of reactions occurs in the cytosol of microbes and can operate either aerobically or anaerobically. Figure 1.10 shows the steps in the glycolytic pathway.

Important features of glycolysis are as follows:

1. The enzyme hexokinase uses the energy of ATP to add a phosphate group to glucose to form glucose-6-phosphate. Similarly, the enzyme phosphofructo-kinase uses ATP to add a phosphate group to fructose-6-phosphate to form fructose-1,6-diphosphate. This six-carbon compound is then split by the enzyme aldolase into two three-carbon moieties, dihydroxyacetone phosphate and glyceraldehyde-3-phosphate. These two compounds are interconvertible by the action of triose isomerase.

2. The oxidation of glyceraldehyde-3-phosphate results in the removal of a pair of electrons by NAD^+ and the addition of a phosphate group to form 1,3-dipho-sphoglyceric acid. This high-energy compound can be used for ATP synthesis by substrate-level phosphorylation. Similarly, the removal of H_2O from 2-phosphoglycerate results in the high-energy compound phosphoenolpyruvate, which can also be used to synthesize ATP by substrate-level phosphorylation.

3. For each molecule of glucose metabolized, two molecules of ATP are used up and four molecules of ATP are formed. Therefore, for each molecule of glucose metabolized by glycolysis, there is a net yield of two ATP molecules.

The overall equation for the glycolytic pathway is

$$\text{glucose} + 2\text{ADP} + 2\text{NAD}^+ + 2P_i \rightarrow 2 \text{ pyruvate} + 2\text{NADH} + 2\text{H}^+ + 2\text{ATP} \quad (1.1)$$

In the absence of oxygen, the electrons removed from glyceraldehyde-3-phosphate can be used to reduce pyruvic acid to lactic acid or ethanol or other products. In organisms having electron transport systems, the electrons can be used to

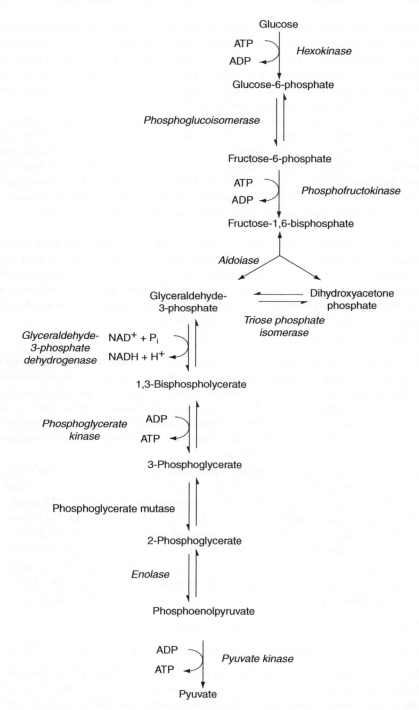

FIGURE 1.10 The glycolytic pathway.

generate a proton motive force. That is, NADH $+ H^+$ can be used to produce energy via oxidative phosphorylation.

The Citric Acid Cycle Although the previous pathways provide energy, some of the critical intermediates, and reducing power for biosynthesis, none provides all of the critical biosynthetic intermediates. Furthermore, the energy yield obtainable from the dissimilation of pyruvate by one of the previous pathways is limited. A significantly greater yield can be attained in the presence of oxygen from the further oxidation of pyruvate to carbon dioxide via the citric acid cycle, also known as the Krebs cycle or the tricarboxylic acid (TCA) cycle. This cycle provides the remaining critical intermediates and large amounts of additional energy.

Although the citric acid cycle in its complete form is found in aerobic microorganisms, even those that do not use oxygen in energy metabolism display most, if not all, of the citric acid cycle reactions. For examples obligate anaerobes typically contain all of the reactions of the citric acid cycle, with the exception of the α-ketoglutarate dehydrogenase. This is a physiological necessity since the critical intermediates for biosynthesis must be supplied for all organisms, irrespective of the way in which they obtain energy. Such a cycle is termed *amphibolic* because it participates in both dissimilative energy metabolism and the production of biosynthetic intermediates.

The sequence of reactions of the citric acid cycle is shown in Fig. 1.11. Pyruvate does not enter this pathway directly; it must first undergo conversion into acetyl coenzyme-A (acetyl-CoA). This reaction is catalyzed by a three-enzyme complex called the pyruvate dehydrogenase complex. This complex contains three types of enzymes: pyruvate dehydrogenase, dihydrolipoic transacetylase, and dihydrolipoic dehydrogenase. The overall reaction is:

$$\text{pyruvate} + NAD^+ + CoA \rightarrow \text{acetyl-CoA} + NADH + H^+ + CO_2 \qquad (1.2)$$

In the citric acid cycle, initially each acetyl-CoA molecule is condensed with oxaloacetic acid to form the 6C citric acid. For every acetyl-CoA entering the cycle:

1. Three molecules of NADH are generated.
2. One molecule of $FADH_2$ is generated in the oxidation of succinic acid to fumaric acid. (FAD is used here because the E_0' volume of the $NAD^+/NADH$ system is not positive enough to allow NAD^+ to accept electrons from succinate.)
3. One molecule of guanosine triphosphate (GTP) is generated by substrate-level phosphorylation. The GTP is energetically equivalent to an ATP (GTP + ADP $\rightarrow$ GDP + ATP).

The overall reaction of the citric acid cycle is as follows:

$$\text{acetyl-CoA (also written acetyl-}S\text{-CoA)} + 2H_2O + 3NAD^+ + FAD + ADP$$
$$+ P_i \rightarrow 2CO_2 + CoASH + 3NADH + 3H^+ + FADH_2 + ATP$$
$$(1.3)$$

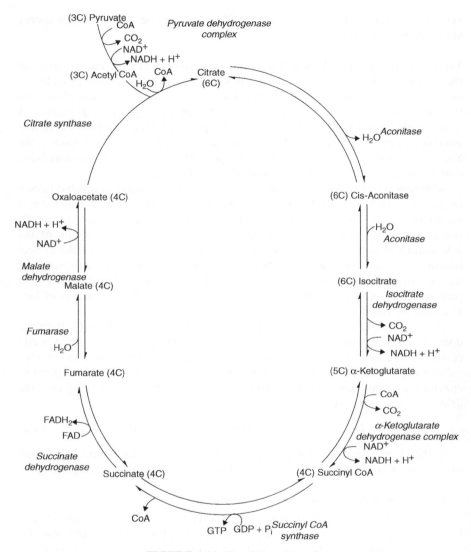

FIGURE 1.11 The citric acid cycle.

Fermentation   A major product in the catabolic pathways discussed above is that of the reduced pyridine nucleotides. A cell contains only a very limited amount of NAD^+ and $NADP^+$. For the central metabolic pathways of dissimilation to continue, a means for continuously regenerating these from the reduced forms must exist. Microorganisms do this either by fermentation or by respiration.

Fermentation is a metabolic process in which the reduced pyridine nucleotides produced during glycolysis or other dissimilatory pathways are used to reduce an organic electron acceptor that is synthesized by the cell itself (i.e., an endogenous electron acceptor). Many microbes utilize derivatives of pyruvate as electron and H^+ acceptors, and this allows $NAD(P)H + H^+$ to be reoxidized to $NAD(P)$. For example, when yeast cells are grown under anaerobiosis, they carry out an alcoholic fermentation. After making pyruvate by glycolysis, they remove a molecule of CO_2 from pyruvate to form acetaldehyde:

$$\text{pyruvic acid} \rightarrow \text{acetaldehyde} + CO_2 \tag{1.4}$$

The acetaldehyde is the acceptor for the electrons of the $NADH + H^+$ produced during glycolysis and becomes reduced to ethanol, thus regenerating NAD^+:

$$\text{acetaldehyde} + NADH + H^+ \rightarrow \text{ethanol} + NAD^+ \tag{1.5}$$

Other microorganisms use different fermentations to regenerate NAD^+. Lactic acid fermentation is a common type of fermentation characteristic of lactic acid bacteria and some *Bacillus* species. For example *Lactobacillus lactis* carries out a lactic acid fermentation by using pyruvic acid itself as the electron acceptor:

$$\text{pyruvate} + NADH + H^+ \rightarrow \text{lactic acid} + NAD^+ \tag{1.6}$$

Just as the alcoholic fermentation is of great importance to the alcoholic beverage industry, the lactic acid fermentation is important for the dairy industry. The many other types of fermentations carried out by bacteria lead to various end products, such as propionic acid, butyric acid, butylene glycol, isopropanol, and acetone. Fermentation is an inefficient process for extracting energy by the cell because the end products of fermentation still contain a great deal of chemical energy. For example, the high energy content of the ethanol produced by yeasts is indicated by the fact that ethanol is an excellent fuel and liberates much heat when burned.

In summary, fermentation is the transformation of pyruvic acid to various products in the absence of a terminal electron acceptor. Both the electron donor and acceptor are organic compounds and ATP is generated solely via substrate-level phosphorylation. Fermentation releases little energy (2 ATP per molecule of glucose), and most of it remains in fermentation products. The latter depends on the type of microorganism involved in fermentation.

Respiration   Respiration is the other process for regenerating $NAD(P)^+$ by using $NAD(P)H$ as the electron donor for an electron transport system. It is much more efficient than fermentation for yielding energy. Not only is $NAD(P)^+$ regenerated, but the electron transport system generates a proton motive force that can be used to power the synthesis of additional ATP molecules. For example, when yeast cells are grown aerobically with glucose, the NADH molecules produced during glycolysis can donate their electrons to an electron transport system that has oxygen as the terminal electron acceptor (aerobic respiration). This system allows not only regeneration of NAD^+ but also the generation of enough of a proton motive force to drive the synthesis of an additional six molecules of ATP. Further breakdown occurs when pyruvic acid is oxidized to acetyl-CoA by pyruvate dehydrogenase.

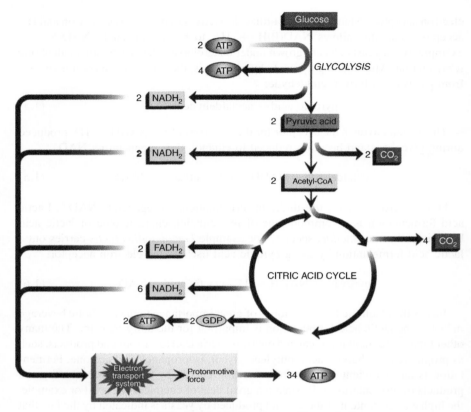

FIGURE 1.12 ATP production by aerobic respiration.

Each of the two molecules of NADH so formed can serve as the electron donor for an electron transport system, creating a proton motive force that can be used for synthesizing six molecules of ATP. Oxidation of the acetyl-CoA by the citric acid cycle yields six more NADH molecules, which can be used to make 18 ATP. In addition, two molecules of $FADH_2$ are produced that can provide enough energy for the synthesis of four molecules of ATP. Two additional ATPs are made by substrate-level phosphorylation. Therefore, the net yield of ATP from complete dissimilation of one glucose molecule is 38 molecules (Fig. 1.12). This is in sharp contrast to the yield of ATP from fermentation when yeast cells are grown anaerobically, where the yield is only two molecules of ATP per molecule of glucose. The complete breakdown of glucose to six molecules of CO_2 results in a net yield of 38 ATP molecules.

1.7.2   Anabolic Metabolic Pathway

Anabolism (biosynthesis) includes all the energy-consuming processes that result in the formation of new cells. It is estimated that 3000 mmol of ATP is required to make 100 mg of dry mass of cells. Moreover, most of this energy is used for protein synthesis (Brock and Madigan, 1991). Cells use energy (ATP) to make building blocks, synthesize macromolecules, repair damage to cells (maintenance energy), and maintain movement and active transport across the cell membrane. Most of the ATP generated by catabolic reactions is used for biosynthesis of biological macro-molecules such as proteins, lipids, polysaccharides, purines, and pyrimidines. Most of the precursors of these macromolecules (amino acids, fatty acids, monosacchar-ides, nucleotides) are derived from intermediates formed during glycolysis, the Krebs cycle, and other metabolic pathways (Entner–Doudoroff and pentose phosphate pathways). These precursors are linked together by specific bonds (e.g., peptide bond for proteins, glycoside bond for polysaccharides, phosphodiester bond for nucleic acids) to form cell biopolymers. This is the pathway by which organisms synthesize protoplasm (construct new cell mass). A fraction of the organic molecules taken up by the organism is modified enzymatically to form part of the biological protoplasm. This synthesis process requires an input not only of organic molecules, but also inorganic molecules [e.g., ammonia (NH_4), phosphorus, and micronutrients], energy, protons, and electrons. The organic components of organism mass are highly complex and very numerous, but principally are proteins, fats (lipids), and carbohydrates. The formation of these compounds (anabolism) follows a wide variety of biochemical pathways too complex to trace.

The primary purpose of the energy reaction is to provide the energy for cell synthesis. The bacteria must synthesize hundreds of different chemical compounds to make a cell. It is not surprising to find that the bacteria use the same basic chemical structures repeatedly, greatly simplifying the synthesis of new cells. It is too difficult to analyze every compound produced in each cell; but it is possible to use total measurements of the organic fraction of bacteria for the synthesis reactions. The primary method for evaluation of synthesis has been to develop an empirical equation of the cell mass from the carbon, hydrogen, oxygen, and nitrogen analyses of bacteria. The techniques for evaluating the empirical formula of bacteria protoplasm have already been presented. It has been found that the bacteria produce the same cell protoplasm regardless of the chemical nature of the substrate, as long as all nutrients are available for normal cell production. The nutrients and the environment determine the overall synthesis reaction. The energy in the cell mass must come from the substrate being metabolized. Since the heat of combustion determination for bacterial cell mass oxidizes nitrogen to nitrogen gas, the heat of combustion values measured are high compared to the energy required by the bacteria to form a unit mass of protoplasm. Most bacteria use ammonia nitrogen as their source of cell nitrogen. Only a few specialized nitrogen-fixing bacteria are able to use nitrogen gas as their source of cell nitrogen. The total energy requirement for the synthesis of bacteria protoplasm will be the energy for synthesis of the cell components plus the energy content of the cell mass produced.

1.7.3 Biomass Synthesis Yields

In the evaluation and modeling of biological treatment systems, we should distin-guish the yield observed and the synthesis yield (or true yield). The biomass yield observed is based on the actual measurements of biomass production and substrate consumption, which are actually less than the synthesis yield because of cell loss concurrent with cell growth.

In full-scale wastewater treatment processes the term *solids production* (or *solids yield*) is also used to describe the amount of VSS generated in the treatment process. The term is different from the synthesis biomass yield values, because it contains other organic solids from the wastewater that are measured as VSS, but they are not biological solids. The synthesis yield is the amount of biomass produced immediately upon consumption of the growth substrate or oxidation of the electron donor in the case of autotrophic bacteria. The synthesis yield is seldom measured directly and is often interpreted from evaluating biomass production data for reactors operating under different conditions. Synthesis yield values for bacterial growth are affected by the following factors: (1) the energy that can be derived from the oxidation–reduction reaction; (2) the growth characteristics of the carbon source; (3) the nitrogen source; and (4) environmental factors such as temperature, pH, and osmotic pressure. The synthesis yield can be estimated if the stoichiometry or the amount of energy produced in the oxidation–reduction reaction is known.

The activated sludge process removes substrate, which exerts an oxygen demand by converting the food into new cell material and degrading this substrate while generating energy. This cell material ultimately becomes sludge, which must be disposed of. Despite the problems in doing so, researchers have attempted to develop enough basic information on sludge production to permit a reliable design basis. A net yield of 0.5 kg mixed liquor VSS (MLVSS) kg^{-1} BOD$_5$ removed could be expected for a completely soluble organic substrate. Most researchers agree that depending on the inert solids in the system and the sludge retention time, 0.40 to 0.60 kg MLVSS kg^{-1} BOD$_5$ removed will normally be observed.

The amount of sludge that must be wasted each day is the difference between the amount of increase in sludge mass and the suspended solids (SS) lost in the effluent.

$$\text{mass to be wasted} = \text{increase in MLSS} - \text{SS lost in effluent} \qquad (1.7)$$

The net activated sludge produced each day is determined by

$$Y_{\text{obs}} = \frac{Y}{1 + k_d \theta_c} \qquad (1.8)$$

$$\text{Px} = Y_{\text{obs}} \, Q \, (S_0 - S) \qquad (\text{kg}/1000 \text{ g}) \qquad (1.9)$$

where Px is the net waste activated sludge produced each day in terms of VSS (kg d^{-1}), Y_{obs} the yield observed (kg MLVSS kg^{-1} BOD$_5$ removed), Q the wastewater flow rate (m^3 d^{-1}), S the soluble BOD$_5$ in aeration tank and effluent (mg L^{-1}), k_d the decay rate of microorganisms (d^{-1}), and θ_c the mean cell residence time (d).

The increase in MLSS may be estimated by assuming that VSS is some fraction of MLSS. It is generally assumed that VSS is 60 to 80% of MLVSS. Thus, the increase in MLSS in Eq. (1.9) may be estimated by dividing Px by a factor of 0.6 to 0.8 (or multiplying by 1.25 to 1.667). The mass of suspended solids lost in the effluent is the product of the flow rate $(Q - Q_w)$ and the suspended solids concentration (X_e).

TABLE 1.7 Typical Bacteria Synthesis Yield Coefficients for Common Biological Reactions in Wastewater Treatment

Growth Condition	Electron Donor	Electron Acceptor	Synthesis Yield
Aerobic	Organic compound	Oxygen	$0.40\,g\ VSS\ g^{-1}\ COD$
Aerobic	Ammonia	Oxygen	$0.12\,g\ VSS\ g^{-1}\ NH_4\text{-}N$
Anoxic	Organic compound	Nitrate	$0.30\,g\ VSS\ g^{-1}\ COD$
Anaerobic	Organic compound	Organic compound	$0.06\,g\ VSS\ g^{-1}\ COD$
Anaerobic	Acetate	Carbon dioxide	$0.05\,g\ VSS\ g^{-1}\ COD$

Typical synthesis yield coefficients are given in Table 1.7 for common electron donors and acceptors in wastewater treatment.

1.7.4 Coupling Energy-Synthesis Metabolism

The bacteria couple the energy-synthesis reactions into a single set of reactions rather than in separate reactions. Substrate metabolism results in a continuous processing of nutrients to create energy for the manufacture of cell mass and the cell mass produced from the use of that synthesis energy. Since the cell mass contains the same amount of energy per unit weight, the energy requirement to produce that unit of cell mass is also constant. It was reported that 62% of the substrate energy was conserved as a cell mass, with 38% being used to produce the energy for synthesis. The data on cell mass yields, based on glucose metabolism, have shown variations in the conversion of glucose and ammonia to cell mass energy ranging from 50 to 70%. A major part of the problem with glucose metabolism is the production of organic storage products in addition to the production of cell mass. Another part of the variation in energy-synthesis relationships can be traced to analytical problems in harvesting and weighing small quantities of bacteria. Still, another part of the problem is related to maintenance energy expended during the growth period. *Maintenance energy*, also termed *endogenous respiration*, is the energy used to maintain cell integrity and depends on the active bacteria mass, time and temperature. The longer the growth period for the bacteria, the greater is the effect of endogenous respiration. The net effect of endogenous respiration is to reduce the proteins contained in the new cell mass.

Close coupling of the energy synthesis–endogenous respiration reactions allows the energy from the endogenous respiration reaction to pass without notice until studies are carried out over long periods under substrate-limiting conditions. Since most bacteriological studies are carried out in excess substrate over short growth periods, endogenous respiration is masked. Temperature also affects endogenous respiration. Endogenous respiration increases as the temperature of metabolism increases. For this reason endogenous respiration has a greater impact on bacteria grown at 37°C than on bacteria grown at 20°C. Additional research is needed on evaluation of the impact of endogenous respiration by bacteria.

Based on 62% energy conversion to cell mass, normal metabolism requires a total of $31.6\,kJ\,g^{-1}$ cell mass produced. The energy requirements for cell synthesis are the same for aerobic metabolism as for anaerobic metabolism. The cell mass contains the same amount of energy, and the synthesis reactions require the same amount of energy to produce a unit of cell mass. The difference between aerobic metabolism and anaerobic metabolism lies in the amount of energy produced under the two environments. Aerobic metabolism produces more energy than anaerobic metabolism from the same amount of substrate metabolized. The net effect is that more cell mass is produced aerobically than anaerobically. Aerobic metabolism of glucose should produce 0.49 g VSS cell mass g^{-1} glucose metabolized. Anaerobic metabolism of glucose to lactic acid should produce only 0.04 g VSS cell mass g^{-1} glucose metabolized.

A major problem with evaluating energy reactions in biological systems is the coupling of the energy reactions with synthesis reactions. The energy reactions do not exist as independent reactions. The thermodynamic data on biologically important organics are not as extensive as for hydrocarbons that have been used in energy systems. Because of problems using heat energy, most energy measurements for biological systems have used Gibbs free energy measurements. Bacteria must follow chemical thermodynamics from both a heat-energy and a free-energy point of view. Fundamental concepts show that heat energy and free energy are related:

$$\Delta H = \Delta G + T \Delta S \qquad (1.10)$$

where ΔH is the change in heat energy, ΔG the change in free energy, T the absolute temperature and S the change in entropy.

In biological aerobic treatment of organic compounds in wastewaters, the two material cycles together constitute the metabolism of the organism and are of paramount importance. This is because one of the principal objectives of wastewater treatment is removal of energy (contained in the organic compounds) from the wastewater. Viewed over the biological treatment system as a whole, this objective is attained biologically in two ways: (1) through energy losses (as heat) to the surroundings resulting from the partial capture of energy in catabolism and the partial loss in the use of this energy for anabolism (both due to inefficiencies in energy transfers), and (2) through transformations of the organic compounds (dissolved or suspended) in the wastewater to organic molecules incorporated in biological protoplasm (anabolism).

1.8 FUNCTIONS OF BIOLOGICAL WASTEWATER TREATMENT

The type of electron acceptor available for catabolism determines the type of decomposition (i.e., aerobic, anoxic, or anaerobic) used by a mixed culture of microorganisms. Each type of decomposition has peculiar characteristics that affect its use in wastewater treatment.

1.8.1 Aerobic Biological Oxidation

From our discussion of bacterial metabolism, you will recall that molecular oxygen (O_2) must be present as the terminal electron acceptor for decomposition to proceed by aerobic oxidation. The bacterial oxidation reactions normally occur in a water environment with oxygen being supplied as dissolved oxygen in the water. These reactions with dissolved oxygen are aerobic reactions. Aerobic metabolism is very important in the environment with the production of the most oxidized form of carbon and hydrogen, as well as yielding the most energy for the bacteria. It should be recognized that dissolved oxygen does not react directly with the organic compound being metabolized in most cases. Oxidation occurs indirectly by removing two hydrogen atoms from the molecule to form a carbon–carbon double bond and adding water across the double bond. The two hydrogen atoms are metabolized through a series of enzyme reactions, ultimately reacting with dissolved oxygen to regenerate the water.

As in natural water bodies, the oxygen is the only terminal electron acceptor used. Hence, the chemical end products of decomposition are primarily carbon dioxide, water, and new cell material (Pelczar and Reid 2003), as shown in Table 1.8. Odiferous gaseous end products are kept to a minimum. In healthy natural water systems, aerobic decomposition is the principal means of self-purification.

A wider spectrum of organic material can be oxidized aerobically than by any other type of decomposition. This fact, coupled with the fact that the final end products are oxidized to a very low energy level, results in a more stable end product than can be achieved by the other decomposition systems.

Glucose has long been used as a simple carbohydrate for bacterial metabolism. Maximum energy is obtained when glucose is oxidized to carbon dioxide and water.

$$C_6H_{12}O_6 + 6O_2 \rightarrow 6CO_2 + 6H_2O \tag{1.11}$$

TABLE 1.8 Representative End Products of Waste Decomposition

Substrates	Aerobic and Anoxic Decomposition	Anaerobic Decomposition
Proteins and other organic nitrogen compounds	Amino acids Ammonia $\rightarrow$ nitrites[a] Alcohols $\rightarrow CO_2 + H_2O$ Organic acids	Amino acids Hydrogen sulfide Methane carbon dioxide Alcohols Organic acids
Carbohydrates	Alcohols $\rightarrow CO_2 + H_2O$ Fatty acids	Carbon dioxide Fatty acids Methane Fatty acids + glycerol
Fats and related substances	Fatty acids + glycerol Alcohols $\rightarrow CO_2 + H_2O$ Lower fatty acids	Carbon dioxide Alcohols Lower fatty acids Methane

[a] Under anoxic conditions the nitrates are converted to nitrogen gas.

In this equation the energy in glucose is transformed by the oxidation reaction to carbon dioxide, water, and released heat energy. A mole of glucose always contains the same amount of energy no matter how it was formed. The same is true of carbon dioxide and water. Thus, the amount of energy released from the oxidation reaction will always be the same.

Bacteria can oxidize many different organic compounds. Various bacteria are able to metabolize alcohols, aldehydes, and ketones to carbon dioxide and water. Short-chain soluble organic compounds are more easily metabolized than long-chain insoluble organic compounds. Straight-chain compounds are metabolized faster than branched compounds. With acclimation bacteria can degrade many substituted organic compounds. The chemical structure of the organic compounds determines how easy or how difficult it is for the bacteria to metabolize the chemicals. Although bacterial metabolism of amino acids results in the production of the reduced form of nitrogen, ammonia, there are aerobic bacteria that can oxidize ammonia to nitrites with the production of energy.

Another group of aerobic bacteria obtain their energy from the oxidation of reduced sulfur compounds. Hydrogen sulfide, H_2S, is the most reduced form of sulfur. Hydrogen sulfide can be oxidized to sulfuric acid:

$$H_2S + 2O_2 \rightarrow H_2SO_4 + heat \qquad (1.12)$$

Sulfur-oxidizing bacteria obtain about $26.5 \, kJ \, g^{-1} \, S$ from reaction (1.12). Although there are bacteria capable of the complete reaction, some sulfur-oxidizing bacteria produce only partial metabolism, stopping at pure sulfur or at thiosulfates. The sulfur-oxidizing bacteria have primarily been classified as *Thiobacillus*.

Iron-oxidizing bacteria are important environmental bacteria, converting soluble ferrous iron, Fe^{2+}, to insoluble ferric iron, Fe^{3+}. Some bacteria convert metallic iron, Fe^0, to ferric iron under aerobic conditions. Energy yield depends on the end products formed. One problem with iron oxidation is that the ferrous iron can be oxidized with dissolved oxygen to ferric iron without the help of bacteria.

Because of the large amount of energy released in aerobic oxidation, most aerobic organisms are capable of high growth rates. Consequently, there is a relatively large production of new cells comparied with other oxidation systems. This means that more biological sludge is generated in aerobic oxidation than in the other oxidation systems.

Aerobic decomposition is the method of choice for large quantities of dilute wastewater (BOD_5 less than $500 \, mg \, L^{-1}$) because decomposition is rapid, efficient, and has a low odor potential. For high-strength wastewater (BOD_5 is greater than $1000 \, mg \, L^{-1}$), aerobic decomposition is not suitable because of the difficulty in supplying enough oxygen and because of the large amount of biological sludge produced. In small communities and in special industrial applications where aerated lagoons are used, wastewaters with BOD_5 up to $3000 \, mg \, L^{-1}$ may be treated satisfactorily by aerobic decomposition.

1.8.2 Biological Nutrients Removal

Biological Nitrification Nitrification is the term used to describe the two-step biological process in which ammonia (NH_4^+-N) is oxidized to nitrite (NO_2^--N) and nitrite is oxidized to nitrate (NO_3^--N). The reasons that nitrification is needed in wastewater treatment are primarily as follows: (1) the effect of ammonia on receiving water with respect to DO concentrations and fish toxicity, (2) the need to provide nitrogen removal to control eutrophication, and (3) the need to provide nitrogen control for water-reuse applications, including groundwater recharge.

Aerobic autotrophic bacteria are responsible for nitrification in activated sludge and biofilm processes. Nitrification, as noted above, is a two-step process involving two groups of bacteria. In the first stage, ammonia is oxidized to nitrite by one group of autotrophic bacteria. In the second stage, nitrite is oxidized to nitrate by another group of autotrophic bacteria. It should be noted that the two groups of autotrophic bacteria are distinctly different.

The initial energy step of nitrification is.

$$2NH_4^+ + 3O_2 \rightarrow 2NO_2^- + 4H^+ + 2H_2O \qquad (1.13)$$

The energy yield is about $22.2 \, kJ \, g^{-1} N$. A second group of aerobic bacteria can oxidize the nitrous acid to nitric acid, the most oxidized form of nitrogen:

$$2NO_2^- + 2O_2 \rightarrow 2NO_3^- \qquad (1.14)$$

Total oxidation reaction:

$$NH_4^+ + 2O_2 \rightarrow NO_3^- + 2H^+ + H_2O \qquad (1.15)$$

Based on the total oxidation reaction above, the oxygen required for complete oxidation of ammonia is $4.57 \, g \, O_2 \, g^{-1} N$ oxidized with $3.43 \, g \, O_2 \, g^{-1}$ used for nitrite production and $1.14 \, g \, O_2 \, g^{-1} \, NO_2$ oxidized. When synthesis is considered, the amount of oxygen required is less than $4.57 \, g \, O_2 \, g^{-1} N$. In addition to oxidation, oxygen is obtained from fixation of carbon dioxide and nitrogen into cell mass.

The energy yield for this reaction is only $7.1 \, kJ \, g^{-1} N$. The second group of bacteria does not obtain as much energy as the first group of bacteria, but that does not diminish their importance. The bacteria that oxidize ammonia to nitric acid are known as *nitrifying bacteria*. The group of nitrifying bacteria that oxidize ammonia to nitrous acid are designated as the *nitroso*-bacteria, called ammonia-oxidizing bacteria; and the group of nitrifying bacteria that oxidize the nitrous acid to nitric acid are designated as the *nitro*-bacteria, called nitrite-oxidizing bacteria. The production of nitrous acid will create problems for the nitrifying bacteria unless there is adequate alkalinity to neutralize the nitrous acid as fast as it is formed. Sodium or calcium bicarbonates are the major forms of alkalinity in the natural environment to neutralize the nitrous acid. If ammonium bicarbonate is the form of ammonia being oxidized, its alkalinity will be destroyed as well as the sodium or calcium bicarbonate alkalinity required to neutralize the nitrous acid. The neutralization reaction that is essential for nitrification is

$$NH_4HCO_3 + 1.5O_2 + NaHCO_3 \rightarrow NaNO_2 + 3H_2O + 2CO_2 \qquad (1.16)$$

The carbon dioxide produced as an end product will depress the environmental pH slightly unless an excess of alkalinity is available to keep the pH from dropping. Since the nitrous acid has been neutralized, there is no need for additional alkalinity for the oxidation of nitrous acid to nitric acid. Nitrifying bacteria use part of the excess carbon dioxide as their source of carbon for cell synthesis. As a net result, the nitrifying bacteria do not compete with the other bacteria for the carbon required for cell protoplasm; but they will compete for oxygen and for nitrogen. The wastewater nitrogen concentration, BOD concentration, alkalinity, temperature, and potential for toxic compounds are major issues in the design of biological nitrification processes. Nitrifying bacteria need CO_2 and phosphorus, as well as trace elements for cell growth.

The aerobic environment in activated sludge systems will stimulate the growth of nitrifying bacteria in the presence of excess NH_3-N. As indicated previously, nitrifying bacteria are autotrophic bacteria capable of obtaining their energy for cell synthesis from the oxidation of NH_3-N. Although there are two major groups of nitrifying bacteria, their overall metabolic activity in activated sludge systems is considered as a single metabolic reaction. Since the end product of the energy reaction is nitric acid (HNO_3), sufficient alkalinity must be available to neutralize the HNO_3 to maintain a suitable pH in the environment for continued growth of the nitrifying bacteria and the carbonaceous bacteria. Like the carbonaceous bacteria the nitrifying bacteria undergo endogenous respiration.

The mixture of carbonaceous bacteria and nitrifying bacteria in activated sludge floc adversely affects the nitrifying bacteria ability to come into contact with DO and NH_3-N for rapid metabolism. Nitrification in conventional activated sludge systems is dependent on the time available for aerobic conditions in the aeration tank.

Biological Denitrification   The biological reduction of nitrate to nitric oxide, nitrous oxide, and nitrogen gas is termed *biological denitrification*. Some microorganisms can use nitrate (NO^-_3) as the terminal electron acceptor in the absence of molecular oxygen. Members of the genera *Alcaligenes, Pseudomonas, Methylobacterium, Bacillus, Paracoccus*, and *Hyphomicrobium* were isolated as part of the denitrifying microbial flora from wastewater treatment plants. Denitrification, the anaerobic respiration with nitrite or nitrate as electron acceptor, is used in wastewater to convert the product(s) of nitrification into gaseous nitrogen compounds (mainly dinitrogen), and thus to remove them from the wastewater. Nitrates yield a little less energy for metabolism than docs dissolved oxygen. Only 83% of the oxidation energy potential in the oxygen in nitrates will be released during the metabolism of nitrates and organic compounds. The cations associated with the nitrates tie up the 17% of the oxidation energy, preventing its use in oxidizing the organic compounds being metabolized. As with DO denitrification in the presence of organic matter results in the synthesis of new bacteria cell mass. Only 83% of the energy contained in the nitrates is available for the bacteria to use for their metabolism. While the metabolism of nitrates is the same as that of DO, the synthesis of new cell mass with nitrates is 83% of the synthesis obtained by bacteria with DO.

The alkaline earth cations normally associated with the nitrates form the corresponding hydroxides that quickly react with carbon dioxide to form the corresponding bicarbonate salts. The 17% of the energy not available to the bacteria is used to produce an equivalent amount of alkalinity. This is why denitrification generates 3.57 mg of alkalinity for every 1.0 mg of nitrate-nitrogen reduced to nitrogen gas. Most of the bacteria that use nitrates for their energy metabolism also can use dissolved oxygen. A general energy reaction indicating organic metabolism with nitrate reduction is

$$\text{organic matter} + \text{NaNO}_3 \rightarrow \text{NaHCO}_3 + 0.5\text{N}_2 + \text{H}_2\text{O} + \text{heat} \qquad (1.17)$$

These nitrate-reducing bacteria have been designated as facultative bacteria, since they can move from aerobic metabolism to anaerobic metabolism and back again, depending on the availability of dissolved oxygen. Because of the higher energy yields obtained with dissolved oxygen, the facultative bacteria always use dissolved oxygen in their metabolism before using nitrates. It is important to notice that the nitrate reduction reaction results in the production of nitrogen gas, not ammonia, as the reduced nitrogen end product. This reaction is very important in the loss of nitrogen from both the aquatic environment and the soil environment. If the bacteria use nitrates as their source of cell nitrogen, they must reduce the nitrates to ammonia for synthesis. Since ammonium ions are usually available in the environment, the bacteria will not have to utilize nitrates as their source of cell nitrogen. Nitrates will be used for cell synthesis only when ammonium ions are unavailable. The bacteria must use additional energy to reduce the nitrates to ammonia. This is energy the bacteria would rather use for additional cell synthesis.

The end products from denitrification are nitrogen gas, carbon dioxide, water, and new cell material. The amount of energy made available to the cell during denitrification is about the same as that made available during aerobic decomposition. As a consequence, the rate of production of new cells, although not as high as in aerobic decomposition, is relatively high. Denitrification is of importance in wastewater treatment where nitrogen must be removed to protect the receiving body. In this case, a special treatment step is added to the conventional process for removal of carbonaceous material. Denitrification is discussed in detail later.

The other important aspect of denitrification is the final clarification of the treated wastewater. If the environment of the final clarifier becomes anoxic, the formation of nitrogen gas will cause large globs of sludge to float to the surface and escape from the treatment plant into the receiving water. Thus, it is necessary to ensure that anoxic conditions do not develop in the final clarifier.

The nitrogen transformations in biological treatment processes are presented in Fig. 1.13. Assimilating nitrate reduction involves the reduction of nitrate to ammonia for use in cell synthesis. Assimilation occurs when $\text{NH}_4\text{-N}$ is not available and is independent of DO concentration. On the other hand, dissimilating nitrate reduction or biological denitrification is coupled to the respiratory electron transport chain, and

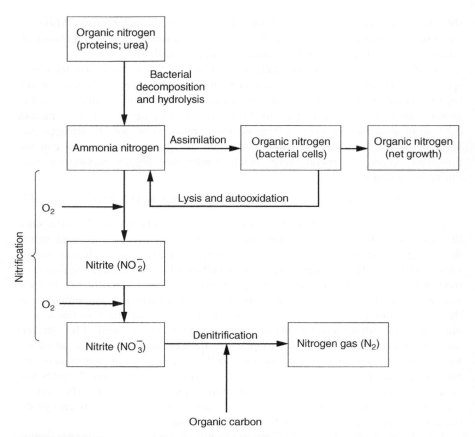

FIGURE 1.13 Nitrogen transformations in biological treatment processes. [From Sedlak (1991).]

nitrate or nitrite is used as an electron acceptor for the oxidation of a variety of organic or inorganic electron donors. Nitrification consumes alkalinity and denitrification generates alkalinity.

Biological Phosphorus Removal   The removal of phosphorus by biological means is known as biological phosphorus removal. Phosphorus removal from wastewater is important to prevent eutrophication because phosphorus is a limiting nutrient in most freshwater systems. Phosphorus removal is therefore an integral part of modern wastewater treatment plants for nutrient removal from municipal and industrial wastewater. Phosphorus can be precipitated by the addition of iron or aluminum salts and can subsequently be removed with the excess sludge. Chemical precipitation is a very reliable method for phosphorus removal but increases significantly the sludge production and thus creates additional costs. Furthermore, the use of chemical precipitants often introduces heavy metal contamination into the sewage and increases the salt concentration of the effluent. Alternatively, phosphorus removal can be achieved by enhanced biological phosphorus removal (EBPR). The principal advantages of biological phosphorus removal are reduced chemical costs and less sludge production compared to that with chemical precipitation.

This process is characterized by cycling the activated sludge through alternating anaerobic and aerobic conditions. The groups of microorganisms that are largely responsible for P removal are known as the *phosphorus-accumulating organisms* (PAOs). These organisms are able to store phosphate as intracellular polyphosphate, leading to P removal from the bulk liquid phase via PAO cell removal in the waste activated sludge. Phosphorus-accumulating organisms are encouraged to grow and consume phosphorus in systems that use a reactor configuration that provides PAOs with a competitive advantage over other bacteria. Phosphorus removal in biological systems is based on the following observations: (1) Numerous bacteria are capable of storing excess amounts of phosphorus as polyphosphates in their cells; (2) under anaerobic conditions, PAOs will assimilate fermentation products (e.g., volatile fatty acids) into storage products within the cells with the concomitant release of phosphorus from stored polyphosphates; and (3) under aerobic conditions, energy is produced by the oxidation of storage products and polyphosphate storage within the cell increases.

Numerous pathways have been proposed to generate the reducing equivalents necessary for anaerobic PAO metabolism. One possibility is that some of the aforementioned pathways exist only in specific microbial groups of PAOs; another possibility is that these organisms could contain multiple or all pathways. Martin et al. (1994) identified the genes necessary for glycolysis and the operation of the full TCA cycle (Fig. 1.14).

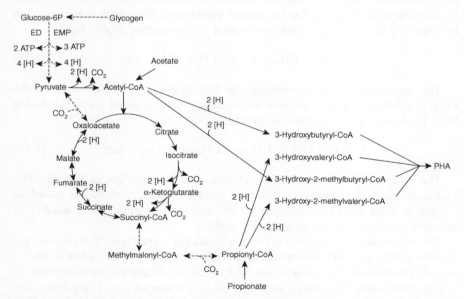

FIGURE 1.14 Proposed anaerobic metabolic pathways of PAOs for the production of reducing equivalents and precursors for PHA synthesis.

In the anaerobic stage, the bacteria responsible for EBPR are supposed to gain energy from polyphosphate hydrolysis accompanied by subsequent P_i release for uptake of short-chain fatty acids and their storage in the form of poly (hydroxyalkanoates) (PHAs). Two different models were postulated for production of the reducing equivalents for this anaerobic metabolism. In the subsequent aerobic stage, PAOs possess a selective advantage compared with other microorganisms that were not able to take up fatty acids under the preceding anaerobic conditions by using the stored PHAs in an otherwise carbon-poor environment. In parallel, PAOs restore their polyphosphate pools by aerobic uptake of available phosphate from the wastewater. After sedimentation in the secondary clarifier, a part of the biomass is recycled to the anaerobic stage and mixed with new wastewater, whereas the excess sludge containing the intracellular polyphosphates is removed from the system.

1.8.3 Anaerobic Biological Oxidation

Not all bacteria can use dissolved oxygen for their energy reactions. Many bacteria use oxygen in chemical compounds for their energy metabolism reactions. Bacteria that obtain energy without using dissolved oxygen in their metabolism are called *anaerobes*. To achieve anaerobic decomposition, molecular oxygen and nitrate must not be present as terminal electron acceptors. Sulfate, carbon dioxide, and organic compounds that can be reduced serve as terminal electron acceptors. The anaerobic bacteria do not obtain as much energy per unit of substrate metabolized as the aerobic bacteria. The amount of energy obtained depends on the total metabolic reactions that the different bacteria create. The anaerobic bacteria oxidize their organic compounds by the same initial pathway that the aerobic bacteria use. They both begin oxidation by removing two hydrogen atoms to create a carbon–carbon double bond:

$$(-CH_2 - CH_3) - H \rightarrow -CH = CH_2 + heat \tag{1.18}$$

The enzymes required for removing the two hydrogen ions are essentially the same in aerobic bacteria as in anaerobic bacteria. Water is added across the double bond to create a more oxidized compound:

$$(-CH = CH_2) + H_2O \rightarrow -CH_2 - CH_2OH + heat \tag{1.19}$$

The difference between aerobic and anaerobic bacteria lies in how the two hydrogen atoms are processed. Whereas aerobic bacteria always use dissolved oxygen to react with the hydrogen atoms, anaerobic bacteria use a number of different reactions with different energy yields.

Sulfates can serve as a source of oxygen for energy metabolism. Sulfate-reducing bacteria (SRB) are strict anaerobes that convert sulfates to sulfides while oxidizing organic compounds. The sulfate-reducing bacteria are unique in their preference for organic compounds that contain large quantities of hydrogen ions. Long-chain fatty acids are the preferred organic compounds for metabolism. SRB can also metabolize short-chain organic acids. Lactic acid is more readily metabolized than glucose, although the two compounds have the same ratios of carbon–hydrogen–oxygen. The oxidation reaction for lactic acid by sulfate-reducing bacteria is given by.

$$C_3H_6O_3 + 1.5SO_4^{2-} \rightarrow 1.5HS^- + 1.5HCO^-_3 + 1.5CO_2 + 1.5H_2O + heat \quad (1.20)$$

The energy yield is about $73.2 \, kJ \, mol^{-1}$ lactic acid. The energy generation for the sulfate-reducing bacteria is quite low compared with that of denitrifying bacteria. For this reason, the sulfate-reducing bacteria are not competitive when nitrates are in the environment. The sulfate-reducing bacteria belong to the *Desulfo* group of bacteria. They are very important in environmental microbiology since the shift from sulfates to sulfides causes a change from an oxidized environment with the sulfates to a strongly reduced environment with the sulfides. Sulfate reduction also produces an increase in alkalinity and prevents loss of sulfides as a gas by keeping the sulfides as the hydrosulfides in proportion to the pH of the environment. All bacteria need sulfur in their protoplasm; but very few bacteria can use sulfates as their ultimate electron acceptor in metabolism. Two important sulfur-containing amino acids, cystine and methione, are synthesized in bacteria protoplasm.

Oxidized organic compounds can be metabolized for energy, producing lower-molecular-weight organic compounds. If nitrates or sulfates are not available, the bacteria will use oxidized organic compounds as their electron acceptors. Metabolism attempts to produce the most oxidized state for the end products. Glucose is metabolized to many different organic acids, depending on the specific bacteria and the environmental conditions in which the bacteria are living. Glucose can be metabolized to lactic acid by the lactic acid bacteria:

$$C_6H_{12}O_6 \rightarrow 2C_3H_6O_3 + heat \quad (1.21)$$

The energy yield for the production of lactic acid is only $87.8 \, kJ \, mol^{-1}$ glucose. The low energy yield for this reaction is created by the high energy content of the lactic acid. Essentially, glucose is simply broken into two smaller molecules with some internal rearrangement of atoms. It has long been known that glucose can be converted into many different end products by specific bacteria, including formic acid, acetic acid, propionic acid, butyric acid, valeric acid, ethanol, propanol, butanol, acetaldehyde, acetyl methyl carbinol, acetone, 2,3-butylene glycol, carbon dioxide, and hydrogen gas. The bacteria simply produce the end products that yield the maximum amount of energy for the minimum amount of substrate metabolized. Metabolism ceases when the energy reactions reach their lowest level, although the organic end products still contain considerable energy that neither the facultative nor any other anaerobic bacteria can utilize.

Metabolic reactions proceed until the oxidants are balanced by the reductants. Cell protoplasm is a major part of the reductants, with the energy for synthesis obtained from the oxidation reactions. The organic end products of anaerobic metabolism would accumulate in the environment if it were not for the acetogenic and methane bacteria. The acetogenic bacteria metabolize the low-molecular-weight alcohols, aldehydes, ketones, and acids to acetic acid, hydrogen, and carbon dioxide. Since hydrogen is reduced and carbon dioxide is oxidized, the acetogenic bacteria can also combine these two end products to form acetic acid. The methane bacteria can take

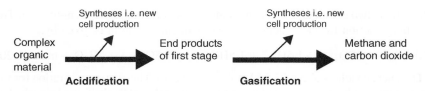

FIGURE 1.15 Simple schematic representation of the anaerobic digestion process.

the end products of the acetogenic bacteria and make methane and carbon dioxide as their end products.

The anaerobic oxidation of organic matter generally is formerly considered to be a two-step process. In the first step, complex organic compounds are fermented to low-molecular-weight fatty acids (volatile fatty acids). In the second step, the organic acids are converted to methane. Methane production is the final step in a cascade of biochemical reactions taking place within anaerobic digesters treating the organic components of sludge and wastewaters. However, no individual microorganism is capable of carrying out all of these reactions independently. Consequently, anaerobic treatment processes are complex ecosystems comprising several diverse microbial guilds that work together in a coordinated manner to convert the organic components to methane and carbon dioxide. Early concepts of anaerobic digestion recognized that the transformation process would involve at least two stages, initial acidification of the complex organic matter followed by gas formation from simpler intermediates (Fig. 1.15).

Today, more and more microbiologists consider that three basic steps are involved in the overall anaerobic oxidation of a waste: (1) hydrolysis, (2) fermentation, and (3) methanogenesis. The three steps are illustrated schematically in Fig. 1.16. The starting point on the schematic for a particular application depends on the nature of the waste to be processed.

Hydrolysis　Hydrolysis is the first step in most fermentation processes. In this step, particulate material is converted to soluble compounds, which can then be hydrolyzed further to simple monomers, which are used by bacteria. For some industrial wastewater treatment, hydrolysis may be the first step in the anaerobic process.

Fermentation　The second step is fermentation (also referred to as *acidogenesis*). In the fermentation process, amino acids, sugars, and some fatty acids are degraded further, as shown on Fig. 1.16. Organic substrates serve as both the electron donors and acceptors. The principal products of fermentation are acetate, hydrogen, CO_2, and propionate and butyrate. The propionate and butyrate are fermented further to produce hydrogen, CO_2, and acetate. Thus, the final products of fermentation (acetate, hydrogen, and CO_2) are the precursors of methane formation (methanogenesis). The free-energy change associated with the conversion of propionate and butyrate to acetate and hydrogen requires that hydrogen be at low concentrations in the system.

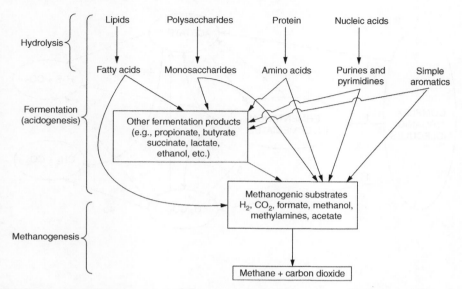

FIGURE 1.16 Anaerobic process schematic of hydrolysis, fermentation, and methanogenesis. [From McCarty and Smith (1997).]

Methanogenesis   Methanogenesis is the third step, which is carried out by a group of microorganisms known collectively as methanogens. Two groups of methanogenic microorganisms are involved in methane production. One group, termed *aceticlastic methanogens,* split acetate into methane and carbon dioxide. The second group, termed *hydrogen-utilizing methanogens,* uses hydrogen as the electron donor and CO_2 as the electron acceptor to produce methane, as shown in Fig. 1.17. Bacteria within anaerobic processes, termed *acetogens,* are also able to use CO_2 to oxidize hydrogen and form acetic acid. However, the acetic acid will be converted to methane, so the impact of this reaction is minor. About 72% of the methane produced in anaerobic digestion is from acetate formation.

As indicated in Fig. 1.17, one group of methane bacteria uses carbon dioxide and hydrogen to produce methane and water:

$$CO_2 + 4H_2 \rightarrow CH_4 + 2HOH + \text{heat} \tag{1.22}$$

This reaction yields 253 kJ mol^{-1} methane produced. This is a very high energy yield for an anaerobic reaction. It depends on the large amount of energy contained in the hydrogen gas. The methane produced by this reaction contains considerable energy that can be released by oxidation. This group of methane bacteria competes with the acetogenic bacteria for carbon dioxide and hydrogen. The efficiency of metabolism favors the methane bacteria. Both groups of bacteria exist together in the environment, indicating that neither organism has a real advantage over the other organism. The second group of methane bacteria uses acetic acid to produce methane and carbon dioxide:

$$CH_3COOH \rightarrow CH_4 + CO_2 + \text{heat} \tag{1.23}$$

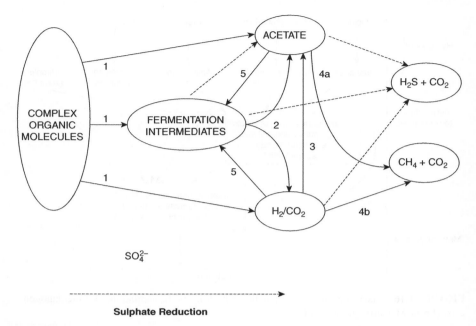

FIGURE 1.17 Flow in anaerobic digesters: 1, hydrolytic/fermentative bacteria; 2, obligate hydrogen-producing bacteria; 3, homoacetogenic bacteria; 4a, acetoclastic methanogens; 4b, hydrogenophilic methanogens; 5, fatty acid–synthesizing bacteria, Dashed lines represent the action of sulfate-reducing bacteria from a wide range of species. [From Ferry (1998).]

The energy yield of this reaction is about $41 \, kJ \, mol^{-1}$ methane produced. The acetate-metabolizing methane bacteria do not obtain as much energy per gram of methane produced as the carbon dioxide–reducing methane bacteria. Since the two groups of methane bacteria do not compete for the same nutrients, they both exist together in the environment.

It has been found the acetate-metabolizing methane bacteria are more sensitive to environmental factors than the hydrogen-metabolizing methane bacteria. As a net result, the acetate-metabolizing methane bacteria are good indicators of the health of the anaerobic environment.

The methane bacteria play a very important role in the final steps of anaerobic metabolism. They complete the stabilization of organic matter with the release of methane gas to the atmosphere. Because only small amounts of energy are released during anaerobic oxidation, the amount of cell production is low. Thus, sludge production is low. Anaerobic fermentation and oxidation processes are used primarily for the stabilization of sludge produced during aerobic and anoxic decomposition and high-strength organic wastes. However, applications for dilute waste streams have also been demonstrated and are becoming more common. Anaerobic fermentation processes are advantageous because of the lower biomass yields and because energy, in the form of methane, can be recovered from the biological conversion of organic substrates.

For treating high-strength industrial wastewaters, anaerobic treatment has been shown to provide a very cost-effective alternative to aerobic processes, with savings in energy, nutrient addition, and reactor volume. Because the effluent quality is not as good as that obtained with aerobic treatment, anaerobic treatment is commonly used as a pretreatment step prior to discharge to a municipal collection system or is followed by an aerobic process to meet discharge standards.

1.8.4 Biological Removal of Toxic Organic Compounds and Heavy Metals

Removal of Toxic Organic Compounds Most of the organic compounds in domestic wastewater and some in industrial wastewaters are of natural origin and can be degraded by common bacteria in aerobic or anaerobic processes. However, some synthetic organic chemicals, termed *xenobiotic compounds*, pose unique problems in wastewater treatment, due to their resistance to biodegradation and potential toxicity to the environment and human health. These compounds belong to several categories, including phenols; aliphatic, polycyclic, and chlorinated aromatic hydrocarbons, phthalates, phosphate esters; ethers; terpenes; sterols; aldehydes; acids; and their esters. Hydrophobic organic compounds are generally removed effectively by wastewater treatment. The removal of organic compounds by biological treatment depends primarily on waste composition, type of treatment, and solids retention time. There is great concern over the impact of toxic industrial pollutants on wastewater treatment processes and upon receiving waters such as lakes and rivers. Organic compounds that are difficult to treat in conventional biological treatment processes are termed *refractory* or *recalcitrant*. In addition, there are naturally occurring substances, such as those found in petroleum products, which are of similar concern.

Since the 1970s, information and knowledge related to the biodegradation of toxic and refractory compounds has increased significantly, based on work with specific industrial wastewaters (i.e., petrochemical, textile, pesticide, pulp and paper, and pharmaceutical industries). In addition, since the 1980s, significant progress has also been made on the biodegradation of organic substances found at hazardous waste sites. Work in both of these fields has expanded knowledge on the capabilities and limitations of biodegradation. Most organic compounds can eventually be biodegraded, but in some cases the rates may be slow, unique environmental conditions may be required (i.e., redox potential, pH, temperature), fungi may be needed instead of prokaryotes, or specific bacteria capable of degrading the xenobiotic compounds may be needed.

Toxic organic pollutants can be removed by biological wastewater treatment processes through the following mechanisms: sorption to sludge biomass and to the added activated carbon, volatilization, chemical oxidation, chemical flocculation, and biodegradation.

Importance of Specific Microorganisms and Acclimation The ability to degrade toxic and recalcitrant compounds will depend primarily on the presence of appropriate microorganisms and acclimation time. In some cases, special seed sources are needed to provide the necessary microorganisms. Once the critical microorganism is present, long-term exposure to the organic compound may be needed to induce and sustain the enzymes and bacteria required for degradation. Acclimation times can vary from hours to weeks, depending on the microorganism population and organic compound. For example, the complete removal of dichlorobenzene (DCB) from a municipal activated sludge plant required three weeks of acclimation. The intermittent addition of DCB resulted in much lower treatment efficiencies. After four weeks of constant exposure to dinitrophenol in a laboratory activated sludge process, seeded from a municipal wastewater plant, dinitrophenol degradation increased from 0 to 98%. When dinitrophenol was not added to the process, the ability to degrade dinitrophenol was eventually lost. Thus, it appears that a relatively constant supply of toxic and recalcitrant organic compounds can lead to better biodegradation performance than can intermittent additions.

The biodegradability of organic compounds is often assessed via substrate disappearance or by BOD or chemical oxygen demand (COD) removal. More accurate approaches include recovery of radiolabeled parent substrate and/or metabolic products, and mineralization products (measuring CO_2 or CH_4 production). Some assay systems for biodegradability tests include (1) measurement of oxygen consumption via manometric and electrolytic systems; and (2) measurement of CO_2 evolution, using infrared or chemical methods.

Biodegradation of organic compounds by wastewater microorganisms is variable and generally low for chlorinated compounds. Exposure of wastewater microbial communities to toxic xenobiotics results in the selection of resistant microorganisms that have the appropriate enzymes to use the xenobiotic as the sole source of carbon and energy. This process is called *acclimation* or *adaptation*. Most microorganisms need a period of acclimation before the onset of metabolism. Prior exposure to the xenobiotic helps reduce the acclimation period.

Biodegradation Pathways   Three principal types of degradation pathways have been observed: (1) the compound serves as a growth substrate; (2) the organic compound provides an electron acceptor; and (3) the organic compound is degraded by cometabolic degradation. In cometabolic degradation, the compound that is degraded is not part of the microorganism's metabolism. Degradation of the compound is brought about by a nonspecific enzyme and provides no benefit to the cell growth. Complete biodegradation of toxic and recalcitrant organic compounds to harmless end products such as CO_2 and H_2O or methane may not always occur; instead, biotransformation to a different organic compound is possible. Care must be taken to determine if the organic compound produced is innocuous, or is just as harmful as, or more harmful than, the initial compound.

Many toxic and recalcitrant organic compounds are degraded under anaerobic conditions, with the compound serving as a growth substrate with fermentation and ultimate methane production. Typical examples include nonhalogenated aromatic and aliphatic compounds such as phenol, toluene, alcohols, and ketones. Some chlorinated compounds could be degraded under anaerobic conditions, including tetrachloroethene,   trichloroethene,   carbon   tetrachloride,   trichlorobenzene, pentachlorophenol, chlorohydrocarbons, and poly chlorinated biphenyes (PCBs). The chlorinated compound serves as the electron acceptor, and hydrogen produced from fermentation reactions provides the main electron donor. Hydrogen replaces chlorine in the molecule, and such reactions have generally been referred to as *anaerobic dehalogenation* or *anaerobic dechlorination*. For example, dechlorination of tetrachloroethene proceeds sequentially with a loss of chlorine in each step via trichloroethene to dichloroethene to vinyl chloride and finally, to ethene.

With proper environmental conditions, seed source, and acclimation time, a wide range of toxic and recalcitrant organic compounds have been found to serve as growth substrates for heterotrophic bacteria. Such compounds include phenol, benzene, toluene, polyaromatic hydrocarbons, pesticides, gasoline, alcohols, ketones, methylene chloride, vinyl chloride, munitions compounds, and chlorinated phenols. However, many chlorinated organic compounds cannot be attacked readily by aerobic heterotrophic bacteria and thus do not serve as growth substrates. Some of the lesser chlorinated compounds, such as dichloromethane, 1,2-dichloroethane, and vinyl chloride, can be used as growth substrates by aerobic bacteria.

A number of chlorinated organic compounds are degradable by cometabolic degradation, including trichloroethene, dichloroethene, vinyl chloride, chloroform, dichloromethane, and trichloroethane. Cometabolic degradation is possible by bacteria that produce nonspecific monooxygenase or dioxygenase enzymes. These enzymes mediate a reaction with oxygen and hydrogen and change the structure of the chlorinated compound. The reaction of the nonspecific oxygenase enzyme with the organic chlorinated compound typically produces an intermediate compound that is degraded by other aerobic heterotrophic bacteria in the biological consortia.

Removal of Heavy Metals Heavy metals sources in wastewater treatment plants include mainly industrial discharges and urban stormwater runoff. Toxic metals may adversely affect biological treatment processes as well as the quality of receiving waters. They are inhibitory to both anaerobic and aerobic processes in wastewater treatment. The removal of heavy metals in biological treatment processes is mainly by adsorption and complexation through the interaction between the metals and the microorganisms. In addition, transformations and precipitation of metal ions are also possible to occur. Microorganisms combine with heavy metal ions and adsorb them to cell surfaces because of interactions between the metal ions and the negatively charged microbial surfaces. Metal ions may also be complexed by the carboxyl groups in microbial polysaccharides and other polymers, or absorbed by protein materials in the biological cell.

A significant amount of soluble metal removal has been observed in biological processes (activated sludge, trickling filter, oxidation ponds), with removal efficiency ranging from 50 to 98%, depending on the initial metal concentration, the biological reactor solids concentrations, and the system sludge retention time (SRT). In anaerobic processes the reduction of sulfate to hydrogen sulfide can promote the precipitation of metal ions as sulfides. For example, adding ferric or ferrous chloride to anaerobic digesters can remove sulfide toxicity by forming iron sulfide precipitates.

In general, the removal of heavy metals by microorganisms may be due to solubilization, precipitation, chelation, biomethylation, or volatilization. The heavy metals may be removed for the following reasons: (1) production of strong acids, such as H_2SO_4, by chemoautotrophic bacteria (e.g., *Thiobacillus*), which dissolve minerals; (2) production of organic acids (e.g., citric acid), which not only dissolve but also chelate metals to form metal–organic molecules; (3) production of ammonia or organic bases, which precipitate heavy metals as hydroxides; (4) extracellular metal precipitation (e.g., sulfate-reducing bacteria produce H_2S, which precipitates heavy metals as insoluble sulfides); (5) production of extracellular polysaccharides, which can chelate heavy metals and thus reduce their toxicity; (6) bacteria (e.g., sheathed filamentous bacteria) that fix Fe and Mn on their surface in the form of hydroxides or some other insoluble metal salts; and (7) biotransformation by bacteria that have the ability to biomethlylate or volatilize (e.g., Hg), oxidize (e.g., As), or reduce (e.g., Cr) heavy metals.

1.8.5   Removal of Pathogens and Parasites

Pathogens and parasites can be removed and/or inactivated in aeration and sedimentation tanks of the activated sludge process. During the aeration phase, environmental (e.g., temperature, sunlight) and biological (e.g., inactivation by antagonistic microorganisms) factors, possibly aeration, have an impact on pathogen and parasite survival. Floc formation during the aeration phase is also instrumental in removing undesirable microorganisms. During the sedimentation phase, certain microorganisms (e.g., parasites) undergo sedimentation, while floc-entrapped microbial pathogens settle readily in the tank. As compared with other biological treatment processes, activated sludge is relatively efficient in removing pathogenic microorganisms and parasites from incoming primary effluents.

1. *Bacteria.* Activated sludge is generally more efficient than trickling filters for the removal of indicator (e.g., coliforms) and pathogenic (e.g., *Salmonella*) bacteria. The removal efficiency may vary from 80% to more than 99%. Bacteria are removed through inactivation, grazing by ciliated protozoa, and adsorption to sludge solids or encapsulation within sludge flocs, or both, followed by sedimentation.

2. *Viruses.* The activated sludge process is the most efficient biological process for virus removal from sewage. It appears that most of the virus particles are solids-associated and are ultimately transferred to sludge. The ability of activated sludge to remove viruses is related to the capacity to remove solids. Thus, many of the viruses found in the effluents are solids-associated. Viruses are also inactivated by environmental and biological factors.

In summary, virus removal and inactivation by activated sludge may be due to the following: (1) virus adsorption to or encapsulation within sludge solids (this results in the transfer of viruses to sludge); (2) virus inactivation by sewage bacteria (some activated sludge bacteria may have some antiviral activity); or (3) virus ingestion by protozoans (ciliates) and small metazoans (e.g., nematodes).

Protozoan cysts, such as *Entamoeba histolytica* and *Giardia* cysts, are not inactivated in the aeration tank of an activated sludge process. They are, however, entrapped in sludge flocs and are thus transferred to sludge after sedimentation. Under laboratory conditions, the activated sludge process removes 80 to 84% of *Cryptosporidium parvum* oocysts. In-plant reduction of *Cryptosporidium* by the activated sludge process varied from 84.6 to 96.8%. The removal efficiency was higher for *Giardia* than for *Cryptosporidium*. However, the removal of protozoan parasites by biological treatment is very variable. The removal efficiency was estimated at 0 to 90% for *Cryptosporidium* and 60 to 90% for *Giardia* cysts in a wastewater treatment plant that incorporates both primary and secondary stages.

Because of their size and density, eggs of helminth parasites (e.g., *Taenia*, *Ancylostoma*, *Necator*) are removed by sedimentation during primary treatment of wastewater and during the activated sludge treatment; thus, they are largely concentrated in sludge.

1.9 ACTIVATED SLUDGE PROCESS

The activated sludge process is the most popular process for treating both domestic and industrial wastewater. It has been used around the world for almost a century, yet is still very much a "black box." Some of the major chemical changes that are taking place can readily be measured (Fig. 1.18), but still, little is known about the microbes that are responsible for these and how their activities are affected by such variables as influent composition, process configuration, and process operation. The application of molecular methods to the activated sludge ecosystem has not only revealed a previously unsuspected level of microbial diversity, but has also questioned many

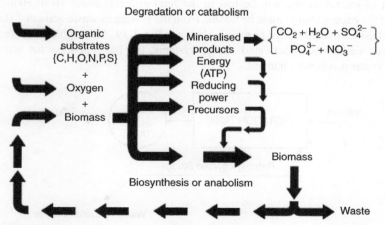

FIGURE 1.18 Main chemical transformations that occur in the activated sludge process.

earlier ideas as to which bacteria were responsible for important processes such as phosphorus removal.

1.9.1 Basic Process

The most widely used biological treatment processes is the activated sludge process, which was developed in England in 1913. It was so named because it involved the production of an activated mass of microorganisms capable of aerobically stabilizing a waste. Many versions of the original processes are in use today, but fundamentally, they are all similar.

Activated sludge is an aerobic, suspended growth system. Activated sludge treatment plants use circular, square, or rectangular aeration tanks. The aeration tank provides a suitable environment for a mixture of bacteria and other microorganisms to aerobically metabolize the biodegradable contaminants in the incoming wastewater. Oxygen is supplied to the microbes by diffused air, mechanical surface aerators, submerged turbines, or impingement jets. The ability of activated sludge to flocculate under quiescent conditions and to separate from the treated wastewaters is an essential characteristic of the activated sludge process. The keys to activated sludge are excess microorganisms, excess dissolved oxygen, sufficient time, and adequate mixing in the aeration tank to promote rapid metabolism of the biodegradable organic compounds. Excess microorganisms can be maintained in the aeration tank as a result of the ability of bacteria to form floc after the nutrients have been metabolized and to settle quickly by gravity under quiescent conditions before being collected and pumped back to the aeration tank as return activated sludge. The continuous stabilization of organic matter in wastewater results in the production of more microorganisms than are needed to maintain the activated sludge at its desired concentration in the aeration tank. The extra microbial production has been termed *excess activated sludge*. The excess sludge must be removed from the activated sludge system to maintain the desired microbial population. A small amount of excess sludge will be lost in the final effluent, about 10 to $30\,\mathrm{mgL}^{-1}$. Most of the excess sludge must be wasted from the system as waste activated sludge.

The basic activated sludge process is shown in Fig. 1.19. Although there have been numerous variations in activated sludge systems, the basic process for activated sludge systems has not changed.

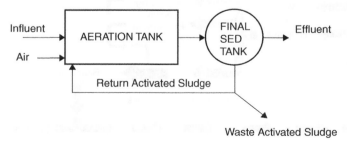

FIGURE 1.19 Schematic diagram of the activated sludge process.

The activated sludge in the aeration tank is called *mixed liquor suspended solids*. The settled sludge returned to the aeration tank is called *return activated sludge* and the sludge removed for wasting is called *waste activated sludge*. The suspended solids carried out in the final effluent are called *effluent suspended solids*.

1.9.2   Microbiology of Activated Sludge

Buswell and Long reported their studies on activated sludge microbiology in 1923. They used daily microscopic examinations of the mixed liquor to obtain gross information on activated sludge organisms. Most of their data dealt with protozoans, since they were easily counted under the microscope. They found that the initial population of small flagellated protozoans and small ciliated protozoans quickly gave way to larger free-swimming ciliated protozoans and stalked ciliated protozoans. As the system became more stable, crawling ciliated protozoans appeared. Only a few rotifers were observed. Nematodes suddenly appeared and then slowly decreased. The overall bacteria were simply classified as zoogleal masses with filamentous bacteria of various types. They thought that both bacteria and protozoans were important in activated sludge.

Bacteria   The overall environment in the aeration tank determines which micro-organisms grow and to what extent they grow. An optimum environment for bacteria includes pH between 7.0 and 8.0; temperature between 20 and 30°C; dissolved oxygen above $1.0\,mg\,L^{-1}$ at all times in all parts of the aeration tank, sufficient agitation to keep the suspended solids in uniform suspension; a readily biodegradable substrate with adequate carbon, nitrogen, phosphorus, and trace nutrients; and adequate time for complete metabolism. The bacteria best able to metabolize the substrate and produce new cell mass will automatically predominate. Normal wastewater load variations will allow the bacteria population to adjust to the changing organic loads. The predominant bacteria will be motile rod-shaped bacteria that can metabolize the maximum amount of organic contaminants to the greatest extent.

All types of aerobic bacteria will grow to the extent that they can obtain nutrients. If the environment is changed, the bacteria predomination will change. It is important to recognize that the only way to change the bacteria predomination in a given activated sludge system is to change the environment in the aeration tank.

Activated sludge treating municipal wastewaters will have bacteria acclimated to proteins, carbohydrates, and lipids. The relative population of acclimated bacteria will depend upon the rate of addition of the three groups of organic compounds. The treatment of unusual organic compounds in industrial wastewaters can pose a challenge in accumulating the desired acclimated bacteria for efficient treatment. In addition to providing a good environment in the aeration tank, it is important to maintain the specific bacteria necessary for metabolism of the industrial contaminants.

The bacteria in activated sludge are capable of metabolizing most organic compounds found in nature. The few complex organic compounds that cannot be metabolized in a reasonable time period are considered to be nonbiodegradable.

Lignin and bacteria polysaccharides are two complex organic compounds that cannot be metabolized in activated sludge systems in a reasonable period of time.

The growth of filamentous bacteria is normal in activated sludge and will not be a problem unless the filamentous bacteria population increases sufficiently to adversely affect the settling rate of the activated sludge. Excessive growth of filamentous bacteria will cause activated sludge to bulk. Bulking sludge is light, fluffy, and slow to flocculate and settle in the final sedimentation tanks. Filamentous bacteria are able to predominate over the normal bacteria when oxygen is limiting, in high-carbohydrate wastewaters, under nitrogen limitation, at low pH, and in excessively long SRT systems. About 95% of the filamentous bulking problems in activated sludge are the result of an inadequate oxygen supply during stabilization of the organic compounds in wastewaters.

It has been proposed that an anaerobic selector be used to prevent the growth of filamentous bacteria. With the anaerobic selector, the incoming wastewaters and the return activated sludge are mixed without aeration to allow the facultative bacteria to begin to grow under anaerobic conditions. If the filamentous bacteria are strict aerobes, they will not grow and will continue to die off under anaerobic conditions.

The total aerobic bacterial counts in standard activated sludge are on the order of 10^8 CFU/mg of sludge. When using culture-based techniques, it was found that the major genera in the flocs are *Zooglea, Pseudomonas, Flavobacterium, Alcaligenes, Achromobacter, Corynebacterium, Comomonas, Brevibacterium, Acinetobacter,* and *Bacillus* spp., as well as filamentous microorganisms. Some examples of filamentous microorganisms are the sheathed bacteria (e.g., *Sphaerotilus*) and the gliding bacteria (e.g., *Beggiatoa, Vitreoscilla*), which are responsible for sludge bulking. Table 1.9 displays some bacterial genera found in standard activated sludge using culture-based techniques. The majority of the bacterial isolates were identified as *Comamonas–Pseudomonas* species.

TABLE 1.9 Distribution of Aerobic Heterotrophic Bacteria in Standard Activated Sludge

Genus or Group	% Total Isolates
Comamonas–Pseudomonas	50.0
Alcaligenes	5.8
Pseudomonas (fluorescent group)	1.9
Paracoccus	11.5
Unidentified (gram-negative rods)	1.9
Aeromonas	1.9
Flavobacterium–Cytophaga	13.5
Bacillus	1.9
Micrococcus	1.9
Coryneform	5.8
Arthrobacter	1.9
Aureobacterium–Microbacterium	1.9

The cocci referred to as the "G-bacteria" and often seen in activated sludge systems in large numbers are phylogenetically diverse and contain mainly novel gram-positive and gram-negative bacteria. They are seen microscopically as tetrads or aggregates in activated sludge. They dominate in systems with poor phosphorus removal because they outcompete phosphorus-accumulating organisms by accumulating polysaccharides instead of polyphosphates. Two strains of G-bacteria were identified as *Tetracoccus cechii* and belong to the alpha group of proteobacteria. The general understanding of their physiology is poor, so their role in EBPR plants is still not certain. All seem to possess an ability to synthesize intracellular storage polymers, but the conditions affecting their production await clarification. It is likely that there are many more G-bacteria in activated sludge systems.

Zoogloea are exopolysaccharide-producing bacteria that produce typical finger-like projections and are found in wastewater and other organically enriched environments. These projections consist of aggregates of *Zooglea* cells surrounded by a polysaccharide matrix. They are found in various stages of wastewater treatment, but their numbers comprise only 0.1 to 1% of the total bacterial numbers in the mixed liquor.

Activated sludge flocs also harbor autotrophic bacteria such as nitrifiers (e.g., *Nitrosomonas, Nitrobacter*), which convert ammonium to nitrate. Nitrifying bacteria use carbon dioxide as their primary source of cell carbon. The growth of nitrifying bacteria is much slower than the heterotrophic bacteria in activated sludge systems. Although the only real competition between the nitrifying bacteria and the heterotrophic bacteria is for DO, the greater growth of heterotrophic bacteria limits the ability of the nitrifying bacteria to obtain nutrients. Dense floc keeps the nitrifying bacteria from the necessary nutrients for rapid growth. The complete nitrification requires a SRT value in aeration of 3 to 5 days at 20°C.

Fungi Activated sludge does not usually favor the growth of fungi, although some fungal filaments are observed in activated sludge flocs. Fungi may grow abundantly under specific conditions of low pH, toxicity, and nitrogen-deficient wastewater. The predominant genera found in activated sludge are *Geotrichum, Penicillium, Cephalosporium, Cladosporium,* and *Alternaria.* Sludge bulking may result from the abundant growth of *Geotrichum candidum*, which is favored by low pH from acid wastes. Fungi are also capable of carrying out nitrification and denitrification, suggesting that they could play a role in nitrogen removal in wastewater under appropriate conditions. Some advantages of a fungi-based treatment system are the ability of fungi to carry out nitrification in a single step, and their greater resistance to inhibitory compounds than bacteria.

Protozoans Protozoans are significant predators of bacteria in activated sludge as well as in natural aquatic environments. Protozoans were observed regularly in activated sludge, there was a clear succession of protozoans during the development of activated sludge treating municipal wastewater. The initial growth of amoeboid protozoans and small flagellated protozoans gave way to small free-swimming ciliated protozoans and then, to larger free-swimming ciliated protozoans. Finally, stalked ciliated protozoans and crawling ciliated protozoans predominated as the activated sludge reached normal operating conditions.

Ciliates appear to be the most abundant protozoans in activated sludge plants. They are subdivided into free, creeping, and stalked ciliates. Free ciliates feed on free-swimming bacteria. The most important genera found in activated sludge are *Chilodonella, Colpidium, Blepharisma, Euplotes, Paramecium, Lionotus, Trachelophyllum,* and *Spirostomum.* Creeping ciliates graze on bacteria on the surface of activated sludge flocs. Two important genera are *Aspidisca* and *Euplotes.* Stalked ciliates are attached by their stalk to the flocs. The predominant stalked ciliates are *Vorticella, Carchesium, Opercularia,* and *Epistylis.*

The growth of protozoans in activated sludge systems is aerobic, requiring positive DO levels in the aeration tanks. The protozoans obtain their energy for cell synthesis by eating the biodegradable nutrients contained in bacteria. The lack of protozoans in the mixed liquor suspended solids (MLSS) is a clear sign of toxicity. Toxicity can be created by toxic chemicals in the incoming wastewater or by a lack of DO. The activated sludge environment allows all of the different groups of protozoans to survive at their appropriate level. When the organic level is high and the residual DO is low, the flagellated protozoans will predominate over the other groups. As the available nutrients decrease, the predomination of protozoans shifts accordingly. The activated sludge system is a dynamic system with all of the microorganisms shifting as the environment changes. Routine microscopic examination of the protozoans in the MLSS on a daily basis is good practice for activated sludge operators. By recording the relative numbers of each group of protozoans and the structure of the bacteria floc, the operator can see how the change in microorganisms affects the activated sludge system.

Some operation conditions heavily influence the microfauna assemblage. The dilution rate of the system is important, because the species that cannot reproduce quickly enough to compensate for such a loss will be removed from the system. Thus, activated sludge with fast flow rates will tend to favor species with rapid rates of reproduction, usually the smaller protista, such as heterotrophic flagellates or small ciliates ($< 30\,\mu m$) Activated sludge with slow flow rates host a greater diversity of organisms, including small metazoans which have slow rates of reproduction. Overloaded systems lead to a higher demand for dissolved oxygen, and low levels of free oxygen will favor those heterotrophic flagellates, amoebas, and small ciliates (Fig. 1.20). When the organic loading decreases, the diversity of organisms increases.

In wastewater treatment, protozoans play a major role, but the full extent of their contribution is not fully quantified. Their major role is probably in maintaining a slime layer in trickling filter systems and in aiding flocculation in activated sludge systems.

Rotifers   Rotifers are metazoans (i.e., multicellular organisms) with sizes varying from 100 to 500 mm. Their body, anchored to a floc particle, frequently "stretches out" from the floc surface. The rotifers found in wastewater treatment plants belong to two main orders: Bdelloidea (e.g., *Philodina* spp., *Habrotrocha* spp.) and Monogononta (e.g., *Lecane* spp., *Notommata* spp.).

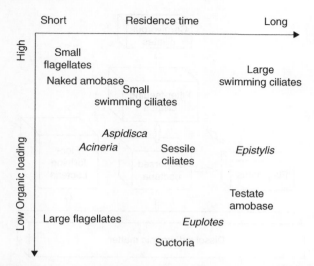

FIGURE 1.20 Effect of organic loading and SRT on the protozoan assemblage in activated sludge.

The role of rotifers in activated sludge is twofold: (1) They help remove freely suspended bacteria (i.e., nonflocculated bacteria) and other small particles and contribute to the clarification of wastewater, and they are also capable of ingesting *Cryptosporidium* oocysts in wastewater and can thus serve as vectors for the transmission of this parasite; and (2) they contribute to floc formation by producing fecal pellets surrounded by mucus. The presence of rotifers at later stages of activated sludge treatment is due to the fact that these animals display a strong ciliary action that helps in feeding on reduced numbers of suspended bacteria (their ciliary action is stronger than that of protozoans).

The complex metabolism and the large size of rotifers allows them to eat the bacteria on the surface of floc particles and even some small floc particles. Rotifers require 3 to 4 mgL^{-1} DO for good growth. For this reason the presence of rotifers in MLSS samples indicates an activated sludge effluent with few soluble biodegradable organic compounds.

Nematodes and Other Worms Other higher animals found in activated sludge include nematodes and round worms. Nematodes are complex animals that consume large numbers of bacteria to survive. Although nematodes are seen in various activated sludge systems, nematodes do not normally occur in activated sludge systems. Nematodes are very motile worms, breaking up floc particles with their rapid thrashing motion. Occasionally, bristle worms will be seen in activated sludge. For the most part, worms are not normally found in activated sludge and indicate that the environment is not normal.

In the aeration tank of biological processes, a true trophic web is established. A simplified diagram is illustrated in Fig. 1.21. The growth of decomposers, prevalently

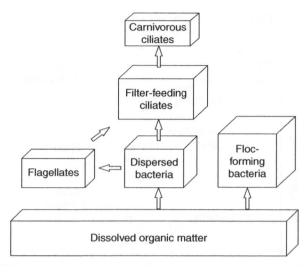

FIGURE 1.21 Simplified diagram of a true trophic web in activated sludge.

heterotrophic bacteria, depends on the quality and quantity of dissolved organic matter in the mixed liquor. For predators, on the other hand, growth depends on the available prey. Dispersed bacteria are thus food for heterotrophic flagellates and bacterivorous ciliates, which, in turn, become the prey of carnivorous organisms. The relationships of competition and predation create oscillations and successions of populations until dynamic stability is reached. This is strictly dependent on plant management choices based on design characteristics aimed at guaranteeing optimum efficiency. Although the ciliates are widely distributed, and many species are able to tolerate precarious environmental conditions, the particular conditions found in sewage treatment processes limit their presence to a restricted number of species.

1.9.3 Biochemistry of Activated Sludge

Basic biochemical reactions produced by the bacteria in activated sludge follow a common reaction pattern with carbohydrates, proteins, lipids and similar organic compounds being oxidized to organic acids before being oxidized to carbon dioxide and water plus ammonia from proteins. The purpose of bacteria metabolism is to yield energy for the synthesis of new cells. The energy reactions are closely coupled with the synthesis reactions. A new cell mass is generated as quickly as energy is produced. It is not surprising that the primary intermediates in the energy reactions, acetate and formate, are the primary intermediates in the synthesis reactions.

It is important to recognize that the biochemistry of activated sludge is the same as the biochemistry of pure cultures of bacteria and pure cultures of protozoans and higher animals. The basic difference is that activated sludge is a mixture of bacteria, protozoans, and higher animals, with the most efficient microorganisms predominating in the activated sludge environment. Much of the biochemical research on pure cultures has applications in activated sludge systems. However, we must be careful in translating the data from the field of microbiology to the field of biological wastewater treatment.

1.9.4 Main Problems in the Activated Sludge Process

Sludge bulking is one of the major problems affecting biological wastewater treatment. There are several types of problems regarding solid separation in activated sludge. These problems are summarized in Table 1.10.

Filamentous Bulking Bulking is a problem consisting of slow settling and poor compaction of solids in the clarifier of an activated sludge system. Filamentous bulking is usually caused by the excessive growth of filamentous microorganisms in activated sludge. Filamentous microorganisms are normal components of the activated sludge flocs. Their overgrowth may be due to one or a combination of the following factors: (1) wastewater composition: high-carbohydrate wastes (e.g., brewery and corn wet-milling industries) appear to be conducive to sludge bulking; (2) substrate concentration [food microorganism (F/M) ratio]: low substrate concentration (i.e., low F/M ratio) appears to be the most prevalent cause of filamentous bulking; (3) pH: the optimum pH in the aeration tank is 7 to 7.5, and pH values below 6.0 may favor the growth of fungi (e.g., *Geotrichum, Candida, Trichoderma*) and cause filamentous bulking; (4) sulfide concentration: high sulfide concentration in the aeration tank causes the overgrowth of sulfur filamentous bacteria such as *Thiothrix and Beggiatoa*; (5) dissolved oxygen level: the growth of certain filamentous bacteria (e.g., *Sphaerotilus natans, Haliscomenobacter hydrossis*) is favored by relatively low dissolved oxygen levels in the aeration tank; (6) nutrient deficiency: deficiencies in nitrogen, phosphorus, iron, or trace elements may cause bulking; and (7) temperature: increased temperature supports the growth of filamentous bacteria associated with low dissolved oxygen concentrations.

Foaming/Scum Formation Foaming is a common problem encountered in many wastewater treatment plants. This problem is due to the proliferation of *Gordonia* and *Microthrix* in aeration tanks of activated sludge units. The following are types of foams and scums that are found in activated sludge (Jenkins et al. 1984): (1) undegraded surface-active organic compounds; (2) poorly biodegradable detergents, which produce white foams; (3) scums due to rising sludge resulting from denitrification in the clarifier; and (4) brown scums due to excessive growth of *Actinomycetes*.

Scum formation in activated sludge plants causes several problems: (1) excess scum can overflow into walkways and cause slippery conditions, leading to hazardous situations for plant workers; (2) excess scum may pass into activated sludge effluent, resulting in increased BOD and suspended solids in the effluent; (3) foaming causes problems in anaerobic digesters; (4) foaming can produce nuisance odors,

TABLE 1.10   Causes and Effects of Activated Sludge Separation Problems

Problem	Cause	Effect
Dispersed growth	Microorganisms do not form flocs but are dispersed, forming only small clumps or single cells.	Turbid effluent; no zone settling of sludge.
Slime (jelly) viscous bulking (also possibly referred to as nonfilamentous resulting bulking)	Microorganisms are present in large amounts of extracellular slime.	Reduced settling and compaction rates; virtually no solids separation in severe cases in overflow of sludge blanket from secondary clarifier.
Pin floc (or pinpoint floc)	Small, compact, weak, roughly spherical flocs are formed, the larger of which settle rapidly; smaller aggregates settle slowly.	Low sludge volume index (SVI) and a cloudy, turbid effluent.
Bulking	Filamentous organisms extend from flocs into the bulk solution and interfere with compaction and settling of activated sludge.	High SVI; very clear supernatant.
Rising sludge (blanket rising)	Denitrification in secondary clarifier releases poorly soluble N_2 gas, which attaches to activated sludge flocs and floats them to the secondary clarifier surface.	A scum of activated sludge forms on the surface of the secondary clarifier.
Foaming/scum formation	Caused by (1) nondegradable surfactants and (2) the presence of *Nocardia* spp. and sometimes (3) the presence of *Microthrix parvicella*.	Foams float large amounts of activated sludge solids to the surface of treatment units; foam accumulates and putrefies; solids can overflow into secondary effluent or onto walkways.

Source: Adapted from Jenkins et al. (1984).

especially in warm climates; and (5) potential infection of wastewater workers with opportunistic pathogenic *actinomycetes*, such as *Nocardia asteroides*.

Foaming is associated primarily with the mycolic acid–containing *Actinomycetes* group, which belongs to the family Nocardiaceae. Genera from this group that have been observed in foams are *Gordonia* (*G. amarae*, formerly *Nocardia amarae*),

Nocardia (*N. asteroides*, *N. caviae*, *N. pinensis*), *Skermania piniformis* (formerly known as *Nocardia pinensis*), *Tsukamurella*, and *Rhodococcus*. There is a relationship between foam-causing organisms and the initiation and stability of foam in activated sludge. FISH (fluorescence in situ hybridization) can detect mycolic acid–containing *Actinomycetes* (mycolata) Foam microorganisms use several growth substrates, varying from sugars to high-molecular-weight polysaccharides, proteins, and aromatic compounds.

The causes and mechanism of foam production are not well understood. Some possible mechanisms are the following: (1) gas bubbles produced by aeration or metabolism (e.g., N_2) may assist in flotation of foam microorganisms; (2) the hydrophobic nature of cell walls of foam microorganisms aids their transport to the air-water interface; (3) biosurfactants produced by foam microorganisms assist in foam formation; (4) foams are associated with relatively long retention times, warm temperatures, and with wastewaters rich in fats.

Numerous measures for controlling foams in activated sludge have been proposed as follows: (1) chlorination of foams (chlorine sprays) or return activated sludge; (2) increase in sludge wasting; (3) use of biological selectors; (4) reducing air flow in the aeration basin; (5) reduction in pH, and oil and grease levels; (6) addition of anaerobic digester supernatant to wastewater; (7) water sprays to control foam buildup; (8) antifoam agents, iron salts, and polymers; (9) physical removal of the foam; (10) use of antagonistic microflora; and (11) potential use of actinophages (i.e., actinomycete-lysing phage).

1.10 SUSPENDED- AND ATTACHED-GROWTH PROCESSES

Biological treatment processes are typically divided into two categories: suspended-growth systems and attached-growth systems. Suspended systems are more commonly referred to as activated-sludge processes, of which several variations and modifications exist. Attached-growth systems differ from suspended-growth systems in that microorganisms attached themselves to a medium, which provides an inert support. Trickling filters and rotating biological contactors are most common forms of attached-growth systems. The definitions of treatment processes used for biological wastewater treatment are listed in Table 1.11.

1.10.1 Suspended-Growth Processes

In suspended-growth processes, the microorganisms responsible for treatment are maintained in liquid suspension by appropriate mixing methods. The most common suspended-growth process used for municipal wastewater treatment is the activated-sludge process. Many suspended growth processes used in municipal and industrial wastewater treatment are operated with a positive dissolved oxygen concentration (aerobic), but applications exist where suspended-growth anaerobic (no oxygen present) reactors are used, such as for high-organic-concentration industrial wastewaters and organic sludge.

TABLE 1.11 Definitions of Treatment Processes Used for Biological Wastewater Treatment

Term	Definition
Suspended-growth processes	Biological treatment processes in which the microorganisms responsible for the conversion of the organic matter or other constituents in the wastewater to gases and cell tissue are maintained in suspension within the liquid.
Attached-growth processes	Biological treatment processes in which the microorganisms responsible for the conversion of the organic matter or other constituents in the wastewater to gases and cell tissue are attached to some inert medium, such as rocks, slag, or specially designed ceramic or plastic materials. Attached-growth treatment processes are also known as fixed-film processes.
Combined processes	Term used to describe combined processes (e.g., combined suspended- and attached-growth processes).

In the aeration tank, contact time is provided for mixing and aerating influent wastewater with the microbial suspension, generally referred to as mixed liquor suspended solids or mixed liquor volatile suspended solids. Mechanical equipment is used to provide the mixing and transfer of oxygen into the process.

The mixed liquor then flows to a clarifier, where the microbial suspension is settled and thickened. The settled biomass, described as *activated sludge* because of the presence of active microorganisms, is returned to the aeration tank to continue biodegradation of the influent organic material. A portion of the thickened solids is removed daily or periodically, as the process produces excess biomass that would accumulate along with the nonbiodegradable solids contained in the influent wastewater. If the accumulated solids are not removed, they will eventually find their way to the system effluent.

An important feature of the activated sludge process is the formation of floc particles, ranging in size from 50 to 200 mm, which can be removed by gravity settling, leaving a relatively clear liquid as the treated effluent. Typically, greater than 99% of the suspended solids can be removed in the clarification step. The characteristics and thickening properties of the flocculent particles will affect the clarifier design and performance.

1.10.2 Attached-Growth Processes

In an attached-growth treatment process, a biofilm consisting of microorganisms, particulate material, and extracellular polymers is attached and covers the support packing material, which may be plastic, rock, or other material. In attached-growth processes, the microorganisms responsible for the conversion of organic material or nutrients are attached to an inert packing material. The organic material and nutrients are removed from the wastewater flowing past the attached growth, also known as a *biofilm.* Packing materials used in attached growth processes include rock, gravel, slag, sand, redwood, and a wide range of plastic and other synthetic materials. Attached-growth processes can also be operated as aerobic or anaerobic processes. The packing material can be submerged completely in liquid or not submerged, with air or gas space above the biofilm liquid layer.

The most common aerobic attached-growth process used is the trickling filter, in which wastewater is distributed over the top area of a vessel containing nonsubmerged packing material. Historically, rock was used most commonly as the packing material for trickling filters, with typical depths ranging from 1.25 to 2 m. Most modern trickling filters vary in height from 5 to 10 m and are filled with a plastic packing material for biofilm attachment. Air circulation provides oxygen for the microorganisms growing as an attached biofilm. Influent wastewater is distributed over the packing and flows as a nonuniform liquid film over the attached biofilm. Excess biomass sloughs from the attached growth periodically and clarification is required for liquid/solids separation to provide an effluent with an acceptable suspended solids concentration. The solids are collected at the bottom of the clarifier and removed for waste-sludge processing.

1.10.3 Hybrid Systems

The optimal growth conditions differ for each type of microorganism involved in biological treatment (nitrifiers, heterotrophs, etc.), and several compromises have to be made to enable all the bacteria to achieve as high a degree of activity as possible. The use of hybrid systems can help to achieve that degree of activity. Hybrid systems can be defined by two types of processes: systems that use (1) a biofilm reactor, usually a trickling filter (TF), and an activated sludge process in series, or (2) a biomass support system (fixed or mobile) immersed in an activated sludge reactor (Wang et al. 1987)

Secondary treatment processes combining fixed growth (trickling filter) and suspended growth (activated sludge) systems in series are popular. These processes offer simplicity of operation and process stability of fixed-film processes with the high-quality effluent associated with suspended-growth processes, and they may also offer economic advantages in comparison to other treatment options. Besides this stable performance, sludge with good settling properties is produced with those processes (Harrison et al. 1999).

Biomass support systems consist of immersing various types of support media in an activated sludge reactor to favor the growth of fixed bacteria. The support can be fixed in the reactor or can consist of mobile media such as foam pads and small carriers. These hybrid systems should allow a reduction in the aeration tank volume following the introduction of biomass support to meet a certain objective, and thus an increase in the treatment system stability and performance (Gebara 2005). The main advantages of these systems are improved nitrification and an increase in sludge settleability (Wanner et al., 2002; Muller 1986). These types of hybrid systems are used primarily for the up-gradation of activated sludge systems, either to increase the effective biomass (higher treatment capacity) or to implement nitrification.

1.10.4   Comparison Between Suspended- and Attached-Growth Systems

It is important to make a comparison between suspended- and attached-growth processes. The main characteristics of both types of processes are given in Table 1.12.

To summarize briefly the difference between the two types of processes: Fixed-film processes (e.g., trickling filter and rotating biological contactor) seem to be less efficient than suspended-growth processes (e.g., activated sludge), but they are more stable. The main difficulty with AS is to grow a biomass that will separate well. Attached microorganisms possess some advantageous properties compared to

TABLE 1.12   Comparison Between Suspended- and Attached-Growth Systems in Wastewater Treatment

Suspended-Growth Systems	Attached-Growth Systems
Microorganisms are suspended in the wastewater by means of mixing and/or aeration.	Microorganisms are retained within the biofilm attached to the media.
Sensitive to the adverse effects of toxicants in the influent.	Fair protection against the adverse effects of toxicants in the influent.
Inter- and intraphase mass transfer is insignificant. Vigorous mixing and/or aeration reduce the thickness of the liquid film surrounding the flocs and the size of the flocs, which, in turn, reduce the effects of mass transfer. Therefore, suspended-growth systems are treated as homogeneous systems.	Inter- and intraphase mass transfer is significant because the biofilm structure tends to retard the rate of transport of substrate through it. The liquid–biofilm interface forms another resistance to the transport of substance across it. Therefore, the biofilm systems are heterogeneous systems.
The system performance is intimately linked to the performance of the secondary clarifier because the maintenance of the desirable biomass concentration in the reactor depends on the recirculation of concentrated microbial solids from the secondary clarifier with proper thickening function.	The system performance is not affected by the performance of the secondary clarifier. The biomass in the reactor is maintained through the attachment of microorganisms on the media surface and the subsequent growth of biofilm.
Possible wash-out of biomass.	Elimination of wash-out restrictions.
Secondary clarification is required to reduce the effluent suspended solids concentration to the acceptable level.	Secondary clarification in some cases may be eliminated because the suspended solids level in the system effluent is very low. This is possible because most of the biomass is retained within the biofilms rather than suspended in wastewater.
Unified design approaches such as the F/M and SRT approaches are now well developed and widely employed for practical applications.	Unified design approaches are not fully developed yet because the biofilm systems are generally complex.

Source: Adapted from Shieh (1958) and Bryers (2002).

suspended microorganisms, such as: (1) increased persistence in the system, (2) faster growth rate, (3) increased metabolic activity, and (4) greater resistance to toxicity (Senthilnathan and Ganczarczyk 1998). A wide variety of microorganisms are found in the aerobic suspended and attached growth treatment processes used for the removal of organic material. Aerobic heterotrophic bacteria found in these processes are able to produce extracellular biopolymers that result in the formation of biological flocs (or biofilms for attached-growth processes) that can be separated from the treated liquid by gravity settling with relatively low concentrations of free bacteria and suspended solids.

Aerobic attached-growth processes, depending on the biofilm thickness, generally have a much more complex microbial ecology than that of activated sludge with films containing bacteria, fungi, protozoans, rotifers, and possibly annelid worms, flatworms, and nematodes. An ecological comparison between the activated sludge process and a trickling filter process is made in Fig. 1.22.

Biomass diversity is greater for the trickling filter process than for activated sludge, which means a process that is more stable and less subject to environmental conditions. Most important, the two forms of biomass, fixed and suspended, differ in their main parameter, the solids retention time, and this may be very advantageous in cases where fast and slow degradable components have to be combined (e.g., organic removal with nitrification) (Wanner et al. 2002).

The increasing standards for nutrient and xenobiotic removal, along with more rigorous noise and odor control, have stimulated the development of new intensive advanced technology processes (Lazarova and Manem 2003). One of these intensive

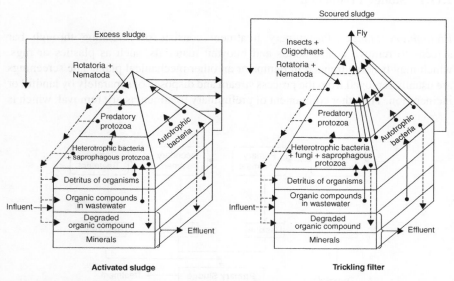

FIGURE 1.22 Comparison of biotas in activated sludge and microbial film. [From Iwai and Kitao (1999).]

processes that is attracting increasing attention is the fluidized-bed reactor, which consists of a biofilm growing on small carriers kept in suspension in the fluid by the drag forces associated with the upward flow of water. Their main advantages include (1) high removal efficiency of carbon and nitrogen through large amounts of fixed biomass with a low hydraulic retention time, (2) no clogging, (3) better oxygen transfer, and (4) reduced sludge production (Lazarova and Manem 2003). The development of intensive processes may be of interest, but there is a growing need for the development of extensive processes (low cost and low operational requirements) for on-site and small community wastewater treatment.

1.11 SLUDGE PRODUCTION, TREATMENT AND DISPOSAL

As mentioned above, the objective of wastewater treatment is to remove solids and to reduce its biochemical oxygen demand before returning the treated wastewater to the environment. Sewage sludge, increasingly referred to as biosolids, is an inevitable product of wastewater treatment. Conventional wastewater treatment processes comprise separate process streams for the liquid and solid fractions (sludge). Sludge is produced at various stages within the wastewater treatment process (Fig. 1.23). Usually, these solids are combined and treated as a whole. Dedicated sludge treatment may not be available at all wastewater treatment plants, particularly smaller plants. In these circumstances it is normal practice to transport the sludge to a larger plant for subsequent treatment.

1.11.1 Sludge Production

Preliminary Sludge Preliminary treatment consists of screening through bar screens to remove coarse solids and buoyant materials, such as plastics or rags, which may become trapped in pumps or an other mechanical plant. The screenings are usually removed from the process stream and disposed of separately by landfill or incineration. The other component of preliminary treatment is grit removal, which is

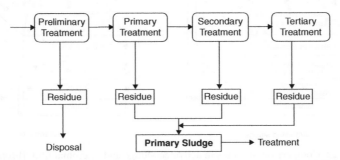

FIGURE 1.23 Schematic representation of wastewater treatment showing sludge production.

accomplished in chambers (or channels) or by centrifugation, taking advantage of the greater settling velocities of these solids. The sand, broken glass, nuts, and other dense material that is collected in the grit chamber is not true sludge in the sense because it is not fluid; the material is largely inorganic in nature. However, it still requires disposal. Because grit can be drained of water easily and is relatively stable in terms of biological activity (it is not biodegradable), it is usually disposed of to landfill without further treatment.

Primary Sludge   Primary treatment is designed to reduce the load on subsequent biological (secondary) treatment processes. Although the design of primary sedimentation tanks differs, they achieve the removal of settleable solids, oils, fats, and other floating material, and a proportion of the organic load. Efficiently designed and operated primary treatment processes should remove 50 to 70% of suspended solids and 25 to 40% of the BOD (organic load). Sludge from the bottom of the primary clarifiers contains 3 to 8% solids, which is approximately 70% organics. This sludge has a high organic content and is usually treated to stabilize the material prior to disposal.

Secondary Sludge   Biological processes are used to convert dissolved biodegradable organic substances and colloidal material into inorganic and biological solids (biomass). Solids separation is the final stage of many of these treatment systems, which produces a sludge whose nature will depend on the upstream treatment process.

This sludge consists of microorganisms and inert materials that have been wasted from the secondary treatment processes. Thus, the solids are about 90% organic. When the supply of air is stopped, this sludge also becomes anaerobic, creating noxious conditions if not treated before disposal. The solids content depends on the source. Wasted activated sludge is typically 0.5 to 2% solids, whereas trickling filter sludge contains 2 to 5% solids. In some cases, secondary sludge contains large quantities of chemical precipitates because the aeration tank is used as the reaction basin for the addition of chemicals to remove phosphorus. Sludge arising from secondary treatment is usually combined with primary sludge and treated as a whole.

Tertiary Sludge   Tertiary treatment will only be required for treatment plants subject to specific discharge conditions. The characteristics of sludge from the tertiary treatment processes depend on the nature of the process. For example, phosphorus removal results in a chemical sludge that is difficult to handle and treat. When phosphorus removal occurs in the activated sludge process, the chemical sludge is combined with the biological sludge, making the latter more difficult to treat. Nitrogen removal by denitrification results in a biological sludge with properties very similar to those of waste activated sludge. The sludge obtained from the various stages is usually in the form of a liquid containing 0.5 to 6% dry solids. The typical composition of raw (untreated) and anaerobically digested sludge is shown in Table 1.13.

TABLE 1.13 Chemical Composition and Properties of Untreated and Digested Sludge

Constituent	Untreated: Range	Primary Sludge: Typical	Digested: Range	Primary Sludge: Typical
Total dry solids (TS) (%)	2.0–8.0	5.0	6.0–12.0	10.0
Volatile solids (% of TS)	60–80	65	30–60	40
Grease and fats (% of TS)				
Ether soluble	6–30		5–20	18
Ether extract	7–35			
Protein (% of TS)	20–30	25	15–20	18
Nitrogen (N, % of TS)	1.5–4	2.5	1.6–6.0	3.0
Phosphorus (P_2O_5, % of TS)	0.8–2.8	1.6	1.5–4.0	2.5
Potassium (K_2O, % of TS)	0.0–0.4	0.1	0.0–3.0	1.0
Cellulose (% of TS)	8.0–15.0	10.0	8.8–15.0	10.0
Iron (not as sulfide)	2.0–4.0	2.5	3.0–8.0	4.0
Silica (SiO_2, % of TS)	15.0–20.0		10.0–20.0	
pH	5.0–8.0	6.0	6.5–7.5	7.0
Alkalinity (mg L^{-1} as $CaCO_3$)	500–1,500	600	2,500–3,500	3,000
Organic acids (mg L^{-1} as HAc)	200–2,000	500	100–600	200
Energy content (kJ kg^{-1})	23,000–29,000	25,500	93,00–14,000	11,500

Source: Metcalf & Eddy, Inc. (2006).

1.11.2 Sludge Treatment Processes

The aim of sludge treatment is to reduce the water and organic content of the sludge and render it suitable for further disposal or reuse. The nature and extent of any sludge treatment depends on the methods of final disposal or beneficial use. The principal methods used for sludge treatment are listed in Table 1.14.

Thickening (concentration), conditioning, dewatering, and drying are used primarily to remove moisture from solids; digestion (aerobic or anaerobic), composting, and incineration or gasification (for energy recovery) are used primarily to treat or stabilize the organic material in the solids.

1. *Thickening.* to remove as much water as possible before final dewatering or digestion of the sludge. It is usually accomplished by flotation or gravity.
2. *Stabilization.* to break down the organic solids through biochemical oxidation processes so that they are more stable and more dewaterable, and to reduce the mass of sludge.
3. *Conditioning.* to treat the sludge with chemicals or heat so that the water can readily be separated. Several methods are available for conditioning sludge to facilitate the separation of the liquid and solids. One of the most commonly used is the addition of coagulants such as ferric chloride, lime, or organic polymers. Another conditioning approach is to heat the sludge at high temperatures (175 to 230 °C) and pressures (1000 to 2000 kPa).

TABLE 1.14 Biosolids Processing and Application Methods

Treatment Method	Function
Preliminary treatment	
Grinding	Particle-size reduction
Screening	Removal of fibrous materials
Degritting	Grit removal
Blending	Homogenization of solids streams
Storage	Flow equalization
Thickening	
Gravity thickening	Volume reduction
Flotation thickening	Volume reduction
Centrifugation	Volume reduction
Gravity-belt thickening	Volume reduction
Rotary-drum thickening	Volume reduction
Stabilization	
Alkaline stabilization	Stabilization
Anaerobic digestion	Stabilization, mass reduction
Aerobic digestion	Stabilization, mass reduction
Autothermal aerobic digestion	Stabilization, mass reduction
Composting	Stabilization, product recovery
Conditioning	
Chemical conditioning	Improve dewaterability
Other conditioning methods	Improve dewaterability
Dewatering	
Centrifuge	Volume reduction
Belt-filter press	Volume reduction
Filter press	Volume reduction
Sludge drying beds	Volume reduction
Reed beds	Storage, volume reduction
Lagoons	Storage, volume reduction
Heat drying	
Direct dryers	Weight and volume reduction
Indirect dryers	Weight and volume reduction
Incineration	
Multiple-hearth incineration	Volume reduction, resource recovery
Fluidized-bed incineration	Volume reduction
Coincineration with solid waste	Volume reduction
Application of biosolids to land	
Land application	Beneficial use, disposal
Dedicated land disposal	Disposal, land reclamation
Landfilling	Disposal

4. *Dewatering.* to separate water by subjecting the sludge to vacuum, pressure, or drying. The most popular method of sludge dewatering is the use of sludge drying beds. The other methods include vacuum filter and continuous belt filter presses.

TABLE 1.15 Typical Nutrient Content of Sewage Sludge (Dry Weight, %)

Constituents	Range	Typical Value
Nitrogen	0.1–17.6	3.0
Phosphorus	0.1–14.3	1.5
Sulfur	0.6–1.5	1.0
Potassium	0.02–2.6	0.3

5. *Reduction.* to convert the solids to a stable form by wet oxidation or incineration, to decrease the volume of sludge. To minimize the amount of fuel used, the sludge must be dewatered as completely as possible before incineration. The exhaust gas from an incinerator must be treated carefully to avoid air pollution.

Detailed descriptions of these processes are outside the scope of this chapter.

1.11.3 Sludge Disposal and Application

Sludge characteristics that affect their suitability for application to land and for beneficial use include organic content (usually measured as volatile solids), nutrients, pathogens, metals, and toxic organic compounds. Sewage sludge contains valuable amounts of plant nutrients (nitrogen and phosphorus) and trace elements, typical nutrient values of wastewater sludge are shown in Table 1.15.

Trace elements are inorganic chemical elements in very small quantities. They can be essential or detrimental to plants and animals. The term *heavy metals* is several of the trace elements present in sludge. Concentrations of heavy metals may vary widely (U.S. EPA 1990), as indicated in Table 1.16. For the application of biosolids to land,

TABLE 1.16 Typical Metal Content in Wastewater Solids (Dry Weight, mg kg^{-1})

Metal	Range	Median
Arsenic	1.1–230	10
Cadmium	1–3410	10
Chromium	10–99,000	500
Cobalt	11.3–2,490	30
Copper	84–17,000	800
Iron	1,000–154,000	17,000
Lead	13–26,000	500
Manganese	32–9,870	260
Mercury	0.6–56	6
Molybdenum	0.1–214	4
Nickel	2–5300	80
Selenium	1.7–17.2	5
Tin	2.6–329	14
Zinc	101–49,000	1,700

concentrations of heavy metals may limit the application rate and the useful life of the application site.

For this reason, sludge has historically been applied to agricultural land as part of an integrated farm management plan. Other options for disposal include energy recovery and land reclamation activities. It is worthwhile to note that the disposal of sewage sludge is subject to strict controls designed to protect soil quality while encouraging the use of sludge in agriculture.

REFERENCES

Baudart J., Coallier J., Laurent P., Prevost M. (2002) Rapid and sensitive enumeration of viable diluted cells of members of the family Enterobacteriaceae in freshwater and drinking water. *Applied and Environmental Microbiology*, **68**: 5007–5063.

Brock T. D., Madigan M. T. (1991) *Biology of Microbiology*, 6th ed., Prentice-Hall, Englewood Cliffs, NJ.

Bryers J. D. (1987) Application of captured cell systems in biological treatment. In: Wise D.L. (ed.) *Bioenviromental Systems*, Vol. IV, CRC Press, Boca Raton, FL, pp. 27–53.

Davis M. L., Cornwell D. A. (1998) *Introduction to Environmental Engineering*, 3rd ed., McGraw-Hill, New York, p. 343.

Dorigo U., Volatier L., Humbert J. (2005) Molecular approaches to the assessment of biodiversity in aquatic microbial communities. *Water Research* **39**, 2207–2218.

Ferry J. G. (1999) Enzymology of one-carbon metabolism in methanogenic pathways. *FEMS Microbiological Review* **23**, 13–38.

Gebara F. (1999) Activated sludge biofilm wastewater treatment system. *Water Research* **33**, 230–238.

Harrison J. R., Daigger G. T., Filbert J. W. (1984) A survey of combined trickling filter and activated sludge processes. *Journal of the Water Pollution Control Federation* **56**, 1073–1079.

Iwai S, Kitao T. (1994) *Wastewater Treatment with Microbial Films*, Technomic Publishing, Lancaster, PA.

Jenkins D., Richard M. G., Daigger G. T. (1984) *Manual on the Causes and Control of Activated Sludge Bulking and Foaming*, Water Research Commission, Pretoria, South Africa.

Keer J. T., Birch L. (2003) Molecular methods for the assessment of bacterial viability. *Journal of Microbiological Methods* **53**, 175–183.

Kogure K., Simidu U., Taga N. (1984) An improved direct viable count method for aquatic bacteria. *Archives of Hydrobiology* **102**, 117–122.

Lazarova V., Manem J. (1994) Advances in biofilm aerobic reactors ensuring effective biofilm activity control. *Water Science and Technology* **29**, 319–327.

Madigan M. T., Martinko J. M., Parker J. (1997) *Brock Biology of Microorganisms*. 8th ed., Prentice Hall, Upper Saddle River, NJ.

Martin H. G., Ivanova N., Kunin V., Warnecke F., Barry K., McHardy A. C., Yeates C., He S., Salamov A., Szeto E., Dalin E., Putnam N., Shapiro H. J., Pangilinan J. L., Rigoutsos I.,

Kyrpides N. C., Blackall L. L., McMahon K. D., Hugenholtz P. (2006) Metagenomic analysis of two enhanced biological phosphorus removal (EBPR) sludge communities. *Nature Biotechnology* **24**, 1263–1269.

McCarty P. L., Smith D. P. (1986) Anaerobic wastewater treatment. *Environmental Science and Technology*, **20**, 1200–1226.

Metcalf & Eddy, Inc. (2003) *Wastewater Engineering: Treatment and Reuse*, 4th ed., McGraw-Hill, New York.

Muller N. (1998) Implementing biofilm carriers into activated sludge process: 15 years of experience. *Water Science and Technology* **37**, 167–174.

Pelczar M. J., Reid R. D. (1958) *Microbiology*, McGraw-Hill, New York.

Sedlak R. I. (1991) *Phosphorus and Nitrogen Removal from Municipal Wastewater*, 2d ed., The Soap and Detergent Association, Lewis Publishers, New York.

Senthilnathan P. R., Ganczarczyk J. J. (1990) Application of biomass carriers in activated sludge process. In: Tyagi R.D., Vembu K.V. (eds.), *Wastewater Treatment by Immobilized Cells*, CRC Press, Boca Raton, FL, pp. 103–141.

Shieh W. K. (1987) Biofilm kinetics: mass transfer effects and their implication to process design, operation and control. In: Wise D.L. (ed.), *Bioenvironmental Systems*, Vol. IV, CRC Press, Boca Raton, FL, pp. 155–179.

Sutton S. D. (2002) Quatification of microbial biomass. In: Bitton G. (ed.), *Encyclopedia of Environmental Microbiology*, Wiley-Interscience, New York, pp. 2652–2660.

U.S. Environmental Protection Agency (EPA) (1984) *Environmental Regulations and Technology: Use and Disposal of Municipal Wastewater Sludge*, EPA/625/10-84-003, EPA, Washington, DC.

Wang J. L., Shi H. C., Qian Y. (2000) Wastewater treatment by a hybrid biological reactor (HBR): effect of loading rates. *Process Biochemistry* **36**, 297–303.

Wanner J., Kucman K., Grau P. (1988) Activated sludge process combined with biofilm cultivation. *Water Research* **22**, 207–215.

2

SLUDGE PRODUCTION: QUANTIFICATION AND PREDICTION FOR URBAN TREATMENT PLANTS AND ASSESSMENT OF STRATEGIES FOR SLUDGE REDUCTION

MATHIEU SPÉRANDIO, ETIENNE PAUL, AND YOLAINE BESSIÈRE

Université de Toulouse; INSA,UPS,INP; LISBP, 135 Avenue de Rangueil, F-31077 Toulouse, France; INRA, UMR792, Ingénierie des Systèmes Biologiques et des Procédés, F-31400 Toulouse, France; CNRS, UMR5504, F-31400 Toulouse, France

YU LIU

Division of Environmental and Water Resources Engineering, School of Civil and Environmental Engineering, Nanyang Technological University, Singapore

2.1 INTRODUCTION

Prediction of excess sludge production is an important issue for the design and modeling of wastewater treatment plants but is somewhat difficult because of the numerous processes involved and the variability of the factors that influence it. Even today, evaluation of wastewater treatment plants (WWTPs) shows that inadequate facility design for sludge handling and a lack of appreciation of wasting requirements are encountered. Operators face difficulties in predicting and even in quantifying (by measurement) the sludge production of their WWTPs. Two questions then arise: What type of model can give an accurate estimation? What experimental approaches are suitable for obtaining representative measurements? Such quantification is

Biological Sludge Minimization and Biomaterials/Bioenergy Recovery Technologies, First Edition.
Edited by Etienne Paul and Yu Liu.
© 2012 John Wiley & Sons, Inc. Published 2012 by John Wiley & Sons, Inc.

clearly crucial if the issue of excess sludge reduction is to be addressed. A good knowledge of the reference sludge production is essential to demonstrate the extent of the reduction due to a specific treatment.

In this chapter we address the following issues: (1) sludge composition in relation to its origin, (2) fundamentals of mechanisms involved in excess sludge production, (3) sludge quantification and prediction by models, (4) change in sludge fractions depending on sludge retention time (SRT) or influent wastewater characteristics, and (5) model-based evaluation of strategies for excess sludge minimisation.

2.2 SLUDGE FRACTIONATION AND ORIGIN

2.2.1 Sludge Composition

In a conventional wastewater treatment plant, sludge is produced mainly by primary settling in a tank and a secondary biological process, commonly an activated sludge process. Primary sludge is composed of suspended solids coming from raw waste-water, whereas secondary biological sludge is the result of floc formation due to the growth and aggregation of microorganisms. It should be noted that in a number of plants, raw sewage is fed directly to the activated sludge process without primary settling (only prescreening). Finally, if a polishing treatment is applied (e.g., a sand filter), a tertiary sludge can also be produced. Figure 2.1 presents typical flocs that can be encountered in biological sludge and a schematic of a typical WWTP.

Sludge concentration is globally quantified by measuring the total suspended solids (TSS), which are divided into volatile suspended solids (VSS) and inorganic suspended solids (ISS). More accurately, sludge is composed of numerous organic materials, which can be classified as biologically active or inactive. Based on organic matter fractionation, different approaches have been developed for predicting sludge composition and sludge quantity.

Active Organic Fractions Basically, aerobic biological sludge is composed of active bacterial cells, mainly heterotrophic biomass (concentration noted X_H) and a few autotrophic nitrifiers (concentration noted X_A), produced, respectively, from the biodegradation of organic compounds (soluble and particulate, S_B and X_B respectively)

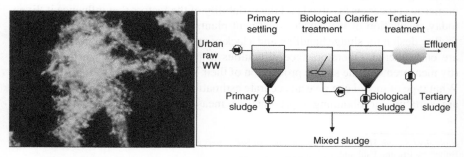

FIGURE 2.1 Sludge production at a conventional biological treatment plant.

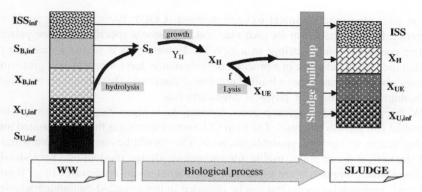

FIGURE 2.2 Schematic representation of sludge fractionation theory.

and ammonia oxidation. Obviously, other microbial communities are neglected in this definition because they do not contribute significantly to the quantity of biomass (VSS) even though they can play an important role in the processes. For example, protozoans are active predators for bacteria in aerobic conditions, which may explain the variation in the bacterial decay rate under different conditions (aerobic, anoxic), but the contribution of protozoans to the total VSS is assumed to be negligible in the quantitative model for predicting sludge mass.

Inactive Organic Fractions Additionally, inactive solids are found in activated sludge. First, organic solids from the influent can accumulate in the sludge. Second, biological residues are also generated (secreted) during bacterial growth and decay. These fractions are noted, respectively, as $X_{U,inf}$ and $X_{U,E}$. Initiated in the early 1960s, the idea that an inactive biomass should be included in activated sludge modeling (Symons and McKinney 2001; Kountz and Forney 1992; McKinney 1998; Washington and Symons 1962) was implemented in the commonly used activated sludge models developed in the 1980s (Marais and Ekama 2009; Dold et al. 1980; Henze et al. 1987). The mathematical expressions proposed in this chapter are inspired largely by this theoretical model framework.

Inactive Mineral Fractions The inorganic fraction of sludge (ISS) is composed not only of inert minerals coming from the influent but also of minerals related to bacterial cells (ashes), and finally, of precipitates generated in the process. A specific section is dedicated to the quantitative estimation of this fraction. Finally, Fig. 2.2 illustrates the fractionation that is assumed for sludge quantification. Based on this theoretical fractionation, it becomes clear that the correct estimation of sludge production requires a detailed characterization of the incoming domestic sewage.

2.2.2 Wastewater Characteristics

Diversity of Organics and Simplified Fractionation Approaches It is obvious that wastewaters contain a large diversity of molecules, each making a small contribution to the total measured chemical oxygen demand (COD). Each molecule could be supposed to be degraded at its own rate and to follow a specific behavior pattern during coagulation and settling in a WWTP. However, as it seems unrealistic to predict individual behavior in a process, organic matter has for practical engineering purposes been separated into a limited number of fractions. These fractions are based on biological, chemical, or physical characteristics.

With regard to the biological process, biodegradable organic matter determines the microbial cell growth potential. The total COD concentration is then fractionated into biodegradable and unbiodegradable fractions. This should be considered as a simplified theoretical assumption, usable for estimating sludge production. Very slowly biodegradable compounds are present in small amounts in wastewater (e.g., lignocellulose, humic substances) but can be included in the so-called "unbiodegradable" fraction, as the retention time of solids in WWTPs is generally too short (5 to 30 d) for their degradation to be considered. But this assumption is no longer valid if a process is run at very high solids, retention time (see Chapter 8 for an example).

In addition, these fractions are divided into soluble and particulate fractions, which should define the behavior of organic components during physicochemical processes such as settling, coagulation, and flocculation. In reality, the large diversity of molecules provides a broad distribution of physical–chemical properties, which change during each treatment process.

A conventional scientific question in wastewater characterization for sludge prediction is "How can the soluble and the particulate be defined?", and a common practical engineer's answer is, "It depends on the separation process you want to predict!" In fact, the practical interest is to distinguish among settleable coagulable and noncoagulable fractions, which gives a direct view of what would be retained by each type of process. But a more satisfactory definition could be proposed by distinguishing soluble, colloidal, and particulate forms (Fig. 2.3).

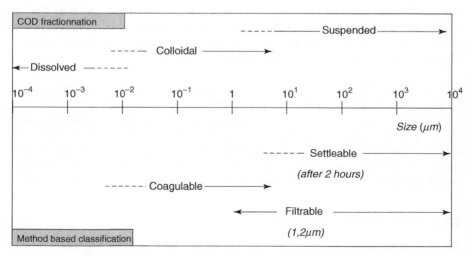

FIGURE 2.3 Physical fractions of compounds in wastewaters.

In this chapter, organic matter (in COD units) is fractionated according to the theoretical framework developed for activated sludge modeling (Marais and Ekama 2009; Dold et al. 1980; Henze et al. 1987) with the recently standardized notations proposed by Corominas et al. (2010):

$$COD_T = S_{inf} = S_B + S_U + X_B + X_U \tag{2.1}$$

where S_B is the soluble (readily) biodegradable COD, S_U the soluble unbiodegradable COD, X_B the particulate (slowly) biodegradable COD, and X_U the particulate unbiodegradable COD. For the coagulation process, the insoluble fraction can be divided into a colloidal and a particulate fraction. The contribution of each is also defined as a fraction of the total COD:

$$COD_T = (f_{BS} + f_{US} + f_{BP} + f_{UP})S_{inf} \tag{2.2}$$

The urban wastewater fractionation is summarized in Fig. 2.4.

Methods for Wastewater Fractionation A number of technical procedures have been developed in the last decade to quantify the various fractions of the organic matter contained in wastewaters. However, it is still difficult to define a standard approach, as the method is generally chosen depending on the objective of characterization.

On the one hand, dynamic modeling is based on an accurate distinction between readily biodegradable compounds and slowly biodegradable compounds because the consumption of electron acceptors (oxygen or nitrate) is related directly to the degradation rate of these compounds. On the other hand, sludge production is much more sensitive to the distinction between total biodegradable and total unbiodegradable compounds (see the following models). For this reason, in this section it is more important to focus on the determination of fractions that are supposed to be unbiodegradable, especially the particulate unbiodegradable fraction. More details

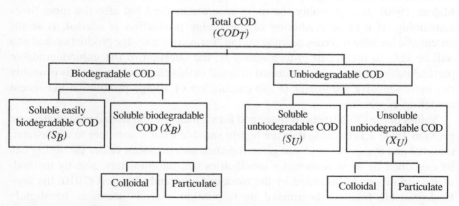

FIGURE 2.4 COD fractionation for urban wastewater. [From Marais and Ekama (2009), Dold et al. (1980), and Henze et al. (1987).]

on the comparison of fractionation methods can be found elsewhere (Gillot and Choubert 2010).

Unbiodegradable fraction is difficult to determine directly and is often estimated from the difference between total COD and biodegradable COD:

$$COD_U = COD_T - COD_B \qquad (2.3)$$

Then, physical techniques are generally used to distinguish between soluble and particulate substances:

$$COD_U = S_U + X_U \qquad (2.4)$$

To assess the total biodegradable COD fraction of a given wastewater (COD_B), three types of biological assays have been developed:

1. Monitoring of the oxygen consumed versus time during specific respirometric batch experiments (Spérandio et al. 1998)
2. Ultimate BOD tests (Roeleveld and van Loosdrecht 2010)
3. Measurement of the COD evolution (total and soluble) versus time in continuously aerated batch reactors (Lesouef et al. 1996)

These tests can be performed with either the total sample or a filtrated sample to distinguish between soluble or particulate fractions. Filtration cutoff size is generally chosen as 0.45 μm.

Because of the high variability of results obtained by these techniques, it was also proposed to estimate the particulate unbiodegradable fraction (f_{UP}) by trial and error. This method consists of fitting a model to the data collected on a lab-scale activated sludge process (or sequencing batch reactor) (Henze 1992; Melcer 1960). It is probably the most accurate method but also the most time-consuming. If a rapid prediction of the sludge production is needed, it seems unrealistic because it comes down to saying "measure the sludge production and you will be able to predict it!" More seriously, the question of the unbiodegradable particulate fraction (f_{UP}) is discussed in detail in this chapter because it is probably the most sensitive parameter in the calculation of sludge production via recent modeling approaches.

Values of the COD fractions measured for various raw and settled wastewaters are given in Table 2.1. Because data are highly variable from wastewater to wastewater, minimal and maximal values are given together with the mean value. Variability can be explained by local wastewater specificities but, unfortunately, also by methodology variations. As indicated by the work of Gillot and Choubert (2010) the non-biodegradable fraction determined by respiration analysis seems to be slightly underestimated compared to values obtained from long-term batch tests with

TABLE 2.1 COD Fractions of Domestic Wastewaters in Various Countries

Origin	S_U	S_B	X_B	X_U	Reference
Raw wastewater					
France	—	6–14	41–66	—	Spérandio (1991)
South Africa	5	20	62	13	Ekama et al. (1986)
Denmark	2–8	20–24	40–49	18–19	Henze (1992)
Switzerland	10–20	7–32	45–60	8–11	Kappeler and Gujer (1992), Henze (1992)
France	—	1–18	15–57	24–63	Ginestet et al. (2002)
Hungary	9	29	43	20	Henze et al. (1987)
Norway	10–15	25–35	15–20	10–15	Barlindhaug and Odegaard (1996)
Settled wastewater					
France	11	6	48	19	Spérandio (1991)
France	6–10	25–33	41–44	8–13	Lesouef et al. (1996)
Switzerland	10	16	40	9	Sollfrank and Gujer (2003)
Denmark	3	29	43	11	Henze (1992)
France	—	1–16	33–74	10–50	Ginestet et al. (2002)
South Africa	8	28	60	4	Ekama et al. (1986)

TABLE 2.2 Comparison of Results Obtained by Different Techniques for Determining Biodegradable and Unbiodegradable COD Fractions of Domestic Wastewaters

	Respirometry (Low Food/Microorganism) Short Term (<1 d)	BOD Test (High Food/Microorganism) Long Term (5–30 d)	Long-Term COD Measurement in Batch Reactors (at least 30 d)
COD_B/COD_T	0.55–0.8	0.55–0.8	0.8–0.9
COD_U/COD_T	0.2–0.45	0.2–0.45	0.1–0.2

Source: Gillot and Choubert (2010).

COD measurements and mass balances (Table 2.2). This is no doubt due to the difference in exposure conditions [food/microorganism for the biochemical oxygen demand (BOD) test] and to the inaccuracy of short-term respirometric techniques for estimating the slowly biodegradable compounds.

Influent Inorganics Wastewater also contains mineral suspended solids (ISS), which can be estimated by the difference between the TSS and VSS measurements. ISS are the suspended substances that remain after drying at 500°C. Table 2.3 shows the proportion of inorganic suspended solids in the TSS found in different raw and settled wastewaters. Inorganic suspended solids generally make up to 15 to 30% of total suspended solids. This fraction varies temporarily with flow rate and rain events.

TABLE 2.3   Inorganic Suspended Solids as a Percentage of Total Suspended Solids in Raw and Settled wastewater

Origin	TSS (mg L^{-1})	ISS (% TSS)	References
Raw wastewater			
France	200–400	14–32	Camacho (2001); Dignac (1998); Grulois et al. (1996)
Japan	46–49	14–15	Yasui and Shibata (1994)
United States	100–350	21–30	Olstein (2003)
Typical	290	19	Dold (2007)
Settled wastewater			
France, Evry	94–200	18–31	Camacho (2001)
France, Toulouse	175	14–19	Massé (1976)

2.3   QUANTIFICATION OF EXCESS SLUDGE PRODUCTION

2.3.1   Primary Treatment

Sludge production from primary treatment depends theoretically on the particulate organic matter concentration of the wastewater and the removal efficiency of the primary settler. Based on typical data on WWTP (Dold 2007; Jimenez et al. 1958), it can be observed that a primary settling tank removes 55 to 60% of total suspended solids. A typical set of data for raw and primary settled wastewater is presented in Table 2.4 and is shown schematically in Fig. 2.5.

From a mass balance on a primary settling tank, total sludge production from primary settling (PPS) is given in TSS units by.

$$PPS_{TSS} = \eta_{PS} Q_{inf} X_{TSS} \qquad (2.5)$$

The contributions of organics and inorganics can be differentiated:

$$PPS_{TSS} = PPS_{VSS} + PPS_{ISS} = \eta_{PS} Q_{inf} (X_{VSS} + X_{ISS}) \qquad (2.6)$$

Organic sludge production is then related to influent particulate fractions

$$PPS_{VSS} = \frac{\eta_{PS} Q_{inf} (1 - f_{CX})(f_{UP} + f_{BP}) S_{inf}}{f_{cv,u,inf}} \qquad (2.7)$$

where f_{CX} is the fraction of insoluble compounds that are colloidal. The sludge production ratio of primary settling can be expressed in kg VSS per kg of influent COD:

$$Y_{PSS} = \frac{PPS_{VSS}}{Q_{inf} S_{inf}} \qquad (2.8)$$

$$Y_{PSS} = \frac{\eta_{PS} (1 - f_{CX})(f_{UP} + f_{BP})}{f_{cv,u,inf}} \qquad (2.9)$$

If coagulation is performed before settling, it can be assumed that most colloidal compounds are converted into particulates. Moreover, a higher efficiency (denoted

TABLE 2.4 Example of Typical Influent Characteristics for Raw, Presettled, and Coagulated-Settled Sewage

	Raw Sewage	Presettled Wastewater, $\eta_{PS} = 60\%$	Coagulated-Settled Wastewater, $\eta_{CPS} = 90\%$
Concentrations			
COD_T	800	530	260
S_U	40	40	40
S_B	160	160	160
X_B (with colloidal)	480	264	48
X_U (with colloidal)	120	66	12
X_B (without colloidal)	360	144	36
X_U (without colloidal)	90	36	9
Fractions			
f_{US}	0.05	0.08	0.15
f_{BS}	0.2	0.30	0.62
f_{BP}	0.6	0.50	0.18
f_{CX}	0.25	0.45	0.25
f_{UP}	0.15	0.12	0.05
$(f_{US} + f_{BS})$ soluble fraction	0.25	0.38	0.77
ISS	75	30	7.5
VSS	281	113	28
TSS	356	143	36

Source: Adapted from Dold (2007) for European wastewaters, considering colloidal matter treatment.

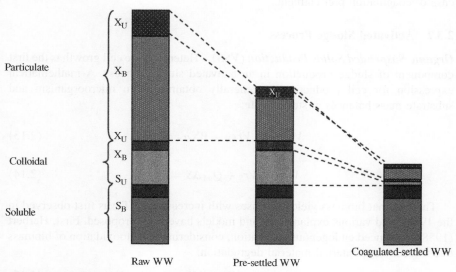

FIGURE 2.5 Schematic representation of typical set of raw, presettled, and coagulated-settled sewage. [Adapted from Dold (2007) for European wastewaters, considering colloidal matter treatment.]

TABLE 2.5   Calculation of Typical Sludge Production Due to a Primary Settling Tank and Physicochemical Treatment (Coagulation + Settling) Considering the Wastewater Characteristics Given in Table 2.4

Scenario	kg VSS kg^{-1} Influent COD	kg TSS kg^{-1} Influent COD
Primary settling tank, Y_{PSS}	0.211	0.267
Physicochemical treatment (coagulation + settling) Y_{CPSS}	0.422	0.506

η_{CPS}, ranging from 80 to 90%) for suspended solid removal is reached thanks to flocculation:

$$PCPS_{ISS} = \eta_{CPS} Q_{inf} X_{ISS} \tag{2.10}$$

$$PCPS_{VSS} = \frac{\eta_{CPS} Q_{inf} (f_{UP} + f_{BP}) S_{inf}}{f_{cv,u,inf}} \tag{2.11}$$

$$Y_{CPSS} = \frac{\eta_{CPS} (f_{UP} + f_{BP})}{f_{cv,u,inf}} \tag{2.12}$$

Calculations of sludge production during primary settling or a physicochemical treatment (coagulation + settling) are given for a typical domestic wastewater in Table 2.5. It can be pointed out that sludge production is logically twice as great in the case of coagulation pretreatment.

2.3.2   Activated Sludge Process

Organic Suspended Solids Production (VSS)   Heterotrophic cell growth is the first component of sludge production in an activated sludge process. A mathematical expression for cell production is generally obtained from microorganism and substrate mass balances at steady state:

$$V \frac{dX_H}{dt} = V r_{XH} - P X_H = 0 \tag{2.13}$$

$$V \frac{dS}{dt} = V r_S + Q_{inf} \Delta S = 0 \tag{2.14}$$

The fact that biomass yield decreases with increasing SRT was first observed in the 1950s, and various explanations and models have been proposed. First, Herbert (1958) introduced endogenous respiration, considering an autooxidation of biomass due to decay and internal material degradation:

$$r_{XH} = \mu X_H - b X_H \tag{2.15}$$

$$r_{XH} = Y_H r_S - b X_H \tag{2.16}$$

TABLE 2.6 Parameter Set for Calculations of Organic Excess Sludge Production (VSS)

Parameter	Value	Reference	Unit
Y_H: heterotrophic biomass yield	0.666	Henze et al. (1987)	g COD/g COD
b: decay constant of active biomass (20°C)	0.24	Marais and Ekama (2009)	d^{-1}
f: inert fraction of biomass	0.20	Washington and Symons (1962)	
$f_{cv,h}$: conversion factor for heterotrophic biomass	1.42	Marais and Ekama (2009)	g COD/g VSS
$f_{cv,u}$: conversion factor for unbiodegradable solids	1.55	Dold (2007)	g COD/g VSS

Sludge retention time (SRT) is defined as the ratio between the mass of sludge in the system (MX_V) and the amount of sludge removed from the system per day (PX_V). In a single sludge system, all the particulate components of the sludge have the same retention time:

$$SRT = \frac{MX_V}{PX_V} \tag{2.17}$$

$$SRT = \frac{MX_H}{PX_H} \tag{2.18}$$

According to Eqs. (2.13) and (2.14) and with consideration of the biodegradable fraction of organic matter in wastewater [$\Delta S = (1 - f_{UP} - f_{US})S_{inf}$], the active heterotrophic biomass production rate becomes

$$PX_H = \frac{Y_H}{1 + b \cdot SRT} (1 - f_{US} - f_{UP}) Q_{inf} S_{inf} \tag{2.19}$$

Remark: Pirt (2001) proposed another concept based on the assumption that a fraction of the substrate is not used for growth but for the maintenance of cells. It should be noted that combined with mass balances, both Pirt's and Herbert's models lead to similar mathematical expressions for observed sludge, but the models differ in the fraction of active biomass.

Based on the observation of activated sludge systems operated during about three months without sludge wastage, Washington and Symons (1962) noted that a fraction of suspended matter accumulated in such systems (only fed with acetate). This accumulation was considered to be due to endogenous residue generation linked to decay. This assumption leads to a new basic mass balance for $X_{U,E}$:

$$V\frac{dX_{U,E}}{dt} = VfbX_H - PX_{U,E} \tag{2.20}$$

The accumulation was estimated to be 0.09 to 0.11 g VSS g^{-1} COD, which gives a value of $f = 0.20$, considering a biomass yield of 0.47 g VSS g^{-1} COD. At the steady state, considering the definition of SRT, this approach leads to a new expression for endogenous biomass production:

$$PX_{U,E} = \frac{Y_H bf \cdot SRT}{1 + b \cdot SRT}(1 - f_{US} - f_{UP})Q_{inf}S_{inf} \tag{2.21}$$

Based on Eq. 2.21, Marais and Ekama (2009) identified the value of the decay coefficient as a function of temperature for the activated sludge process:

$$b = 0.24 \times 1.029^{T-20} \tag{2.22}$$

In the treatment of real domestic wastewater, the fact that unbiodegradable organic matter ($X_{U,inf}$) accumulates in the system should also be introduced.

$$V\frac{dX_{U,inf}}{dt} = Q_{inf}f_{UP}S_{inf} - PX_{U,inf} = 0 \tag{2.23}$$

Thus,

$$PX_{U,inf} = Q_{inf}f_{UP}S_{inf} \tag{2.24}$$

Remark: It should be noted that the assumption of an "inert" fraction in influent was proposed to predict the sludge production correctly for systems with conventional SRT (fewer than 30 days). It was then suggested that this assumption was valid for a limited range of SRT (Henze et al. 2000), as the compounds which are taken to be "unbiodegradable" could become biodegradable at high SRT (> 30 d for extended-aeration activated sludge processors and membrane bioreactors) due to biomass adaptation.

Finally, the observed organic sludge yield (Y_{obs}) is defined as the mass of sludge removed from the system per day (PX_V) divided by the mass of organic matter (COD) removed in the process per day:

$$Y_{obs} = \frac{PX_V}{Q_{inf}(S_{inf} - S_{eff})} = \frac{PX_V}{Q_{inf}(1 - f_{US})S_{inf}} \tag{2.25}$$

The production of suspended solids in VSS (PX_V) is the sum of the individual contributions: (1) active heterotrophic biomass (PX_H), (2) endogenous residue ($PX_{U,E}$) and (3) inactive particulates from the influent ($PX_{U,inf}$) (given in COD units) converted into VSS by specific conversion factors.

$$PX_V = \frac{PX_H}{f_{cv,h}} + \frac{PX_{U,E}}{f_{cv,u,e}} + \frac{PX_{U,inf}}{f_{cv,u,inf}} \tag{2.26}$$

Thus, a general expression for the observed sludge production yield can be expressed as

$$Y_{obs} = \left((1 - f_{UP} - f_{US}) \left(\frac{Y_H}{1 + b \cdot SRT} \frac{1}{f_{cv,h}} + \frac{Y_H bf \cdot SRT}{1 + b \cdot SRT} \frac{1}{f_{cv,u,e}} \right) + \frac{f_{UP}}{f_{cv,u,inf}} \right) \Big/ (1 - f_{US})$$

(2.27)

Remark: Eq. (2.27) can be used either for real domestic wastewater or for synthetic substrate by choosing adequate f_{UP} and f_{US} values. For example, for systems fed with only a soluble, completely biodegradable synthetic substrate, $f_{UP} = 0$ and $f_{US} = 0$.

Relation Between SRT and SUR Because biomass production results from food consumption by cells, sludge production is also related to the specific *substrate utilization rate* (SUR), defined as the ratio between the mass of organic matter (COD) removed in the process per day and the mass of sludge in the system:

$$SUR = \frac{Q_{inf}(S_{inf} - S_{eff})}{MX_V}$$

(2.28)

A useful expression can be obtained from Eqs. (2.26) to (2.28):

$$Y_{obs} \cdot SUR \cdot SRT = 1$$

(2.29)

Equation (2.30) shows further that a general relation exists between SUR and SRT, and this relation varies with the influent characteristics (f_{UP}, f_{US}):

$$\frac{1}{SRT} = SUR \left[(1 - f_{UP} - f_{US}) \left(\frac{Y_H}{(1 + b \cdot SRT) f_{cv,h}} + \frac{Y_H bf \cdot SRT}{(1 + b \cdot SRT) f_{cv,u,e}} \right) + \frac{f_{UP}}{f_{cv,u,inf}} \right] (1 - f_{US})$$

(2.30)

Remark: With the assumption that no endogenous and no inert mass are accumulated ($f = 0$, $f_{UP} = 0$), this expression has been simplified to a linear form in a number of studies ($1/SRT = Y \cdot SUR - b$). However, Marais and Ekama (2009) demonstrated that it is impossible to find a unique set of values for Y_H and b that can describe the experimental observations, and this simplification leads to an underestimation of b by at least 50% at low SRT and up to 90% at SRTs between 6 and 30 days.

Figure 2.6 shows the variation of sludge production yield with SRT, and also shows the typical relation between 1/SRT and SUR. As the sludge production yield depends on the wastewater characteristics, two options are compared: with a typical domestic wastewater ($f_{UP} = 0.15$) or a synthetic wastewater without any particulate matter ($f_{UP} = 0$). For SRT varying from 1 to 50 days, sludge production yield decreases from 0.4 to 0.2 and from 0.4 to 0.1 kg VSS kg^{-1} COD, respectively, for domestic or synthetic wastewaters. Y_{obs} decreases significantly for SRT, varying from 1 to 25 days but reaches a "plateau" at high SRT. This is explained by the fact that inert matter becomes the major part of sludge at high sludge age, and no significant effect of retention time is observed if this matter is not hydrolyzed. The relation between 1/SRT and SUR is relatively linear at SRT values less than 10 days

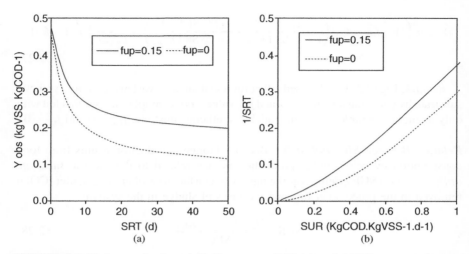

FIGURE 2.6 Sludge production yield Y_{obs} versus SRT (a) and 1/SRT versus substrate utilization rate SUR (b) calculated with a conventional set of parameters (Table 2.6) for domestic ($f_{UP} = 0.15$) and synthetic ($f_{UP} = 0$) wastewater.

and SUR values higher than 0.5 kg COD kg^{-1} VSS d^{-1}, but progressively "incurves" at high sludge age and very low SUR. These confirm the important role of inert matter coming from the influent (f_{UP}) in the sludge production yield.

Remark: Concerning the f and b parameters, two types of data can be found in the literature, basically because two options are proposed for modeling decay: the death-regeneration concept used in activated sludge model 1 (ASM1) (Dold et al. 1980; Henze et al. 1987) and the endogenous respiration concept used in ASM3. In the latter case, which is chosen in this book, biomass decay leads to the release of a fraction of inert matter (f), and the other fraction of biomass ($1 - f$) is taken to be directly oxidized. In the death–regeneration concept, dead biomass is converted to inerts (f') and the other fraction ($1 - f'$) is converted to a new substrate, which will be degraded by heterotrophic biomass. It has been shown that both concepts lead to exactly the same numerical relation if (b, f) and (b', f') are chosen according to the following expression (e.g., if $b = 0.24$ d^{-1} and $f = 0.2$, then $b' = 0.62$ d^{-1} and $f' = 0.08$):

$$b = b' - Y_H(1 - f')b' \qquad (2.31)$$

$$f = \frac{f'}{1 - Y_H(1 - f')} \qquad (2.32)$$

Inorganic Suspended Solids Production In the same way as for organic compounds, a fractionation approach can be proposed for mineral suspended solids

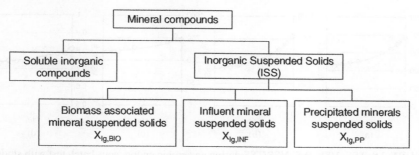

FIGURE 2.7 Fractionation of mineral compounds of mixed liquor in the activated sludge process.

production from activated sludge (Fig. 2.7). Total mineral compounds can be divided into soluble and particulate minerals, the latter constituting the inorganic suspended solids (ISS). The concentration of ISS is measured by burning a sample of suspended solids at 500°C. In this chapter it is assumed that ISS are composed of the mineral content of the biomass, denoted $X_{Ig,bio}$, the entrapped inorganic content coming from influent inorganic suspended solids noted $X_{Ig,inf}$, and possibly a fraction of minerals formed by precipitation, which is noted $X_{Ig,PP}$. This last fraction is especially important when mineral coagulants are used for chemical phosphorus precipitation. Basically, it can be considered that total ISS is the sum of the three:

$$ISS = X_{Ig,bio} + X_{Ig,inf} + X_{Ig,PP} \qquad (2.33)$$

The contribution of each fraction depends on the influent characteristics and operating conditions, and their quantitative prediction would probably merit more research attention because solubilization and precipitation are not yet considered in the models (Wentzel et al. 2002; Ekama and Wentzel 2004).

The term $X_{Ig,bio}$ is the mineral content of the biomass. It is related to properties of heterotrophic biomass and endogenous residue via conversion factors:

$$X_{Ig,bio} = f_{ISS} \left(\frac{X_H}{f_{cv,h}} + \frac{X_{U,E}}{f_{cv,e}} \right) \qquad (2.34)$$

Experimentally, about 10% of the total mass of cells is found to be composed of minerals (P_2O_5, K_2O, CaO, MgO) that remain after drying at 500°C. This gives an acceptable value for f_{ISS} of 0.1 g ISS g^{-1} VSS. A slightly different approach was proposed by Ekama and Wentzel (2004), considering a higher f_{ISS} value for X_H (0.15) but assuming that $X_{U,E}$ did not contain an inorganic fraction, but this assumption has not yet been demonstrated.

These parameters can be deduced from the variation of total suspended solids and inorganic suspended solids during batch experiments. Figure 2.8 shows simulated

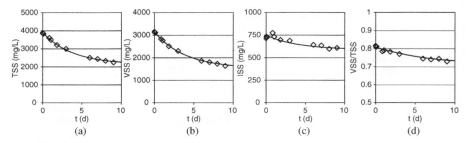

FIGURE 2.8 TSS, VSS, ISS, VSS/TSS during an aerobic endogenous batch test with sludge coming from an aerobic activated sludge process (high load). Measured and modelled data. $f_{ISS,XH} = 0.1$, $f_{ISS,XU} = 0.1$, $X_{Ig,inf}(0) = 468$ mg L^{-1}, $X_H(0) = 2650$ mg COD L^{-1}, $X_{U,E}(0) = 1850$ mg COD L$_{-1}$.

and experimental data obtained in an aerobic batch endogenous test lasting 10 d. The model correctly indicated the diminution of each parameter due to biomass decay and a diminution of the VSS/TSS ratio. It should be noted that the concentration of entrapped inorganics ($X_{Ig,inf}$) was assumed to be constant, and consequently, its contribution to the ISS increased.

At the steady state in activated sludge, a mass balance on mineral compounds gives the production rate of inorganic solids:

$$PX_{ISS} = f_{ISS,XH} \frac{PX_H}{f_{cv,h}} + f_{ISS,XU} \frac{PX_{U,E}}{f_{cv,e}} + Q_{inf} \eta_{ISS} ISS_{inf} + PX_{ISS,PP} \qquad (2.35)$$

ISS_{inf} is the concentration of particulate inorganics in the influent. A certain entrapment efficiency, η_{ISS}, of incoming inorganic suspended solids in the sludge is considered.

The ratio between VSS and TSS can be deduced from

$$\frac{VSS}{TSS} = \frac{PX_V}{PX_V + PX_{ISS}} \qquad (2.36)$$

As shown in Fig. 2.9, the ISS/COD ratio can vary for different wastewaters, depending on the pretreatment, and leading to different VSS/TSS ratios for the mixed liquor. It is predicted that the diminution of the VSS/TSS ratio with SRT is due to an accumulation of ISS in the sludge, whereas organic matter is progressively degraded. This seems logical, but the influence of SRT on the VSS/TSS ratio also depends greatly on the efficiency of ISS entrapment in the sludge, as shown on Fig. 2.9b. Practical experience indicates that the decrease in the VSS/TSS ratio with increasing SRT is not very significant (see below), which is probably explained by the fact that a large amount of incoming inorganic suspended solids is not entrapped or is solubilized in the system at a high sludge age. As little information is available on this phenomenon, an entrapment efficiency of 50% was assumed in this work.

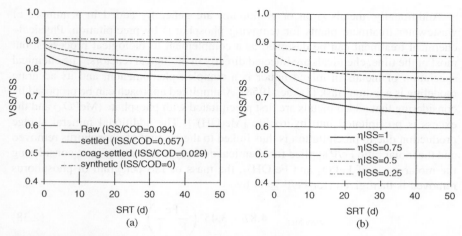

FIGURE 2.9 VSS/TSS as a function of SRT: (a) for different wastewaters with varying amounts of ISS ($\eta_{ISS} = 0.5$); (b) for different entrapment efficiencies with the same wastewater (raw, ISS/COD = 0.094; no precipitation).

2.3.3 Phosphorus Removal (Biological and Physicochemical)

Biological phosphorus removal is obtained by alternating anaerobic and aerobic or anoxic zones. The sludge production of enhanced biological phosphorus removal (EBPR) processes should be considered specifically. The mineral fraction of phosphate-accumulating bacteria is higher than that of ordinary heterotrophic organisms because of the accumulation of polyphosphate as an internal energy reserve. Polyphosphate has an elementary composition estimated as follows: $K_{0.25}Mg_{0.25}Ca_{0.05}PO_3$, which corresponds to a g ISS/g P ratio of 3.11. Hence, the amount of ISS associated with polyphosphate can be related to the amount of phosphorus accumulated in the sludge. The approach presented here is similar to those of Paul et al. (1996) and Ekama and Wentzel (2004). It is considered that the global phosphorus content of sludge depends on the ratio of phosphorus-accumulating organisms (PAOs) to ordinary heterotrophic organisms (OHOs) in the sludge and the polyphosphate content of PAOs. In EBPR systems, based on storage of organic carbon in a pre-anaerobic zone, it is assumed that the amount of PAOs is linked to the easily degradable fraction of biodegradable organic matter. Then the following expression can be proposed:

$$PX_{ISS} = \left(f_{ISS,XH} + 3.11 f_{P,PAO} \frac{f_{BS}}{1 - f_{US} - f_{UP}} \right) \frac{PX_H}{f_{cv,h}} + f_{ISS,XU} \frac{PX_{U,E}}{f_{cv,u}} + Q_{inf} \eta_{ISS} ISS_{inf}$$

(2.37)

This expression is valid if P removal is only biological (no physical–chemical removal). The proportion of phosphorus in PAO ($f_{P,PAO}$) depends on the efficiency of phosphorus uptake. Paul et al. (1996) proposed a value of 0.30, whereas Ekama and Wentzel (2004) proposed different values for anoxic (0.16) and aerobic (0.35) bioreactors.

Additionally, metals (iron or aluminum) are generally added in a number of wastewater treatment plants for removing phosphorus by precipitation. Physical–chemical treatment can be designed as a complement to biological processes, but most of the time, chemicals are injected directly in biological reactors. The chemical speciation of metals in mixed liquor is a complex phenomenon, and its accurate modeling is a tedious task (Takacs 1958). A simplified approach can be proposed by considering that added metals are first precipitated with phosphate ($MePO_4$) and the excess is precipitated into hydroxide [$Me(OH)_3$]. The additional mineral sludge production due to precipitation is thus linked to the amount of phosphorus removed and the molar ratio Fe/P applied for chemical dosage. In the case of iron, considering the molar mass of $FePO_4$ and $Fe(OH)_3$, the mass of ISS per gram of phosphorus removed is then given (for Fe/P $\geq$ 1) by

$$f_{ISS,MeP} = 4.87 + 3.45^* \left(\frac{Fe}{P-1} \right) \tag{2.38}$$

For a system with enhanced biological phosphorus removal, the amount of excess sludge produced by chemical precipitation is given by

$$PX_{ISS,PP} = f_{ISS,MeP} \left[Q_{inf} \eta_P S_{P,inf} - \left(f_{P,XH} + f_{P,PAO} \frac{f_{BS}}{1 - f_{US} - f_{UP}} \right) \frac{PX_H}{f_{cv,h}} \right] \tag{2.39}$$

For a system without enhanced biological phosphorus removal this expression is simplified:

$$PX_{ISS,PP} = f_{ISS,MeP} \left(Q_{inf} \eta_P S_{P,inf} - f_{P,XH} \frac{PX_H}{f_{cv,h}} \right) \tag{2.40}$$

From these expressions and the set of data given in Table 2.7, it is possible to calculate the production of inorganic material as a function of sludge retention time

TABLE 2.7 Typical Set of Parameters for Calculations of Inorganic Excess Sludge Production

Parameter	Value	Reference	Unit
$f_{ISS,XH}$: mass of ISS per unit mass of active heterotrophic biomass	0.1	The authors' own work	g ISS g^{-1} VSS
$f_{ISS,XU}$: mass of ISS per unit mass of endogenous residue	0.1	The authors' own work	g ISS g^{-1} VSS
$f_{ISS,MeP}$: mass of ISS per unit mass of precipitate	4.87	The authors' own work (for Fe/P = 1)	g ISS g^{-1} P
$f_{P,PAO}$: mass of phosphorus as polyphosphate per unit mass of PAO	0.30	Paul et al. (1996)	g P g^{-1} VSS
$f_{P,XH}$: mass of phosphorus per unit active heterotrophic biomass	0.025	Paul et al. (1996)	g P g^{-1} VSS
η_P: phosphorus removal efficiency (objective)	0.9	The authors' own work	

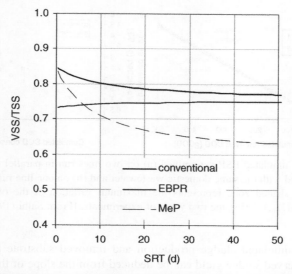

FIGURE 2.10 VSS/TSS as a function of SRT for various processes: conventional ASP, biological phosphorus removal (EBPR), and physical–chemical (MeP) phosphorus removal assuming that Fe/P = 1(b).

as well as the VSS/TSS ratio of the mixed liquor, for conventional, EBPR, and combined biological–physical processes (Fig. 2.10).

2.4 PRACTICAL EVALUATION OF SLUDGE PRODUCTION

2.4.1 Sludge Production Yield Variability with Domestic Wastewater

In an activated sludge system, sludge production is quantified experimentally by a mass balance on suspended solids:

$$PX_V = Q_W VSS_W + Q_{eff} \cdot VSS_{eff} + V \frac{dX_V}{dt} + \frac{dMX_{settler}}{dt} \qquad (2.41)$$

Generally, this mass balance is cumulated over a given period:

$$MX_V = Q_W \, \Delta t \, VSS_W + Q_{eff} \, \Delta t \, VSS_{eff} + V \, \Delta X_V + \Delta MX_{settler} \qquad (2.42)$$

The mass balance should be integrated over a long stable period (three to four times the SRT is a reasonable value) to obtain good accuracy. Similarly, the COD removed is also determined daily and integrated over the same period:

$$MCOD_{removed} = Q_{inf} \, \Delta t \, S_{inf} - (Q_{eff} + Q_W) \Delta t \, S_{S,eff} \qquad (2.43)$$

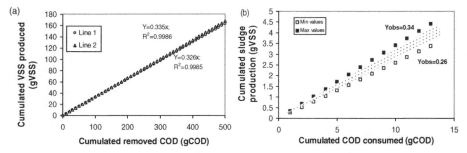

FIGURE 2.11 Cumulated ESP determined (a) on two lines run in parallel under identical conditions and fed with the same domestic wastewater and (b) on one line run during a two-year study. The shaded zone represents the maximum variation of the observed sludge production yield (Y_{obs}) during the two years of experiments. [From Salhi (1999).]

Finally, if cumulated sludge production and removed substrate are measured frequently, observed sludge yield can be deduced from the slope of the graph MX_V versus $MCOD_{removed}$ plotted over a long time period (Fig. 2.11):

$$Y_{obs} = \frac{MX_V}{MCOD_{removed}} \tag{2.44}$$

Figure 2.11 shows the results of a series of experiments on two identical bench-scale activated sludge processes fed with the domestic wastewater from the town of Toulouse (Salhi 1999). The two lines were run in parallel with the same conditions (aerobic/anoxic alternance, SRT = 12 d, T = 16 to 20°C).

The slope of the curves gives information on the repeatability and variability of Y_{obs} measurement on a given system with real wastewater. The results demonstrated that the repeatability was very good for two lines operated at the same time with the same influent (0.335 and 0.326 g VSS g^{-1} COD). However, the variability of measurements performed at different times during two years was much higher (from 0.26 to 0.34 g VSS g^{-1} COD). This can be explained by the variability of the COD characteristics of wastewater during the different seasons with temperatures and the practices of the inhabitants.

2.4.2 Influence of Sludge Age: Experimental Data Versus Models

Experimental data were obtained in the United States and France and the main characteristics (MLSS, SRT) are reported in Table 2.8. These values are used in Fig. 2.12, where sludge production yield (Y_{obs}) is plotted versus SRT. As expected, a decreasing trend is observed with increasing SRT. The dispersion of data can be explained by variations in the wastewater characteristics and by mass balance uncertainties. However, a satisfactory accuracy of Y_{obs} estimation can be noted when the standard composition of wastewater is used (Table 2.6) in activated sludge processes as in membrane bioreactors.

TABLE 2.8 Review of Literature for Sludge Production Yield in Activated Sludge Process

Country	References	Influent	SRT (d)	Y_{obs} (g VSS g⁻¹ COD)	Y_{obs} (TSS) (g TSS g⁻¹ COD)	SUR (g COD g⁻¹ VSS d⁻¹)	VSS (g L⁻¹)	TSS (g L⁻¹)	VSS/TSS
United States	Schultz and Cronin (1997)	Domestic wastewater	6	—	0.336				
			15	—	0.292				
			8	—	0.252				
			12	—	0.284				
			10	—	0.316				
			7	—	0.488				
France, Toulouse	Massé et al. (2005)	Domestic wastewater	9.2	0.302	0.345	0.360	1.4	1.6	0.88
			14.3	0.276	0.322	0.253	1.8	2.1	0.86
			32	0.244	0.293	0.128	2.5	3	0.83
			12	0.320	0.380	0.260	—	—	0.84
			10	0.280	0.373	0.357	—	—	0.75
			44	0.159	0.230	0.143	1.797	2.6	0.69
France, Evry	Salhi (1999); Déléris (2001); Camacho (2001)	Settled wastewater	19	0.230	0.300	0.229	1.150	1.5	0.77
			9	0.252	0.320	0.441	0.709	0.9	0.79
			28	0.225	0.270	0.159	1.417	1.7	0.83
			12	0.287	0.360	0.290	0.957	1.2	0.80
			14	0.297	0.370	0.241	1.204	1.5	0.80
			14	0.268	0.360	0.267	0.893	1.2	0.74
			80	0.132	0.180	0.095	2.273	3.1	0.73
			26	0.203	0.250	0.189	2.111	2.6	0.81
			17	0.261	0.330	0.225	0.870	1.1	0.79

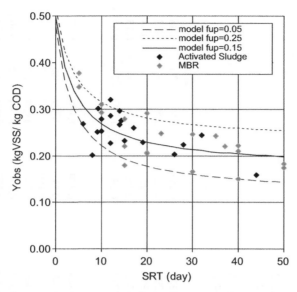

FIGURE 2.12 Y_{obs} versus SRT for activated sludge processes and membrane bioreactors treating domestic wastewaters. Modeling with Eq. (2.27) with $f_{UP} = 0.05$, 0.15, and 0.25, and $f_{US} = 0.05$.

Most of the data collected on different ASPs fed by different domestic wastewaters can be estimated by considering that the inert particulate fraction (f_{UP}) is close to 0.15, as an average value. Eighty-seven percent of the data is found between two extreme predictions, assuming $f_{UP} = 0.05$ and $f_{UP} = 0.25$, whereas 50% of data are obtained between $f_{UP} = 0.1$ and $f_{UP} = 0.2$. Concerning influent characteristics, it appears that the inert particulate fraction (f_{UP}) may induce marked changes in the sludge production yield observed for the activated sludge process. This effect is more pronounced when SRT is increased to reach $\pm10\%$ at 40 days for a variation of 25% in f_{UP}. Therefore, the influent unbiodegradable particulate fraction should be determined accurately for predictive purposes. Furthermore, as f_{UP} is expected to decrease from 0.15 to about 0.125 during settling (Table 2.4), primary treatment should reduce the production yield in the activated sludge from about 4% for SRT of 10 d and up to 6% for plants operated with an SRT of 40 d. But such a small difference is difficult to demonstrate practically because, conversely, primary sludge increases the overall WWTP sludge production (see the following section).

Analysis of an activated sludge process running with the same wastewater at different sludge ages allows us to evaluate the influence of this parameter more accurately. On two case studies (pilot plants fed by wastewater from Evry and Toulouse in France), the organic, total, and inorganic sludge production yields were quantified at different periods (Fig. 2.13).

The fractionation of COD was different for each wastewater ($f_{UP} = 0.14$ and $f_{UP} = 0.19$), resulting in slightly different VSS production yields (Fig. 2.13a). However, due to a greater quantity of entrapped inorganic solids in the Evry process, ISS production

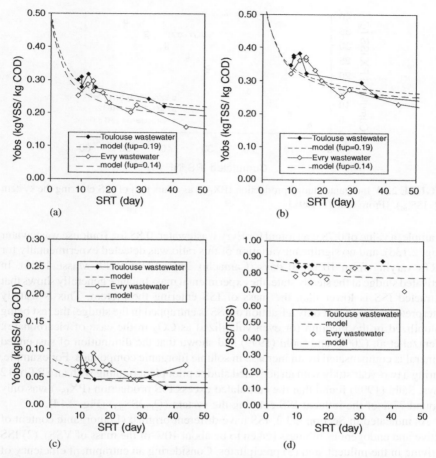

FIGURE 2.13 Two French case studies (Toulouse and Evry): organic (a), total (b), inorganic (c), and sludge production yield VSS/TSS ratio (d) versus SRT. [From Salhi (1999), Déléris (2001), Massé (1976), and Camacho (2001).]

yield was higher (Fig. 2.13c) and TSS production yields were finally similar (Fig. 2.13b). The prediction of the influence of SRT on the different parameters was very good, except for very high sludge ages. At high sludge age, the experimental values in pilot plants were generally lower than the values predicted. This was probably due to a slow hydrolysis of particulate and endogenous residue at a very high SRT (Lubello et al. 2003; Ramdani et al. 1965). This mechanism may be particularly applicable to the case of membrane bioreactors, which can be operated at a very high sludge age.

2.4.3 ISS Entrapment in the Sludge

The VSS/TSS ratio in activated sludge found on the bench-scale pilot was relatively constant at various SRTs for a given process fed with the same wastewater. For

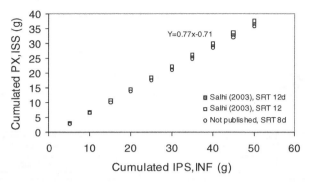

FIGURE 2.14 Inorganic sludge production (PX_{ISS}) as a function of ISS entering the system ($Q \cdot ISS_{inf}$). [From Salhi (1999).]

example, a value of 0.78 was found for Evry wastewater, 0.85 for Toulouse wastewater (Fig. 2.13d), and no significant variation of this ratio was detected experimentally for SRTs varying from 10 to 50 days (Camacho 2001; Salhi 1999; Massé 1976). In activated sludge at the steady state, the experimental mass balance generally shows that extracted ISS is lower than the mass of ISS entering the system. This is usually interpreted to mean that only a fraction of ISS is entrapped in the sludge, the rest being solubilized in the medium (or even volatilized as CO_2 in the case of bicarbonate). Wentzel et al. (2002) and Salhi (1999) had shown that the diminution of suspended mineral is compensated by an increase in soluble inorganic compounds. For example, during a two-year study with an activated sludge pilot plant running with an SRT of 12 days, Salhi (1999) found that the cumulated excess ISS production (PX_{ISS}) was only around 77% of the influent ISS entering the system ($Q_{inf}ISS_{inf}$) (Fig. 2.14).

As indicated in Section 2.3.2, ISS have different origins: (1) inorganic content of active and endogenous biomass (taken to be about 10% of the mass of VSS), (2) ISS arriving in the influent, and (3) precipitates. Considering an entrapment efficiency of 50%, a modeling approach (Fig. 2.15) demonstrates that the ratio between excess ISS (PX_{ISS}) and influent ISS ($Q_{inf}ISS_{inf}$) decreases with increasing SRT. This figure confirms that the ratio will be around 75% for an activated sludge process working at an SRT of 12 d (Salhi 1999). Thus, it can be supposed that 50% of entering ISS is probably a reasonable figure for the entrapment efficiency (η_{ISS}). Wentzel et al. (2002) proposed a value of 20% but assumed that the ISS content of biomass was 0.17 g ISS g^{-1} VSS, whereas it is estimated to be 0.1 g ISS g^{-1} VSS in this chapter.

2.4.4 Example of Sludge Production for a Different Case Study

Primary treatment removes a part of both biodegradable and nonbiodegradable suspended solids. For this reason, primary treatment reduces the activated sludge ESP but increases the total sludge production of a WWTP. For example, based on the wastewater characteristics defined in Table 2.4, the total excess sludge production of an activated sludge process without pretreatment is 30% lower than in a WWTP, including primary settling, and 47% lower than in a system with primary coagulation and settling (Table 2.9

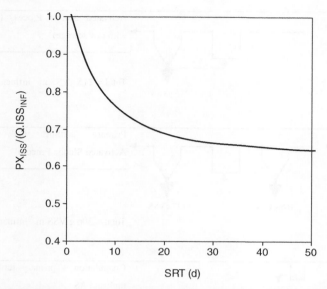

FIGURE 2.15 Evolution of ratio between excess ISS and incoming ISS in activated sludge as a function of SRT. Assumptions: $ISS/COD = 0.06$, $f_{UP} = 0.19$, $\eta_{ISS} = 0.5$, $SRT = 12$ d.

TABLE 2.9 Total Excess Sludge Production of Various WWTPs with or Without Primary Treatment[a]

	Activated Sludge Process (Fed with Raw Sewage)	Primary Settling Tank + Activated Sludge Process	Coagulation + Primary Settling Tank and AS
Primary treatment			
g VSS m^{-3} influent	0	168	337
g TSS m^{-3} influent	0	214	405
Activated sludge			
g VSS g^{-1} COD influent	0.269	0.259	0.223
g TSS g^{-1} COD influent	0.335	0.306	0.259
g VSS m^{-3} influent	215	137	58.0
g TSS m^{-3} influent	268	162	67
Total			
g VSS m^{-3} influent	215	306	395
g TSS m^{-3} influent	268	376	472
g VSS g^{-1} COD influent	0.269	0.383	0.494
g TSS g^{-1} COD influent	0.335	0.470	0.590

[a] Activated sludge process operated with an SRT of 10 d for a typical domestic wastewater with the characteristics as in Table 2.4.

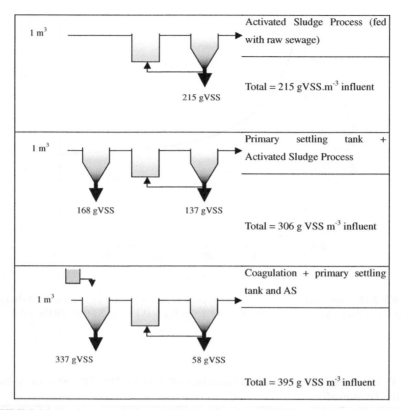

FIGURE 2.16 Total excess sludge production of various WWTPs, with or without primary treatment. Activated sludge process operated with an SRT of 10 d for a typical domestic wastewater with characteristics as in Table 2.4.

and Fig. 2.16). These results have been confirmed by Jimenez et al. (1958) with a pilot study including a membrane bioreactor. Of course, this observation has to be tempered, as a system with primary (coagulation) settling is usually equipped with an anaerobic digester on the sludge line, which can lead to a reduction of 80% in primary sludge VSS.

2.5 STRATEGIES FOR EXCESS SLUDGE REDUCTION

2.5.1 Classification of Strategies

Various excess sludge reduction (ESR) strategies are proposed in the literature. Methodologies are based on the choice of specific operating conditions for the activated sludge processes (e.g., high SRT, predation) or using specific destruction techniques on the mixed liquor produced (oxidation, thermal, enzymatic, mechanical treatments, etc.). Because sludge composition varies with the nature of the

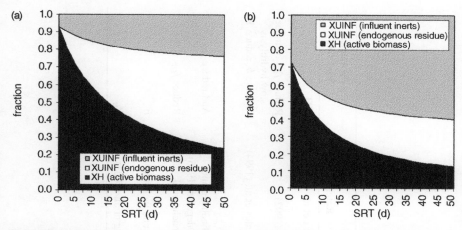

FIGURE 2.17 Theoretical composition of mixed liquor suspended solids (MLSS) as a function of SRT and influent characteristics. (a) $f_{UP} = 0.05$ and (b) $f_{UP} = 0.20$.

wastewater and the operating conditions of the WWTP, the efficiency of these techniques also varies. As illustrated in Fig. 2.17, a model-based analysis of the sludge composition indicates that the proportions of inert compounds (endogenous or originating from influent) and active biomass depend on the SRT and influent characteristics. Thus, the effect of each ESR approach can be evaluated theoretically.

ESR methodologies can be distinguished in terms of target and mechanisms (Table 2.10). For example, some of them are used to limit bacterial growth (addition of uncouplers, heating at low temperature, increase in the SRT), whereas others mainly play a role in increasing the biodegradability of inert compounds (oxidation with chemicals, heating at high temperature $\approx 170°C$). Consequently, regarding Fig. 2.17, it seems logical that a strategy that consists of reducing the microbial growth yield will have more effect on a system working at a low SRT with a wastewater containing a small amount of inert suspended solids (e.g., mostly soluble biodegradable substrate) than on a system operated at a high sludge age with a lot of particulate inerts.

To appreciate the efficiency of ESR strategies, an impact indicator can be calculated, ΔY_{obs}, which is the relative reduction of sludge production yield:

$$\Delta Y_{obs}(\%) = \frac{Y_{obs,ref} - Y_{obs}}{Y_{obs,ref}} \cdot 100 \qquad (2.45)$$

where the reference value ($Y_{obs,ref}$) corresponds to results obtained with a conventional activated sludge process in a reference condition.

2.5.2 Increasing the Sludge Age

To reduce the sludge production observed, the first strategy could be to increase the SRT. The variation in ΔY_{obs} is plotted versus SRT in Fig. 2.18 for the same data as

TABLE 2.10 Example of Classification of Excess Sludge Reduction Strategies

Operation	Mechanisms	Target	Reference	Key Parameters in Modeling
Increase SRT (e.g., MBR)	Increase biomass decay and slow hydrolysis	Bacteria and slowly hydrolysable compounds	Laera et al. (1959)	SRT
Oxidation Chemicals	Improve biodegradability of inerts	Accumulated organic residues from biomass and influent	Liu (1992)	Reduce f_{UP} or model slow hydrolysis
Thermal	Increase biomass decay and reduce bacterial growth yield (low T)	Active biomass	Canales et al. (1994)	Increase b, reduce Y_H
	and improve biodegradability of inerts (high T)	Accumulated organic residues from biomass and influent	Barlindhaug and Odegaard (1996)	And reduce f_{UP}
Mechanical	Improve biodegradability of inerts	Accumulated organic residues from biomass and influent	Camacho et al. (2002)	Reduce f_{UP}
Protozoan reactor	Increase bacterial decay by encouraging predators	Active biomass and residue	Lee and Welander (2009)	b
Addition of uncouplers	Reduce bacterial growth yield	Active biomass and residue	Yang et al. (2003)	Y_H

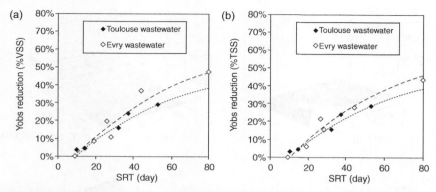

FIGURE 2.18 Variation in Y_{obs} versus SRT as a percentage of an activated sludge process at SRT = 10 d: (a) in VSS, (b) in TSS. [Data from Salhi (1999), Déléris (2001), and Massé (1976) for Toulouse wastewater, and from Camacho (2001) for Evry wastewater.]

presented previously (wastewater from Evry and Toulouse, France), compared to a reference yield obtained for SRT = 10 d. Here, it is observed that an increase in SRT from 10 to 40 d decreases the sludge production by 25%, and an increase in SRT from 10 to 80 d decreases the sludge production by 40 to 45%. The reduction is relatively similar for VSS and TSS, which means that organic and inorganic suspended solids are either oxidized or solubilized simultaneously. The reduction in Y_{obs} is slightly lower for the Toulouse wastewater, which contains more particulate inert compounds ($f_{UP} = 0.19$). This is logical, as the increase in SRT mainly reduces the active biomass, which makes up a lower fraction of MLSS in this wastewater.

2.5.3 Model-Based Evaluation of Advanced ESR Strategies

In previous sections we stressed that various mechanisms are responsible for excess sludge production: bacterial growth, accumulation of influent inert compounds, and accumulation of endogenous residues. In this section, simulations are conducted to assess the possible effect of different strategies, depending on the target: (1) reduction in active biomass, and (2) reduction in inert biomass.

Reduction in Heterotrophic Biomass   Heterotrophic biomass accumulation can be reduced either by increasing the decay rate (imposed by b) or by decreasing the intrinsic cell yield (Y_H). The biomass decay rate can be increased using various techniques: thermal, oxidative, predation, and so on. The effect of the decay constant on ESP is more significant for a short sludge age (fewer than 10 days), where a variation of 25% induces a relative modification of Y_{obs} of 8%, whereas for a longer SRT, the modification in sludge production yield does not exceed 4%. The reduction in excess sludge production reaches a maximum value of 16% when biomass decay is doubled compared to the reference value, this maximum reduction being obtained for

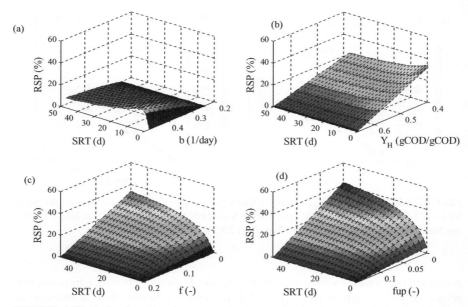

FIGURE 2.19 Evaluation of various strategies on a reduction in excess sludge production.

6 d of SRT (Fig. 2.19a). This moderate effect of decay rate on total sludge production is due primarily to the fact that increasing decay reduces the biomass production but simultaneously increases the accumulation of inert compounds due to cell lysis. To limit the accumulation of inert matter observed when increasing the decay rate, a possible strategy would be to increase the degradation of endogenous residue simultaneously, as discussed below.

Another strategy is to reduce the biomass intrinsic growth yield, Y_H, which means increasing the amount of substrate that is oxidized. To do this, the use of an uncoupler molecule can be proposed, which increases maintenance energy requirements. Mayhew and Stephenson (2004) experimentally observed a decrease of 30% of the heterotrophic biomass yield when an uncoupler (2,4-dinitrophenol) was used. Canales et al. (1994) also found an increase in maintenance energy by applying a thermal treatment in association with a membrane bioreactor. Figure 2.19b points out that a variation of 25% of heterotrophic biomass yield, Y_H, induces a modification of more than 13% (for high SRT) and up to 20% (for low SRT) of the sludge production yield. As shown in Fig. 2.19b, this decrease in Y_H may induce a reduction in sludge production ranging from 15 to 20% for SRTs of 50 to 6 d, respectively. However, the environmental impact of the uncoupler should be investigated thoroughly with regard to the reduction in excess sludge production (RSP) reached. Another strategy could be to encourage internal reserve storage to minimize the cell growth yield, but the effect on Y_{obs} would also be relatively low (5 to 8%).

As shown in Table 2.11, strategies that target biomass growth are expected to induce a decrease in the active biomass fraction. For example, doubling the decay rate

TABLE 2.11 Simulated Active Biomass Fraction to Reach 15% Reduction in Sludge Production for an ASP with a 10-Day SRT[a]

Strategy	Value of Key Parameter	% of Active Biomass
Reduction in bacterial growth	$b = 0.48 \text{ d}^{-1}$	30
	$Y_H = 0.5 \text{ g COD g}^{-1} \text{ COD}$	38
Reduction of inerts	$f = 0.045$	51
	$f_{UP} = 0.06$	57

[a] RSP = 15%; $\%X_{H,\text{ref},10\text{days}} = 43\%$.

leads to a theoretical decrease of the active fraction from 43% to 30% of total VSS. The direct consequence may be a decrease in removal performance, as the F/M ratio would be increased.

Reduction of Inert Compounds and Endogenous Residue It is clear that the accumulation of inert compounds becomes the most important technical target of excess sludge reduction strategy when focusing on WWTPs treating real domestic wastewater, especially if they are designed and operated at a high sludge age. Considering previous results, a limit on excess sludge reduction occurs when associated treatments aim either at modifying the decay constant or at modifying the cell growth yield, even for X_U-free wastewater. When the wastewater-suspended inert fraction is significant (domestic wastewater), the bottleneck lies in this inert matter accumulation. Moreover, increasing an SRT would lead to a physical limitation of the settling systems due to the associated increase in solids concentration. Therefore, targeting inert matter is the strategy to develop if the objective, with an SRT value of 15 d or more, is to reduce ESP by 30% or more. Figure 2.19c and d show that either a reduction in endogenous residue (reduction of f) or a reduction in wastewater inert compounds (reduction of f_{UP}) can decrease the excess sludge production by up to 40% at a high sludge age. From a practical point of view, it is difficult to avoid the production (or arrival) of these residues ($X_{U,\text{inf}}$ and $X_{U,E}$), but their reduction can be obtained by increasing their degradation or biodegradability.

As a limit value, the conjunction of any method (e.g., chemical, mechanical) able to make these fractions fully biodegradable with a relevant retention time would lead to a process producing no organic sludge. It is therefore appropriate to direct efforts toward finding processes that enable the biodegradability of these fractions to be increased. Treatments such as thermal treatment (Weemaes and Verstraete 1998), ozonation-coupled treatment (Déléris et al. 2000), or biological self-digestion (Saiki et al. 2002) could be interesting candidate processes for such a purpose. With these techniques, experiments have proved that a nearly complete ESP reduction is achievable.

2.6 CONCLUSIONS

The fundamental processes involved in excess sludge production have been detailed for the prediction of accurate design and modeling: active heterotrophic biomass production, endogenous residue production, and accumulation of organic inerts from the influent. In addition, the accumulation of inorganic suspended solids has also been described accurately, leading to an overall theoretical approach that matches experimental observations correctly: the effect of influent characteristics and the influence of SRT. From a practical point of view, it points out the importance of good wastewater characterization and good accuracy in mass balances for the correct evaluation of ESP. Finally, a model-based approach has demonstrated the potential of "inert reduction" in excess sludge reduction strategies compared with "growth limitation" strategies.

2.7 NOMENCLATURE

Parameter	Description	Unit
μ:	Heterotrophic growth rate	d^{-1}
b:	Decay constant of active biomass (endogenous respiration concept)	d^{-1}
b':	Decay constant of active biomass (death-regeneration concept)	d^{-1}
b_{XUE}:	Decay constant of endogenous particulate "residue"	d^{-1}
f:	Inert fraction of biomass (endogenous respiration concept)	-
f':	Inert fraction of dead biomass (death-regeneration concept)	-
f_{BP}:	Biodegradable particulate fraction of wastewater COD	-
f_{BS}:	Biodegradable soluble fraction of wastewater COD	-
$f_{cv,h}$:	Conversion factor for heterotrophic biomass	g COD g^{-1} VSS
$f_{cv,u,e}$:	Conversion factor for endogenous residue	g COD g^{-1} VSS
$f_{cv,u,inf}$:	Conversion factor for influent inert particulate	g COD g^{-1} VSS
f_{CX}:	Colloidal fraction of wastewater slowly biodegradable COD	-
$f_{ISS,MeP}$:	Mass of ISS per unit mass of precipitate	g ISS g^{-1} P
$f_{ISS,XH}$:	Mass of ISS per unit mass of active heterotrophic biomass	g ISS g^{-1} VSS
$f_{ISS,XU}$:	Mass of ISS per unit mass of endogenous residue	g ISS g^{-1} VSS
$f_{P,PAO}$:	Mass of phosphorus as polyphosphate per unit mass of PAO	g P g^{-1} VSS
$f_{P,XH}$:	Mass of phosphorus per unit mass of active heterotrophic biomass	g P g^{-1} VSS

f_{UP}:	Inert particulate fraction of wastewater COD	-
f_{US}:	Inert soluble fraction of wastewater COD	-
$MCOD_{removed}$	Mass of organic matter removed	g COD
MX_V	Mass of suspended solids produced	g VSS
PCPS:	Sludge Production from Primary Coagulation +Settling	g VSS d^{-1}
PPS:	Sludge Production from Primary Settling	g VSS d^{-1}
PX_H:	Heterotrophic biomass production rate	g COD d^{-1}
PX_{ISS}:	Inorganic solids production rate	g ISS d^{-1}
PX_{UE}:	Endogenous residue production rate	g COD d^{-1}
PX_{UINF}:	Influent unbiodegradable solids production rate	g COD d^{-1}
PX_V:	Total organic sludge production rate	g VSS d^{-1}
Q_{INF}:	Influent flow rate	m^3 d^{-1}
Q_{EFF}:	Effluent flow rate	m^3 d^{-1}
Q_W:	Waste flow rate	m^3 d^{-1}
r_S:	Substrate degradation rate	g COD m^{-3} d^{-1}
r_{XH}:	Heterotrophic biomass evolution rate	g COD m^{-3} d^{-1}
S:	Substrate concentration in bioreactor	g COD m^{-3}
S_B:	Soluble readily biodegradable COD concentration	g COD m^{-3}
S_{EFF}:	Effluent COD	g COD m^{-3}
S_{INF}:	Influent COD	g COD m^{-3}
S_U:	Soluble unbiodegradable COD concentration	g COD m^{-3}
T	Temperature	°C
t	Time	d
X_A	Autotrophic biomass concentration	g COD m^{-3}
X_B	Insoluble slowly biodegradable COD concentration	g COD m^{-3}
X_H	Heterotrophic biomass concentration	g COD m^{-3}
X_U	Insoluble unbiodegradable COD concentration	g COD m^{-3}
X_{UE}	Endogenous particulate "residue"	g COD m^{-3}
X_{UINF}	Influent particulate "inerts"	g COD m^{-3}
$X_{Ig,BIO}$	ISS concentration associated with active biomass	g ISS m^{-3}
$X_{Ig,INF}$	ISS concentration associated with entrapped ISS from influent	g ISS m^{-3}
$X_{Ig,PP}$	ISS concentration associated with precipitation	g ISS m^{-3}
Y_{CPSS}	Primary (coagulation + settling) sludge production yield (per unit inlet COD)	g VSS g^{-1} COD
Y_H	Heterotrophic intrinsic biomass yield	g VSS g^{-1} COD or g COD g^{-1} COD
Y_{obs}	Observed biomass yield	g VSS g^{-1} COD

Y_{PSS}	Primary (settling) sludge production yield (per unit inlet COD)	g VSS g^{-1} COD
η_{CPS}	Removal efficiency of primary coagulation +settling	-
η_{ISS}	Inorganic suspended solids entrapment efficiency	-
η_P	Phosphorus removal efficiency (objective)	-
η_{PS}	Removal efficiency of primary settling on suspended particle	-

REFERENCES

Barlindhaug J., Odegaard H. (1996) Thermal hydrolysis for the production of carbon source for denitrification. *Water Science and Technology* **34**(1–2), 371–378.

Camacho P. (2001) Etude de procédés de réduction de la production de boues par couplage de traitement physique ou chimique et biologique. Thesis, Toulouse University, INSA, Toulouse, France.

Camacho P., Geaugey V., Ginestet P., Paul, E. (2002) Feasibility study of mechanically disintegrated sludge and recycle in the activated-sludge process. *Water Science and Technology* **46**(10), 97–104.

Canales, A., Pareilleux, A., Rols, J. L., Goma, G., Huyard, A. (1994) Decreased sludge production strategy for domestic wastewater treatment. *Water Science and Technology* **30**(8), 97–106.

Corominas L., Rieger L., Takacs I., Ekama G., Hauduc H., Vanrolleghem P. A., Oehmen A., Gernaey K. V., van Loosdrecht M. C. M., Comeau Y. (2010) New framework for standardized notation in wastewater treatment modelling. *Water Science and Technology* **61**(4), 841–857.

Déléris, S. (2001) Réduction de la production de boue lors du traitement des eaux résiduaires urbaines. Analyse du traitement combiné: ozonation et traitement biologique. Thesis, Toulouse University, INSA, Toulouse, France.

Déléris S., Paul E., Audic J. M., Roustan M., Debellefontaine H. (2000) Effect of ozonation on activated sludge solubilization and mineralization. *Ozone Science and Engineering* **22**(5), 473–486.

Dignac M. F. (1998) Caractérisation chimique de la matière organique au cours du traitement des eaux usées par boues activées. Ph.D. dissertation, Université Paris VI, France.

Dold P. L. (2007) Quantifying sludge production in municipal treatment plants. Proceedings of WEFTEC, pp. 1522–1549.

Dold P. L., Ekama G. A., Marais G. V. R. (1980) A general-model for the activated sludge process. *Progress in Water Technology* **12**, 47–77.

Ekama G. A., Wentzel M. C. (2004) A predictive model for the reactor inorganic suspended solids concentration in activated sludge systems. *Water Research* **38**(19), 4093–4106.

Ekama G. A., Dold P. L., Marais G. V. R. (1986) Procedures for determining influent COD fractions and the maximum specific growth rate of heterotrophs in activated sludge systems. *Water Science and Technology* **18**(6), 91–114.

Gillot S., Choubert J.-M. (2010) Biodegradable organic matter in domestic wastewaters: comparison of selected fractionation techniques. *Water Science and Technology* **62**(3), 630–639.

Ginestet P., Maisonnier A., Spérandio M. (2002) Wastewater COD characterization: biodegradability of physico-chemical fractions. *Water Science and Technology* **45**(6), 89–97.

Grulois P., Famel J. C., Hangouet J. P., Fayoux C. (1996) Rien ne se perd, rien ne se crée, tout se transforme...en boues! L' Eau, l'industrie, les nuisances 195, 42–46.

Henze M. (1992) Characterisation of wastewater for modelling of activated sludge processes. *Water Science and Technology* **25**(6), 1–15.

Henze M., Grady C. P., Gujer W., Marais G. V. R., Matsuo T. (1987) A general model for single-sludge wastewater treatment systems. *Water Research* **21**(5), 505–515.

Henze M., Gujer W., Mino T., van Loosdrecht M. (2000) *Activated Sludge Models ASM1, ASM2, ASM2D and ASM3*, IWA Publishing, London.

Herbert D. (1958) Some pinciples in continuous culture. *Recent progress in microbiology*, 381–396.

Jimenez J., Grelier P., Meinhold J., Tazi-Pain A. (2010) Biological modelling of MBR and impact of primary sedimentation. *Desalination* **250**(2), 562–567.

Kappeler J., Gujer W. (1992) Estimation of kinetic parameters of heterotrophic biomass under aerobic conditions and characterization of wastewater for activated sludge modelling. *Water Science and Technology* **25**(6), 125–139.

Kountz R. R., Forney C. J. (1959) Metabolic energy balances in a total oxidation activated sludge system. *Sewage and Industrial Wastes* **31**(7), 819–826.

Laera G., Pollice A., Saturno D., Giordano C., Sandulli R. (2009) Influence of sludge retention time on biomass characteristics and cleaning requirements in a membrane bioreactor for municipal wastewater treatment. *Desalination* **236**(1–3), 104–110.

Lee N. M., Welander T. (1996) Use of protozoa and metazoa for decreasing sludge production in aerobic wastewater treatment. *Biotechnology Letters* **18**(4), 429–434.

Lesouef A., Payraudeau M., Rogalla F., Kleiber B. (1992) Optimizing nitrogen removal reactor configurations by on-site calibration of the IAWPRC activated-sludge model. *Water Science and Technology* **25**(6), 105–123.

Liu Y. (2003) Chemically reduced excess sludge production in the activated sludge process. *Chemosphere* **50**(1), 1–7.

Lubello C., Caffaz S., Gori R., Munz G. (2009) A modified activated sludge model to estimate solids production at low and high solids retention time. *Water Research* **43**(18), 4539–4548.

Marais G. V. R. Ekama G. A. (1976) The activated sludge process: 1. Steady state behaviour. *Water SA* **2**(4), 163–200.

Massé A. (2004) Bioréacteur à membranes immergées pour le traitement des eaux résiduaires urbaines:spécificité physico-chimiques du milieu biologique et colmatage. Thesis, Toulouse University, INSA, Toulouse, France.

Mayhew M., Stephenson T. (1998) Biomass yield reduction: Is biochemical manipulation possible without affecting activated sludge process efficiency? *Water Science and Technology* **38**(8–9 pt 7), 137–144.

McKinney R. E. (1960) Complete mixing activated sludge. *Water and Sewage Works* **111**, 246–259.

Melcer H. (2003) *Methods for Wastewater Characterization in Activated Sludge Modeling*, Water Environment Federation, Alexandria, VA, and IWA Publishing, London.

Olstein M. (1996) *Benchmarking Wastewater Treatment Plant Operations*, Water Environment Research Foundation, Alexandria, VA.

Paul E., Laval M. L., Spérandio M. (2001) Excess sludge production and costs due to phosphorus removal. *Environmental Technology* **22**(11), 1363–1371.

Pirt S. J. (1965) The maintenance energy of bacteria in growing cultures. Royal Society of London Proceedings Series B 163, 224–231.

Ramdani A., Dold P., Déléris S., Lamarre D., Gadbois A., Comeau Y. (2010) Biodegradation of the endogenous residue of activated sludge. *Water Research* **44**(7), 2179–2188.

Roeleveld P. J., van Loosdrecht M. C. M. (2002) Experience with guidelines for wastewater characterisation in The Netherlands. *Water Science and Technology* **45**(6), 77–87.

Saiki Y., Imabayashi S., Iwabuchi C., Kitagawa Y., Okumura Y., Kawamura H. (1999) Solubilization of excess activated sludge by self-digestion. *Water Research* **33**(8), 1864–1870.

Salhi M. (2003) Procédés couplés boues activées-ozonation pour la réduction de la production de boues: étude, modélisation et intégration dans la filière de traitement des eaux. Thesis, Toulouse University, INSA, Toulouse, France.

Sollfrank U., Gujer W. (1991) Characterisation of domestic wastewater for mathematical modelling of the activated sludge process. *Water Science and Technology* **23**(4), 1057–1066.

Spérandio M. (1998) Développement d'une procédure de compartimentation d'une eau résiduaire urbaine et application à la modélisation dynamique de procédés à boues activées. Thesis, Toulouse University, INSA, Toulouse, France.

Spérandio M., Urbain V., Ginestet P., Audic M. J., Paul E. (2001) Application of COD fractionation by a new combined technique: comparison of various wastewaters and sources of variability. *Water Science and Technology* **43**(1), 181–190.

Symons J. M., McKinney R. E. (1958) Biochemistry of nitrogen in the synthesis of activated sludge. *Sewage and Industrial Wastes* **30**(7), 874–890.

Takacs, I. (2008) Experiments in activated sludge modelling. Thesis, Gent University, Ghent, Belgium.

Washington D. R., Symons J. M. (1962) Volatile sludge accumulation in activated sludge systems. *Journal of the Water Pollution Control Federation* **34**, 767–790.

Weemaes M. P. J., Verstraete W. H. (1998) Evaluation of current wet sludge disintegration techniques. *Journal of Chemical Technology and Biotechnology* **73**(2), 83–92.

Wentzel M. C., Ubisi M. F., Lakay M. T., Ekama G. A. (2002) Incorporation of inorganic material in anoxic/aerobic-activated sludge system mixed liquor. *Water Research* **36**(20), 5074–5082.

Yang X. F., Xie M. L., Liu Y. (2003) Metabolic uncouplers reduce excess sludge production in an activated sludge process. *Process Biochemistry* **38**(9), 1373–1377.

Yasui H., Shibata M., (1994) An innovative approach to reduce excess sludge production in the activated sludge process. *Water Science and Technology* **30**(9), 11–20.

3

CHARACTERIZATION OF MUNICIPAL WASTEWATER AND SLUDGE

ETIENNE PAUL, XAVIER LEFEBVRE, AND MATHIEU SPERANDIO

Université de Toulouse; INSA,UPS,INP; LISBP, 135 Avenue de Rangueil, F-31077 Toulouse, France; INRA, UMR792, Ingénierie des Systèmes Biologiques et des Procédés, F-31400 Toulouse, France; CNRS, UMR5504, F-31400 Toulouse, France

DOMINIQUE LEFEBVRE

Université Paul Sabatier, Laboratoire de Biologie Appliquée à l'Agroalimentaire et à l'Environnement, Auch, France

YU LIU

Division of Environmental and Water Resources Engineering, School of Civil and Environmental Engineering, Nanyang Technological University, Singapore

3.1 INTRODUCTION

Prediction of both primary sludge and waste activated sludge (WAS) production is undoubtedly one of the major tasks and challenges in the design and operation of a wastewater treatment plant (WWTP). Such a prediction is based on detailed characterization of influent organic and inorganic components that are essential for applications of empirical or sophisticated mechanistic models (e.g., the activated sludge models). For the purpose of characterization, chemical oxygen demand (COD) has been chosen to represent organic matter in both wastewater and sludge. Various lumped COD components and their relative fractions with respect to total COD (COD_{tot}) have been defined to account for significant field observations

Biological Sludge Minimization and Biomaterials/Bioenergy Recovery Technologies, First Edition.
Edited by Etienne Paul and Yu Liu.
© 2012 John Wiley & Sons, Inc. Published 2012 by John Wiley & Sons, Inc.

(e.g., settling, dynamic oxygen demand, excess sludge production, treatment efficiency). Extensive attention has thus been given to the prediction of changes in these fractions along various physicochemical and biological treatment units.

Undoubtedly, determination of the biodegradable COD (BCOD) and of unbiodegradable particulate COD in influent is a major challenge for the prediction of excess sludge production because the former is utilized for microbial growth, and the latter is accumulated in the sludge. However, it should be realized that such information may not be sufficient, due to the fact that other inert components (soluble and particulate) are produced during biological transformations. Obviously, the newly produced inert compounds must be taken into account, and they, in fact, make the wastewater characterization task much more complicated. Moreover, the inert soluble COD is related directly to the outlet COD leaving a WWTP.

Definition of COD fractions is somewhat arbitrary and depends on wastewater characterization methods. Various regional and national organizations have put in much effort to standardize the characterization methods for various COD fractions (WERF 2003). However, COD fractionation is linked to a specific mathematical model and its hypothesis, and also depends on plant configuration [e.g., sludge retention time (SRT)] and the wastewater treatment objectives (e.g., nutrient removal, sludge reduction). In addition, some new technological development should be taken into account in COD fractionation: (1) membrane bioreactors; (2) new wastewater treatment concepts (e.g., use of direct influent filtration or chemically enhanced sedimentation to maximize the removal of organic matter for anaerobic digestion and therefore to reduce energy input for aeration in the activated sludge treatment) (Odegaard 1998; van Nieuwenhuijzen et al. 2001); (3) new treatment strategies, such as sludge reduction; and (4) new treatment objectives (e.g., incorporation of agroindustrial waste/wastewater in the main stream). Therefore, wastewater characterization must adapt to these new contexts, and the existing test protocols may no longer be valid when such new situations are faced.

Sophisticated methods have been developed in laboratories for characterization of wastewater fractions, whereas simple and reproducible methods are preferred for routine wastewater characterization at a full-scale plant. This means that COD fractionation must comply with the demand of both researchers and practitioners. In addition to wastewater characterization, there is a strong demand on sludge characterization. Indeed, information about sludge composition and structure is essential for prediction of methane production and the potential of sludge valorization. WAS is formed mainly under aerobic/anoxic units, while it has to be degraded under anaerobic condition for recovery of biogases.

There is an increasing demand for reducing excess sludge production as well as for recovering useful materials and energy from excess sludge. For these purposes, sludge undergoes specific digestion with disintegration pretreatments (e.g., thermal, mechanical, oxidative) on the wastewater or sludge treatment line. Sound changes in the sludge physical, chemical, and biological properties may occur during the additional treatment, and released materials may affect the treatment efficiency. Physical, chemical, and biological methods have been widely used for supernatant and sludge fractionation after disintegration. However, due to differences in protocols for organic

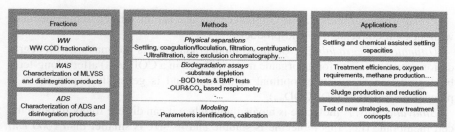

FIGURE 3.1 Characterization and applications of wastewater, WAS, and ADS.

matter characteristics and uses of various definitions, it appears to be impossible to compare results reported in the literature. For example, the definition of soluble fraction depends strongly on its determination by physical methods. Similarly, improved biodegradability may be due to an increase in the biodegradation rate or an increase in the biodegradation extent; obviously, both need to be distinguished in practice.

In this chapter we briefly overview existing methods for characterization of COD fractions of both wastewater and sludge, with a focus on methods for prediction of sludge production and sludge composition which are highly helpful for further assessment of sludge digestion capacity and characterization of sludge disintegration products (Fig. 3.1). Characterization of the mixed liquor volatile suspended solids (MLVSS) after application of a disintegration technique is also considered. Some definitions are given in Section 3.2 to specify the meaning of some important properties and transformations. Then COD fractions of wastewater, WAS, and anaerobically digested sludge (ADS) are described in relation to conventional models, ASMs, and anaerobic digestion models (Section 3.3). Physical (Section 3.4) and biological (Section 3.5) fractionation methods are then presented. Finally, in the last part of this chapter we focus on the application of these methods to wastewater (Section 3.6) and sludge (Section 3.7) characterization.

3.2 DEFINITIONS

Biodegradation. Biodegradation is the partial simplification or complete mineralization of the molecular structure of molecules by complex, genetically regulated physiological reactions catalyzed largely by microorganisms and consortia of microorganisms (Madsen 1991, 2001; Alexander 1999). The microorganisms or consortia with essential enzymatic functions are able to transform the molecules along complex metabolic pathways for energy generation and biosynthesis. Another term related to biodegradation is biomineralization, in which organic matter is totally converted to minerals. These biotransformations are based on the bioaccessibility and bioavailability of target molecules to microorganisms. Thus, the physicochemical state of carbon in the organic matrix (floc) is crucial for biotransformation (Aquino et al. 2008).

Primary biodegradation. The Original compound is transformed to intermediates without total conversion to end products.

Ultimate biodegradability. Ultimate biodegradability is the maximal biodegradation extent obtained for an organic material (e.g., in a COD unit) after a long-term biodegradation assay under optimal conditions, and is generally expressed as a percentage in total COD (COD_{tot}).

Bioavailability. A molecule is bioavailable when it can diffuse freely through the cell membrane (i.e., this molecule is soluble and its size is smaller than 1000 Da) (Madigan et al., 2003). Some active transport processes allow specific larger molecules to enter into the cell.

Bioaccessibility. Compounds and components in wastewater or sludge are present in the form of a complex particulate matrix, leading to transport limitation. Moreover, complexes can be formed between various compounds or molecules, resulting in reduced bioaccessibility. In the case of sludge, there is a decrease in the pollutant's *effective concentration* which is balanced proportionately by a lingering reservoir of this pollutant in the biological floc. Various sequestration mechanisms can be involved: complexation into bound residues, diffusion into floc pores, and adsorption.

Hydrolysis. The substrate may be in a polymerized form (e.g., proteins, polysaccharides). The large size of polymeric substances prevents them from diffusing across the bacterial membrane, and they must be hydrolyzed before biological utilization. Batstone (2000) reviewed the various enzymatic mechanisms of sludge hydrolysis: (1) enzyme secretion and then reaction with the substrate after adsorption; (2) enzyme secretion in the vicinity of the particulate substrate on which the microorganism had previously been adsorbed; and (3) enzyme remains attached to the microorganism, which adsorbs to the particle. Mechanisms (1) and (2) suggest a close contact between the polymer and the enzyme or the microorganism, which raises the question of the bioaccessibility of the polymer. Hydrolysis of particulate substrates is a surface-related process. Colonization of a particle surface by a biofilm is necessary for complete degradation (Spérandio and Paul 2000).

The measurement of COD biodegradability, bioavailability, and bioaccessibility is essential to better assess the real potential of sludge production during biological stabilization of organic matters. Such information is also important for selecting the suitable treatment process for enhancing the ultimate biodegradability.

3.3   WASTEWATER AND SLUDGE COMPOSITION AND FRACTIONATION

Wastewater and sludge characterization appears to be a key issue for prediction of the transformations of their organic components in the physicochemical and biological processes. The conventional municipal wastewater and primary or secondary sludge is composed of different types of molecules. A fine biochemical and physical characterization is not applicable in routine operation, although it has been suggested by some researchers (Huang et al. 2010). Instead, use of COD fractionation is preferable, together with kinetic and stoichiometric parameters (e.g., soluble, colloidal, and kinetic particulates). It should be noted that COD alone cannot differentiate biodegradable and unbiodegradable matters, nor can it provide information on how to distinguish settleable, coagulable, and soluble matters.

A WWTP is composed of various interconnected treatment units. As such, the output from an upstream unit becomes input to the downstream unit. WAS and primary sludge generated during the process is further directed to the anaerobic digestion process. Therefore, coherence among all the operation units must be ensured (Ekama et al. 2007). Additional sludge treatment has often been employed to improve its biodegradability and reduce excess sludge production. Such treatment may affect the physical and biological fractionation of COD, and resulting changes must be analyzed to better understand the mechanism of action of the additional sludge treatment.

3.3.1   Wastewater COD Fractions

COD_{tot} in a wastewater can be divided into various fractions regarding its physical state or the potential of biodegradability. For a conventional municipal wastewater, COD_{tot} can be expressed as (Corominas et al. 2010)

$$COD_{tot} = (f_{BS} + f_{US} + f_{BX} + f_{UX}) \cdot COD_{inf} \tag{3.1}$$

$$COD_{tot} = COD_{inf} = S_B + S_{U,inf} + X_B + X_{U,inf} \tag{3.2}$$

in which S_B is soluble (readily) biodegradable COD, $S_{U,inf}$ is soluble unbiodegradable COD, X_B is (slowly) biodegradable particulate COD, $X_{U,inf}$ is unbiodegradable particulate COD, and f_{BS}, f_{US}, f_{BX}, and f_{UX} are the corresponding COD fractions of these components. According to Dold (2007), for real wastewater, these fractions are useful, as total COD may vary substantially from plant to plant, while the COD fractions seem to be more consistent among WWTPs. Heterotrophic (X_{OHO}) and autotrophic (X_{ANO}) biomasses in the influent may also be considered. A schematic representation of these COD fractions is shown in Fig. 3.2. When the objective is to

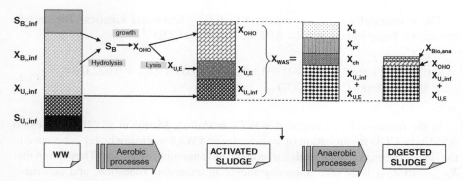

FIGURE 3.2 Schematic representation of wastewater and sludge COD fractionation theory for aerobic activated sludge treatment and anaerobic digestion of WAS.

predict sludge production, determination of the unbiodegradable particulate fraction and the entire biodegradable fraction that will be transformed to biomass active cells and cell debris is crucial. The quantitative determination of each fraction is addressed later in the chapter.

According to the wastewater type and the sludge retention time in a WWTP, some COD fractions can be further divided into subcomponents. For example, $X_{U,inf}$ often contains some very slowly biodegradable COD that must be accounted for at an SRT higher than 30 days (Nowak et al. 1999), whereas slowly hydrolyzable soluble COD should also be considered when required (Orhon and Çokgör 1997).

3.3.2 WAS COD Fractions

When COD biodegradation occurs in a conventional biological process, active heterotrophic cells (X_{OHO}) are produced; meanwhile, unbiodegradable COD is generated from the biomass growth and decay (Washington and Symons 1962): for example, unbiodegradable particulate COD from cell decay ($X_{U,E}$) and unbiodegradable soluble COD ($S_{U,E}$) (Fig. 3.2). The fraction of biomass yielding $X_{U,E}$ is called f and an f value of 0.2 has commonly been used, due to endogenous respiration. The activated sludge process has been operated in a wide SRT range: several days to 100 Part of $X_{U,inf}$ and $X_{U,E}$ will be more biodegradable at a high SRT, especially after sludge treatment by disintegration, for example.

3.3.3 ADS Organic Fractions

During anaerobic digestion of sludge, complex particulate matter (X_{WAS}) in WAS or primary sludge is first disintegrated to carbohydrate (X_{ch}), protein (X_{pr}), and lipid (X_{li}) particulate substrates, as well as particulate and soluble inert materials, as shown in Fig. 3.2. The following equation is derived according to a mass balance on COD:

$$X_{WAS} = 0.1S_U + 0.25X_U + 0.2X_{ch} + 0.2X_{pr} + 0.25X_{li} \qquad (3.3)$$

The extracellular steps are assumed to follow first-order kinetics. The carbon content of X_{WAS} should thus be $0.02786 \, kmol \, C \, kg \, COD^{-1}$:

$$0.03.0.1S_U + 0.03.0.2X_U + 0.0313.0.2X_{ch} + 0.03.0.2X_{pr} + 0.022.0.3X_{li} \\ = 0.02786 \, kmol \, C \cdot kg^{-1} \, COD \qquad (3.4)$$

In the framework of integrated WWTP modeling, Ekama et al. (2007) assessed ASM-type COD fractionation of wastewater and WAS to ensure better coherence in the link between activated sludge treatment and anaerobic digestion. They found that $X_{U,inf}$ and $X_{U,E}$ were also unbiodegradable in anaerobic digestion, and anaerobic biodegradation can thus be predicted from the WAS composition under conventional operating conditions of anaerobic digestion.

The division between the different fractions is somehow arbitrary and may vary with the operating conditions of the WWTP (e.g., SRT and the type of wastewater). For example, to better predict excess sludge production in an activated sludge process run at a high SRT, a very slow hydrolysis rate should be considered at least on the $X_{U,E}$ COD fraction (Jones et al. 2007; Lubello et al. 2009; Ramdani et al. 2010) or a new COD fraction must be added to the models (Nowak et al. 1999). Fractionation is also influenced by the model to be used and the experimental methods employed to quantify fractions.

3.4 PHYSICAL FRACTIONATION

3.4.1 Physical State of Wastewater Organic Matter

In urban wastewater, the major part of the organic matter is in particulate or colloidal form (see also Table 3.1). It may be separated in the primary or secondary settlers or may be degraded by heterotrophic bacteria after hydrolysis. As the result, the COD of wastewater compounds can be grouped into different categories according to size for the prediction of various transformations and separations: for example, the settling and coagulation efficiency of influent compounds, the extent of biological hydrolysis of wastewater molecules, and oxygen demand profiles. Figure 3.3 shows a typical physical fractionation of wastewater. For the purpose of fractionation, various separation techniques have been used (e.g., settling, centrifugation, filtration).

3.4.2 Methods for Physical Fractionation of Wastewater Components

Settleable Fraction Ginestet (2000) developed a laboratory settling method to simulate the normal working conditions of a primary settler, in which a 1-L graduated Imhoff cone is used to determine the settleable fraction of wastewater. After 2 h of

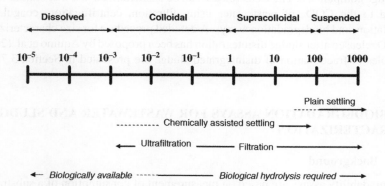

FIGURE 3.3 Physical state of the matter and physical fractionation of wastewater with respect to operational units and biological transformations.

settling, the settleable fraction is withdrawn from the bottom of the cone, and the remaining supernatant is recovered as the unsettleable fraction, from which liquid at the top of the cone which contains floating particles must be removed. Coagulation using ferric chloride ($FeCl_3$) has also been used to assess the extent of organic material to be removed by chemically assisted settling (Ginestet et al. 2002).

Soluble Fraction   To differentiate the fractionation between soluble and particulate COD, filtration with a 0.45-μm pore size filter has been recommended (Roeleveld and van Loosdrecht 2002), although some colloidal organic matter can pass through the filter. Therefore, filtration at 0.1 μm or, alternatively, coagulation with $Zn(OH)_2$ has been proposed.

Narrower Ranges for Wastewater Physical Characterization   As presented earlier, new challenges in wastewater treatment require sound physicochemical character-ization methods. For this, ultrafiltration (Engström and Gytel 2000; Sophonsiri and Morgenroth 2004; Doğruel et al. 2006; Dulekgurgen et al. 2006) or size-exclusion chromatography (Levine et al. 1985, 1991) has been employed to differentiate wastewater components within much narrow ranges. The filtered fraction (< 0.45 μm) consists of the colloidal ($100 \text{ kDa} < x < 0.45$ μm) and actual dissolved ($x < 100 \text{ kDa}$) fractions, which can be treated further by ultrafiltration with mem-branes having different nominal cutoffs (e.g., 100, 10, and 1 kDa) for determination of the molecular-weight distribution of the sample. The soluble fraction is often defined as < 1 nm (≤ 1000 amu) (Fig. 3.2).

Physical Characterization After Sludge Disintegration   The combined treatment for excess sludge reduction can generate a significant amount of COD_S, which ultimately ends up in the outlet of the plant unless it is biodegradable or adsorbed by sludge (Salhi et al. 2003). Physical fractionation has been used widely to characterize the COD released after the sludge disintegration treatment (Müller et al. 1998; Paul et al. 2006). This fractionation also helps to understand the effect of the disintegration technique on the sludge components. The COD release can be characterized in a way similar to that applied to the COD_S of wastewater using filtration, centrifugation, coagulation/ flocculation, and biodegradation assays. A detailed procedure for size characterization of COD released after sludge disintegration has been proposed by Aquino et al. (2008). Examples of fractionation of disintegrated sludge are presented in Section 3.7.

3.5   BIODEGRADATION ASSAYS FOR WASTEWATER AND SLUDGE CHARACTERIZATION

3.5.1   Background

Biodegradability assays are based on measurement of consumption of a substrate or the formation of one or more products involved in the biological reaction. Figure 3.4 describes various methods for biodegradation assay.

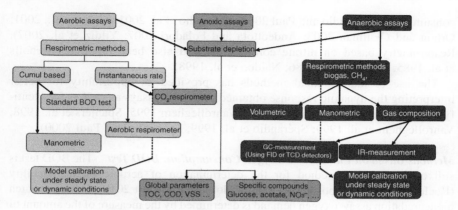

FIGURE 3.4 Methods for biodegradation assays.

3.5.2   Methods Based on Substrate Depletion

In a biodegradability assay, COD has been used instead of total organic carbon (TOC) and volatile suspended solids (VSS) due to the fact that COD-based mass balance can be performed more easily, while COD is also related to the redox state of compounds. The COD mass balance in batch or continuous culture experiments had been reported for the characterization of wastewater or sludge COD fractions (Ekama et al. 1986, 2007; Lesouef et al. 1992; Zeeman et al. 1997; Orhon et al. 1999; Parker 2005). Most often, these experiments are complemented by the use of steady-state or dynamic models for identifying both kinetic parameters and lumped component fractions (Kappeler and Gujer 1992; Ekama et al. 2007).

3.5.3   Methods Based on Respirometry

Background   Respirometry can be applied to aerobic, anoxic, and anaerobic environments for the study of microbial metabolisms. Oxygen/nitrate consumption or carbon dioxide/methane production is measured, which serves as an indicator of biodegradation. The indicator is chosen according to the objective and the electron acceptor used in the given environment, whereas the incubation temperature must be defined (e.g., 20°C, 35°C, 55°C). Two types of respirometry techniques have been employed: (1) a respirometry technique based on the cumulative consumption or production of a component involved in respiration, such as the well-known biological oxygen demand (BOD) test (Roeleveld and van Loosdrecht 2002; Gillot and Choubert 2010), and the biological methane production test (Owen et al. 1979; Owens and Chynoweth 1993; Rozzi and Remigi 2001); and (2) a respirometry technique based on the online measurement of oxygen consumption versus time (Spanjers and Vanrolleghem, 1995). In this, the oxygen uptake rate is calculated through an oxygen mass balance, and the total oxygen consumption can be calculated by integrating the oxygen consumption rate within a period of substrate consumption (Spérandio and Paul 2000; Spérandio et al. 2001; Ziglio et al., 2001; Orhon and Okutman 2003; Andeottola and Foladori 2007; Yildiz et al. 2007). Respirometry based on nitrate consumption had also been reported (Nicholls et al. 1985; Ekama et al. 1986; Naidoo et al. 1998).

The use of mathematical methods has provided an opportunity for better interpreting the dynamic response obtained during bioassays as well as for identifying model parameters (Spranjers and Vanrolleghem 1995; Spanjers et al. 1998; Vanrolleghem et al. 1999; Spérandio et al. 1999; Spérandio and Paul 2000).

Methods Based on Cumulative Oxygen Consumption: BOD Test The BOD test is still a widely used method for the determination of aerobic biodegradability (Roeleveld and van Loosdrecht 2002; Gillot and Choubert 2010). During a batch biodegradation assay, oxygen demand is determined by the measure of the amount of oxygen consumed in a closed bottle. The usual BOD testing apparatus is described in the Standard Methods for the Examination of Water and Wastewater (APHA 1998). Other systems can also be used for the BOD test, such as the manometric system (e.g., the Sapromat); http://www.reoterm.com.br/central/Autoclaves_Bloco_Agitadores/Sapromat/SAPROMAT.pdf, which is good for monitoring oxygen demand in long-term experiments with a rather constant oxygen concentration. In the manometric system, CO_2 produced by aerobic respiration is trapped by a soda solution, and the pressure drop due to oxygen consumption is compensated by the injection of oxygen produced through water electrolysis.

Triplicate BOD assay has been recommended to improve the assay reliability as well as for inhibition of nitrification by Ally thiourea (ATU). The biological tests should be performed on wastewater or sludge samples as soon as possible after collection, or if not possible, the sample must be stored in a closed bottle in the absence of air at 4°C. Ultimate BOD must be measured on long-term experiments (30 days). Part of the biomass formed during the assay may be transformed to unbiodegradable compounds; thus, a systematic error in the determination of BCOD would be introduced. A correction factor (f_{BOD}) of 0.1 to 0.2 has been recommended for the ultimate BOD measured (Roeleveld and van Loosdrecht 2002). Gillot and Choubert (2010) reported repeatability tests on the determination of BCOD of wastewaters using the long-term BOD test with 11 grab samples taken at the inlets of various municipal WWTPs located in the Ile de France (France). Analysis of the duplicate tests on the same wastewater showed a variation of less than 11%, with an average value of 4% (SD = 3%, $n = 21$). It was thus concluded that in the range of COD tested (from 350 to 1078 mgL^{-1}), results from the BOD test had good repeatability. The fraction BCOD/COD$_{tot}$ was found to vary between 0.58 and 0.76, with an average of 0.69 (SD = 0.06, $n = 8$), whereas the ratios of BOD$_5$ to COD$_{tot}$ fell between 0.42 and 0.59. It should be noted that the BCOD/COD$_{tot}$ ratio indeed is a good indicator of aerobically biodegradable COD.

OUR-Based Respirometry Several respirometric methods for online oxygen uptake rate (OUR) measurement are currently available (Spanjers et al. 1998).

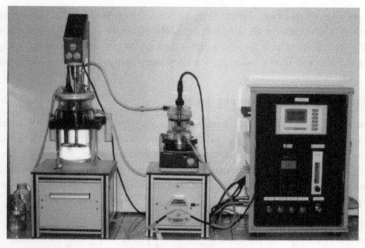

FIGURE 3.5 Respirometer combining an aerated contactor and a measurement cell. [From Spérandio (1998) and Spérandio and Paul (2000).]

Mass balance on oxygen in an aerated batch reactor shows that

$$\text{OUR} = k_L a(C_L^* - C_L) - \frac{dC_L}{dt} \tag{3.5}$$

However, as there is a significant change in the $k_L a$ value due to variation in physicochemical properties of the medium (e.g., biosurfactants released due to cell activity or lysis), a hybrid respirometry technique has been developed (Spérandio 1998), which consists of an aerated contactor combined with a measurement cell. In this system, liquid in the measurement cell is sequentially circulated to the contactor (Fig. 3.5), and when circulation is stopped and the cell becomes a non-aerated closed reactor, OUR is calculated according to

$$\text{OUR} = -\frac{dC_L}{dt} \tag{3.6}$$

Using the hybrid-sequenced respirometry, the BCOD of wastewater can be obtained from the assays performed at low S_0/X_0 (e.g., 0.2 g COD g^{-1} MLVSS):

$$\text{BCOD}_{\text{resp}} = \frac{\int \text{OUR}\, dt\, V_{\text{tot}}}{(1 - Y_{\text{OHO}})V_{\text{WW}}} \tag{3.7}$$

where Y_{OHO} is the heterotrophic yield coefficient (e.g., 0.63 g COD$_{X\text{OHO}}$ g^{-1} COD$_{\text{biodegraded}}$), V_{tot} is the total liquid volume of the respirometer, and V_{WW} is the volume of wastewater added.

Respirometry Based on CO_2 Measurement Production of carbon dioxide is a measure of mineralization of an organic molecule (Sturm 1973; Larson et al. 1992). The carbon dioxide–based respirometry had also been used for characterization of wastewater or for accurate measurement of Y_{OHO} (Spérandio et al. 1999). CO_2 can be detected by various methods, including infrared spectroscopy, gaschromatography, and chemical adsorption by alkaline solution [e.g., $Ba(OH)_2$]. Due to the high solubility of CO_2 in water, which is also highly dependent on water pH, the CO_2-based respirometric method is not widely used in wastewater and sludge characterization.

3.5.4 Anaerobic Biodegradation Assays

Background In anaerobic biodegradation assays, organic substrate is degraded and biogases (e.g., CO_2, CH_4, H_2, H_2S, NH_3) and other volatile compounds are produced, together with a small amount of newly synthesized biomass. Given the elemental composition ($C_nH_aO_b$) of organic materials, it is possible to determine the theoretical biological methane potential (BMP_{theo} in L CH_4 g^{-1} COD) by Buswell's stoichiometric equation:

$$C_nH_aO_b + \left(n - \frac{a}{4} - \frac{b}{2}\right)H_2O \rightarrow \left(\frac{n}{2} + \frac{a}{8} - \frac{b}{4}\right)CH_4 + \left(\frac{n}{2} - \frac{a}{8} + \frac{b}{4}\right)CO_2 \quad (3.8)$$

$$BMP_{theo} = \frac{(n/2 + a/8 - b/4)(22.4)}{(n + a/4 - b/2)(32)} \quad (3.9)$$

where 22.4 is the volume of 1 mol of gas at STP conditions. For example, at 30°C and 101.325 kPa, 394 mL of methane is theoretically produced from 1 g of biodegradable COD. The anaerobic biodegradability of an organic matter is often expressed as COD_{CH4} produced divided by COD degraded.

A variety of test procedures for the determination of anaerobic biodegradability have been reported (Angelidaki and Sanders 2004; Lesteur et al. 2010). Measuring the substrate consumption (through direct or indirect determination of COD, VSS, and TOC) usually requires more complex analysis than simply measuring methane or CO_2 in biogases. At the temperatures used for the determination of the BMP (e.g., 35°C or 55°C), methane is practically nonsoluble in water. However, this is not the case for CO_2 that has a high solubility in water (Spérandio et al. 1999). Therefore, determination of the BMP is preferable.

BMP Test The BMP test is carried out in a batch mode over a period of around 30 days. Produced biogas from a known amount of sludge is measured. The methane content in biogases can be determined online by trapping carbon dioxide with a Ba $(OH)_2$ or KOH solution. Biogas composition can also be determined by gas chromatography (GC) (Rozzi and Remigi 2001) or by infrared spectrophotometer. GC with thermal conductivity detection (TCD) allows determination of both methane and carbon dioxide, whereas GC with flame ionization detection (FID) allows determination of methane only (Angelidaki et al. 1993). A blank test is conducted without the sample to determine the part of the biogas emitted by anaerobic inoculum. Generally, the inoculum may be taken from an anaerobic sludge digester. It is of primary importance to use an acclimated inoculum with the right microbial populations to avoid inhibition effects [mainly by volatile fatty acids (VFAs) and

NH$_3$], as well as for complete degradation of biodegradable organic matters (Angelidaki et al. 1993). Angelidaki and Sanders (2004) proposed a method that allows calculating the amount of active inoculum required to avoid VFA accumulation:

$$\frac{X_B V_w k_H}{V_{\text{react}}} = \frac{V_{\text{inoc}} \text{VSS}_{\text{inoc}} q_{S,\text{inoc}}}{V_{\text{react}}} \tag{3.10}$$

where X_B is the concentration of biodegradable hydrolyzable COD, V_W the volume of the waste to be tested (here, sludge) (L), k_h the first-order hydrolysis constant (d^{-1}), V_{react} the batch BMP reactor volume (L), V_{inoc} the volume of inoculum required (L), COD$_{\text{inoc}}$ the COD of the VSS of the methanogenic inoculum (g COD L^{-1}), and $q_{S,\text{inoc}}$ the inoculum methanogenic activity (g g^{-1} COD$_{\text{VSS}}$ d^{-1}). The value of the hydrolysis constant can be found elsewhere (Batstone et al. 2002).

A synthetic medium with all necessary nutrients can be used in the test. In particular, the pH must be kept around 7 (between 6.0 and 8.3 and preferably between 7 and 8). A low pH may lead to VFA accumulation, while free ammonia inhibition may occur at high pH. The culture temperature at 35°C (or 55°C for thermophilic growth) is also important for ensuring optimal growth of methanogenic bacteria. In addition, temperature also has a strong effect on hydrolysis reactions, with a standard free energy of activation of 46 ± 14 kJ mol^{-1} (Angelidaki and Sanders 2004). At high temperatures, unstable fermentation may lead to a lower biogas potential. On the other hand, high concentrations of sulfate or nitrate in wastewater or sludge can result in low methane production potential. The BMP results obtained under the standard temperature and pressure can be expressed as L CH$_4$ kg^{-1} VSS, L CH$_4$ kg^{-1} COD, or kg COD$_{\text{CH4}}$ kg^{-1} COD.

Although the BMP test has not yet standardized, it is a highly reproducible method, as shown in Fig. 3.6, in which the BMP measurement was repeated on a WAS sample based on its total COD or soluble (COD$_S$) and particulate (COD$_X$) fractions. In fact, the COD mass balance in these tests was as high as 92 to 98%, and the sum

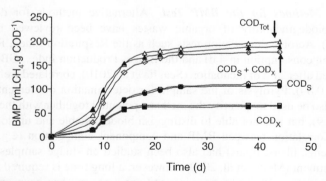

FIGURE 3.6 Repeatability tests on soluble, particulate, and total fractions of WAS from a WWTP near Toulouse, France.

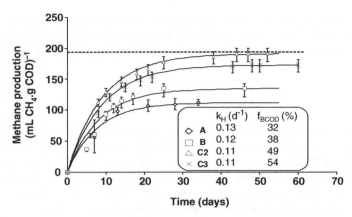

FIGURE 3.7 BMP tests for various WAS from different WWTPs near Toulouse, France.

$BMP_{COD,S} + BMP_{COD,X}$ was found to be very close to $BMP_{COD,tot}$. It was also verified that no methane was produced between 45 and 180 d.

Additional kinetic information can be deduced from the time course of methane production (Fig. 3.7). It allows defining anaerobic kinetic parameters. In anaerobic digestion, a series of successive reactions take place, including hydrolysis and acidogenesis, followed by methanogenesis. If hydrolysis is the limiting step, the methane production rate reflects the corresponding hydrolysis rate. The hydrolysis rate constant (k_H) (or knowing k_H, the BMP_{tot}) can thus be estimated:

$$BMP_{tot} = \frac{1}{1 - e^{-k_H t}} \cdot BMP_t \qquad (3.11)$$

On the contrary, if methane production is the controlling step, acidogenesis and methanogenesis rates can be assessed.

Alternative Methods for the BMP Test   Alternative methods for determining anaerobic biodegradability of organic wastes have been reviewed by Lesteur et al. (2010). Aerobic degradation tests such as the Respiration Index, RI4 (cumulative oxygen consumption in 4 d) and the Biogas Production Index, GB21, a BMP test measured after 21 d of incubation (Scaglia et al. 2010), correlated well with each other ($R^2 = 0.89$). Pyrolysis of the sample for determination of elemental composition can also be used to quantify the methane potential together with the Bushwell, equation (3.9), but it is not able to distinguish biodegradable and unbiodegradable fractions. Correlation between BMP and component composition (e.g., carbohydrates, proteins, fibers, lipids) had also been studied on sludge samples subject to thermal treatment (Mottet et al. 2010). However, a long time is required to measure all the components. Recently, near-infrared spectroscopy has been employed to predict the BMP for municipal solid waste (Lesteur et al. 2011).

3.6 APPLICATION TO WASTEWATER COD FRACTIONATION

3.6.1 Global Picture of Fractionation Methods and Wastewater COD Fractions

Wastewater characterization is a key step determining the reliability of models used to predict treatment and separation efficiencies, oxygen requirement, sludge production, sludge reduction potential, and so on. Extensive effort has been dedicated to the development and standardization of the experimental procedures for determination of the wastewater fraction. It appears that the organic fractions with respect to the operation unit and transformation in a WWTP can be reasonable estimated by a combined physical and biological technique. Nevertheless, the types of physical (e.g., filtration, ultrafiltration, settling, centrifugation) and biological (i.e., batch or continuous, long or short term, etc.) techniques are not yet, fixed and numerous methods and protocols are currently available in the literature. Figure 3.8 presents three major methods for determination of COD fraction in municipal wastewater. Method A is based on a long-term BOD test (Roeleveld and van Loosdrecht 2002; Gillot and Choubert 2010); method B is conducted with OUR-based respirometry at both high and low S_0/X_0 ratios and mathematical identification of kinetic parameters of an ASM model (Sperandio and Paul 2000); method C is based on the COD mass balance obtained from two or three batch assays with consideration of the generation of soluble and particulate microbial products (Orhon and Artan 1994). In addition to the methods presented in Fig. 3.8, steady-state and/or dynamic operation of a continuous lab-scale activated sludge system, and calibration of the model COD fractions had also been presented by pioneer researchers in this field (Ekama et al. 1986; Wentzel et al. 1989; Henze 1992).

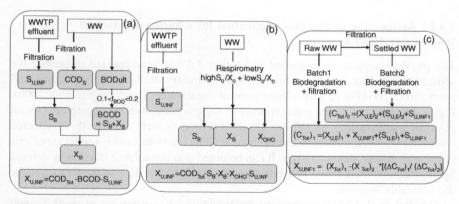

FIGURE 3.8 Three methods for determination of the COD fractions of municipal wastewater. Method A: long-term BOD test (Roeleveld and van Loosdrecht 2002; Gillot and Choubert 2010); method B: OUR-based respirometry at high and low S_0/X_0 ratios coupled with mathematical identification of kinetic parameters using an ASM model (Spérandio and Paul 2000); method C: COD mass balance on batch assays with consideration of the generation of soluble and particulate microbial products (Orhon and Artan 1994).

TABLE 3.1   COD Fractions of Municipal Wastewater in Various Countries

Origin	S_U	S_B	X_B	X_U	Reference
Raw wastewater					
France	—	6–14	41–66	—	Spérandio (1998)
South Africa	5	20	62	13	Ekama et al. (1986)
Denmark	2–8	20–24	40–49	18–19	Henze (1992)
Switzerland	10–20	7–32	45–60	8–11	Kappeler and Gujer (1992)
France	0	1–18	15–57	24–63	Ginestet et al. (2002)
Hungary	—	29	43	20	Henze et al. (1987)
Norway	9	25–35	15–20	10–15	Barlindhaug and Odegaard (1996)
The Netherlands	10–15	9–42	10–48	23–50	Roeleveld and van Loosdrecht (2002)
Settled wastewater					
France	11	6	48	19	Spérandio (1998)
France	6–10	25–33	41–44	8–13	Lesouef et al. (1992)
Switzerland	10	16	40	9	Sollfrank and Gujer (1991)
Denmark	3	29	43	11	Henze (1992)
France	—	1–16	33–74	10–50	Ginestet et al. (2002)
South Africa	8	28	60	4	Ekama et al. (1986)

In many countries, wastewater characterization has been carried out with developed methods for determination of the COD fractions in relation to the ASM models. Table 3.1 summaries the COD fractions of raw and presettled wastewater determined by different methods in various countries.

3.6.2   Application of Physical Separation for Characterization of Wastewater COD Fractions

The physical separation described in Section 3.4 has been applied to predict the separation efficiency of the primary settler (Ginestet et al. 2002; Sophonsiri and Morgenroth 2004) or to give a fingerprint of wastewater (Dulekgurgen et al. 2006). Figure 3.9 shows COD fractions reported by various authors on raw wastewaters with physical fractionation. As similar filtration protocols were used in these selected works in Fig. 3.9, the differences observed in COD fractions mainly reflect variations of the wastewater characteristics. It can be noted that the soluble fraction as defined by the methods used varied between 12 and 64% and 15 to 45% of the $COD_{tot,inf}$ for the settleable fraction.

Ginestet et al. (2002) determined fractionations of wastewater in seven French municipal WWTPs using a physical fractionation including 2-h settling and a coagulation flocculation step (Section 3.4). The results in Fig. 3.10 show again the great variability of the physical characteristics of a wastewater: for example, the settleable fraction, ranging from 21 to 46% of the $COD_{tot,inf}$. The total of settleable and coagulable fractions on average was about 76% of COD_{tot}.

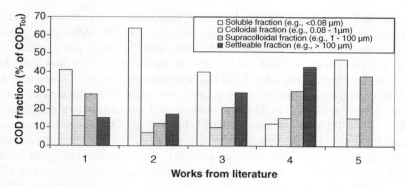

FIGURE 3.9 COD fractions reported in the literature on raw wastewaters with the same physical fractionation. 1, Balmat (1957); 2, Heukelekian and Balmat (1959); 3, Rickert and Hunter (1971); 4, Munch et al. (1980); 5, Hu et al. (2002).

3.6.3 Biodegradable COD Fraction

Long-Term BOD Test Standardized guidelines for wastewater characterization are often based on a long-term BOD test coupled with a 0.1-μm filtration method to distinguish soluble and particulate fractions (Fig. 3.9) (Roeleveld and van Loosdrecht 2002). $S_{U,inf}$ is obtained from the effluent COD of a target wastewater treatment plant. To ensure a more accurate determination of $S_{U,inf}$, it may be necessary to remove the biodegradable COD completely from this effluent. It is the reason that some authors recommended aerating the effluent to eliminate the biodegradable COD completely (Henze et al. 1987; Wentzel et al. 1999) or to use a correction factor of 0.9. S_B is therefore determined as the difference between the soluble COD_{inf} after 0.1-μm filtration and the value obtained for $S_{U,inf}$. The sum $S_B + X_B$ is equal to the BCOD obtained from the long-term BOD test (using the

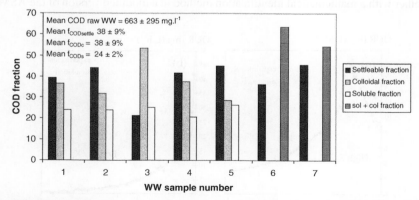

FIGURE 3.10 COD fractionation in seven raw wastewaters with 2 h of settling at 20 to 25°C in Imhoff cones and coagulation with $FeCl_3$ plus 15 min of settling. [From (Ginestet et al. 2002).]

correction factor for inert COD produced, i.e., f_{BOD}) and $X_{U,inf}$ is obtained from the difference between the COD_{tot} and the sum of $S_{U,inf}$ + BCOD. After many years of practice, this method appears to be simple, sufficiently accurate, and applicable for routine analysis (Roeleveld and van Loosdrecht 2002). Similarly, Gillot and Choubert (2010) developed a long-term BOD test complemented with COD measurements after flocculation for minimal wastewater characterization. It should be noted that the S_B value determined by the BOD-based method can be significantly higher than that obtained from OUR-based respirometry (Fall et al. 2011), as elaborated in Section 3.6.4. In addition, direct estimation of $X_{U,inf}$ has been recommended to quantify more accurately the microbial products ($X_{U,E}$) formed during the biodegradation assay (Orhon and Artan 1994; Orhon and Çokgör 1997; Orhon et al. 1997; Orhon and Okutman 2003).

OUR-Based Respirometry   Other methods have also been developed with the intention of dissociate S_B and X_B, while simultaneously estimating the kinetics parameters. One of these methods is described in Fig. 3.8 B. In batch respirometric assays, biological response depends strongly on the ratio of initial COD concentration to initial COD biomass concentration (S_0/X_0) (Ekama et al. 1986; Spérandio and Paul 2000). At a high S_0/X_0 ratio, the S_B is high enough compared to X_0 to allow a short exponential increase in the OUR, due to growth at the beginning of the experiment. On the contrary, at low S_0/X_0, growth will not be significant and the dynamics of OUR mainly reflects hydrolysis. The OUR dynamic is thus related to the consumption of X_B and decay products of X_{OHO}. Figure 3.11 shows the time course of OUR under two experimental conditions. At high S_0/X_0 (Figure 3.11 A), growth parameters and the S_B value can be better estimated, while at low S_0/X_0 (Figure 3.11 B), the best estimation is obtained for X_B and decay parameters. According to such observations, Spérandio and Paul (2000) proposed using these two complementary experiments conducted at different S_0/X_0 ratios to estimate simultaneously the kinetic parameters and the initial concentrations of biodegradable COD fractions in the wastewater (S_B, X_B, X_{OHO}), together with a mathematical identification method in a modified version of the ASM1

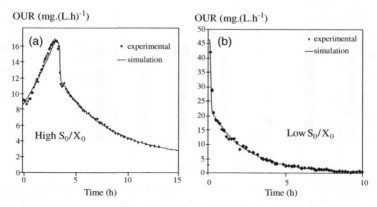

FIGURE 3.11 Time course of OUR for a determination of biodegradable and heterotrophic COD fractions of a municipal wastewater: (a) high S_0/X_0; (b) low S_0/X_0.

model (Henze et al. 1987). Figure 3.11 shows the simulation results of the model (solid line). The model prediction was in good agreement with experimental data. At a high S_0/X_0 ratio (Figure 3.11 A), only wastewater is added to the respirometer, while at a low S_0/X_0 ratio (Figure 3.11 B), less than 0.2 g COD_{WW} g^{-1} MLVSS must be added to limit the biomass growth. For the purpose of parameter identification, the heterotrophic yield (Y_{OHO}) was assumed to be 0.63 g COD g^{-1} COD, and the inert fraction of the biomass was fixed at 0.08. Values of the COD fractions obtained using this method are discussed later in this section.

Comparison of Aerobic Respirometric Methods   Online measurement of the OUR has been considered as the most representative method for biological modeling of a conventional activated sludge treatment plant (SRT < 30 days) since it allows simultaneous determination of kinetics, organic fractions, and biomass metabolic states (Spérandio and Paul 2000). On the contrary, respirometry techniques based on a cumulative consumption of oxygen (BOD) are well appropriated for ultimate biodegradability measurements and easier to use in practice (Roeleveld and van Loosdrecht 2002; Gillot and Choubert 2010).

BCOD and its complementary unbiodegradable COD fraction obtained from the wastewater characterization is essential for better understanding of sludge production and reduction. Gillot and Choubert (2010) compared the results of BCOD obtained with OUR respirometric methods ($BCOD_{resp}$) by various researchers and those obtained from the ultimate BOD test ($BCOD_{BOD}$). No statistical difference was observed between the values of $BCOD_{resp}$ and $BCOD_{BOD}$ due to the large variability of wastewater. However, the results by Gillot and Choubert (2010) showed that the fraction of $BCOD_{resp}$ on average appeared to be slightly lower than the fraction of $BCOD_{BOD}$. This may be explained by the short duration of the respirometric test (around 10 to 15 h). Indeed, very slowly biodegradable materials may not be quantified by OUR-based respirometry unless a much longer-term experiment is carried out. Figure 3.12 presents the results

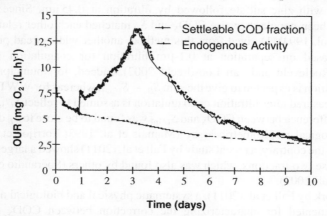

FIGURE 3.12 Time course of the OUR for the 2-h-settleable fraction of wastewater. This settleable COD fraction was previously concentrated in order to be able to dissociate its degradation from the degradation due to endogenous processes.

obtained from a 10-day experiment after injection of concentrated particulate material from a municipal wastewater. Indeed, particulate COD of wastewater is necessary for determination of the OUR from slowly biodegradable COD which can be differentiated from the endogenous OUR. It can be seen that part of COD was slowly degraded after 2 d, while the first increase in the OUR was due to colonization of the particulate matter. After the entire particle surface was colonized, the OUR started to decrease.

3.6.4   Relation Between Physical and Biological Properties of Organic Fractions

The size of compounds in wastewater certainly influences biodegradation rates of wastewater and is responsible for the wide range of biodegradation rates reported on the literature on wastewater treatment (Wentzel et al. 1999). For example, a molecule must be soluble and small enough to be transported across the cell membrane and then metabolized. Physicochemical methods have also been developed for wastewater characterization, as they are easier than biological methods to use. Thus, size fractions has been correlated to biodegradability and even to COD fractions of ASM models (Dold et al. 1986; Lesoeuf et al. 1992; Mamais et al. 1993; Wentzel et al. 1999; Roeleveld and van Loosdrecht, 2002; Dulekgurgen et al. 2006; Gillot and Choubert 2010; Fall et al. 2011).

The first attempt is to quantify COD_S for predicting the readily biodegradable COD (S_B) used in activated sludge model 1 (ASM1). Correlations between COD_S and S_B have been established by using different separation protocols for COD_S. For this purpose, filtration by a 0.45-μm membrane was proposed initially, which can be handled easily in laboratories and full-scale plants. However, Dold et al. (1986) reported an overestimation by 25 to 30% of the S_B fraction, which was based on the value of the COD_S recovered after a unique 0.45-μm filtration. Therefore, other methods had then been tested. For example, Mamais et al. (1993) proposed coagulation with zinc sulfate followed by filtration at 0.45 μm. Since then, this method has been popular because COD_S and S_B matched each other relatively well (Torrijos et al. 1994). Derived from this method, another wide spread protocol for COD_S is based on separation at 0.1-μm filtration (or coagulation + 0.45-μm filtration) (Roeleveld and van Loosdrecht 2002). Indeed, for municipal sewage, 0.1-μm filtration is expected to give the sum $S_B + S_{U,inf}$, whereas for WWTP effluent, the COD measured after filtration or coagulation is assumed to reflect $S_{U,inf}$. In some cases, the difference between COD_S and $S_{U,inf}$ was found to be close to S_B determined from a biological respirometric assay (Mamais et al. 1993; Torrijos et al. 1994). However, to the contrary, a recent study by Fall et al. (2011) showed a large difference between these two fractions, which was also found by others (Spérandio et al. 2001; Ginestet et al. 2002).

In the work by Fall et al. (2011), a systematic physical and biological method had been implemented for characterizing the correction between COD_S and S_B in wastewater at a large WWTP in Mexico. These researchers compared the COD remaining after filtrations at 1 to 2 μm, 0.45 μm, 0.1 μm, and coagulation + filtration

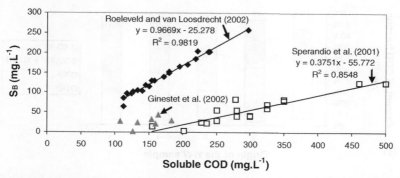

FIGURE 3.13 Correlations between S_B and COD_S. COD_S was measured through 0.45-μm filtration (Spérandio et al. 2001) or coagulation + filtration at 0.45 μm (Ginestet et al. 2002; Roeleved and van Loosdrecht 2002).

at 0.45 μm, with the COD corresponding to S_B obtained by a respirometric method. Depending on the pore-size cutoff, significant differences between the filtered COD measured from the wastewater samples: 1.2 μm > 0.45 ≈ 0.1 μm > (COD_C + 0.45 μm). More surprisingly, a remarkable difference (five-to sixfold) was observed between the "COD_S" obtained by physicochemical methods (170 to 200 mg L^{-1}) and the S_B determined by respirometry (34 mg L^{-1}). Hence, it appears that the COD_S should contain colloidal materials that can easily be enmeshed into flocs and were then rapidly removed from the liquid by adsorption (i.e., they were not accounted for as easily biodegradable material in respirometric tests).

Although a discrepancy was found between COD_S and S_B, there was a correlation between these two variables, as shown in Fig. 3.13, which presents results from three studies dedicated to the COD_S/S_B correlation (Spérandio et al. 2001; Ginestet et al. 2002; Roeleved and van Loosdrecht 2002). However, the slopes appear to be case dependent. This may be due to the lack of reproducibility of the protocols for respective physical and respirometric estimation of COD_S and S_B. In addition, in some wastewater, the fraction of S_B is so low that the correlation might be highly inaccurate [e.g., for results from Ginestet et al. (2002)].

To better understand the effects of settling and chemically assisted settling on the proportion of COD fractions, Ginestet et al. (2002) used the OUR-based respirometry to determine various fractions in raw, settled, and coagulated wastewater (Fig. 3.14). A significant proportion of inert organic material was found in raw wastewater. After coagulation and subsequent settling, the remaining COD is classified as COD_S, which contains a large proportion of X_B and a small portion of S_B.

3.6.5 Unbiodegradable Particulate COD Fractions

Analytical Methods Determination of unbiodegradable particulate COD (X_U) is of great importance in the evaluation of sludge production. Various methods for determination of this fraction have been proposed, as summarized in Table 3.2 and described in Fig. 3.15.

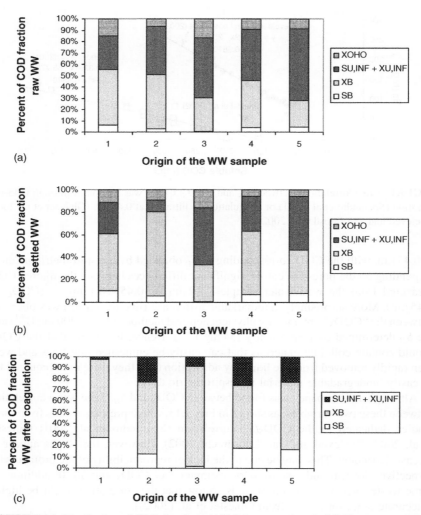

FIGURE 3.14 Distribution of COD fractions (ASM) in raw and settled (2 h) wastewater and after coagulation (= soluble fraction, use of $FeCl_3$ + 15 min of settling) for five French wastewaters. [From Ginestet et al. (2002).]

The unbiodegradable particulate COD fraction of a municipal wastewater is often estimated by the difference between $COD_{tot,inf}$ and $BCOD_{inf}$:

$$COD_{U,inf} = COD_{tot,inf} - BCOD_{inf} \tag{3.12}$$

and soluble and particulate matters can then be distinguished by filtration:

$$X_{U,inf} = COD_{U,inf} - S_{U,inf} \tag{3.13}$$

TABLE 3.2 Various Methods for the Determination of Unbiodegradable Particulate COD ($X_{U,\text{inf}}$) of Urban and Industrial Wastewaters

Test Methods	Wastewater	Approach	Account for Microbial Product	References
Continuous pilot + model calculation	D	Calibration of the AS MLVSS concentration with the MLVSS model prediction	No	Ekama et al. (1986)
Model calibration	D	Calibration of the AS MLVSS concentration with the MLVSS model prediction	No	Henze et al. (1987)
Two-Batch method	D&I	$X_{U,\text{inf}}$ calculated accounting for both soluble and particulate inert products	Yes	Orhon et al. (1994); Orhon and Çokgör (1997)
Batch	D	Model evaluation and mass balance	No	Kappeler and Gujer (1992)
Batch	D	Mass balance	No	Lesouef et al. (1992)
Batch respirometric procedure	D&I	Elimination of the interference of residual microbial products, enabling direct determination of the soluble and total biodegradable COD	Yes	Orhon and Okutman (2003)
Long-term BOD test + $S_{U,\text{inf}}$ on WWTP	D	STOWA procedure. $X_{U,\text{inf}} = \text{COD}_{\text{tot}} - \text{BCOD} - S_{U,\text{inf}}$ Correction for microbial products on BOD test to calculate BCOD	Yes	Roeleveld and van Loosdrecht (2002)

It should be noted that this approach has received criticism. First, as $X_{U,\text{inf}}$ is determined by difference, all errors from determination of the other fractions will be introduced to the $X_{U,\text{inf}}$ value. For example, when short-term OUR-based respirometric assays are used, only part of slowly biodegradable COD can be identified as unbiodegradable COD. Second, these methods do not account for microbial products,

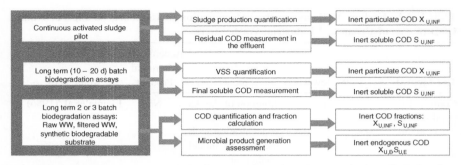

FIGURE 3.15 Methods developed for determination of the inert particulate COD fraction from a municipal wastewater.

which are important for determination of wastewater COD fractions as pointed out by Orhon et al. (1994).

Other methods had also been employed to determine the unbiodegradable particulate fraction as the difference between measured MLVSS and MLVSS calculated from process kinetics in an activated sludge pilot plant (SRT > 5 d) (Ekama et al. 1986). Such estimation depends strongly on the values of Y_{OHO}, b, and f. In addition, this method requires running a continuous pilot plant, and is timeconsuming. To cope with this problem, a new procedure was proposed by Kappeler and Gujer (1992) and Orhon et al. (1994), which is applicable only for wastewater that includes a large amount of particulate matter. In this method, two aerated batch reactors are run in parallel, fed with unfiltered and filtered wastewater, respectively. After depletion of all the biodegradable COD (C_{B1} for reactor 1 and S_{B1} for reactor 2), initial unbiodegradable COD and that produced remain, as newly produced heterotrophic biomass is negligible, due to the small amount of inoculum and BCOD. Figure 3.16 shows the various COD fractions in the two aerated reactors operated in parallel at the beginning of the experiment and after complete depletion of the biodegradable fractions.

$X_{U,inf}$ can be determined from measured soluble and particulate COD fractions in the two batches:

$$(X_{tot})_1 - (X_{tot})_2 = (X_{U,E})_1 + X_{U,inf1} - (X_{U,E})_2 \qquad (3.14)$$

$$X_{U,inf1} = (X_{tot})_1 - (X_{tot})_2 - (X_{U,E})_1 + (X_{U,E})_2 = (X_{tot})_1 - (X_{tot})_2 \left[\frac{C_{B1}}{S_{B1}}\right] \qquad (3.15)$$

The production of endogenous compounds is proportional to the biodegraded substrate:

$$(S_{U,E})_1 = Y_{SU,E} C_{B1} \quad \text{and} \quad (X_{U,E})_1 = Y_{XU,E} C_{B1} \qquad (3.16)$$

$$(S_{U,E})_2 = Y_{SU,E} S_{B1} \quad \text{and} \quad (X_{U,E})_2 = Y_{XU,E} S_{B1} \qquad (3.17)$$

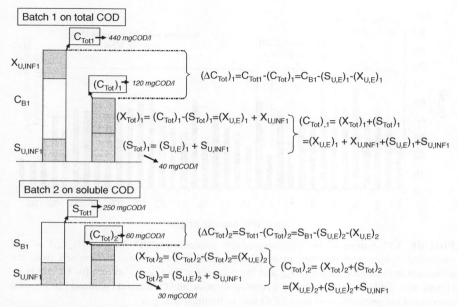

FIGURE 3.16 Two-batch method for determination of COD fractions according to conventional ASM models (Orhon and Artan 1994). Numerical data from the work of Lesouef et al. (1992) allow calculation of $X_{U,inf}$ for a urban wastewater (Orhon and Artan 1994).

Thus,

$$(\Delta C_{tot})_1 = (1 - Y_{SU,E} - Y_{XU,E})C_{B1} \quad \text{and} \quad (\Delta C_{tot})_2 = (1 - Y_{SU,E} - Y_{XU,E})S_{B1} \tag{3.18}$$

which leads to

$$\frac{(\Delta C_{tot})_1}{(\Delta C_{tot})_2} = \frac{C_{B1}}{S_{B1}} \tag{3.19}$$

Consequently, $X_{U,INF1}$ can be calculated as follows:

$$X_{U,inf1} = (X_{tot})_1 - (X_{tot})_2 \frac{(\Delta C_{tot})_1}{(\Delta C_{tot})_2} \tag{3.20}$$

A numerical method was proposed by Orhon and Artan (1994) and applied to the results by Lessouef et al. (1992). Values of soluble and particulate COD obtained for the two batch methods are presented in Fig. 3.16, and $X_{U,inf1}$ was estimated as $80 - 30 \times 320/190 = 29.5 \, \text{g COD m}^{-3}$.

Unbiodegradable Particulate COD Figure 3.17 shows $f_{XU,inf}$ values for the screened wastewater collected from a full-scale treatment plant located in various countries. It needs to be pointed out that $f_{XU,inf}$ was determined by the difference between the total COD_{inf} and the other COD fractions (f_{BCOD} and $f_{SU,inf}$) except for

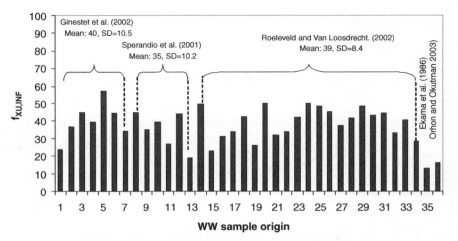

FIGURE 3.17 Values of the unbiodegradable particulate COD fraction ($f_{XU,\text{inf}}$) of raw municipal wastewaters reported in the literature. This fraction was determined from the difference between the total COD_{inf} and fractions other than $f_{XU,\text{inf}}$, except for Ekama et al. (1999), who calibrate this fraction in a continuous pilot, and Orhon and Okutman (2003), who considered the production of inert COD due to biomass decay.

data reported by Ekama et al. (1999) and Orhon and Okutman (2003). Ekama et al. (1999) calibrated this fraction in a continuous pilot, whereas Orhon and Okutman (2003) considered the production of inert COD due to biomass decay. Figure 3.17 suggests that (1) if the mean values of $f_{XU,\text{inf}}$ obtained by different researchers from a large number of WWTPs are comparable (however the standard deviation indeed shows a strong variation of this fraction among plants); and (2) values obtained by Ekama et al. (1986) and Orhon and Okutman (2003) are significantly lower than those obtained by the other researchers. This can be explained by the difference in the determination methods for $f_{XU,\text{inf}}$, in which microbial product release may or may not be taken into account.

Is Unbiodegradable COD Really Inert?   Existing evidence shows that the definition of inert organic material (X_U) depends on the operating conditions of a WWTP. Nowak et al. (1999) thought that sludge production cannot be predicted if inert particulate material is assumed to be constant. This was further confirmed by Ramdani et al. (2010), in whose study WAS generated in a membrane bio reactor was cultivated at an SRT of 5.2 d with acetate as the sole influent carbon source. The use of acetate, a totally biodegradable substrate, allows study of the biodegradability extent of the endogenous fraction of WAS ($X_{U,E}$). Biodegradation assays were then carried out with the WAS produced, in batch tests run under alternating aerated and nonaerated conditions at 35°C for 90 days. Results confirmed that endogenous products were biodegradable on a long-term basis. Hydrolysis subject to first-order kinetics had been proposed to account for such a slow biodegradation rate of $X_{U,E}$ (Lubello et al. 2009; Ramdani et al. 2010).

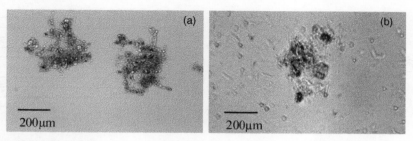

FIGURE 3.18 Morphology of sludge before (a) and after (b) thermal treatment at 65°C.

3.7   ASSESSMENT OF THE CHARACTERISTICS OF SLUDGE AND DISINTEGRATED SLUDGE

3.7.1   Physical Fractionation of COD Released from Sludge Disintegration Treatment

The use of disintegration techniques may modify the sludge structure. For example, Fig. 3.18 shows the morphology of sludge before and after thermal treatment at 65°C. Partial disintegration of the floc led to release of organic and mineral materials to the liquid. Specific protocols have been developed to quantify the effect of such disintegration techniques. Figure 3.19 presents a physical fractionation protocol developed by Camacho (2001) for study of the effects of mechanical, thermal, and oxidative treatment on WAS. Sludge disintegration and solubilization can be distinguished by the use of centrifugation (giving COD_{ace}) or centrifugation with a pre- or postcoagulation (giving COD_C, COD removed by coagulation; COD_{Ce},

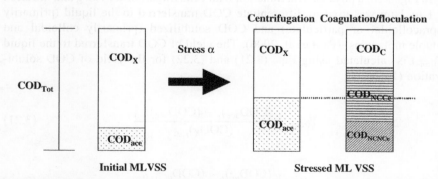

FIGURE 3.19 Physical fractionation reported by Camacho (2001) after treatment for sludge disintegration. COD_{ace}; COD after centrifugation; COD_C; COD removed by coagulation; COD_{Ce}: COD removed by centrifugation after coagulation; COD_{NCCe}; COD removed by centrifugation that cannot be removed by coagulation; COD_{NCNCe}; COD removed neither by centrifugation nor by coagulation.

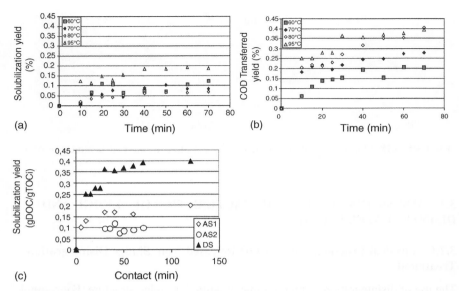

(a)

(b)

(c)

FIGURE 3.20 Comparison of COD solubilization (a) and COD transfer (b) at different temperatures for differents contact times. In (c), solubilization at 95°C is assessed for different sludge origins. AS1, AS2, and AD are AS and ADS from full-scale plants near Toulouse, France. [Paul et al. (2006).]

COD removed by centrifugation after coagulation; or COD_{NCCe}, COD removed by centrifugation that cannot be removed by coagulation; or COD_{NCNCe}, COD removed neither by centrifugation nor by coagulation). COD_{NCNC} is considered to be the true soluble COD fraction.

In Fig. 3.20, a physical fractionation with centrifugation at 3700 g and filtration at 1 to 2 μm was used to differentiate COD transferred to the liquid (primarily supracolloidal or particulate) and COD solubilized (primarily colloidal and soluble molecules) (Paul et al. 2006). The yield of COD transferred to the liquid (Y_{trans}) is calculated using Eqs. (3.21) and (3.22) for the yield of COD solubilization (Y_{sol}).

$$Y_{trans} = \frac{(COD_{ace})_t - (COD_{ace})_{t=0}}{(COD_X)_{t=0}} \qquad (3.21)$$

$$Y_{sol} = \frac{(COD_{af})_t - (COD_{af})_{t=0}}{(COD_X)_{t=0}} \qquad (3.22)$$

It should be noted that the amount of solubilized COD is strongly sludge dependent (Fig. 3.20).

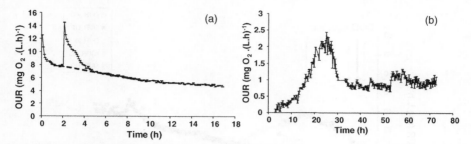

FIGURE 3.21 Time course of the OUR after injection of COD from sludge solubilized by an ozonation treatment. The protocol for the estimation of S_B and X_B is based on two tests in parallel at (a) low S_0/X_0 and (b) high S_0/X_0. [From Salhi et al. (2003).]

3.7.2 Biological Fractionation of COD Released from Sludge Disintegration Treatment

Long-term BOD or BMP tests and short-term OUR-based respirometric tests have been used to quantify the biodegradability of treated sludge (Spérandio and Paul 2000; Salhi et al. 2003). An example of the time courses of the OUR at high and low S_0/X_0 ratios is presented in Fig. 3.21, and identified biodegradable COD fractions are listed in Table 3.3. It appears from the table that all the materials released into the liquid phase due to ozonation of sludge were biodegradable.

Determination of BCOD fractions is not always an easy task. As can be seen in Fig. 3.22, WAS was treated at 65°C for different periods, and the solubilized fraction was injected into the respirometer, and OUR versus time was observed. The large variation in the S_0/X_0 ratio was probably due to the different inactivation degree of X_{OHO}, which was further dependent on the treatment time.

3.7.3 Biodegradability of WAS in Anaerobic Digestion

BMP is one of the characterization methods used widely for the determination of the biodegradability of primary and WAS sludges (Lesteur et al. 2010). It has been shown by many researchers that the ultimate biodegradability is strongly sludge dependent (Mottet et al. 2010). Table 3.4 presents the biodegradability (% of COD_{tot}) of sludges determined by a 50-day BMP test. Primary sludge and WAS used were sampled from five WWTPs near Toulouse to assess the global variability among treatment plants or

TABLE 3.3 Results of Fractionation[a] of the COD Solubilized by an Ozonation Treatment at Increasing Ozone Dosage

Ozone Dosage (mg O_3)	Solubilized COD (mg O_2)	BOD_{resp} (mg O_2)	$BCOD_{resp}$ (mg O_2)
70	250	90	240
90	260	95	255
300	1260	480	1260

[a] The fractionation protocol is that developed by Spérandio and Paul (2000).

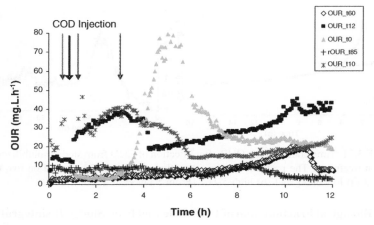

FIGURE 3.22 Time-course OUR in a sequenced respirometer after injection of CODS from WAS previously subjected to a low-temperature (65°C) treatment for different periods.

from one specific full-scale WWTP over 10 months to study variability with the treatment plant. In addition, WAS biodegradability sampled at a lab-scale activated sludge pilot plant at a SRT of 8 days was also tracked over six months. These results clearly showed high variability of biodegradability even for WAS sampled from the same WWTP.

3.7.4 Unbiodegradable COD in Anaerobic Digestion

For the prediction of total in-plant sludge production, a key modeling issue is whether after activated sludge treatment, inert materials remain inert in anaerobic digestion. Ekama et al. (2007) used data from previous investigations (Gossett and Belser 1982; van Haandel et al. 1998a, b), those from their own experiments, and modeling to assess unbiodegradable fractions of COD in anaerobic digestion. For this purpose

TABLE 3.4 Biodegradability of Primary Sludge and WAS Sampled at Full-Scale Plants Near Toulouse and at a Lab-Scale Activated Sludge Pilot Plant

Sludge Origin	Sampling Program	Sludge Ultimate Biodegradability (% of COD_{tot})
Primary sludge	Four samples	55–60
WAS	One sample, five WWTPs	27–55
WAS, same WWTP	One sample/month, 10 months	36–53
WAS, lab-scale pilot plant fed with real municipal wastewater	One sample/month, 6 months	39–51
WAS and mixed sludge	Variability calculated from results in the literature	29–65

they run over a period of about 150-d a 15-d sludge age. A nitrogen removal AS system was run at an SRT of 15 d for 150 d and an AD system fed with WAS at an SRT of 60 d. Experimental results were fitted to ASM1 and the steady-state ADM of Sötemann et al. (2006). The unbiodegradable COD fraction of the WAS (f_{ASUP}) was calculated as follows:

$$(f_{AS'UP}) = 1 - (1 - f')f_{av} \tag{3.23}$$

where f' is the unbiodegradable fraction of heterotrophic bacteria (death–regeneration model concept) and f_{av} is the fraction of heterotrophic bacteria in VSS. According to Ekama et al. (2007), $f_{AS'UP}$ calculated from the ASM was $1 - (1 - 0.08) \times 0.395 = 0.637$, and $f_{AS'UP}$ was found to be 0.627 when the anaerobic digester was run. In fact, these suggest the stability of unbiodegradable COD in AS systems and an AD step. Moreover, the biodegradability of WAS can be calculated with consideration of the active fraction of WAS. This is of considerable importance for the prediction of sludge production in a WWTP including AD. Results obtained by Ekama et al. (2007) are certainly reasonable at a low SRT of < 40 d in an anaerobic digester. However, similar to that observed in aerobic treatment at high SRT, it has been reported that a slow degradation for unbiodegradable COD should be taken into account at a high-digesting SRT (Jones et al. 2007).

3.8 NOMENCLATURE

Parameter	Description	Unit
b	Decay constant of active biomass (endogenous respiration concept)	d^{-1}
C_L	Dissolved oxygen concentration	g COD m^{-3}
C_L^*	Dissolved oxygen concentration at saturation	g COD m^{-3}
COD_{tot}	Total COD	g COD m^{-3}
C_{tot}	Total COD of a wastewater at the beginning of a biodegradation assay	g COD m^{-3}
(C_{tot})	Total COD of a wastewater remaining after complete biodegradation	g COD m^{-3}
f	Inert fraction of biomass (endogenous respiration concept)	
f'	Inert fraction of biomass (death–regeneration concept)	
$f_{AS'UP}$	Unbiodegradable COD fraction of the WAS	
f_{av}	Fraction of heterotrophic bacteria in activated sludge	
f_{BOD}	Correction factor for the estimation of BCOD from the ultimate BOD measurement	
f_{BX}	Biodegradable particulate fraction of wastewater COD	
f_{BS}	Biodegradable soluble fraction of wastewater COD	

f_{UX}	Inert particulate fraction of wastewater COD	
f_{US}	Inert soluble fraction of wastewater COD	
Ig_S	Soluble inorganic compounds	$g\ m^{-3}$
Ig_{tot}	Total inorganic compounds	$g\ m^{-3}$
k_H	Hydrolysis constant	d^{-1}
$k_L a$	Oxygen transfer coefficient	h^{-1}
OUR:	Oxygen uptake rate	$mg\ O_2\ L^{-1}\ h^{-1}$
$q_{S,inoc}$:	Specific consumption rate of the inoculum methanogenic bacteria	$g\ COD\ g^{-1}$ $COD_{VSS}\ d^{-1}$
S_0/X_0	Initial ratio substrate concentration on active biomass concentration	$g\ COD_{WW}\ g^{-1}$ MLVSS
S_B	Soluble readily biodegradable COD concentration	$g\ COD\ m^{-3}$
S_U	Soluble unbiodegradable COD concentration	$g\ COD\ m^{-3}$
$S_{U,E}$	Endogenous soluble "residue"	$g\ COD\ m^{-3}$
$S_{U,inf}$	Soluble unbiodegradable COD concentration	$g\ COD\ m^{-3}$
T	Temperature	$°C$
t	Time	d
V	Volume	L
$X_{bio,ANA}$	Anaerobic organisms concentration (in digester)	$g\ COD\ m^{-3}$
X_{ANO}	Autotrophic nitrifying organisms concentration	$g\ COD\ m^{-3}$
X_B	Insoluble slowly biodegradable COD concentration	$g\ COD\ m^{-3}$
X_{ch}	Carbohydrate particulate COD	$g\ COD\ m^{-3}$
X_{li}	Lipid particulate COD	$g\ COD\ m^{-3}$
X_{OHO}	Heterotrophic biomass concentration	$g\ COD\ m^{-3}$
X_{pr}	Protein particulate COD	$g\ COD\ m^{-3}$
X_U	Insoluble unbiodegradable COD concentration	$g\ COD\ m^{-3}$
$X_{U,E}$	Endogenous particulate "residue"	$g\ COD\ m^{-3}$
$X_{U,inf}$	Unbiodegradable particulate COD in the influent	$g\ COD\ m^{-3}$
Y_{OHO}	Heterotrophic intrinsic biomass yield	$g\ COD\ g^{-1}\ COD$
Y_{sol}	COD solubilization yield after sludge disintegration	$g\ COD\ g^{-1}\ COD$
$Y_{SU,E}$	Yield of production of soluble unbiodegradable COD from biomass decay	$g\ COD\ g^{-1}\ COD$
Y_{trans}	COD yield transferred after sludge disintegration	$g\ COD\ g^{-1}\ COD$
$Y_{XU,E}$	Yield of production of particulate unbiodegradable COD from biomass decay	$g\ COD\ g^{-1}\ COD$

Indices

aCe	Remaining after centrifugation
af	Remaining after filtration
B	Biodegradable
C	Colloidal or can be removed by coagulation
Ce	Removed by centrifugation
inf	Influent
Inoc	Inoculum

NC	Not removed by coagulation
NCe	Not removed by centrifugation
NCNCe	Not removed either by coagulation or by centrifugation
OHO	Ordinary heterotrophic organisms
react	Reactor
resp	Respirometry or respirometer
S	Soluble
theo	Theoretical
tot	Total
U	Unbiodegradable
ult	Ultimate
W	Waste
WW	Wastewater
X	Particulate

REFERENCES

Andeottola G., Foladori P. (2007) Treatability evaluation. In: Quevauviller P., Thomas O., van der Beken A. (eds.), *Wastewater Quality Monitoring and Treatment*, Wiley, Chichester, UK.

Alexander M. (1999) *Biodegradation and Bioremediation*, 2nd ed., Academic Press, San Diego, CA.

APHA (American Public Health Association); American Water Works Association; Water Environment Federation (1998) *Standard Methods for the Examination of Water and Wastewater*, 20th ed., APHA, Washington, DC.

Angelidaki I., Sanders W. (2004) Assessment of the anaerobic biodegradability of macro-pollutants. *Reviews in Environmental Science and Bio/Technology* 3, 117–129.

Angelidaki I., Ellegaard L., Ahring B. K. (1993) A mathematical model for dynamic simulation of anaerobic digestion of complex substrates: focusing on ammonia inhibition. *Biotechnology and Bioengineering* 42, 159–166.

Aquino S. F., Chernicharo C. A. L., Soares H., Takemoto S. Y., Vazoller R. F. (2008) Methodologies for determining the bioavailability and biodegradability of sludges. *Environmental Technology* 29(8), 855–862.

Balmat J. L. (1957) Biochemical oxidation of various particulate fractions of sewage. *Sewage and Industrial. Wastes* 29(7), 757–761.

Barlindhaug J., Odegaard H. (1996) Thermal hydrolysate as a carbon source for denitrification. *Water Science and Technology* 33(12), 99–108.

Batstone D. (2000) High rate anaerobic treatment of complex wastewater. Ph. D. *dissertations*, The University of Queensland. Australia.

Batstone D. J., Keller J., Angelidaki I., Kalyuzhnyi S. V., Pavlostathis S. G., Rozzi A., Sanders W. T. M., Siegrist H., Vavilin V. A. (2002) Anaerobic Digestion Model No.1 (ADM1). In: ITGfMMoAD (ed.,) *Processes*, IWA Publishing, London.

Camacho P. (2001) Etude de procédés de réduction de la production de boues par couplage de traitements physique ou chimique et biologique. INSA, Toulouse, France.

Corominas L., Rieger L., Takacs I., Ekama G., Hauduc H., Vanrolleghem P. A., Oehmen A., Gernaey K. V., van Loosdrecht M. C. M., Comeau Y. (2010) New framework for standardized notation in wastewater treatment modelling. *Water Science and Technology* **61**(4), 841–857.

Doğruel S., Dulekgurgen E., Orhon D. (2006) Effect of ozonation on chemical oxygen demand fractionation and color profile of textile wastewaters. *Journal of Chemical Technology and Biotechnology* **81**, 3–4.

Dold P. L. (2007) Quantifying sludge production in municipal treatment plants. Proceedings of WEFTEC, pp. 1522–1549.

Dold P. L., Bagg W. K., Marais G. V. R. (1986) *Measurement of the Readily Biodegradable COD Fraction (Sbs) in Municipal Wastewater by Ultrafiltration*, UCT Report W57, Department of Civil Engineering, University of Cape Town, Rondebosh, South Africa.

Dulekgurgen E., Dogruel S., Karahan O., Orhon D. (2006) Size distribution of wastewater COD fractions as an index for biodegradability. *Water Research* **40**(2), 273–282. Ekama (1999)

Ekama G. A., Dold P. L., Marais G. R. (1986) Procedures for determining COD fractions and the maximum specific growth rate of heterotrophs in activated sludge systems. *Water Science and Technology* **18**(6), 91–114.

Ekama G. A., Sötemann S. W., Wentzel M. C. (2007) Biodegradability of activated sludge organics under anaerobic conditions. *Water Research* **41**(1), 244–252.

Engström T., Gytel U. (2000) Different treatment methods for effluent from a pulpmill and their influence on fish health and propagation. In: Hahn H. H., Hoffmann E., Ødegaard H. (eds.), Chemical Water and Wastewater Treatment VI: Proceedings of the 9th Gothenburg Symposium, Istanbul, Turkey, October 2–4, 2000, pp. 317–323.

Fall C., Flores N. A., Espinoza M. A., Vazquez G., Loaiza-Návia J., van Loosdrecht M. C. M., Hooijmans C. M. (2011) Divergence between respirometry and physicochemical methods in the fractionation of the chemical oxygen demand in municipal wastewater. *Water Environment Research* **83**(2), 162–172.

Gillot S., Choubert J. M. (2010) Biodegradable organic matter in domestic wastewaters: comparison of selected fractionation techniques. *Water Science and Technology* **62**(3), 630–639.

Ginestet P. (2000) A novel approach for wastewater characterisation: C, N and P typology. Poster presented at the 1st World Congress of the International Water Association, Paris, July 3–7.

Ginestet P., Maisonnier A., Sperandio M. (2002) Wastewater COD characterization: biodegradability of physico-chemical fractions. *Water Science and Technology* **45**(6), 89–97.

Gossett J. M., Belser R. L. (1982) Anaerobic digestion of waste activated sludge. *Journal of the Environmental Engineering Division ASCE 108(EE6)* 1101–1120.

Henze M. (1992) Characterization of wastewater for modelling of activated sludge process. *Water Science and Technology* **25**(6), 1–15.

Henze M., Grady C. P. L., Gujer W., Marais G. V., Matsuo, T. (1987) *Activated Sludge Model No.1*, IAWPRC Scientific and Technical Report 1, IAWPRC, London.

Heukelekian H., Balmat J. L. (1959) Chemical composition of particulate fractions of domestic sewage. Sewage and Industrial. *Wastes* **31**, 413–423.

Hu Z. Q., Chandran K., Smets B. F., Grasso D. (2002) Evaluation of a rapid physical–chemical method for the determination of extant soluble COD. *Water Research* **36**(3), 617–624.

Huang M., Li Y., Gu G. (2010) Chemical composition of organic matters in domestic wastewater. *Desalination* **262**, 36–42.

Jones R., Parker W., Khan Z., Murthy S., Rupke M. (2007) Characterization of sludges for predicting anaerobic digester performance. In: *Proceedings of the WEF Specialty Conference on Residuals and Biosolids Management*, Denver, CO.

Kappeler J., Gujer W. (1992) estimation of heterotrophic parameters under aerobic conditions and characterization of wastewater for activated sludge modelling. *Water Science and Technology* **25**, 125–139.

Larson R. J., Hansmann M. A., Bookland E. A. (1992) Carbon dioxide recovery in ready biodegradation tests: Mass transfer and kinetic considerations. *Chemosphere* **3**(6), 1195–1210.

Lesouef A., Payraudeau M., Rogalla F., Kleiber B. (1992) Optimizing nitrogen removal reactor configuration by onsite calibration of the IAWQ activated sludge model. *Water Science and Technology* **25**(6), 105–123.

Lesteur M., Bellon-Maurel V., Gonzalez C., Latrille E., Roger J. M., Junqua G., Steyer J. P. (2010) Alternative methods for determining anaerobic biodegradability: a review. *Process Biochemistry* **45**, 431–440.

Lesteur M., Latrille E., Bellon Maurel V., Roger J. M., Gonzalez C., Junqua G., Steyer J. P. (2011) First step towards a fast analytical method for the determination of Biochemical Methane Potential of solid wastes by near infrared spectroscopy. *Bioresource Technology* **102**, 2280–2288.

Levine A. D., Tchobanaglous G., Asano T. (1985) Characterization of the size distribution of contaminants in wastewater: treatment and reuse implications. *Journal of the Water Pollution Control Federation* **57**(7), 805–816.

Levine A. D., Tchobanoglous G., Asano T., (1991) Size distributions of particulate contaminants wastewater and their impact on treatability. *Water Research* **25**, 911–922.

Lubello C., Caffaz S., Gori R., Munz G. (2009) A modified activated sludge model to estimate solids production at low and high solids retention time. *Water Research* **43**(18), 4539–4548.

Madsen E. L. (1991) Determining in situ biodegradation. *Environmental Science and Technology* **25**(10), 1663–1673.

Madsen E. L. (2001) Methods for determining biodegradability. In: Hurst C. J., Crawford R. L., Knudsen G. R., McInerney M. J., Stetzenbach L. D. (eds.), *Manual of Environmental Microbiology*, American Society of Microbiology, New York.

Madigan M. T., Martinko J. M., Parker J. (2003) *Brock Biology of Microrganisms*, 3rd ed., Prentice Hall, Upper Saddle River, NJ.

Mamais D., Jenkins D., Pitt P. (1993) A rapid physical–chemical method for the determination of readily biodegradable soluble COD in municipal wastewater. *Water Research* **27**(1), 195–197.

Mottet A., François E., Latrille E., Steyer J. P., Déléris S., Vedrenne F., Carrère H. (2010) Estimating anaerobic biodegradability indicators for waste activated sludge. *Chemical Engineering Journal* **160**(2), 488–496.

Müller J., Lehne G., Schwedes J., Battenberg S., Näveke R., Kopp J., Dichtl N., Scheminski A., Krull R., Hempel D. C. (1998) Disintegration of sewage sludges and influence on anaerobic digestion. *Water Science and Technology* **38**(8–9) 425–433.

Munch R., Hwang C. P., Lackie T. H. (1980) Wastewater fractions add to total treatment picture. *Water and Sewage Works* **127**, 49–54.

Naïdoo V., Urbain V., Buckley C. A. (1998) Characterization of wastewater and activated sludge from European municipal wastewater treatment plants using the NUR test. *Water Science and Technology* **38**(1), 303–310.

Nicholls H. A., Pitman A. R., Osborn D. W. (1985) The readily biodegradable fraction of sewage: its influence on phosphorus removal and measurement. *Water Science and Technology* **17**, 73–87.

Nowak O., Svardal K., Franz A., Kuhn V. (1999) Degradation of particulate organic matter: a comparison of different model concepts. *Water Science and Technology* **39**(1), 119–127.

Odegaard H. (1998) Optimised particle separation in the primary step of wastewater treatment. *Water Science and Technology* **37**(10), 43–53.

Orhon D., Artan N. (1994) *Modelling of Activated Sludge Systems*. Technomic Publishing, Lancaster, PA.

Orhon D., Çokgör E. U. (1997) COD fractionation in wastewater characterization: the state of the art. *Journal of Chemical Technology and Biotechnology* **68**(3), 283–293.

Orhon D., Artan N., Ates E. (1994) A description of three methods for the determination of the inert particulate chemical oxygen demand of wastewater. *Journal of Chemical Technology and Biotechnology* **61**, 73–80.

Orhon D., Ates E., Sözen S., Çokgör E. U. (1997) Characterization and COD fractionation of domestic wastewaters. *Environmental Pollution* **95**(2), 191–204.

Orhon D., Karahan Ö., Sözen S. (1999) The effect of residual microbial products on the experimental assessment of the particulate inert COD in wastewaters. *Water Research* **33**(14), 3191–3203.

Orhon D., Okutman D. (2003) Respirometric assessment of residual organic matter for domestic sewage. *Enzyme and Microbial Technology* **32**(5), 560–566.

Owen M. F., Stuckey D. C., Healy J. B., Young L. Y., McCarthy P. L. (1979) Bioassay for monitoring biochemical methane potential and anaerobic toxicity. *Water Research* **13;** 485–492.

Owens J. M., Chynoweth D. P. (1993) Biochemical methane potential of municipal solid waste components. *Water Science and Technology* **27**, 1–14.

Parker W. J. (2005) Application of the ADM1 model to advanced anaerobic digestion. *Bioresource Technology* **96**(16), 1832–1842.

Paul E., Camacho P., Lefebvre D., Ginestet P. (2006) Organic matter release in low temperature thermal treatment of biological sludge for reduction of excess sludge production. *Water Science and Technology* **54**(5), 59–68.

Ramdani A., Dold P., Déléris S., Lamarre D., Gadbois A., Comeau Y. (2010) Biodegradation of the endogenous residue of activated sludge. *Water Research* **44**, 2179–2188.

Rickert D. A., Hunter J. V. (1971) General nature of soluble and particulate fractions of domestic sewage. *Water Research* **5**(7), 421.

Roeleveld P. J., van Loosdrecht M. C. M. (2002) Experience with guidelines for wastewater characterization in The Netherlands. *Water Science and Technology* **45**(6), 77–87.

Rozzi A., Remigi E. (2001) Anaerobic biodegradability. In : Conference Proceedings 9th World Congress, Anaerobic Digestion, Antwerp, Belgium, 2–6 September. Workshop 3: Harmonisation of anaerobic activity and biodegradation assays.

Salhi M., Deleris S., Debellefontaine H., Ginestet P., Paul E. (2003) More insights into the understanding of reduction of excess sludge production by ozone. *Wastewater Sludge as a Resource*, pp. 39–46.

Scaglia B., Confalonieri R., D'Imporzano G., Adani F. (2010) Estimating biogas production of biologically treated municipal solid waste. *Bioresource Technology* **101**, 945–952.

Sollfrank U., Gujer W. (1991) Characterisation of domestic wastewater for modelling of the activated sludge process. *Water Science and Technology* **23**, 1057–1066.

Sophonsiri C., Morgenroth E. (2004) Chemical composition associated with different particle size fractions in municipal, industrial and agricultural wastewaters. *Chemosphere* **55**, 691–703.

Sötemann S. W., van Rensburg P., Ristow N. E., Wentzel M. C., Loewenthal R. E., Ekama G. A. (2006) Integrated chemical, physical and biological processes modelling of anaerobic digestion of sewage sludge. *Water Science and Technology* **54**(5), 109–117.

Spanjers H., Vanrolleghem P. (1995) Respirometry as a tool for rapid characterization of wastewater and activated sludge. *Water Science and Technology* **31**(2), 105–114.

Spanjers H., Vanrolleghem P. A., Olsson G., Dold P. L. (1998) *Respirometry in Control of the Activated Sludge Process: Principles*, International Water Association, London.

Spérandio M. (1998) Development of a respirometric procedure for wastewater fractionation: *application to the dynamic modelling of activated sludge processes*. Ph.D. dissertation No 488, INSA, Toulouse, France.

Spérandio M., Paul E. (2000) Estimation of wastewater biodegradable COD fractions by combining respirometric experiments in various S_0/X_0 ratios. *Water Research*, **34**(4), 1233–1246.

Spérandio M., Urbain V., Audic J. M., Paul E. (1999) Use of carbon dioxide evolution rate for determining heterotrophic yield and characterizing denitrifying biomass. *Water Science and Technology* **39**(1), 139–146.

Spérandio M., Urbain V., Ginestet P., Audic J. M., Paul E. (2001) Application of COD fractionation by a new combined technique: comparison of various wastewaters and sources of variability. *Water Science and Technology* **43**(1), 181–190.

Sturm R. N. (1973) Biodegradability of nonionic surfactants: screening test for predicting rate and ultimate biodegradation. *Journal of the American Oil Chemists' Society* **50**(5), 159–167.

Torrijos M., Cerro R. M., Capdeville B., Zeghal S., Payraudeau M., Leseouf A. (1994) Sequencing batch reactor: a tool for wastewater characterisation for the IAWPRC model. *Water Science and Technology* **31**(2), 149–160.

van Haandel A. C., Catunda, P. F. C., Araujo L. (1998a) Biological sludge stabilization: 1. Kinetics of aerobic sludge digestion. *Water SA* **24**(3), 223–230.

van Haandel A. C., Catunda P. F. C., Araujo L. (1998b) Biological sludge stabilization:2. Influence of the composition of waste activated sludge on anaerobic digestion. *Water SA*, **24**(3), 231–236.

van Nieuwenhuijzen A. F., van der Graaf J. H. J. M., Mels A. R. (2001) Direct influent filtration as a pretreatment step for more sustainable wastewater treatment systems. *Water Science and Technology* **43**(11), 91–98.

Vanrolleghem P., Spanjers H., Petersen B., Ginestet P., Tacaks I. (1999) Estimating (combinations of) activated sludge model No. *1 parameters and components by respirometry*. *Water Science and Technology* **39**(1), 195–214.

Washington D. R., Symons J. M. (1962) Volatile sludge accumulation in activated sludge systems. *J. Water Pollut. Control Fed.*, **34**(8), 767–790.

Wentzel M. C., Mbewe A., Lakay M. T., Ekama G. A. (1999) *Batch test for characterization of the carbonaceous materials in municipal wastewaters. Water SA* **25**(3), 327–335.

WERF (Water Environment Research Foundation) (2003) *Methods for Wastewater Characterization in Activated Sludge Modeling,* Project 99-WWF-3, WERF, Alexandria, VA.

Yildiz G., Insel G., Cokgor E. U., Orhon D. (2007) Respirometric assessment of biodegradation for acrylic fibre–based carpet finishing wastewaters. *Water Science and Technology* **55**(10), 99–106.

Zeeman G., Sanders W. T. M., Wang K. Y., Lettinga G. (1997) Anaerobic treatment of complex wastewater and waste activated sludge: application of upflow anaerobic solid removal (UASR) reactor for the removal and pre-hydrolysis of suspended COD. *Water Science and Technology* **35**(10), 121–128.

Ziglio G., Andeottola G., Foladori P., Ragazzi M. (2001) Experimental validation of a single-OUR method for wastewater RBCOD characterisation. *Water Science and Technology* **43**(11), 119–126.

4

OXIC-SETTLING-ANAEROBIC PROCESS FOR ENHANCED MICROBIAL DECAY

QINGLIANG ZHAO

State Key Laboratory of Urban Water Resource and Environment, School of Municipal and Environmental Engineering, Harbin Institute of Technology, Harbin, China

JIANFANG WANG

School of Environmental Science and Engineering, Suzhou University of Science and Technology, Suzhou, China

4.1 INTRODUCTION

Biological treatment processes have been used widely in municipal and industrial wastewater treatment facilities, and large amounts of excess sludge are produced in the process. Upgrading of existing plants will result in increased excess sludge production because the requirements of effluent quality requirements are expected to become more stringent. Treatment and disposal of sewage sludge from wastewater treatment plants (WWTPs) accounts for about half, even up to 60%, of the total cost of wastewater treatment (Wei et al. 2003). The conventional disposal method of land filling is becoming more and more difficult, due to limited landfill spaces and secondary pollution problems. Thus, the excess sludge reduction has been one of the major challenges in this field.

Biological Sludge Minimization and Biomaterials/Bioenergy Recovery Technologies, First Edition.
Edited by Etienne Paul and Yu Liu.
© 2012 John Wiley & Sons, Inc. Published 2012 by John Wiley & Sons, Inc.

Strategies for minimizing excess sludge production from an activated sludge process are becoming a very practical and urgent issue. An ideal way to solve sludge-associated problems is to reduce sludge production in the wastewater treatment rather than in the posttreatment of the sludge produced. Microbial metabolism liberates a portion of the carbon from organic substrates in respiration and assimilates a portion into biomass (Liu and Tay 2001). To reduce the production of biomass, wastewater processes must be engineered such that substrate is diverted from assimilation for biosynthesis to fuel exothermic, nongrowth activities.

The oxic-settling-anaerobic (OSA) process is one of strategies developed for sludge reduction in an engineering method based on this principle that can contribute to reduction in excess sludge treatment and disposal challenges in wastewater treatment plants due to economic, environmental, and regulation factors.

In this chapter, the effect of the anaerobic sludge holding tank on the performance of the OSA system is evaluated. Sludge production, performance of pollutant removal, and sludge settlability of the OSA system are presented. Factors affecting sludge production and possible causes of sludge reduction in the OSA process are analyzed.

4.2 DESCRIPTION OF THE OXIC-SETTLING-ANAEROBIC PROCESS

4.2.1 Oxic-Settling-Anaerobic Process

The OSA process is a modification of conventional activated sludge technology in which an anaerobic sludge holding tank is inserted in the sludge return line between the aeration tank and the secondary clarifier, as shown in Fig. 4.1. In the OSA process, thickened sludge from the final clarifiers is returned to the aeration tanks via a sludge holding tank where the sludge is thickened further and then exposed to a low oxidation–reduction potential (ORP) environment. Activated sludge of the OSA process is exposed periodically to an anaerobic or anoxic zone under no-food and low–ORP conditions.

This process has been employed successfully to repress the growth of filamentous organisms (Liu and Tay 2001; Martins et al. 2004). Westgarth et al. (1964) reported for the first time that the insertion of a period of anaerobiosis in a high-rate activated

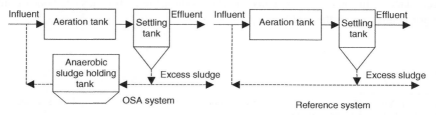

FIGURE 4.1 Schematic diagram of an OSA system and a reference system.

sludge process could reduce the rate of excess sludge production by 50% compared with a conventional process without an anaerobic reactor. Since then, an alternative fasting/feasting approach based on oxic and anaerobic cycling has been considered seriously for minimizing excessive sludge production in the activated sludge process. Chudoba et al. (1992) included an anaerobic sludge zone in the sludge recycle stream of a laboratory-scale activated sludge system and achieved significant sludge reduction, and the sludge volume index (SVI) value in the OSA process was much lower than that observed in a conventional process. With increasing sludge loading rates, sludge production in a conventional activated sludge process increases; however, sludge production in the OSA process shows a reducing trend (Chudoba et al. 1991a). This in turn implies that the OSA process is capable of handling high-strength organic pollutants without serious sludge-associated problems. Another successful application of OSA strategy is in a sequencing batch reactor (SBR) system, in which lower sludge production and excellent settleability were obtained (Ghiglizza et al. 1996). Up to a 50% reduction in excess sludge production without affecting effluent quality and sludge settleability has been reported (Chen et al. 2001; Saby et al. 2003).

4.2.2 Characteristics of the OSA Process

The excess sludge reduction in the OSA process is associated with the insertion of a sludge anaerobic tank that retains thickened sludge from the settling tank with no air supply, which results in an "anaerobic" sludge zone. It is believed that the settler can minimize both substrate residues in the liquid and food storage in the sludge, which induces sludge starvation under anaerobic conditions. This anaerobic sludge zone is different from such zones in biological nutrient removal processes such as the A/O and A/A/O processes, in terms of both substrate level and sludge concentration. In the anaerobic sludge tank, few external organic substrates are left since they have already been utilized in the clarifier prior to entering the sludge holding tank. In the anaerobic zone of a conventional nutrient removal process, however, adequate external substrate is supplied. In addition, the sludge anaerobic tank also contains twice the amount of sludge as that in conventional processes in terms of sludge concentration, which means that a large portion of the sludge is exposed to the anaerobic zone in the OSA process. A higher biomass concentration coupled with a longer retention period of the recycled sludge in the anaerobic sludge tank is necessary to maintain proper anaerobic conditions.

The OSA system has the following benefits compared to other approaches for reducing excess sludge production: (1) it is relatively easy to introduce the anaerobic zone in a conventional activated sludge process; and (2) neither a physical or chemical treatment nor chemicals are needed. The OSA system therefore seems to be an economical modification of an existing plant to reduce excess sludge production. Furthermore, the OSA process not only reduces excess sludge production significantly but also improves COD and nutrient removal as well as sludge settleability. Thus, use of an OSA system to achieve low excess sludge production seems to be a promising alternative.

4.3   EFFECTS OF AN ANAEROBIC SLUDGE TANK ON THE PERFORMANCE OF AN OSA SYSTEM

4.3.1   Fate of Sludge Anaerobic Exposure in an OSA System

The sludge anaerobic tank is the key unit in the OSA system, and a series of biochemical reactions occur in this tank that influence sludge production. It is generally thought that the anaerobic digestion process of organic wastewater or waste biosolids goes through three stages: hydrolysis, acidification, and methane production. Excess sludge consists of refractory organic matter, and it can be decomposed by the anaerobic digesters (Bolzonella et al. 2005). Volatile fatty acids (VFAs) are produced during sludge hydrolysis and acidification (Çokgör et al. 2009). During anaerobic exposure, soluble chemical oxygen demand (COD), nitrogen, and phosphorus are released. The increase in supernatant COD was attributed primarily to the conversion of biomass COD into soluble COD due to sludge decay, as is evident from a corresponding reduction in the mixed liquor suspended solids (MLSS) level. The cell lysis phenomenon is substantiated further by increasing ammonia and phosphorus concentration in the anaerobic sludge holding tank. Previous studies found that significant ammonium nitrogen (NH_4^+-N) and soluble phosphorus were released during sludge anaerobic treatment (Chen et al. 2003, 2007; Saby et al. 2003; Wang et al. 2008a). To evaluate sludge decay in an OSA system, a batch experiment was designed, as shown in Fig. 4.2. The experiment was carried out at an ORP level of $-250\,mV$. Sludge samples were taken from the aeration tank of both the reference and OSA systems. The initial MLSS concentration in the batch reactor was maintained at a level close to the sludge concentration of the holding tank of the OSA system ($9\,g\,L^{-1}$). The initial soluble COD concentration in all batch reactors was $35\,mg\,L^{-1}$. The reactor was well mixed using a magnetic stirrer at $20^{\circ}C$ (An and Chen 2008).

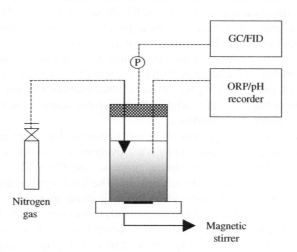

FIGURE 4.2 Experimental setup for the COD balance test of sludge decay.

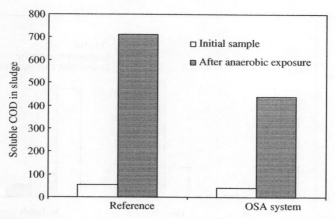

FIGURE 4.3 Change in COD concentration during an anaerobic batch experiment. [From Chen et al. (2003).]

The result shows that the COD concentration increased, achieving nearly 450 mg L^{-1} after 16 h of anaerobic treatment (Fig. 4.3). The COD increase was ascribed primarily to the conversion of biomass COD into soluble COD during the sludge decay, evidenced by a corresponding reduction in MLSS level in the batch reactor. If the reduced biomass was converted entirely into soluble COD without any biochemical reaction involved, the amount of COD generated from the OSA sludge decay should be the same as the increase in the COD concentrations in the reference. However, it was found that the increase in soluble COD of the OSA sludge was only 50 to 60% of that supposed to be generated from the biomass COD reduction. The results showed that the anaerobic exposure affected the assimilation or generation of COD from sludge reduction.

Figure 4.4 shows the average values of the initial and final nitrate, phosphate, and sulfate concentrations when sludges from the OSA system were exposed to anaerobic conditions in a closed batch reactor. Under an ORP level of −250 mV, available electron acceptors such as nitrate and sulfate were depleted, while phosphorus was released under such conditions. There is a significant difference between an OSA process and conventional biological nutrient removal processes where anaerobic tanks contain an adequate amount of substrates to elicit denitrification or phosphorus release. Sludge undergoes starvation under anaerobic conditions in the OSA process. Nitrification, anaerobic phosphorus release, and sulfate reduction eat up some of soluble COD generated from sludge lysis without an external substrate. Less soluble COD released from the OSA sludge was measured than that from the reference sludge when the sludges were exposed to anaerobic environment at the same time (Fig. 4.3). The phenomenon confirmed that part of the soluble COD was used as a carbon source for relevant biochemical reactions in an anaerobic sludge tank. Therefore, the results indicated that denitrifiers, sulfate reducers, and poly-P bacteria were present in the anaerobic sludge tank. Since some of these bacteria are known to be slow growers, they may have an impact on the overall sludge growth in the OSA system (Chudoba et al. 1991b).

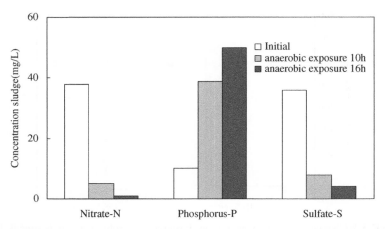

FIGURE 4.4 Nitrate and sulfate reduction and phosphorus release of OSA sludge during anaerobic exposure under an ORP level of $-250\,mV$. [From An and Chen (2008).]

Particle size was also modified after anaerobic exposure in the OSA system. The mean sludge floc size decreased from $87.4\,\mu m$ to $81.6\,\mu m$ after $16\,h$ of anaerobic exposure. This suggests further that the sludge anaerobic exposure enhanced sludge decomposition or sludge decay (An and Chen 2008). Usually, the pH will drop, due to the production of VFAs and their accumulation during sludge anaerobic treatment. Reactions such as denitrification, sulfate reduction, and gas production might have consumed the VFAs produced, thereby preventing a drop in the pH level in the anaerobic tank of an OSA system. A stable pH value favors all biochemical reactions in the anaerobic sludge tank of an OSA system.

4.3.2 Effect of Sludge Anaerobic Exposure on Biomass Activity

Microorganisms in activated sludge processes use oxygen for substrate oxidation. The oxygen uptake rate (OUR) can be used to measure the biological activity, since a higher OUR indicates a higher level of biological activity. By combining that with volatile suspended solids (VSS) measurement, the OUR result can be expressed in terms of a specific OUR (SOUR; $mg\,O_2\,g^{-1}\,VSS\,h^{-1}$), which represents a specific bioactivity. SOUR was investigated for estimating the effect of anaerobic exposure on biomass activity. The reference system showed an average SOUR of $50\,mg\,O_2\,g^{-1}$ $VSS\,h^{-1}$, which is within the normal range of SOUR for an activated sludge process (40 to $70\,mg\,O_2\,g^{-1}\,VSS\,h^{-1}$) (Rittmann and McCarty 2001; An 2004). The OSA system had an average SOUR of $60\,mg\,O_2\,g^{-1}\,VSS\,h^{-1}$, which was a little higher than that of the reference system. The results confirmed that the insertion of a sludge holding tank in the activated sludge process did not affect the activity of microorganisms. This is a significant advantage of the OSA system, as some of the approaches to minimizing excess sludge production are reported to affect the microbial activity adversely.

To determine the impact of the anaerobic tank on bacteria activity in the sludge of an OSA system, cell DNA-staining and cell respiratory activity-detecting techniques were employed. A 4′,6′-diamidino-2-phenylindole (DAPI)–based cell counting technique was used to measure the total number of bacteria, because DAPI can stain DNA in bacterial membranes of all kinds of bacteria both when they are viable and when they dead. A 5-cyano-2,3-ditolyltetrazolium chloride (CTC)–based counting technique was adopted to count respiring or active facultative bacteria, as CTC can produce red fluorescent CTC-formazan granules in respiring cells (Saby et al. 1997). Thus, CTC counting represents the number of active cells rather than a total cell number. Both DAPI- and CTC-stained cells can be counted under an epifluorescence microscope using ultraviolet light of a specific wavelength. The CTC counting can detect directly all types of respiring bacteria present in a sample, independent of conventional cell cultivation.

The total cell number per gram of MLSS appears to be 40 to 50% higher in the OSA sludge than in the reference sludge. The cell density in the sludge of the OSA system seems to be denser than the reference sludge since the former accommodates much high numbers of cells. However, the proportion of the active bacteria determined by CTC staining was four times lower in the OSA sludge than in the reference sludge. The results imply that the bacteria in the OSA sludge may have a lower activity, due to the low ORP condition in the anaerobic tank under which the cell activities might have been affected.

The sludge anaerobic exposure appears to have an important effect on the activity of bacteria in the reference sludge since the proportion of respiring bacteria decreased by 50% after an anaerobic treatment at an ORP of $-250\,\mathrm{mV}$ (Chen et al. 2003). This finding implies that the microbial population in the reference system is different from that in the OSA sludge because the activity of bacteria in the OSA system is not affected in the anaerobic treatment, due to the bacteria's adaptability in an anaerobic environment. On the other hand, the finding shows that insertion of an anaerobic sludge tank in an OSA system may affect the biomass activity and bacteria population.

4.4 SLUDGE PRODUCTION IN AN OSA SYSTEM

It is well known that anaerobic sludge treatment is helpful in reducing the amount of sludge for final disposal. Inserting an anaerobic sludge tank in an activated sludge process may affect the sludge yield. Excess sludge production in an OSA system is discussed.

The observed sludge yield in OSA processing has been reported to be lower (0.13 to 0.29 g VSS g^{-1} COD) than that in a conventional activated sludge process (0.28 to 0.47 g VSS g^{-1} COD) (Chudoba et al. 1992a). Table 4.1 shows the sludge production of a reference system and an OSA system for various organic loadings. The sludge production under the same anaerobic conditions in Saby et al.'s (2003) study was nearly 20% larger than in Chudoba et al.'s work. This difference can be attributed primarily to the difference in hydraulic retention times. In Saby et al.'s

TABLE 4.1 Comparison of Sludge Yield in Reference and OSA Systems

| Parameter | Reference System | | | OSA System (-250 mV) | | |
	Chudoba et al. (1992a)	Saby et al. (2003)	Wang et al. (2008)	Chudoba et al. (1992)	Saby et al. (2003)	Wang et al. (2008)
Organic loading (aeration tank only) (kg COD kg^{-1} TSS d^{-1})	0.34	0.92	0.66	0.83	0.33	0.92	0.66	0.83
Sludge production (kg TSS/kg^{-1} TSS d^{-1})	0.25	0.38	0.40	0.42	0.25	0.24	0.17	0.24
HRT in anaerobic time (h)	—	—	—	—	3	3	10.5	10.5
Reduction efficiency (%)	—	—	—	—	0	36.8	57.5	40

study the aeration and anaerobic tanks were maintained for 6 and 10.4 h, whereas in the Chudoba et al. studies the retention times were only 2 h in the aeration tank and 3 h in the anaerobic tank. The importance of a longer anaerobic exposure time on sludge production had been noted by Westgarth et al. (1964). The hydraulic retention time in the anaerobic tank is important for reducing the sludge production in an OSA system. With the same hydraulic retention, the sludge production in Saby et al.'s study was higher than that in Wang et al.'s (2008a) study, because Saby et al.'s study employed a membrane unit for solid–liquid separation.

Chudoba et al.'s studies showed that a higher loading in the conventional system in turn resulted in a significant increase in sludge production. In contrast to this phenomenon, sludge production showed a reducing trend in their OSA system, even though organic loading was increased from 0.33 to 0.92 kg COD kg^{-1} TSS d^{-1} at an ORP level of -250 mV in the anaerobic tank (Table 4.1). This in turn implies that the oxic-settling-anaerobic process is capable of handling high-strength organic pollutants without serious sludge-associated problems.

4.5 PERFORMANCE OF AN OSA SYSTEM

4.5.1 Organic and Nutrient Removal

A significant amount of attention has been paid to the influence of an anaerobic sludge tank on effluent quality in the OSA process. An (2004) found the effluent COD concentration in an OSA system to be lower than that in a reference system under the same loading (1.32 kg m^{-3} d^{-1}). Saby et al. (2003) found that the COD concentrations in both the settler and aeration tanks in an OSA system were lower than those in the aeration tank of the reference system, which means that the insertion of an anoxic tank actually improves COD removal. COD removal efficiency in the OSA process was slightly higher than that in the reference system under the same loading at 1.97 kg m^{-3} d^{-1} (Wang et al. 2007). An explanation is that when sludge is exposed in a low-ORP environment in the anoxic tank, the sludge may be "starved" under a "stressful" condition, which in turn increases its substrate removal ability in the following aerobic environment with the presence of adequate food in the aeration tank (Chen et al. 2001).

In addition to COD removal, denitrification and phosphorus release were observed in the OSA system. The removal efficiency of total nitrogen and phosphorus could be enhanced to 42.58% and 53.84%, respectively (Wang et al. 2007). Although a higher ammonia concentration was observed in the sludge anaerobic tank of the OSA system, evidently resulting from cell lysis, the OSA system showed excellent nitrification, reaching about 37% of TN (total nitrogen) removal. In contrast, TN removal of the reference system was about 10% (An 2004). This suggested that the nutrient removal of the OSA system was improved due to denitrification in the sludge anaerobic tank.

Phosphorus removal in the reference system was insignificant; while substantial phosphorus removal in the OSA system was detected, 40 to 60%. The higher level of phosphorus removal in the OSA system was due to its alternating aerobic and anaerobic sludge conditions (Capdeville and Nguyen 1990). The phosphorus was released in the sludge anaerobic tank under a lower OPR, and the phosphorus released was taken up later in the aeration tank.

Regarding sulfate, the OSA system had an 80% removal rate, while the reference system did not show any removal. This was obviously due to the presence of sulfate-reducing bacteria in the sludge anaerobic tank (An 2004). In other words, insertion of an anaerobic sludge tank is able to improve the COD and nutrient removal in an OSA system.

4.5.2 Sludge Settleability

The settleability of activated sludge is of great importance in an activated sludge process. A good-settling sludge enables a high solid concentration in return sludge, which ensures a higher sludge concentration in the sludge anaerobic tank. According to Low and Chase (1999), different sludge reduction strategies may affect the growth rate of individual microbial species in different ways, thus altering the microbial population dynamics. This, in turn, may affect the sludge settling characteristics adversely by either changing the surface chemistry of bacterial cells, thus causing poor flocculation, or encouraging a proliferation of filamentous bacteria, leading to sludge bulking.

The settleability of the OSA sludge was found to be better than that of the reference system, in addition to the improvement in COD removal in an OSA system (Saby et al. 2003). Because of alternative aerobic and anaerobic environments in the OSA process, sludge settleability and activity are improved. The SVI of the OSA system averaged 110, while the mean SVI of the reference system was 180. It was also observed that the sludge taken from the OSA system was more cohesive and contained more cells than the sludge taken from the reference system (Saby et al. 2003). These may be related to the release of intracellular polymers under anoxic conditions since they can act as floc bridging agents to improve sludge settleability (Barker and Stuckey 1999).

In essence, the OSA system is the ideal selector system. The mechanism of improving sludge settleability can be explained by the theory of selector systems. In selector-like systems, the microorganisms are subjected to periods with and without an external substrate. In the selector, the microorganisms are subjected to high-growth-rate environments and are able to accumulate substrate as internal storage products in their cells. A sufficiently long period without an external substrate available should then exist to reestablish the storage capacity of the cells. Worldwide, selectors are the engineering tool most commonly used for the prevention of bulking sludge phenomena (Martins et al. 2004). Thus, the OSA process significantly reduces excess sludge production as well as improving sludge settleability due to a similar environment selector.

4.6 IMPORTANT INFLUENCE FACTORS

Oxidation–reduction potential (ORP) and sludge anaerobic exposure time (SAET) are the two important parameters for sludge anaerobic digestion. The use of an anaerobic tank is decisive to sludge reduction in an OSA process. Therefore, ORP and SAET are important process parameters that may affect the overall sludge production in an OSA system. It has been validated that a longer hydraulic retention time (HRT) and higher sludge concentration in the sludge holding tank resulted in a lower ORP, which enhanced excess sludge reduction. Operation of the OSA process with an ORP of −250 mV and an HRT of 12 h in the sludge holding tank was found to be most effective in reducing excess sludge production and improving effluent quality (Chen et al. 2003).

4.6.1 Influence of the ORP on Sludge Production

Figure 4.5 shows the cumulative excess sludge wasted daily when the ORP of the anaerobic tank was controlled at +110, −100, and −250 mV, respectively. Compared with the reference system, the excess sludge production in the OSA system was clearly reduced at each controlled low ORP level, which indicates that a low ORP level in the anoxic tank promotes excess sludge reduction. When the ORP level was at −250 mV, the excess sludge production rate was only 2.3 g d^{-1}, almost half of that in the reference system (4.7 g d^{-1}). Even in the same OSA system, the excess sludge production rate at an ORP level of −250 mV in its anoxic tank was 36% lower than that at an ORP level of +100 mV. Therefore, it can be concluded that the OSA system can reduce excess sludge effectively and that the ORP level in the anoxic tank is one of the keys to achieving an effective reduction of excess sludge (Saby et al. 2003).

4.6.2 Influence of the ORP on Performance of an OSA System

When the ORP was −100 mV, the COD concentration in the anoxic tank was found to be increased significantly over that observed at an ORP of +100 mV, indicating that an ORP below +100 mV in the anoxic tank accelerates COD release. The cause of this release may not be the result of cell decomposition under anoxic conditions, but may also be triggered by a stressful environment with no external food available. It

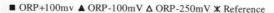

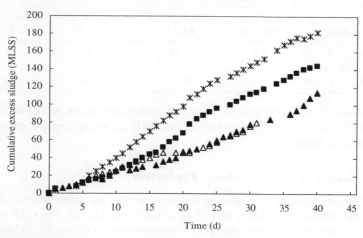

FIGURE 4.5 Effect of the ORP level in an anoxic tank on excess sludge production in an OSA system. [From Saby et al. (2003).]

is believed that this COD release is associated with a reduction in the excess sludge in an OSA system. Saby et al. (2003) observed a drastic drop in COD level in the anoxic tank and an increase in sludge production when the ORP level of the anoxic tank had a sharp increase. It was obvious that the COD release in the anoxic tank is sensitive to the ORP level. This phenomenon indicates that the low ORP levels may play a key role in COD release.

However, lower COD concentrations of effluent were found in OSA systems, which implies that insertion of an anoxic tank actually improves COD removal under the same COD loading rate (Table 4.2). One reason for this is that denitrification and phosphorus release are able to eat up a certain portion of the organic matter generated from the reduction of sludge. In addition, an alternating feasting and fasting environment stimulates microorganisms to increase the substrate removal ability.

TABLE 4.2 Summary of the Water Quality in the Operation of Two Systems (mg L^{-1})

	Aeration Tank Only	With an Anoxic Tank (the OSA System)		
		ORP + 100 mV	ORP − 100 mV	ORP − 250 mV
COD in treated water	30	18	22	7
Soluble COD in sludge	41	27	27	27
Nitrate-N in treated water	34	25	20	11
Phosphate-P in treated water	3.6	3.7	4.5	7.2

Source: Saby et al. (2003).

TABLE 4.3   Summary of Sludge Production Rate at Different SAET in the Two Systems

System Condition	Reference System	OSA with 6-h SAET	OSA with 10-h SAET	OSA with 12-h SAET
Net sludge production rate (g SSd^{-1})	4.7	3.53	2.38	1.98
Y_{obs} (g SS g^{-1} COD)	0.40	0.27	0.19	0.17

It is observed that both denitrification and phosphorus release in the anoxic tank occurred (Table 4.2). With a decrease in the ORP, denitrification and phosphorus release were enhanced.

4.6.3   Influence of SAET on Sludge Production

It is well demonstrated that extending sludge anaerobic retention time (SAET) can enhance the efficiency of sludge hydrolysis at lower ORP levels. The ORP level is a function of both the SAET and the sludge concentration in the sludge holding tank. Usually, the required ORP level should be achieved and maintained by a sufficient sludge retention time or by the injection of pure nitrogen gas. In view of the practical feasibility, the sludge retention time may be much more practical. It is believed that extended sludge exposure to anaerobic conditions enhances the reduction of excess sludge production rate mainly through the endogenous activity.

An (2004) studied the influence of SAET in the sludge anaerobic tank (6, 10, and 12 h) on sludge yield at an ORP level of -250 mV. Compared with the reference system, the excess sludge production in the OSA system was significantly reduced with increasing SAET (Table 4.3). When the SAET in the sludge anaerobic tank was 6 h, the excess sludge production rate was 3.53 g d^{-1}, which was only 75% of that in the reference system (4.7 g d^{-1}). The sludge production rate was further reduced to 2.38 and 1.98 g d^{-1}, at SAETs of 10 and 12 h, respectively. The result suggests that a longer SAET in the sludge anaerobic tank promoted the reduction in excess sludge production.

4.6.4   Influence of SAET on the Performance of an OSA System

It was confirmed that insertion of a sludge anaerobic tank did not affect the effluent quality despite a change in the SAET of the OSA system (An 2004; An and Chen 2008). The COD concentration in the anaerobic tank was increased with an increased SAET. Relative biochemical reactions, including nitrification, anaerobic phosphorus release, and sulfate reduction, were enhanced with increasing anaerobic exposure time, as shown in Fig. 4.4. It demonstrates that a longer SAET may accelerate lysis or decay of sludge in an OSA system.

4.7   POSSIBLE SLUDGE REDUCTION IN THE OSA PROCESS

To apply the OSA process effectively, an understanding of the sludge reduction phenomenon is necessary. Possible approaches to sludge reduction in an OSA system

TABLE 4.4   Expected Sludge Production in Various Biochemical Reactions

Reaction	Aerobic Oxidation	Denitrification	Sulfate Reduction	Phosphorus Release	Methane Production
Y (g VSS/g COD)	0.55[a]	0.3[b]	0.2[b]	0.18[b]	0.05[c]

[a] An and Chen (2008).
[b] Zehnder and Wuhrmann (1976).
[c] Higging and Novak (1997).

may include three aspects: (1) domination of slow growers over the entire microbial population, which may also result in a small sludge growth yield; (2) energy uncoupling metabolism; and (3) possible sludge decay acceleration in the sludge anaerobic tank. Microfauna predation has been one of the possible approaches to sludge minimization in wastewater biological treatment (Huang et al. 2007; Song and Chen 2009); however, predating worms have not been observed in OSA systems. Thus, sludge predation by microorganisms has not been verified to be the cause of reducing sludge production in the OSA process.

4.7.1   Slow Growers

To quantify the number of slow growers, Chen et al. (2003) designed a batch experiment to measure $Y_{s/x}$ (observed cell growth yield, mg MLSS mg^{-1} COD) in both systems periodically. The samples were adopted from a reference system and an OSA system and were placed in a 1-L reactor filled with synthetic wastewater for a 6-h aerobic treatment with the same MLSS level and S_0/X_0 ratio. If domination by slow growers does occur, the value $Y_{s/x}$ in the OSA system should decline, in contrast with that in the reference system. However, no significant changes in $Y_{s/x}$ values in the two systems were found over the entire operation period. This indicates further that slow growers may not become the dominant species in an OSA system. Therefore, excess sludge reduction in an OSA system could not be attributed to the domination of slow growers.

Denitrification, sulfate reduction, phosphorus release, and methane production have been found in the anaerobic tank of an OSA system. The sludge yields in these reactions are much lower than those of aerobic oxidation (Table 4.4). Corresponding microorganisms have lower sludge yields than those of other aerobic heterotrophic bacteria. These microorganisms are able to eat up a certain portion of the organic matter generated from sludge decay and contribute to sludge reduction. The limited reaction is to produce soluble COD by sludge lysis during anaerobic treatment. Thus, they cannot be the major contributors to the significant reduction in sludge yield in OSA systems (An and Chen 2008).

4.7.2   Energy Uncoupling Metabolism

Energy uncoupling or spilling is defined as a discrepancy in the energy balance between catabolism and anabolism (Low et al. 2000). For aerobic microorganisms, adenosine triphosphate (ATP) is generated from the oxidation of exogenous organic substrate. When the microorganisms are subject to anaerobic conditions without a food supply, they are no longer able to produce energy and have to use their ATP reserves as an energy source. During the anaerobic starvation period, the ATP would be exhausted. After microorganisms return to a food-enriched aerobic reactor, they have to rebuild the necessary energy reserves prior to biosynthesis because cellular synthesis could not proceed without a certain intracellular stock of ATP. In this case, the substrate consumption should thus be consumed by catabolic metabolism to satisfy the energy requirements of microorganisms. Therefore, it appears that alternative aerobic–anaerobic cycling of activated sludge would stimulate catabolic activity and make catabolism dissociate from anabolism. The energy uncoupling induced by alternating aerobic and anaerobic treatment comprises the theoretical basis for the aerobic–settling–anaerobic technique designed for excess sludge minimization (Chudoba et al. 1991a; Liu and Tay 2001).

Chen et al. (2001) investigated the effect of sludge fasting and feasting on growth in an activated sludge culture. It was found that when the fasted cultures were treated in a feasting environment, an accumulation of carbohydrate storage did not occur but that specific oxygen uptake rates (SOURs) showed a sharp increase. Both the substrate utilization and biomass growth rates were also accelerated. It was therefore confirmed that sludge feasting did occur after a fasting treatment for fastable cultures. However, an increase in sludge ATP content was not brought about by a feasting treatment. It was concluded that sludge fasting–feasting treatment could not induce a reduction in the growth yield observed (Y_{obs}).

Chen et al. (2003) designed a batch experiment to study energy uncoupling. Sludge samples were taken from the aeration tank, sludge holding tank, and settling tank of an OSA system to test this theory under an ORP level of $-250\,mV$. These samples were treated for 5 h with no external food source under low-ORP conditions.

Certain portions of the treated sludge were then transferred immediately to an aerobic treatment for 6 h under aeration conditions with sufficient food, in which $Y_{s/x}$ was determined based on the changes in both COD and MLSS from the oxic treatment. According to the theory, if energy uncoupling does occur during an alternative exposure between a food-sufficient oxic environment and a food-insufficient anaerobic environment, $Y_{s/x}$ will decline. However, $Y_{s/x}$ throughout the entire operational period of the OSA system was stable, and it showed that the energy uncoupling proposed did not occur in the OSA system. A low ORP value and no external food-may promote sludge reduction by imposing stress on the microbes. Such a stressing effect on the sludge in an OSA system may be less obvious than that on the sludge from a reference system because the microbes in the OSA system have already adapted to a low-ORP environment. It is clear that these consecutive treatments do not induce a reduction of $Y_{s/x}$ throughout the entire operational period of the OSA system, which indicates that the energy uncoupling proposed does not occur in the OSA system. These results further confirm that the energy uncoupling theory is unable to explain the excess sludge reduction in an OSA process (Chen et al. 2003).

4.7.3 Sludge Endogenous Decay

The yield of active biomass in an activated sludge system is determined by the net specific growth rate resulting from the balance of its growth and endogenous decay processes. During periods of high growth rate with an excess supply of substrate, growth dominates and endogenous processes can often be neglected. However, in many environmental systems, microbial growth is substrate limited and endogenous processes significantly influence the amount of active biomass (Lopez et al. 2006). When biomass undergoes death, decay, and cell maintenance, a certain portion of their cell bodies is converted into soluble secondary substrates that can be further oxidized, thereby reducing the amount of biomass produced.

Under some stressful conditions, endogenous processes can result in a significant reduction in overall sludge production and, an increase in electron acceptor utilization. In the OSA process, the repeated passage of activated microorganisms through the anaerobic sludge zone may create conditions of physical stress (Chudoba et al., 1992b). A considerable part of the energy produced under oxic conditions (normally available for biomass growth) would be used for maintenance functions or would be wasted under anaerobic conditions. The anabolic process (biomass growth) would thus be hampered, which might result in the reduction of excess sludge (Chudoba et al. 1991a). Soluble COD is generated from sludge decay under low ORP levels in the anaerobic tank of an OSA system, where there are scarcely external substrates. Sludge reduction in an OSA system results primarily from COD loss through various reactions and the emission of gaseous products produced under anaerobic conditions.

The sludge decay rate also appears to change with cell age, biomass concentration, and substrate level (Rittmann and McCarity 2001). Low et al. (2000) found that increasing biomass concentration from $3\,g\,L^{-1}$ to $6\,g\,L^{-1}$ reduced biomass production by 12%, and an analysis of a similar system showed a reduction in biomass production of 44% when increasing biomass concentration from $1.7\,g\,L^{-1}$ to $10.3\,g\,L^{-1}$ (Low and Chase 1999). The biomass concentration in the anaerobic tank of the OSA system was twice that in the settling tank. An increase in sludge decay might therefore be expected in the sludge holding tank of the OSA system without an external substrate, a long SRT, and a high biomass concentration due to anaerobic exposure of the sludge.

To validate whether biomass reduction during anaerobic treatment was caused by sludge endogenous decay in an OSA system, Chen et al. (2003) compared the amount of total bacteria and respiring bacteria before and after anaerobic treatment. It was found that there was a great difference in terms of the percentage of respiring bacteria, although the total amount of bacteria was almost the same in the reference and OSA sludge. The percentage of respiring bacteria in the sludge from the reference system was nearly 22%, whereas it was 6% from the OSA system. Such a low percentage of respiring bacteria in the OSA system may be associated with periodic exposure to a no-food and anaerobic environment, which eventually results in a prevalence of bacteria with low activities in the microbial population. The results showed that the concentration of active biomass was reduced by decay processes, which include

TABLE 4.5 COD Conversion Factors in Various Biochemical Reactions

Reaction	Reduced/Produced Electron Acceptors	COD Consumed (g)	Reference
Deification	1 g NO_3^--N reduced	4.46	Rittmann and McCarty (2001)
Sulfate reduction	1 g SO_4^{2-}-S reduced	2	Rittmann and McCarty (2001)
Phosphate release	1 g P released	2	Rittmann and McCarty (2001)
Gas production	1 g CH_4 produced	4	Metcalf Eddy, Inc. (2003)

spontaneous cell death and lysis. This observation is verified by the fact that the respiring bacteria percentage (6%) did not change after 16 h of anaerobic exposure. The floc size mean value decreased about 4 to 6 μm after 16 h of anaerobic exposure, implying sludge decay in the OSA system (Chen et al. 2003).

Low excess sludge in an OSA system therefore involves two major functions: (1) enhanced sludge decay, and (2) effective utilization of the secondary substrate through the methanogens, denitrifiers, and sulfate reducers that coexist in the sludge holding tank. To evaluate sludge decay in an OSA system, a batch experiment was designed, as shown in Fig. 4.2. The operational conditions were the same as those of batch experiment I (An and Chen 2008).

The COD removal (ΔCOD) in the batch test can be calculated as initial total COD concentration – final total COD concentration = (initial soluble COD + P × initial VSS) – (final soluble COD + P × final VSS). This expression can be written as follows:

$$S_{T0} - S_{Te} = (S_0 + PX_{v0}) - (S_e + PX_{ve}) \qquad (4.1)$$

where S_{T0} is the initial total COD concentration (mg L^{-1}), S_{Te} the final total COD concentration (mg L^{-1}), S_0 the initial soluble COD concentration (mg L^{-1}), S_e the final soluble COD concentration (mg L^{-1}), X_{v0} the initial total VSS (mg L^{-1}), X_{ve} the final total VSS (mg L^{-1}), and P the COD equivalence of VSS (1.42 mg COD mg^{-1} VSS based on the cell composition of $C_5H_7O_2N$).

By measuring the removal or production of various inorganic species, such as PO_4^{3-}, SO_4^{2-}, NO_3^-, and CH_4, it was possible to determine COD removal in each reaction by employing conversion factors, as shown in Table 4.5.

The initial and final total COD (soluble + particulate) concentrations were determined by Eq. (4.1), and their difference indicated the COD loss in the batch experiments. The amount of COD removed corresponding to the reductions in nitrate and sulfate and release in phosphorus were determined according to Table 4.5. The results of the COD balance analysis are summarized in Table 4.6. The COD balance results reveal that gas production under −250 mV is the major source of sludge reduction.

The endogenous decay coefficient accounts for the loss of cell mass, because internal storage products are oxidized to obtain energy for cell maintenance, cell death, and predation by higher forms of organisms (van Loosdrecht and Henze 1999). The sludge decay coefficient (k_a) in the anaerobic tank of an OSA system was

TABLE 4.6   COD Balance for the Anaerobic Tank in the OSA (ORP = −250 mV)

Test	COD Loss/ S_{T0}-S_{Te} (mg L^{-1})	COD Unaccounted for (%)	Total COD Consumption (mg L^{-1})	Denitrification	Sulfate Reduction	Phosphorus Release	Gas Production
				COD Consumption (mg L^{-1})			
1	536.32	12.4	469.7	152.1	7.2	60.4	250
2	431.32	2.6	420.2	159.2	10.4	70.6	180
3	476.48	4.8	453.6	166.4	9.6	77.6	200

calculated as 0.13, which is far greater than that in an anaerobic bioreactor (a typical anaerobic sludge decay coefficient ranges from 0.02 to 0.04 (Metcalf & Eddy, Inc. 2003). The higher sludge decay coefficient in the anaerobic tank indicates that the low sludge production in the OSA system resulted from the increased sludge decay rate in the sludge anaerobic tank. The increased sludge decay rate facilitates the effective conversion of the secondary substrates into gaseous products, such as methane and nitrogen, in the sludge holding tank, thereby causing a low sludge yield in an OSA process.

4.8   MICROBIAL COMMUNITY IN AN OSA SYSTEM

A series of biochemical reactions that occur in wastewater biological treatment, such as organic oxidation and methane fermentation, nitrification, and denitrification, are mediated by microorganisms. The sludge anaerobic tank inserted in the return sludge circuit of an OSA system plays a key role in reducing the sludge production of the OSA system, which may influence the microbial population. The stability and performance of the process are highly dependent on complex microbial interactions when microorganisms undergo alternating anaerobic and aerobic environments in the OSA process. Thus, microbial population and community should be investigated.

Whether there are phosphorus-accumulating organisms (PAOs) in OSA sludge has been argued. Using the Neisser staining method, Chudoba et al. (1992a) found that OSA biomass contained about 60% polyphospate-accumulating bacteria. However, Chen et al. (2003) reported that poly-P bacteria were not the dominant bacteria in an OSA system, because no significant intake of phosphate was observed under aerobic conditions with sufficient food available, although phosphate release was observed under anaerobic conditions.

Wang et al. (2008b) analyzed precipitate-bound phosphorus and biological phosphorus accumulation in aerobic sludge from reference and OSA systems, as shown in Table 4.7. Total phosphorus (TP) contents of aerobic sludge in the OSA process were twice that of those in the reference process, while the precipitate-bound phosphorus content in both processes was nearly the same. The results indicated that biological phosphorus accumulation led to higher phosphorus removal efficiency in

TABLE 4.7 Total, Precipitate-Bounded, and Biological Phosphorus Accumulation in Dry Aerobic Sludge from Reference and OSA Systems

Phosphorus (mg g^{-1})	Reference System	OSA System
Total phosphorus	14.9	30.5
Precipitate-bounded phosphorus	3.8	3.6
Biological phosphorus accumulation	11.1	26.9

the OSA system. It can be concluded that some phosphate-accumulating bacteria exist in the OSA system which have the capability to take up excess phosphate in the aerobic condition.

4.8.1 Staining Analysis

The abundance of polyphosphate-accumulating bacteria in OSA sludge should be investigated. Special staining and fluorescent in situ hybridization (FISH) without cultivation of individual species can be adopted to analyze the microbial community (Sanz and Köchling 2007). In the enhanced biological phosphorus removal process (EBPR), PAOs store volatile fatty acids (VFAs) as poly-β-hydroxybutyrate (PHB) and release phosphate under anaerobic conditions, followed by accumulation of excess amounts of phosphate in the form of poly-P under aerobic conditions. Therefore, the amount of cellular poly-P granule and PHB granule represented that of PAOs to a certain extent. Staining for lipophilic granules was carried out with Sudan black stain (Murray et al. 1994). The lipophilic granules are referred to as PHB granules in the polyphospate bacteria. A black-blue granule in a clear or light pink background indicates the presence of this storage polymer (Serafim et al. 2002). Thus, if anaerobic sludge shows positive in reaction with Sudan black stain, it demonstrates the existence of PHB in the biomass.

Intracellular poly-P particles and microbial cells are stained by 4′,6′-diamidino-2-phenylindol dihydrochloride. The stained poly-P particles were released from sludge under aerobic conditions emit yellow light under ultraviolet excitation while the stained cell emitted dim blue light (Liu et al. 2005). The samples were observed with an epifluorescence microscope using an excitation wavelength of 330 to 385 nm. Table 4.8 summarizes the oligonucleotide probes used for FISH in the study. FAM-labeled EUB338 was specific for active bacteria, and Cy3-labeled PAOMIX probes comprising equal amounts of probes PAO462, PAO651, and PAO846 were specific for *Rhodocyclus*-associated PAO cluster (Crocetti et al. 2000).

Sudan black staining and DAPI were employed to confirm the storage and release of poly-P granules and PHB granules, respectively. The microscopic results of PHB staining in Fig. 4.6a and b showed that percentages of black-blue granules in sludge obtained from various operation phases (the 85th and 135th days) were relatively stable. Bacteria with PHB-positive reactions were large coccoid cells with a diameter of 2 to 4 μm, accounting for about 30 to 35% of bacteria in anaerobic sludge in an OSA system.

TABLE 4.8 Information Relevant to FISH Oligonucleotides

Probe	Sequence (5′-3′)	Target Site (bp)	Specificity	Formamide (%)	Label
EUB338	GCTGCCTCCCGTAGGAGT	338–355	Most bacteria	20	FAM
PAO462	CCGTCATCTACWCAGGGTATTAAC	462–485	PAO cluster	35	Cy3
PAO651	CCCTCTGCCAAACTCCAG	651–668	PAO cluster	35	Cy3

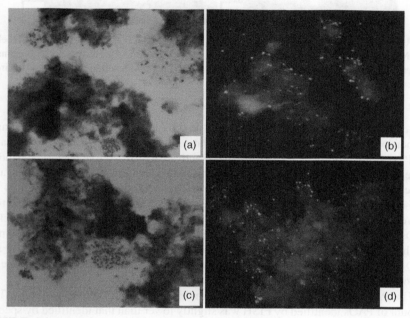

FIGURE 4.6 Images of Sudan black and DAPI staining for sludge in the OSA process. (a) Anaerobic sludge on the 85th day; (b) anaerobic sludge on the 135th day; (c) aerobic sludge on the 85th day; (d) aerobic sludge on the 135th day.

DAPI staining revealed that poly-Ps were accumulated by PAOs in the OSA process. Approximately 35% of bacteria were capable of accumulating poly-P (Fig. 4.6c and d). The finding was consistent with the relative percentage of bacteria with positive PHB staining. Yellow spots of sludge increased slightly from the 85th to the 135th days. Thus, the staining results demonstrated that 35% of the bacteria had characteristics of PAOs in the OSA process. In contrast to aerobic sludge in the OSA system, there were scarcely any yellow spots in that of the CAS system.

4.8.2 FISH Analysis

FISH with specific probes was performed to assess the number of PAOs. The micrographs in Fig. 4.7 show the percentage of PAOMIX-binding cells and active

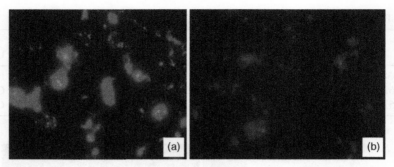

FIGURE 4.7 FISH images of sludge with FAM-labeled EUB338 probe and CY3-labeled PAOMIX probes from the OSA system. (a) Aerobic sludge, 135d, bright area presents domain bacteria; (b) Anaerobic sludge, 135d, bright area represents DAPI staining; bright dots in circle represent PAOs.

bacteria. The amount of PAO probe-positive cells was counted and expressed as a proportion of EUB338-binding cells. The ratio of the area of EUB338 to the area of DAPI staining represents the percentage of active bacteria. Active bacteria in sludge were about 80 to 90% of total microorganisms via image analysis, while the ratio of active bacteria in anaerobic sludge was lowered slightly, by about 4% (Fig. 4.7). The results support the conclusion by Chen et al. (2003) that the amount of active microorganisms was scarcely affected by sludge decay in the anaerobic reactor. PAOs were quantified as about 28% of the total active microorganisms represented by the PAO/EUB338 ratio, and about 31% of the total biomass represented by the PAO/DAPI ratio. The findings showed that PAOMIX-binding bacteria were one of important communities in the OSA sludge.

The PAOs were identified by staining and FISH assay in an OSA system. The amount of PAOs identified by FISH was slightly lower than that identified by special staining (poly-P staining and PHB staining). This may be caused by statistical error. It should be noted that the amount of poly-P-accumulating bacteria shown in Fig. 4.7 was less than that reported by Chudoba et al. (1992a). The dissolved oxygen concentration in the aerobic tank was maintained at 8 mg L^{-1} in Chudoba et al.'s OSA system, while that of the aerobic tank in our OSA system was controlled at 2 to 3 mg L^{-1}. High oxygen concentration might stimulate poly-P accumulation in the OSA system. With higher oxygen concentrations, sufficient oxidization in the aerobic tank may accumulate more energy in the cells. More energy was thus stored by means of the intracellular adenosine triphosphatase (ATP) pool, and the surplus was transferred into poly-Ps accumulated by poly-P bacteria (Chudoba et al. 1992a).

4.9   COST AND ENERGY EVALUATION

The OSA system is a potential technique for reducing sludge production. The decision to apply this system depends primarily on the magnitude of capital

TABLE 4.9 Comparison of the OSA and Reference Processes in Economic terms[a]

	Cost-Increasing Unit			Cost-Saving Unit		
Process	Sludge Anaerobic Tank Construction	Pumping	ORP Control	Digester Volume	Sludge Treatment and Disposal Cost	Disposal Capacity (Landfill)
Reference system	Q: 25,000 m³ d⁻¹; V:10,416 m³ (HRT = 10)	Additional for sludge pumping	Yes	700 m³ d⁻¹ × 15 d =10,500 m³[b]	1.02 × 10⁷ US dollars y⁻¹[c]	210 m³ d⁻¹
The OSA system	No	No	No	1100 m³ d⁻¹ × 15 d =16,500 m³[c]	1.6 × 10⁷ USD y⁻¹[c]	330 m³ d⁻¹

Source: An and Chen (2008).
[a] Based on 100,000 m³ d⁻¹ of flow rate for two systems.
[b] Metcalf & Eddy, Inc. (2003).
[c] Christoulas et al. (2000).

investments, easy operation, energy costs, and sludge disposal costs. An and Chen (2008) made a rough evaluation of cost by comparing the conventional activated sludge and OSA systems in economic terms, based on a treatment capacity of 100,000 m³ d⁻¹, as shown in Table 4.9.

Taking into account the increased costs of sludge disposal, the operational cost and the investment needed for the OSA system may be offset by the decreased operational costs for sludge treatment and disposal. When existing sludge settling basins are available for modification into a sludge holding tank, the OSA process should provide an ideal solution for achieving effective excess sludge reduction in a full-scale application (An and Chen, 2008). However, there is limited literature on accurate economic evaluation, as cost and energy evaluation should be investigated further.

4.10 EVALUATION OF THE OSA PROCESS

The OSA process is a well-proven technology for sludge reduction. The introduction of an anaerobic tank in the OSA process does not influence the effluent quality significantly and the sludge settleability is improved. Alternating oxic and anaerobic cycling improves the sludge settlement and avoids bulking and foaming. It is convenient to modify the conventional activated sludge by inserting an anaerobic tank in engineering practice. No chemical addition reduces operation costs and avoids second pollutants. For many chemicals long-term bioacclimation may be xenobiotic and potentially harmful to the environment. No accumulation of inorganic and inert particles over long-term operation has been found in an OSA system.

Although the good performance and low sludge yield of the OSA process has been investigated in batch- and pilot-scale experiments, there is seldom a report about its application in practice. An obstacle that restraines industrial application is the difficulty in controlling accurately the operational condition of the OSA system.

Biochemical reactions occurring in the anaerobic tank are sensitive to the ORP level. The low ORP level in the anoxic tank is crucial to achieving an effective reduction of excess sludge. Saby et al. (2003) found that ORP disturbance led to an increase in the sludge production rate, which actually resulted in a month-long restoration period to recover the system in a pilot-scale experiment. To maintain the ORP level effectively at −250 mV, pure nitrogen gas was occasionally injected in batch- and pilot-scale experiments. However, the ORP level is usually regulated by controlling operational conditions in engineering practice, while injection of pure nitrogen is seldom employed in large-scale wastewater biological treatment. In practice, low ORP can be created by inceasing sludge concentration and SAET in the anaerobic tank of an OSA system. However, alternating aerobic and anaerobic sludge circulation may sometimes cause a sharp increase in the ORP level. Any improper operation may disturb the low ORP level in the anaerobic tank, which may increase the sludge production inversely. Therefore, the rigorous operational conditions may be a primary reason for limiting application of the OSA process on a large scale.

The release of redundant soluble COD and nutrient release into effluent increases downstream nutrient removal requirements, although a part of the COD generated from sludge decay in the anaerobic tank was utilized by denitrification, phosphorus release, sulfate reduction, and methane gas production. When anaerobic sludge with a low ORP level is returned to the aerobic tank, the total oxygen demand increases sharply and thus raises the aeration costs. In future studies, more attention should be paid to optimizing the operating conditions of an OSA system and strengthening sludge decay in the anaerobic sludge tank. Combining the OSA process with other reduction mechanisms to reduce sludge production and economic costs as well as to enhance nutrient removal is a promising approach.

4.11   PROCESS DEVELOPMENT

4.11.1   Sludge Decay Combined with Other Sludge Reduction Mechanisms

To improve the performance of sludge reduction, other reduction processes combined with the OSA process were reported. 3,3′,4′,5-Tetrachlorosalicylanilide (TCS) is one type of chemical uncouplers used to reduce sludge by energy uncoupling. Too large a dose may create a second pollutant. It was confirmed that the TCS and OSA combined process cut down excess sludge production more effectively, while the TCS dosage could be reduced remarkably. The combined processes reduced sludge yield by 21 to 56% for the same sludge retention time (6.75 h) in a sludge anoxic holding tank with the addition of 0.05, 0.10, and 0.15 g TCS, respectively. The substrate removal capability and nutrient removal efficiency were not affected adversely by the presence of TCS or the insertion of an anoxic sludge holding tank (Ye and Li, 2010).

A novel biological process capable of repeated coupling of aerobes and anaerobes by the use of macroporous microbial carriers was proposed. Baffles were used to separate the entire reactor into small compartments, and alternative aeration divided the neighboring compartments into numerous microenvironments of alternating aerobic and anaerobic conditions along the water-flow direction. In this process, sludge decay is accelerated inside the membrane-attached macroporous microbial carriers for long sludge age and low ORP. The result showed that the sludge production in this system was 0.13 kg SS kg^{-1} COD, which was about 30 to 50% of that of the conventional activated sludge as a control. The existence of protozoans and metazoans in the aerobic units and sludge decay due to alternative aerobic and anaerobic conditions favor sludge reduction (Xing et al. 2008). Numerous alternative aerobic and anaerobic microenvironments are created by macroporous carriers and biomembrane attached on carriers in this process. This decreases sludge production and energy costs and increases the operational feasibility.

4.11.2   Improved Efficiency in Sludge Anaerobic Digestion

The sludge anaerobic tank is crucial to sludge decay, which directly influences the sludge production in an OSA system. Enhancing anaerobic digestion efficiency may reduce sludge production. Several approaches were introduced to improve the efficiency of sludge anaerobic digestion, including combining sludge anaerobic treatment with the addition of chemicals, such as surfactant, ozone, enzyme, uncouplers, or optimizing the operational conditions of the anaerobic reactor.

Surfactant may influence sludge hydrolysis and acidification as well as methanogensis during sludge anaerobic treatment. Jiang et al. (2007) investigated the effect of surfactant [sodium dodecyl sulfate (SDS)] on the fermentation of activated sludge at ambient temperature. It was found that the concentrations of protein, carbohydrate, NH_4^+-N, phosphate and short-chain fatty acids in fermentation liquor increased with the addition of SDS.

It is well documented that excess sludge production can be greatly reduced by partial ozonation of the returned sludge in an activated sludge process. Anaerobic digestion combined with partial ozonation may enhance sludge hydrolysis efficiency and decrease ozone dosage. It was confirmed that combining anaerobic digestion with ozonation achieved higher sludge hydrolysis efficiency. The nondecomposed fraction of VSS compounds in the municipal sludge was only 12% in the ozonation system and 37% in the control system. The biogas production in the test reactor was 1.3 times higher than that in the control reactor (Goel et al. 2003; Yasui et al. 2005).

Previous studies showed that adding enzymes to the anaerobic digestion process could cut down digesting time, improve sludge digestibility, and reduce disposal costs (Wawrzynczyk et al. 2008; Romano et al. 2009). Yang et al. (2010) confirmed that the mixture of two enzymes (protease: amylase = 1:3) resulted in optimum hydrolysis efficiency, and the efficiency of solids hydrolysis increased from 10% to 68.43% at a temperature of 50°C. Correspondingly, the concentration of reducing sugar and NH_4^+-N improved by about 377% and 201%, respectively.

Optimizing operational conditions such as retention time, biomass concentration, and pH is another effective approach to enhancing the efficiency of anaerobic digestion. Yuan et al. (2009) investigated the effect of solids retention time (SRT) and biomass concentration on the generation of VFAs from the nonmethanogenic fermentation of waste activated sludge. It was found that the VFA yield increased with SRT. At the same SRT, VFA yields increased when the biomass concentration decreased. At a SRT of 10 d, the VFA yield increased by 46%, when the biomass concentration decreased from $13\,g\,L^{-1}$ to $4.8\,g\,L^{-1}$. Wu et al. (2009) investigated the effect of pH in the range 3.0 to 11.0 on anaerobic fermentation of primary sludge at room temperature. The experimental results showed that the concentrations of soluble COD, soluble protein and carbohydrate, and short-chain fatty acids under alkaline conditions were significantly higher than those under other pHs. At pH 10.0, the VSS reduction reached 38%.

4.11.3   Combined Minimization of Excess Sludge with Nutrient Removal

It is a promising process to combine minimization of excess sludge with resource recovery. Using waste sludge to biologically produce VFAs has drawn much attention recently because the VFAs can be used as the preferred carbon source of biological nutrient removal microbes (Moser-Engeler et al. 1998; Çokgör et al. 2009; Feng et al. 2009). For low-organic-content wastewater such as municipal wastewater, external carbon source addition is becoming necessary to stimulate nutrient removal sufficiently to meet the increasingly stringent limits on phosphorus in effluent. On-site production of carbon source by sludge fermentation is a widely used method that decreases sludge production as well as operational costs.

Gao et al. (2011) developed a novel process, in which simultaneous sludge reduction and enhanced nutrient removal were expected to be achieved. Pilot-scale experiments conducted in the combined system (Fig. 4.8) included a continuously stirred tank reactor (CSTR) for alkaline pretreatment (first step), an up-flow hydrolysis and acidification column (UHAC) for sludge fermentation (second step), and an A^2O reactor for enhanced nitrogen and phosphorus removal. Such a design with a two-step fermentation would enhance the performance by strong alkaline

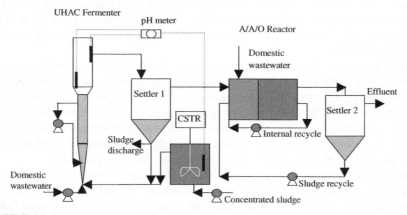

FIGURE 4.8 Schematic layout of the pilot-scale combined reactors. [From Gao et al. (2011).]

pretreatment in the CSTR. Moreover, the UHAC served not only as a fermentor but also as a buffer, where the pH shock of sludge fermentation liquids to the following A^2O reactor would be avoided. The results showed that 38.2% of sludge was hydrolyzed, 19.7% was finally acidified into VFAs, and as much as 42.1% of the sludge was removed. Moreover, after introducing fermentation liquids with higher proportions of acetic acid and propionics acid into the A^2O reactor, the total nitrogen and phosphorus removal efficiencies reached 80.1% and 90.0%, respectively. Sludge reduction and nutrient removal increase could be achieved simultaneously in the system proposed.

Zheng et al. (2010) developed a novel process in which the waste activated sludge alkaline fermentation liquid was used as the main carbon source for phosphorus and nitrogen removal under anaerobic conditions followed by alternating aerobic–anoxic conditions. The use of alkaline fermentation liquid not only affected the transformations of phosphorus, nitrogen, intracellular poly (hydroxyalkanoates), and glycogen, but also led to higher removal efficiencies for phosphorus and nitrogen compared with that for acetic acid as a carbon source. Alkaline fermentation liquid resulted in higher removal efficiencies for phosphorus (95%) and nitrogen (82%). Therefore, the new process might be a more promising choice for simultaneous nutrient removal and sludge reduction.

REFERENCES

An K. J. (2004) Reduction of excess sludge in an OSA process. Ph.D. dissertation, the Hong Kong University of Science and Technology, Hong Kong.

An K. J., Chen G. H. (2008) Chemical oxygen demand and the mechanism of excess sludge reduction in an oxic-settling-anaerobic activated sludge process. *Journal of Environmental Engineering—ASCE* **134**, 469–477.

Barker D. J., Stuckey D. C. (1999) A review of soluble microbial products (SMP) in wastewater treatment systems. *Water Research* **33**, 3063–3082.

Bolzonella D., Pavan P., Battistoni P., Cecchi F. (2005) Mesophilic anaerobic digestion of waste activated sludge: influence of the solid retention time in the wastewater treatment process. *Process Biochemistry* **40**, 1453–1460.

Capdeville B., Nguyen K. M. (1990) Kinetics and modeling of aerobic and anaerobic film growth. *Water Science and Technology* **22**, 149–170.

Chen G. H., Yip W. K., Mo H. K., Liu Y. (2001) Effect of sludge fasting/feasting on sludge growth in activated sludge cultures. *Water Research* **35**, 1029–1037.

Chen G. H., An K. J., Saby S., Brois E., Djafer M. (2003) Possible cause of excess sludge reduction in an oxic-settling-anaerobic activated sludge process (OSA process). *Water Research* **37**, 3855–3866.

Chen Y. G., Jiang S., Yuan H. Y., Zhou Q., Gu G. W. (2007) Hydrolysis and acidification of waste activated sludge at different pHs. *Water Research* **41**, 683–689.

Christoulas D. G., Andreadakis A. D., Kouzeli-Katsiri A., Aftias E., Mamais D. (2000) Alternative schemes for the management of the sludge produced at Psyttalis WWTP. *Water Science and Technology* **42**, 29–36.

Chudoba P., Chevalier J. J., Chang J., Capdeville B. (1991a) Effect of anaerobic stabilization of activated sludge on its production under batch conditions at various S_0/X_0 ratios. *Water Science and Technology* **23**, 917–926.

Chudoba P., Chang J., Capdeville B. (1991b) Synchronized division of activated sludge microorganisms. *Water Research* **25**, 817–922.

Chudoba P., Chudoba J., Capdeville B. (1992a) The aspect of energetic uncoupling of microbial growth in the activated sludge process: OSA system. *Water Science and Technology* **26**, 2477–2480.

Chudoba P., Morel A., Capdeville B. (1992b) The case of both energetic uncoupling and metabolic selection of microorganisms in the OSA activated sludge system. *Environmental Technology* **13**, 761–770.

Çokgör E. U., Oktay S., Tas D. O., Zengin G. E., Orhon D. (2009) Influence of pH and temperature on soluble substrate generation with primary sludge fermentation. *Bioresource Technology* **100**, 380–386.

Crocetti G. R., Hugenholtz P., Bond P. L., Schuler A., Keller J., Jenkins D., Blackall L. L. (2000) Identification of polyphosphate accumulating organisms and design of 16S rRNA-directed probes for their detection and quantitation. *Applied and Environmental Microbiology* **66**, 175–1182.

Feng L. Y., Wang H., Chen Y. G., Wang Q. (2009) Effect of solids retention time and temperature on waste activated sludge hydrolysis and short-chain fatty acids accumulation under alkaline conditions in continuous-flow reactors. *Bioresource Technology* **100**, 44–49.

Gao Y. Q., Peng Y. Z., Zhang J. Y., Wang S. Y., Guo J. H., Ye L. (2011) Biological sludge reduction and enhanced nutrient removal in a pilot-scale system with 2-step sludge alkaline fermentation and A^2O process. *Bioresource Technology* **102**, 4091–4097.

Ghiglizza R., Lodi A., Converti A., Nicolella C., Rovatti M. (1996) Influence of the ratio of the initial substrate concentration to biomass concentration on the performance of a sequencing batch reactor. *Bioprocess Engineering* **14**, 131–137.

Goel R., Tokutomi T., Yasui H. (2003) Anaerobic digestion of excess activated sludge with ozone pretreatment. *Water Science and Technology* **47**, 207–214.

Higging M. J., Novak J. T. (1997) The effect of cations on the settling and dewatering of activated sludge. *Water Environment Research* **69**, 215–224.

Huang X., Liang P., Qian Y. (2007) Excess sludge reduction induced by *Tubifex tubifex* in a recycled sludge reactor. *Journal of Biotechnology* **127**, 443–451.

Jiang S., Chen Y. G., Zhou Q. (2007) Influence of alkyl sulfates on waste activated sludge fermentation at ambient temperature. *Journal of Hazardous Materials* **148**, 110–115.

Liu Y., Tay J. H. (2001) Strategy for minimization of excess sludge production from the activated sludge process. *Biotechnology Advances* **19**, 97–107.

Liu Y., Zhang T., Fang H. H. P. (2005) Microbial community analysis and performance of a phosphate-removing activated sludge. *Bioresource Technology* **96**, 1205–1214.

Lopez C., Pons M. N., Morgenroth E. (2006) Endogenous processes during long-term starvation in activated sludge performing enhanced biological phosphorus removal. *Water Research* **40**, 1519–1530.

Low E. W., Chase H. A. (1999) The effect of maintenance energy requirements on biomass production during wastewater treatment. *Water Research* **33**, 847–853.

Low E. W., Chase H. A., Milner M. G., Curtis T. P. (2000) Uncoupling of metabolism to reduce biomass production in the activated sludge process. *Water Research* **34**, 3204–3212.

Martins M. P. A., Pagilla K., Heijnen J. J., van Loosdrecht M. C. M. (2004) Filamentous bulking sludge: a critical review. *Water Research* **38**, 793–817.

Metcalf & Eddy, Inc. (2003) *Waterwater Engineering: Treatment and Reuse*, (4th eds) McGraw-Hill, New York.

Moser-Engeler R., Udert K. M., Wild D., Siegrist H. (1998) Products from primary sludge fermentation and their suitability for nutrient removal. *Water Science and Technology* **38**, 265–273.

Murray R. G. E., Doetsch R. N., Robinow C. F. (1994) Determinative and cytological light microscopy: methods for general and molecular bacteriology. American Society for Microbiology, Washington, DC.

Rittmann B. E., McCarty P. L. (2001) *Environmental Biotechnology: Principles and Application*. New York, McGraw-Hill.

Romano R. T., Zhang R. H., Teter S., McGarvey J. A. (2009) The effect of enzyme addition on anaerobic digestion of *JoseTall* wheat grass. *Bioresource Technology* **100**, 4564–4571.

Saby S., Sibille I., Mathieu L., Paquin J. L., Block J. C. (1997) Influence of water chlorination on the counting of bacteria with DAPI (4′, 6-diamidino-2-phenylindole) *Applied and Environmental Microbiology* **63**, 1564–1569.

Saby S., Djafer M., Chen G. H. (2003) Effect of low ORP in anoxic sludge zone on excess sludge production in oxic-settling-anoxic activated sludge process. *Water Research* **37**, 11–20.

Sanz J. L., Köchling T. (2007) Molecular biology techniques used in wastewater treatment: an overview. *Process Biochemistry* **42**, 119–133.

Serafim L. S., Lemos P. C., Levantesi C., Tandoi V., Santos H., Reis M. A. M. (2002) Methods for detection and visualization of intracellular polymers stored by polyphosphate-accumulating microorganisms. *Journal of Microbiological Methods* **51**, 1–18.

Song B. Y., Chen X. F. (2009) Effect of *Aeolosoma hemprichi* on excess activated sludge reduction. *Journal of Hazardous Materials* **162**, 300–304.

van Loosdrecht M. C. M., Henze M. (1999) Maintenance, endogenous, respiration, lysis, decay and predation. *Water Science and Technology* **39**, 107–117.

Wang J. F., Jin W. B., Zhao Q. L., Liu Z. G., Lin J. K. (2007) Performance of treating wastewater and anti-impact in oxic-settling-anaerobic (OSA) process for minimization of excess sludge. *Chinese Journal of Environmental Science* **28**, 2488–2493.

Wang J. F., Zhao Q. L., Liu Z. G., Edward L. K. H. (2008a) Influence factors of excess sludge reduction of the oxic-settling-anaerobic technique. *Chinese Journal of Environmental Science* **28**, 427–432.

Wang J. F., Zhao Q. L., Jin W. B., You S. J., Zhang J. N. (2008b) Performance of biological phosphorus removal and characteristics of microbial community in the oxic-settling-anaerobic process by fluorescent in situ hybridization (FISH). *Journal of Zhejiang University Science A* **7**, 1004–1010.

Wawrzynczyk J., Recktenwald M., Norrlow O., Dey E. S. (2008) The function of cation-binding agents in the enzymatic treatment of municipal sludge. *Water Research* **42**, 1555–1562.

Wei Y. S., Van Houtenb R. T., Borgerb A. R., Eikelboomb D. H., Fan Y. B. (2003) Minimization of excess sludge production for biological wastewater treatment. *Water Research* **37**, 4453–4467.

Westgarth W. C., Sulzer F. T., Okun D. A. (1964) Anaerobiosis in the activated sludge process. In: *Proceedings of the Second IAWPRC Conference*, Tokyo, pp. 43–55.

Wu H. Y., Yang D. H., Zhou Q., Song Z. B. (2009) The effect of pH on anaerobic fermentation of primary sludge at room temperature. *Journal of Hazardous Materials* **172**, 196–201.

Xing X. H., Yu A. F., Feng Q., Chu L., Yan S. T., Zhou Y. N. (2008) Principle and practice of a novel biological wastewater treatment technology capable of on-site reduction of excess sludge. *Journal of Biotechnology* **136S**, 647–677.

Yang Q., Luo K., Li X. M., Wang D. B., Zheng W., Zeng G. M., Liu J. J. (2010) Enhance efficiency of biological excess sludge hydrolysis under anaerobic digestion by additional enzymes. *Bioresource Technology* **101**, 2924–2930.

Yasui H., Komatsu K., Goel R., Li Y. Y., Noike T. (2005) Full-scale application of anaerobic digestion process with partial ozonation of digested sludge. *Water Science and Technology* **52**, 245–252.

Ye F. X., Li Y. (2010) Oxic-settling-anoxic (OSA) process combined with 3,3′,4′, 5- tetra-chlorosalicylanilide (TCS) to reduce excess sludge production in the activated sludge system. *Biochemical Engineering Journal* **49**, 229–234.

Yuan Q., Sparling R., Oleszkiewicz J. A. (2009) Waste activated sludge fermentation: effect of solids retention time and biomass concentration. *Water Research* **43**, 5180–5186.

Zehnder A. J. B., Wuhrmann K. (1976) Titatium(III) citrate as a non-toxic oxidation reduction buffering system for the culture of anaerobes. *Science* **194**, 1165–1166.

Zheng X., Chen Y. G., Liu C. C. (2010) Waste activated sludge alkaline fermentation liquid as carbon source for biological nutrients removal in anaerobic followed by alternating aerobic–anoxic sequencing batch reactors. *Chinese Journal of Chemical Engineering* **18**, 478–485.

5

ENERGY UNCOUPLING FOR SLUDGE MINIMIZATION: PROS AND CONS

BO JIANG AND YU LIU

Division of Environmental and Water Resources Engineering, School of Civil and Environmental Engineering, Nanyang Technological University, Singapore

ETIENNE PAUL

Université de Toulouse and Ingénierie des Systèmes Biologiques et des Procédés, Toulouse, France

5.1 INTRODUCTION

Metabolic networks represent the set of biochemical pathways that involve interrelated catabolic and anabolic reactions. Adenosine triphosphate (ATP), a primary bioenergy currency of life, is synthesized through catabolic activity by coupling two reactions: electron transport and oxidative phosphorylation (Terada 1990). According to the chemiosmotic hypothesis (Mitchell 1961), substrates are oxidized via respiration, generating the electrochemical gradient of hydrogen ions [also called the proton motive force (PMF)] across the inner energy-transducing membrane, which in turn becomes the energy source for driving ATP synthesis from adenosine diphosphate (ADP) and orthophosphate (P_i) by ATP synthase. The connected processes of electron transport and oxidative phosphorylation are membrane-associated. In eukaryotes, these two steps are carried out in inner mitochondrial membrane, while in prokaryotic cells, they occur in the cytoplasmic membrane, and photophosphorylation takes place in the chloroplast envelope (Hames and Hooper 2005).

It is known that the PMF produced is not only for ATP synthesis but is also utilized in a variety of physiological activities, including active transport for

Biological Sludge Minimization and Biomaterials/Bioenergy Recovery Technologies, First Edition.
Edited by Etienne Paul and Yu Liu.
© 2012 John Wiley & Sons, Inc. Published 2012 by John Wiley & Sons, Inc.

uphill movement of solutes and nutrients against gradients across the membrane, mechanical work for flagellar rotation of bacteria, and biochemical work for the synthesis of many thousands of macromolecules, such as proteins and polysaccharides (Palmen et al. 1994; McCall et al. 2001; Moat et al. 2002). If more PMF is spent on performing these works, less energy will be available for ATP synthesis. Under normal conditions, electron transport and oxidative phosphorylation are tightly coupled. Thus, inhibition of either of these processes results in reduced ATP output (Roach and Benyon 2003). In this sense, addition of various types of inhibitors of electron transport or oxidative phosphorylation would effectively reduce ATP yield.

Uncouplers, a large family of hydrophobic and weak acidic reagents, can suppress ATP generation due to their ability to dissipate the proton gradient created through respiration chain across the inner cellular membrane. As a consequence, ATP synthesis comes to a halt while the activities of electron transport and ATP synthase are not affected (Hanstein 1976; Terada 1990). Theoretically, microbial growth yield depends strongly on the availability of bioenergy in terms of ATP. For example, synthesis of 1 mg of dry mass of cells would require about 30 μmol of ATP (Stouthamer 1973). Energy uncoupling for reducing the production of excess sludge has been studied intensively, and some typical chemical uncouplers have been employed in laboratory and pilot-scale systems. In this chapter, we introduce electron transport and oxidative phosphorylation processes and strategies for control of ATP synthesis, with special focus on the mechanisms of energy uncoupling and its applications in reducing excess sludge production; the potential advantages and disadvantages are also discussed. This chapter can offer in-depth insights into an energy uncoupling–assisted activated sludge process for minimization of excess sludge production.

5.2 OVERVIEW OF ADENOSINE TRIPHOSPHATE SYNTHESIS

5.2.1 Electron Transport System

The electron transport system (ETS) of eukaryotes consists of four protein complexes: NADH dehydrogenase (complex I), succinate dehydrogenase (complex II), coenzyme Q–cytochrome c reductase (complex III), cytochrome c oxidase (complex IV), and four mobile electron carriers: NADH, succinate, coenzyme Q (also called ubiquinone), and cytochrome c. These four protein complexes are tightly bound to the mitochondrial membrane and can transfer electrons from one electron carrier to another. The electron carriers are not associated with any of these complexes or membrane, but can shuttle electrons between complexes (Zannoni 2004).

The ETS is a coordinated series of coupled redox reactions in sequence. Complex I accepts electrons from the primary electron donor NADH and passes to coenzyme Q, resulting in the oxidation of NADH to NAD^+, reduction of coenzyme Q to UQH_2, and a net movement of four protons into the intermembrane space. Complex II, an alternative entry site of ETS, oxidizes succinate to fumarate and passes electrons to FAD, which is subsequently reduced to $FADH_2$. $FADH_2$

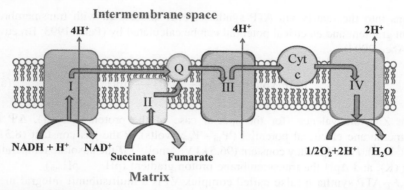

FIGURE 5.1 ETS in the mitochondria. Electrons are transferred from NADH or FADH$_2$ to O$_2$ by a series of complexes and electron carriers. At the same time, a 10-proton gradient is created across the inner mitochondrial membrane. [Adapted from Garrett and Grisham (2008).]

further transfers electrons to coenzyme Q and reduces coenzyme Q to UQH$_2$ in a similar manner to complex I. Afterward, complex III accepts electrons from UQH$_2$, the common product of both complex I and II, and transports to the soluble protein cytochrome c. As a result, cytochrome c is reduced, which in turn is the electron donor to complex IV. Meanwhile, four protons are transported into the intermembrane space. Complex IV is the final electron acceptor in aerobic respiration, which receives electrons from cytochrome c, transfers them to O$_2$, and ultimately converts H$^+$ and O$_2$ to H$_2$O. Complex IV brings about a net flux of two protons into the intermembrane space. Compared to eukaryotes, prokaryotes have an aerobic respiratory chain similar to the mitochondrial counterpart but with more complexity. Nevertheless, they can also create an electrochemical gradient across the transmembrane via proton pump(s). The entire electron transport process in mitochondria is shown in Fig. 5.1.

5.2.2 Mechanisms of Oxidative Phosphorylation

Oxidative phosphorylation is a biochemical process in which ATP is synthesized using energy released through ETS. The chemiosmotic hypothesis states that the potential energy of electron transport is conserved by pumping protons from the matrix into the intermembrane space (or periplasmic space of prokaryotes), creating an electrochemical gradient across the membrane, serving as the energy reservoir for ATP synthesis. The chemiosmotic hypothesis developed initially by Mitchell (1961) has been accepted as an important contribution towards understanding biological energy transfer.

The electrochemical gradient across the cellular membrane [also referred to as the proton motive force (PMF)] created by electron transport comprises a proton gradient ΔpH due to proton concentration difference and an electrical potential $\Delta\psi$ resulting from charge separation. The PMF could be harnessed to phosphorylate ATP from adenosine diphosphate (ADP) and orthophosphate (P$_i$) by the backflow of protons into the matrix via ATP synthase. PMF associated with transmembrane proton gradient and electrical potential can be calculated by (Petty 1993; Breeuwer and Abee 2004)

$$PMF(volts) = Z \Delta\psi - 2.303 \frac{RT}{F} \Delta pH \qquad (5.1)$$

where Z is the valence (for the special case of the proton, $Z = +1$), $\Delta\Psi$ the transmembrane electrical potential ($\Psi_{in} - \Psi_{out}$, volts), R the gas constant (8.314 J mol^{-1} K^{-1}), F the Faraday constant (96.5 kJ V^{-1} mol^{-1}), T the absolute temperature scale (K), and ΔpH the transmembrane proton gradient (pH$_{in}$ − pH$_{out}$).

$F_o F_1$-ATP synthase (also called complex V) is a multisubunit integral membrane protein consisting of two linked distinct functional domains: the catalytic core F_1 (including five subunits: alpha, beta, gamma, delta, epsilon) projecting inward from the inner membrane and a connecting hydrophobic proton channel protein F_o (including up to three different subunits) embedded in the membrane (Terada 1990). F_1 and F_o complexes function akin to two rotary motors rotating in opposite directions. The F_o complex resides in the membrane and the proton gradient across the membrane causes F_o to rotate—just like water turning a mill wheel. Subsequently, the coupled F_1 is triggered to rotate in the opposite direction, inducing the synthesis of ATP. These two complexes can also act in reverse to hydrolyze ATP to pump protons against the electrochemical gradient, resulting in an increase of PMF across the membrane (Yoshida et al. 2001; Moat et al. 2002).

ATP, the major bioenergy currency of a living cell, is expended in a wide variety of physiological functions. An ATP molecule consists of a purine base (adenine), a pentose sugar (ribose), and three phosphate groups (Fig. 5.2). Two outermost highenergy phosphate anhydride bonds (β and γ) are responsible for the high-energy content of this molecule. Once these bonds are broken down, the energy will be liberated. The standard free energy released through hydrolysis of the phosphate anhydride bond γ from ATP is 30.5 kJ mol^{-1} (i.e., ATP $\leftrightarrow$ ADP + P$_i$; $\Delta G^0 = -30.5$ kJ).

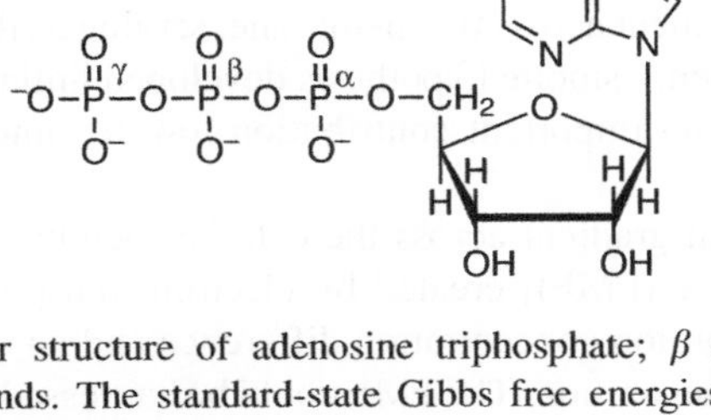

FIGURE 5.2 Molecular structure of adenosine triphosphate; β and γ are high-energy phosphate anhydride bonds. The standard-state Gibbs free energies of the β and γ bonds are −32.2 and −30.5 kJ, respectively.

5.3 CONTROL OF ATP SYNTHESIS

5.3.1 Diversion of PMF from ATP Synthesis to Other Physiological Activities

The PMF generated through ETS is not only for ATP synthesis, but also for other useful work, such as active transport, mechanical work, and biochemical work. More PMF is consumed in this work, and less ATP will be produced. Tempest and Neijssel (1992) found that the anabolism rate of bacterial species was lowered dramatically under carbon substrate excess and nutrient limitation conditions. One possible reason is the overproduction of metabolites. Tavares et al. (1999) studied the physiological responses of xylose-grown *Debaryomyces hansenii* under different nutrient stresses (C in terms of xylose, NH_4^+, K^+, PO_4^{3-}, and O_2 limitation) and discovered that the K^+-limiting condition was the most severe nutritional stress, provoking a drastic decrease in metabolic rates, leading to the lowest biomass yield of 0.22 g g^{-1}. At the same time, the highest xylose and O_2 specific consumption rates were observed. Microorganisms might adopt phenotype adjustment as one of their strategies to adapt to unfavorable environments. Under nutrient limitation conditions, they may alter the cellular structure and chemical composition (e.g., the cell envelope of bacteria) to make sure that as much as cell material as possible could be synthesized at a certain concentration of the limiting nutrient (Harder and Dijkhuizen 1983). They may also acquire the specific ability to synthesize more assimilation systems or change the existing enzyme systems into "high-affinity" uptake systems to increase the transport rate of a limiting nutrient (Teixeira De Mattos and Neijssel 1997). It can be concluded that cells might channel part of their energy to meet the requirements for limiting nutrient uptake rather than for complete biomass synthesis. It has also been reported that the bacterial biomass yield was greatly decreased in the presence of heavy metals (e.g., copper, zinc, cadmium) (Cabrero et al. 1998; Liu 2000a,b; Henriques et al. 2007), indicating that bacteria might consume extra energy under toxin stress conditions other than growth, such as stimulated excretion of extracellular polymeric substances. Other extreme conditions, such as high temperature and high or low pH, have also been proved to promote species shift and biomass production reduction (Greenman et al. 1983; Zakharov and Kuzmina 1992; Ogbonda et al. 2007).

5.3.2 Inhibition of Oxidative Phosphorylation

There are several well-known chemicals that can restrain ATP synthesis by inhibiting electron transport or oxidative phosphorylation at specific sites. ETS inhibitors perform by binding on the electron transport chain, blocking respiration along electron entry routes. Each ETS inhibitor binds specifically to a carrier or a complex. For example, rotenone (used as an organic pesticide and insecticide) and 5-ethyl-5-isoamylbarbituric acid (amytal, used as a sedative) inhibit complex I (Gutman et al. 1970; Li et al. 2003); malonate competitively inhibits complex II (Dervartanian and Veeger 1964); antimycin A blocks the electron transfer in complex III between

TABLE 5.1   Typical Inhibitors of Electron Transport and Oxidative Phosphorylation

Inhibitors	Functions and Effects
Rotenone, amytal, piericidin A	ETS inhibitor. Inhibits NADH dehydrogenase (complex I).
Malonate, oxaloacetate	ETS inhibitor. Inhibits succinate dehydrogenase (complex II).
Antimycin A, BAL (British anti-lewisite)	ETS inhibitor. Blocks coenzyme Q–cytochrome c reductase (complex III).
Cyanide, azide, carbon monoxide (CO), hydrogen sulfide (H_2S)	ETS inhibitor. Inhibits cytochrome c oxidase (complex IV) by preventing electron transfer to oxygen.
Oligomycin, DCCD	F_oF_1-ATP synthase inhibitor. Blocks the flow of protons through F_o complex.
Atractyloside	Transport inhibitor. Blocks the transport of ATP and ADP across the inner cellular membrane.
Bongkrekic acid	Transport inhibitor. Inhibits the ATP–ADP translocase.
Valinomycin	Ionophore. Catalyzes the electrical movement of K^+ to dissipate the electrochemical potential.
Nigericin	Ionophore. Catalyzes the exchange of proton for potassium across the inner cellular membrane.

cytochrome b and c_1 segments (Baum et al. 1967); cyanide, azide, and carbon monoxide inhibit the action of complex IV (Tsubaki 1993). Inhibition of any electron carrier/complex by an ETS inhibitor will lead to the blockage of electron transport from NADH or $FADH_2$ to O_2. F_oF_1-ATP synthase inhibitors belong to another class of chemicals that hinder phosphorylation by binding to ATP synthase to block the proton channel. Oligomycin (an antibiotic) and dicyclohecylcarbdiimide (DCCD) are two common ATP synthase inhibitors that can block the movement of protons through F_o (Shchepina et al. 2002). There are many other drugs and toxins that are able to interfere with electron transport and oxidative phosphorylation processes, including transport inhibitors (e.g., atractyloside and bongkrekic acid) (Henderson and Lardy 1970) and ionophores (e.g., valinomycin and nigericin) (Cammann 1985). Some typical inhibitors and their functions and effects are summarized in Table 5.1.

5.3.3   Uncoupling of Electron Transport and Oxidative Phosphorylation

Uncouplers, an important category of chemical reagents, have the power to abolish the tight linkage between electron transport and oxidative phosphorylation. In general, chemical uncouplers are organic weak acids that carry protons and can freely penetrate cellular membrane. As a result, the proton gradient created by electron transport is disrupted and ATP synthesis is strongly suppressed (Fig. 5.3); that is, the energy generated through electron transport is dissipated as heat instead of phosphorylation of ADP and P_i to ATP. It should be noted that uncouplers do not bind to any of the proteins of the ETS or the F_1F_o-ATP synthase, but can shuttle back and forth across the inner cellular membrane (Lehninger and Wadkins 1962). In the

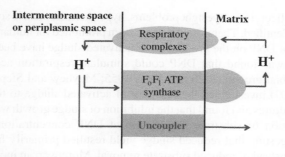

FIGURE 5.3 Schematic presentation of dissipation of the proton gradient across the membrane by a chemical uncoupler. [Adapted from Terada (1990).]

presence of a chemical uncoupler, the respiration rate is stimulated markedly, as the cell attempts to pump more protons out of the matrix to restore a proton gradient for driving ATP generation.

5.4 ENERGY UNCOUPLING FOR SLUDGE REDUCTION

5.4.1 Chemical Uncouplers Used for Sludge Reduction

Nitrophenol-like Compounds Nitrophenols, dinitrophenols, and trinitrophenols are all phenolic compounds with nitro group(s) on the benzene ring, including *o*-nitrophenol (2-nitrophenol, 2-NP, or ONP), *m*-nitrophenol (3-nitrophenol, 3-NP, or MNP), *p*-nitrophenol (4-nitrophenol, 4-NP, or PNP), 2,4-dinitrophenol (DNP), and 2,4,6-trinitrophenol (TNP), as shown in Fig. 5.4.

DNP has been used widely in the manufacture of dyes, pesticides/insecticides, explosives, and wood preservatives (Karim and Gupta 2006). In the 1930s, DNP was touted extensively as an effective diet tablet. As a protonophore, DNP can destroy the proton gradient across the cellular membrane by transporting protons from the high concentration side to the low concentration side, leading to inhibited ATP synthesis. As a consequence, the Krebs substrates, even the stored fats, are oxidized rapidly to attenuate the energy deficit caused by DNP. Although DNP is a potent drug for weight

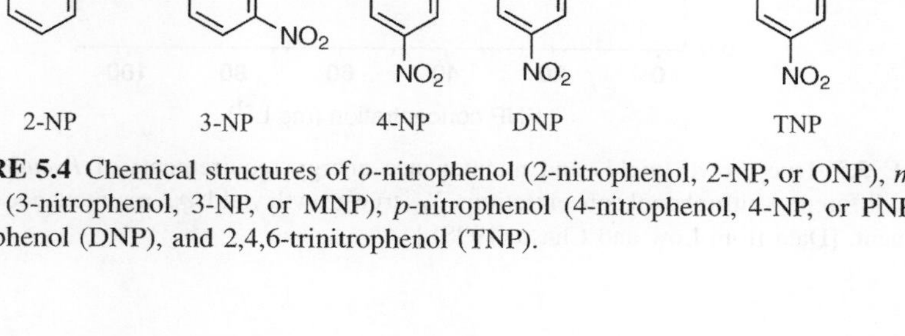

OH	OH	OH	OH	OH
2-NP	3-NP	4-NP	DNP	TNP

FIGURE 5.4 Chemical structures of *o*-nitrophenol (2-nitrophenol, 2-NP, or ONP), *m*-nitrophenol (3-nitrophenol, 3-NP, or MNP), *p*-nitrophenol (4-nitrophenol, 4-NP, or PNP), 2,4-dinitrophenol (DNP), and 2,4,6-trinitrophenol (TNP).

reduction, side effects (e.g., eyesight problems, hyperthermia, muscle soreness, insomnia) have been identified. Therefore, DNP has been prohibited for human consumption.

The effects of DNP on the production of activated sludge have been investigated for decades. It was found that DNP could stimulate respiration accompanied by inhibited microbial growth (Rich and Yates 1955; Mayhew and Stephenson 1998). Chen et al. (2007) investigated the response of activated sludge to the presence of DNP in batch cultures and found that the inhibition of sludge growth was more severe than the inhibition of substrate degradation at DNP concentrations higher than $10\,mg\,L^{-1}$, suggesting that reduced sludge yield resulted primarily from decreased sludge growth instead of reduced substrate removal. Moreover, an increased specific oxygen uptake rate was observed at a DNP concentration of 1 to $20\,mg\,L^{-1}$, indicating that the electron transport process was stimulated.

p-Nitrophenol (PNP) has been used primarily for the synthesis of medicines (e.g., paracetamol), dyes, and pesticides. Low and Chase (1998) investigated biomass production in the presence of PNP in a monoculture of *Pseudomonas putida*. It was found that the true growth yield (Y_G) of biomass was reduced with an increase in PNP concentration. For example, 62% of sludge reduction was achieved at the PNP dosage of $100\,mg\,L^{-1}$, whereas the specific substrate uptake rate was also increased, implying an enhanced respiration caused by PNP. More important, cells would tend to satisfy their maintenance energy requirements prior to utilizing energy for anabolism at the reduced availability of energy (Fig. 5.5).

Chlorophenol-like Compounds   Chlorophenols, dichlorophenols, trichlorophenols, tetrachlorophenols, and pentachlorophenol all belong to the family of phenolic

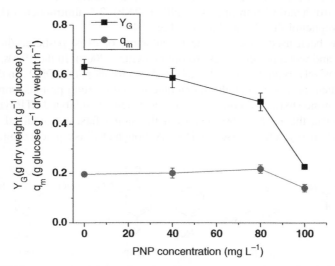

FIGURE 5.5 True growth yields and maintenance energy requirements of *Pseudomonas putida* at different *p*-nitrophenol concentrations. Y_G, true growth yield; q_m, maintenance energy requirement. [Data from Low and Chase (1998).]

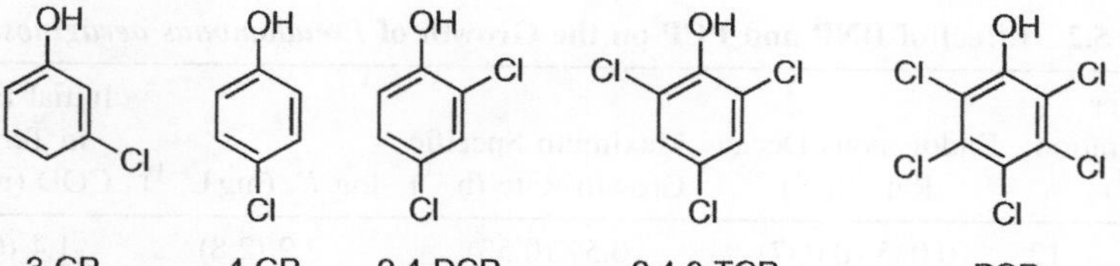

3-CP　　　4-CP　　　2,4-DCP　　　　2,4,6-TCP　　　　　　PCP

FIGURE 5.6 Chemical structures of m-chlorophenol (3-chlorophenol, 3-CP, or MCP), p-chlorophenol (4-chlorophenol, 4-CP, or PCP), 2,4-dichlorophenol (2,4-DCP), 2,4,6-trichlorophenol (2,4,6-TCP), and pentachlorophenol (PCP).

compounds with different numbers and positions of covalently bonded chlorine atoms on the benzene ring. Many compounds in this group have been used as intermediates for the manufacture of insecticides, herbicides, preservatives, antiseptics, disinfectants, or the precursors for higher chlorophenols. Chlorophenols are also considered as protonophoric uncouplers, whereas the uncoupling activities are enhanced by increasing chlorine substitutions (Tissut et al. 1987; Argese et al. 1999). The compounds that have been investigated for sludge minimization include m-chlorophenol (3-chlorophenol, 3-CP, or MCP), p-chlorophenol (4-chlorophenol, 4-CP, or PCP), 2,4-dichlorophenol (2,4-DCP), 2,4,6-trichlorophenol, (2,4,6-TCP), and pentachlorophenol (PCP) (Fig. 5.6).

Chen et al. (2000) studied the response of activated sludge to the presence of 2,4-dichlorophenol (2,4-DCP) in a batch culture, and observed that both the substrate degradation and sludge growth were slightly affected at the 2,4-DCP concentrations of 1 to 20 mg L^{-1}. 2,4-DCP at the concentration higher than 5 mg L^{-1} would affect the physicochemical properties and flocculation ability of the activated sludge. The sludge hydrophobicity tended to decrease at the 2,4-DCP concentration higher than 2 mg L^{-1}, probably due to EPS production promoted by 2,4-DCP. Cultures supplemented with 2,4-DCP exhibited higher specific oxygen uptake rates than those of control free of 2,4-DCP, indictaing a higher level of energy dissipation for metabolic regulation, and the extra oxygen consumed may be used for non-growth-associated activities.

Lin et al. (2010) looked into the effects of 2,4-DCP on the characteristics of activated sludge and sludge reduction in membrane bioreactors (MBRs). In the presence of 2,4-DCP, the sludge growth rate was reduced significantly, accompanied by slightly reduced COD removal rate. In addition, a high specific oxygen utilization rate was observed at increased 2,4-DCP dosage due to the chemical uncoupling effect of 2,4-DCP, as discussed earlier. In a bioreactor fed continuously with 3 mg L^{-1} of 2,4-DCP for 45 days, the microbial community remained almost unchanged as compared to control free of 2,4-DCP, while sludge settleability in terms of SVI was slightly increased. These in turn suggest that a metabolic uncoupler would have a negligible impact on system performance and sludge settleablility.

The feasibility of 2,4,6-trichlorophenol (2,4,6-TCP) for sludge reduction had been examined in sequencing batch reactors (Zheng et al. 2007, 2008). Long-term

TABLE 5.2   Effect of DNP and PCP on the Growth of *Pseudomonas aeruginosa*[a]

Uncoupler Concentration (mg L^{-1})		Endogenous Decay Rate (h^{-1})	Maximum Specific Growth Rate (h^{-1})	log K_s (mg L^{-1})	Initial Biomass in Terms of COD (mg L^{-1})
PNP	12	0.035 (0.037)	0.57 (0.53)	2.9 (2.8)	1.4 (0.9)
	49	0.052 (0.045)	0.58 (0.55)	2.6 (2.5)	0.7 (0.7)
	78	0.049 (0.037)	0.59 (0.57)	2.9 (2.9)	2.5 (2.1)
	140	0.054 (0.039)	0.54 (0.50)	2.5 (2.4)	3.8 (3.4)
	300	0.071 (0.044)	0.50 (0.57)	2.2 (2.7)	1.0 (0.9)
	420	0.053 (0.036)	0.41 (0.47)	1.2 (2.3)	0.02 (1.0)
	700	0.135 (0.045)	0.48 (0.52)	1.8 (2.2)	0.2 (0.7)
PCP	15	0.036 (0.029)	0.45 (0.45)	3.2 (3.3)	0.8 (0.9)
	38	0.041 (0.032)	0.45 (0.49)	2.3 (2.5)	0.9 (1.0)
	85	0.045 (0.032)	0.30 (0.49)	1.3 (2.5)	0.02 (1.6)

Source: Data from Ray and Peters (2008).
[a] K_s is the half-saturation constant in the Monod equation. Data in parentheses are estimates from corresponding nonstressed controls.

experimental results demonstrated that sludge production was reduced by 47% at 2 mg L^{-1} of 2,4,6-TCP, while COD removal efficiency was only slightly affected due mainly to reduced biomass concentration. Microscopic observations further revealed that filamentous microorganisms appeared, and some protozoans were found to disappear in an activated sludge system fed with 2,4,6-TCP. DGGE analysis also showed a shift of microbial populations which was in accordance with microscopic examination. In fact, the disappearance of protozoans induced by 2,4,6-TCP may be responsible for the aggravation of sludge settleability.

Ray and Peters (2008) investigated the impact of DNP and PCP on microbiological activity of *Pseudomonas aeruginosa* in batch cultures. Biomass growth yields were reduced, while substrate utilization was not inhibited at the DNP concentrations of 49 to 140 mg L^{-1} and 15 and 38 mg L^{-1} for PCP. A portion of carbon and energy sources diverted from growth may be used to induce the synthesis of heat shock protein for stress management and protection. When the DNP concentration was increased further to 300 to 700 mg L^{-1} and PCP to 85 mg L^{-1}, the growth yields and substrate utilization rates were diminished significantly (i.e., inhibition to microbial activity would occur at such high DNP and PCP concentrations) (Table 5.2).

Yang et al. (2003) compared the effectiveness of *p*-chlorophenol, *m*-chlorophenol, *m*-nitrophenol, and *o*-nitrophenol in sludge reduction as well as their effects on the performance of the activated sludge process through a series of batch experiments. Compared to the control test, all four uncouplers studied were very effective in reducing sludge production, and the reduction rates were positively related to the applied concentration of each metabolic uncoupler. Among these four compounds, *m*-chlorophenol was the most effective by compromising sludge reduction and process performance (Fig. 5.7).

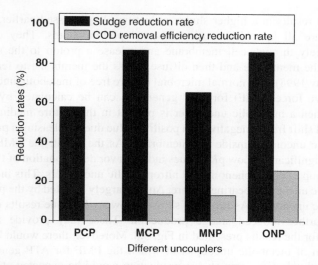

FIGURE 5.7 Effects of *p*-chlorophenol, *m*-chlorophenol, *m*-nitrophenol, and *o*-nitrophenol on the activated sludge process in terms of sludge reduction and COD removal efficiency at uncoupler concentration of 20 mg L^{-1}. [Data from Yang et al. (2003).]

Figure 5.8 further shows the relationship between the acidity constant (pK_a) of metabolic uncouplers and sludge reduction at an uncoupler concentration of 20 mg L^{-1}. In fact, PCP, MCP, MNP, and ONP can be grouped into two clusters, chlorophenols and nitrophenols. In a chemical sense, a stronger uncoupler has a smaller pK_a value. It appears from Fig. 5.8 that a chemical uncoupler with a lower pK_a led to a higher sludge reduction. These suggest that a metabolic uncoupler with a lower pK_a value is more effective in dissociating energy metabolism and

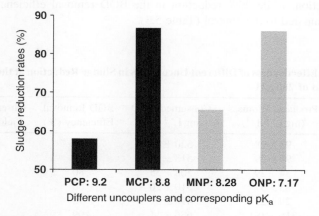

FIGURE 5.8 Effect of pK_a of metabolic uncoupler on sludge reduction at the uncoupler concentration of 20 mg L^{-1}. [Data from Yang et al. (2003).]

subsequently results in a higher sludge reduction. As discussed earlier, metabolic uncouplers are all lipophilic weak acids and protonophores. They can diffuse relatively freely through cell membrane and release a proton to the solution on one side of the membrane and then diffuse across the membrane to fetch another proton (Zubay 1998). In a normal microbial culture free of metabolic uncoupler, the proton motive force (PMF) for ATP generation can be calculated by Eq. (5.1). However, when a metabolic uncoupler is present in the culture medium, ΔpH in Eq. (5.1) will shift from a negative to a positive value due to releasing a proton ion of the metabolic uncoupler inside the membrane. As the result, the PMF would be diminished significantly. Low pK_a values indeed favor deprotonation of the phenolic hydroxyl group in chlorophenolic and nitrophenolic uncouplers. This indicates that in a metabolic uncoupler-bearing culture, ΔpH is largely affected by the pK_a value of the metabolic uncoupler. As Eq. (5.1) shows, a lower pK_a value results in a weaker PMF and further reduced sludge production. These may provide a plausible explanation for the results presented in Fig. 5.8. Moreover, there would be a critical concentration of metabolic uncoupler at which the PMF for ATP generation disappears completely (i.e., zero sludge production would be expected at the critical concentration of uncloupler). This is supported by experimental findings. For example, zero sludge production was observed at a 2,4-aminophenol concentration higher than 20 mg L^{-1} (data not shown), whereas no excess sludge was produced at a p-nitrophenol concentration of 120 mg L^{-1} (Low and Chase 1998).

Hiraishi and Kawagishi (2002) investigated the effects of different chemical uncouplers on microbial biomass production, metabolic activity, and community structure in an activated sludge system. It was found that five congeners of chlorophenols and nitrophenols (3-chlorophenol, 4-chlorophenol, 2-nitrophenol, 3-nitrophenol, and 4-nitrophenol) at 200 μM exerted severe effects on the biomass production but had no or minor effects on the respiratory chain in terms of BOD removal rates and enzyme activities in a short-term culture period. Among these five uncouplers, 4-nitrophenol (4-NP) was found to be the most effective, led to 90% of sludge reduction, while 20% reduction in the BOD removal efficiency was also observed compared to the control (Table 5.3).

TABLE 5.3 **Effectiveness of Different Uncouplers in Sludge Reduction at the Uncoupler Concentration of 200 μM**

Uncoupler	Produced Biomass (mg L^{-1} d^{-1})	Consumed BOD (mg L^{-1} d^{-1})	BOD Removal Efficiency (%)	Observed Growth Yield (mg mg^{-1})
3-CP	91 ± 28	520 ± 27	82	0.18
4-CP	91 ± 29	518 ± 25	81	0.18
2-NP	34 ± 29	508 ± 35	80	0.067
3-NP	83 ± 57	510 ± 20	80	0.16
4-NP	29 ± 22	498 ± 37	78	0.059
Control	316 ± 191	636 ± 11	99	0.49

Source: Data from Hiraishi and Kawagishi (2002).

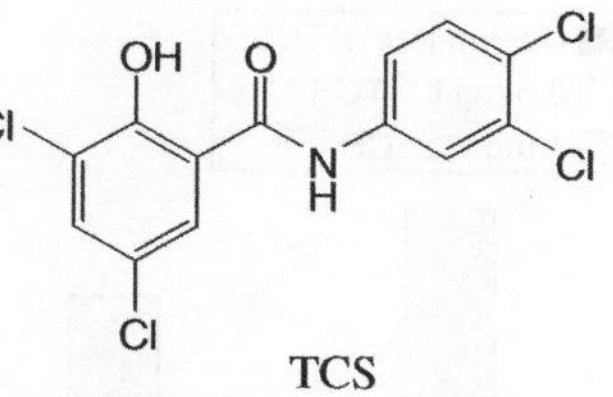

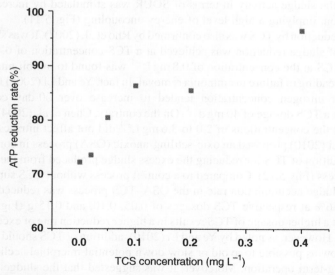

FIGURE 5.9 Chemical structure of 3,3',4',5-tetrachlorosalicylanilide.

3,3',4',5-Tetrachlorosalicylanilide 3,3',4',5-Tetrachlorosalicylanilide (TCS), a representative halogenated salicylanilide, has been known as an antibacterial agent added widely to shampoos, surgical and laundry soaps, rinses, polishes, and deodorants (Fig. 5.9). It has also been identified as a bacteriostat additive in cooling fluids, textiles, and many industrial products. So far, intensive research has been conducted to look into the ability of TCS for sludge reduction in the activated sludge process.

Chen et al. (2000) explored the feasibility of using TCS to reduce activated sludge production in both batch and continuous cultures. At a TCS concentration of 0.8 ppm, the growth yield of activated sludge was reduced by 40% and 69% in batch and continuous cultures, respectively; meanwhile, no significant reduction in the COD removal efficiency was observed. In addition, a batch experiment of pure culture *Escherichia coli* also showed that TCS would be able to reduce the cell density but did not change the cell viability at the concentration studied. The ATP content of *E. coli* was reduced significantly with the increase in TCS concentration, indicating that a high TCS concentration induced high energy dissipation (Fig. 5.10).

FIGURE 5.10 Effects of TCS on ATP reduction rates of *E. coli* after a 3-h culture. [Data from Chen et al. (2000).]

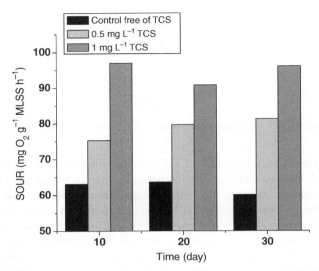

FIGURE 5.11 SOUR profile of activated sludge at different dosages of TCS. [Data from Chen et al. (2002).]

Chen et al. (2002) investigated the long-term effects of TCS on activated sludge production in a batch mode for 30 d. At the TCS dosages of 0.5 and 1 mg L^{-1} d^{-1}, the excess sludge production rates were reduced by 22% and 44%, respectively, compared to the control experiment free of TCS, whereas the substrate removal efficiency and sludge settleability were not affected significantly over 30-d operation. It was also found that the sludge activity in terms of SOUR was stimulated by increased TCS concentration, implying a high level of energy uncoupling (Fig. 5.11).

Sludge reduction by TCS was also confirmed by Rho et al. (2007). It was shown that over 60% of sludge reduction was achieved at a TCS concentration of 0.4 mg L^{-1}. However, TCS at the concentration of 0.8 mg L^{-1} was found to inhibit nitrification, eventually leading to failure in ammonia removal. In fact, Ye and Li (2005) found that the effluent nitrogen concentration tended to increase over 60-day continuous operation at a TCS dosage of 40 mg d^{-1}. On the contrary, Chen et al. (2004) reported that TCS at the concentrations of 2.0 to 3.6 mg L^{-1} did not affect nitrification.

Ye and Li (2010) proposed an oxic-settling-anoxic (OSA) process in combination with the addition of TCS for reducing the excess sludge produced from the activated sludge process (Fig. 5.12). Compared to a control process without TCS supplementation, the sludge accumulation rate in the OSA–TCS process was reduced by 21%, 37%, and 56% at respective TCS dosages of 0.05, 0.10, and 0.15 g (Fig. 5.13). It appears that a higher dosage of TCS results in a higher reduction rate of excess sludge production. However, as noted by Ye and Li (2010), addition of TCS should be kept at a level as low as possible to avoid or slow down potential microbial acclimation to TCS in long-term operation. Moreover, it was suggested that the sludge reduction rate was higher when TCS was added every 2 days rather than on a daily basis at the same total TCS dosage (Ye et al. 2008). At a TCS dosage of 0.05 to 0.15 g, a TOC

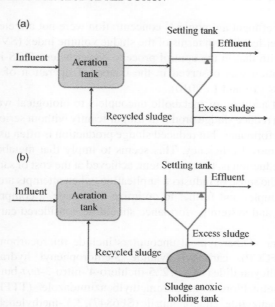

FIGURE 5.12 Conventional activated sludge process (a) and combined OSA–TCS process (b). [Adapted from Ye and Li (2010).]

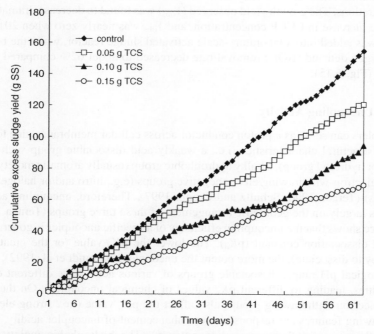

FIGURE 5.13 Sludge accumulation in a conventional activated sludge process (control) and a combined OSA–TCS process. [Data from Ye and Li (2010).]

removal rate and effluent ammonia-N concentration were not affected significantly, whereas sludge settleability in terms of the sludge volume index (SVI) was found to be comparable with that in the control process. Nevertheless, TCS-induced shift in microbial population was observed in the course of operation of the TCS–OSA combined process (Ye and Li 2010).

It appears that addition of metabolic uncouplers to biological wastewater treatment systems can reduce sludge production significantly without serious perturbation on the system performance, but reduced sludge production is often associated with a lowered COD removal efficiency. This seems to imply that metabolic uncoupler-induced sludge reduction is, to some extent, achieved at the cost of sacrificing system performance. In the sense of industrial application, when attempts are made to select a metabolic uncoupler and further to optimize its dosage, a compromise between sludge reduction and system performance should be considered carefully.

Other Uncouplers   Other typical uncouplers include fluorocarbonylcyanide phenylhydrazone (FCCP), carbonyl cyanide 3-chlorophenyl hydrazone (CCCP), 3,4′,5-trichlorosalicylanilide (DCC), 2′,5-dichloro-4′-nitro-3-*tert*-butylsalicylanilide (S-13), 4,5,6,7-tetrachloro-2′-trifluoromethylbenzimidazole (TTFB), 3,5-di-*tert*-butyl-4-hydroxybenzylidenemalononitrile (SF6847), 3,3′-methylenebis-(4-hydroxy-coumarin) (dicumarol), and flufenamic acid (Fig. 5.14).

Hiraishi and Kawagishi (2002) tested the effect of CCCP on biomass production and substrate removal efficiency in 24-h batch cultures fed with different CCCP concentrations. The growth yield observed (Y_{obs}) was found to decrease dramatically with the increase in CCCP concentration, and Y_{obs} was nearly zero when 20 μM of CCCP was added into a laboratory-scale activated sludge reactor, while the biological oxygen demand (BOD) removal rate decreased to about 62% compared to the control (Fig. 5.15).

5.4.2   Uncoupling Activity

Uncouplers can serve as a proton conductor across cellular membranes, due to their unique structural characteristics (i.e., a weakly acid dissociable group such as an amino or hydroxyl group), a bulky hydrophobic group (usually aromatic moiety), and strong electron-withdrawing/electronegative groups (e.g., nitro and/or halogen substituents) (Terada 1990; Schultz and Cronin 1997). Therefore, uncoupling activity depends largely on the geometric arrangement of these three groups (Terada 1990). Evidence shows that the uncoupling efficiency of a specific uncoupler is governed by its acid dissociation constant (pK_a). The lower the pK_a value (or the greater the tendency to dissociate), the more potent the uncoupler is (Brandt et al. 1992). In the physiological pH range, dissociable groups of various acids have different deprotonabilities, leading to different pK_a values of chemical uncouplers. On the other hand, electron-withdrawing groups also affect the pK_a value (i.e., strong electron-withdrawing features are responsible for enhancement of uncoupler acidity, which can further increase their uncoupling potency). The hydrophobic moiety of an uncoupler renders it membrane-soluble so that the uncoupler can shuttle back

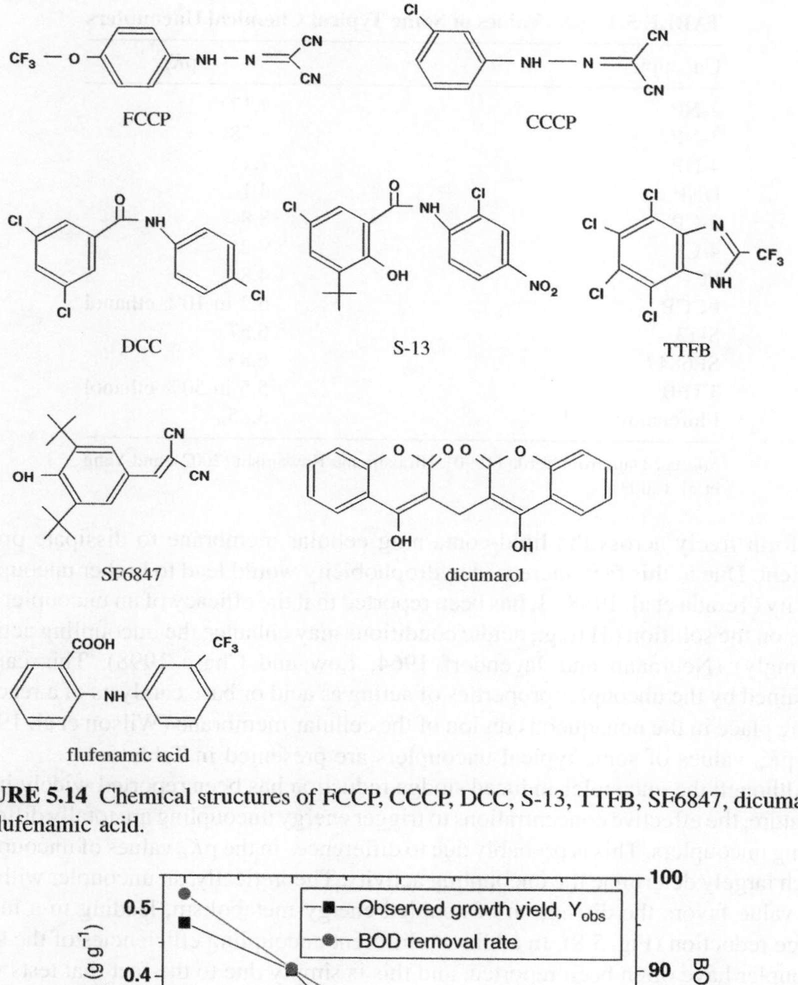

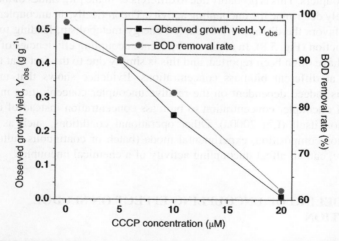

FIGURE 5.14 Chemical structures of FCCP, CCCP, DCC, S-13, TTFB, SF6847, dicumarol, and flufenamic acid.

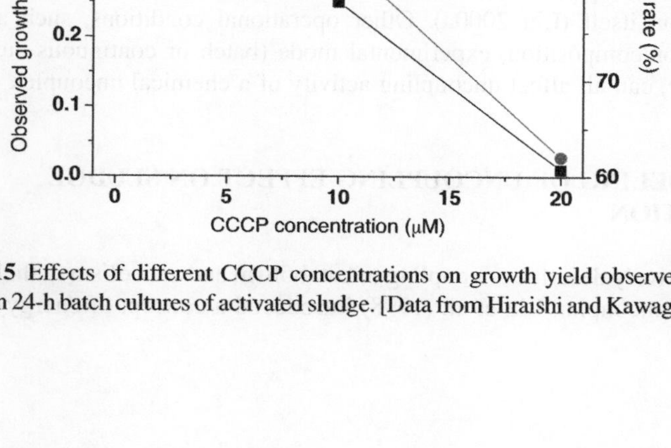

FIGURE 5.15 Effects of different CCCP concentrations on growth yield observed and BOD removal rate in 24-h batch cultures of activated sludge. [Data from Hiraishi and Kawagishi (2002).]

TABLE 5.4   pK_a Values of Some Typical Chemical Uncouplers

Uncoupler	pK_a
2-NP	7.17
3-NP	8.28
4-NP	7.15
DNP	4.1
3-CP	8.8
4-CP	9.2
PCP	4.8
FCCP	6.2 in 10% ethanol
S-13	6.57
SF6847	6.83
TTFB	5.5 in 50% ethanol
Flufenamic acid	3.85

Source: Data from Terda (1990), Hiraishi and Kawagishi (2002), and Yeng et al. (2003).

and forth freely across the lipid-containing cellular membrane to dissipate proton gradient. Due to this fact, increased hydrophobicity would lead to higher uncoupling activity (Terada et al. 1988). It has been reported that the efficacy of an uncoupler also relies on the solution pH (e.g., acidic conditions may enhance the uncoupling activity strikingly) (Neumann and Jagendorf 1964; Low and Chase 1998). This can be explained by the uncoupler properties of acting as acid or base catalysts of a reaction taking place in the nonaqueous region of the cellular membrane (Wilson et al. 1971). The pK_a values of some typical uncouplers are presented in Table 5.4.

Although the uncoupler-induced sludge reduction has been reported widely in the literature, the effective concentrations to trigger energy uncoupling are totally different among uncouplers. This is probably due to differences in the pK_a values of uncouplers, which largely determine the uncoupling activity. Theoretically, an uncoupler with low pK_a value favors the disruption of coupled energy metabolism, leading to a higher sludge reduction (Fig. 5.8). In addition, different uncoupling efficiencies of the same uncoupler have often been reported, and this is simply due to the fact that tests were conducted at different biomass concentrations. Evidence shows that uncoupling efficiency is indeed dependent on the relative uncoupler concentration in terms of the ratio of uncoupler concentration to biomass concentration instead of uncoupler concentration itself (Liu 2000a). Other operational conditions, such as substrate concentration/composition, experimental mode (batch or continuous cultures), and temperature, can all affect uncoupling activity of a chemical uncoupler.

5.5   MODELING OF UNCOUPLING EFFECT ON SLUDGE PRODUCTION

To quantitatively describe uncoupling of catabolism and anabolism in the presence of a chemical uncoupler, Liu et al. (1998) introduced a concept of energy uncoupling coefficient:

$$E_u = \frac{(Y_{obs})_{max} - Y_{obs}}{(Y_{obs})_{max}} \quad (5.2)$$

where E_u is the energy uncoupling coefficient; $(Y_{obs})_{max}$ the maximum observed growth yield under normal culture condition; and Y_{obs} the growth yield observed in the presence of uncoupler. Liu (2000a) further proposed an empirical model describing the effect of the relative uncoupler concentration on the growth yield observed for activated sludge:

$$\frac{1}{Y_{obs}} = \frac{1}{(Y_{obs})_{max}} + \frac{1}{(Y_w)_{min}} \frac{C_u/X_0}{C_u/X_0 + K_{u/X}} \quad (5.3)$$

where C_u is the initial uncoupler concentration in the culture medium, $(Y_w)_{min}$ the minimal energy spilling–related growth yield, X_0 the biomass concentration; and $K_{u/X}$ a C_u/X_0-related constant. Thereafter, several other energy uncoupling models have also been developed from the Monod model or Eq. (5.3).

In a steady-state biological process, sludge retention time (θ) and endogenous respiration rate (k_d) are involved in calculation of the growth yield observed:

$$\frac{1}{Y_{obs}} = \frac{1}{Y_t} + \frac{k_d}{Y_t}\theta \quad (5.4)$$

where Y_t is the true growth yield. In consideration of the maintenance-associated uncoupling, Eq. (5.4) is rearranged as (Chen et al. 2008)

$$\frac{1}{Y_{obs}} = \frac{1}{Y'_{max}} + \frac{k_d}{Y'_{max}}\theta \quad (5.5)$$

where Y'_{max} is the maximum sludge yield observed with a consideration of maintenance energy requirement. In the presence of chemical uncoupler, Eq. (5.5) can be modified further to

$$\frac{1}{Y_{obs}} = \frac{1}{(Y'_{max})_c} + \frac{k_d}{(Y'_{max})_c}\theta \quad (5.6)$$

where $(Y'_{max})_c$ represents the maximum sludge yield observed with consideration of both maintenance energy requirement and the effect of chemical uncoupling.

In substrate-sufficient cultures in the presence of a chemical uncoupler, Saini and Wood (2008) proposed the following empirical model, which is derived from Eq. (5.3):

$$\frac{1}{Y_{obs}} = \frac{1}{(Y_{obs})_{max}} + \frac{1}{(Y_w)_{min}} \frac{S_0/X_0}{S_0/X_0 + K_{S/X}} + \frac{1}{(Y_{wu})_{min}} \frac{C_u/X}{C_u/X + K_{u/X}} \quad (5.7)$$

where $(Y_{obs})_{max}$ is the maximum growth yield observed under substrate-limited and uncoupler-free conditions, $(Y_w)_{min}$ the minimal energy spilling–related growth yield, $(Y_{wu})_{min}$ the minimal energy spilling–related growth yield under uncoupler addition conditions, $K_{s/x}$ a S_0/X_0-related saturation constant, $K_{u/x}$ a C_u/X-related saturation constant, X_0 the initial biomass concentration; X the biomass concentration at the uncoupler addition point, and S_0 the initial substrate concentration.

5.6 SIDEEFFECTS OF CHEMICAL UNCOUPLERS

The dissipation of energy via uncoupling biochemical processes can promote sludge reduction, and the effectiveness of metabolic uncouplers in reducing excess sludge production has been proven. However, it should be realized that most metabolic uncouplers are xenobiotic and potentially harmful to the environment. Among the metabolic uncouplers currently used to reduce excess sludge production, TCS is gentler and environmentally sound. In fact, TCS has often been used as a component in the formulation of soaps, rinses, shampoos, and so on (Budavari 1989).

Other technical problems associated with use of metabolic uncouplers are unexpected high dissolved oxygen consumption and potential microbial acclimation to metabolic uncouplers during long-term operation. According to Zubay (1998), the dissolved oxygen consumption rate can increase by a factor 50 after addition of a metabolic uncoupler to a suspension of mitochondria. Similarity was also observed in the activated sludge processes (Mayhew and Stephenson 1998; Strand et al. 1999). For example, the specific oxygen utilization rates were increased from $8\,g\,O_2\,g^{-1}$ VSS d^{-1} without TCP addition to approximately $20\,g\,O_2\,g^{-1}$ VSS d^{-1} when TCP was supplemented. It has thus been proposed that the combined pure oxygen aeration and metabolic uncouplers process would be a solution for uncoupler-induced oxygen overconsumption (Liu and Tay 2001; Liu 2003).

Many uncouplers belong to aromatic compounds (i.e., these chemicals are potentially recalcitrant, carcinogenic, mutagenic, and toxic). The U.S. Environmental Protection Agency (EPA) has listed 2-NP, 4-NP, DNP, DCP, 2,4,6-TCP, and PCP as priority pollutants, and classified 2,4,6-TCP and PCP as probable human carcinogens (Richard 2009). Thus, precautions need to be taken in dealing with these chemical uncouplers, whereas residual uncouplers in the effluent also pose a challenge for large-scale application.

Most uncouplers are poorly soluble in water. Some are moderately soluble in alkaline solution (such as nitrophenols and CCCP), but some may only be stable when the pH value is below 8. Due to their hydrophobic property, uncouplers are usually made up as stock solution in organic solvents, such as ethanol, dimethyl-formamide, dimethyl sulfoxide, and methyl cellosolve (Heytler 1979). However, it should be realized that organic solvents may eventually enter the treatment process in this way.

Adaptation of activated sludge microorganisms to uncouplers is another issue of concern that may be encountered in long-term operation of the activated sludge process. Initially, nonacclimated activated sludge has no ability to degrade external

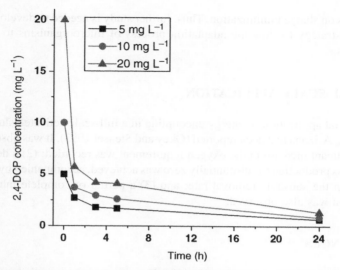

FIGURE 5.16 Concentration profiles of 2,4-dichlorophenol during 24-h cultures at different initial concentrations in MBRs. [Data from Lin et al. (2010).]

metabolic uncouplers. However, to sustain a lower sludge yield, metabolic uncouplers need to be dosed continuously to the aeration tank. As a result, microbial acclimation to uncouplers would gradually develop over time. For example, the residual 2,4-DCP concentration in the bioreactor was negligible after a 24-h reaction (Fig. 5.16). This in turn implies that 2,4-DCP could be biologically degraded by the activated sludge microorganisms.

Gage and Neidhardt (1993) reported that wide-type *E. coli* could adapt to DNP by increasing the synthesis rates of 53 proteins, which in turn may ensure their survival and growth when faced with such environmental challenges. The adaptation rate was accelerated with the presence of pyrroloquinoline quinine (PQQ) in the growth medium. In *E. coli*, *emr*A and *emr*B, which confer resistance to CCCP and TCS, were cloned and found to be responsible for encoding multidrug resistance pumps (Lewis et al. 1994). Cubonava et al. (2003) compared the composition of membrane-associated proteins from wild-type and TCS-resistant mutant strains of methanoarchaeon *Methanothermobacter thermautotrophicus* by SDS-PAGE analysis, and found that the protein size or concentrations of subunits A, B, and *c* (proteolipid) of the A_1A_0-ATPasesynthase were not changed. However, a 670-kDa membrane-associated protein complex was revealed in the mutant strain (but not in the wild type) which was composed of at least five different putative subunits of 95, 52, 42, 29, and 22 kDa. Uncoupler-resistant mutants cannot inactivate uncouplers but do possess the ability to exclude uncouplers from the energized coupling membrane (i.e., the protonophoric efficiency of uncouplers remains unchanged in the mutants) (Krulwich et al. 1990; Lewis et al. 1994). Adaptation is an ineluctable problem when applying chemical uncouplers to minimize excess sludge production. As noted by Strand et al. (1999), long-term microbial acclimation could eventually negate the effect of uncouplers on sludge minimization. Thus, further study is needed to develop optimal operation strategy to slow the adaptation process of microorganisms to chemical uncouplers.

5.7 FULL-SCALE APPLICATION

An industrial application of energy uncoupling in a full-scale activated sludge plant in Phoenix, Arizona had been reported (Okey and Stensel 1993). It was observed that (1) a significant increase in the oxygen requirement was recorded; (2) a decrease in net biomass production to substantially zero was achieved, accompanied by a modest decrease in the substrate removal rate; and (3) a partial or complete inhibition of nitrification was also observed.

REFERENCES

Argese E., Bettiol C., Giurin G., Miana P. (1999) Quantitative structure–activity relationships for the toxicity of chlorophenols to mammalian submitochondrial particles. *Chemosphere* **38**(10), 2281–2292.

Baum H., Rieske J. S., Silman H. I., Lipton S. H. (1967) On the mechanism of electron transfer in complex III of the electron transfer chain. *Proceedings of the National Academy of Sciences USA* **57**(3), 798–805.

Boyer P. D., Cross R. L., Momsen W. (1973) A new concept for energy coupling in oxidative phosphorylation based on a molecular explanation of the oxygen exchange reactions. *Proceedings of the National Academy of Sciences USA* **70**(10), 2837–2839.

Brandt U., Schubert J., Geck P., Vonjagow G. (1992) Uncoupling activity and physicochemical properties of derivatives of fluazinam. *Biochimica et Biophysica Acta* **1101**(1), 41–47.

Breeuwer P., Abee T. (2004) Assessment of the membrane potential, intracellular pH and respiration of bacteria employing fluorescence techniques. *Molecular Microbial Ecology Manual* **8**, 1563–1580.

Budavari S. (1989) *Encyclopedia of Chemicals, Drugs and Biologicals*, 10th ed., The Merck Index, Rahway, NJ.

Cabrero A., Fernandez S., Mirada F., Garcia J. (1998) Effects of copper and zinc on the activated sludge bacteria growth kinetics. *Water Research* **32**(5), 1355–1362.

Cammann K. (1985) Ion-selective bulk membranes as models for biomembranes-active ion-transport as a consequence of stationary state situations at asymmetric biomembranes. *Topics in Current Chemistry* **128**, 219–259.

Chen G. H., Mo H. K., Liu Y. (2002) Utilization of a metabolic uncoupler, 3,3',4',5-tetrachlorosalicylanilide (TCS) to reduce sludge growth in activated sludge culture. *Water Research* **36**(8), 2077–2083.

Chen G. H., Mo H. K., Saby S., Yip W. K., Liu Y. (2000) Minimization of activated sludge production by chemically stimulated energy spilling. *Water Science and Technology* **42**(12), 189–200.

Chen G. W., Yu H. Q., Liu H. X., Xu D. Q. (2006) Response of activated sludge to the presence of 2,4-dichlorophenol in a batch culture system. *Process Biochemistry* **41**(8), 1758–1763.

Chen G. W., Yu H. Q., Xi P. G. (2007) Influence of 2,4-dinitrophenol on the characteristics of activated sludge in batch reactors. *Bioresource Technology* **98**(4), 729–733.

Chen G. W., Yu H. Q., Xi P. G., Xu D. Q. (2008) Modeling the yield of activated sludge in the presence of 2,4-dinitrophenol. *Biochemical Engineering Journal* **40**(1), 150–156.

Chen Y. X., Ye F. X., Feng X. S. (2004) The use of 3,3',4',5-tetrachlorosalicylanilide as a chemical uncoupler to reduce activated sludge yield. *Journal of Chemical Technology and Biotechnology* **79**(2), 111–116.

Cubonava L., Majernik A., Smigan P. (2003) Biochemical characteristics of a mutant of the methanoarchaeon. *Methanothermobacter thermautotrophicus* resistant to the protonophoric uncoupler TCS. 3rd International Symposium of Anaerobic Microbiology (ISAM). Kosice, Slovakia.

Dervartanian D. V., Veeger C. (1964) Studies on succinate dehydrogenase: I. Spectral properties of the purified enzyme and formation of enzyme-competitive inhibitor complexes. *Biochimica et Biophysica Acta Enzymological Subjects* **92**(2), 233–247.

Gage D. J., Neidhardt F. C. (1993) Adaptation of *Escherichia coli* to the uncoupler of oxidative phosphorylation 2,4-dinitrophenol. *Journal of Bacteriology* **175**(21), 7105–7108.

Garrett R., Grisham, C. M. (2008) *Biochemistry*, 4th ed, Cengage Learning. Stanford, CT.

Greenman J., Holland K. T., Cunliffe W. J. (1983) Effects of pH on biomass, maximum specific growth rate and extracellular enzyme production by three species of cutaneous propionibacteria grown in continuous culture. *Journal of General Microbiology* **129**(5), 1301–1307.

Gutman M., Singer T. P., Beinert H., Casida J. E. (1970) Reaction sites of rotenone, piericidin A, and amytal in relation to the nonheme iron components of NADH dehydrogenase. *Proceedings of the National Academy of Sciences USA* **65**(3), 763–770.

Hames B. D., Hooper, N. M. (2005) *Biochemistry*, 3rd ed., Taylor & Francis, Oxford; UK.

Hanstein W. G. (1976) Uncoupling of oxidative phosphorylation. *Biochimica et Biophysica Acta* **456**(2), 129–148.

Harder W., Dijkhuizen L. (1983) Physiological responses to nutrient limitation. *Annual Review of Microbiology* **37**, 1–23.

Henderson P. J., Lardy H. A. (1970) Bongkrekic acid: an inhibitor of the adenine nucleotide translocase of mitochondria. *Journal of Biological Chemistry* **245**(6), 1319–1326.

Henriques I. D. S., Kelly Ii R. T., Dauphinais J. L., Love N. G. (2007) Activated sludge inhibition by chemical stressors: a comprehensive study. *Water Environment Research* **79**(9), 940–951.

Heytler P. G. (1979) Uncouplers of oxidative phosphorylation. In: *Methods in Enzymology.* Academic Press, Waltham, Massachusetts. pp. 462–472.

Hiraishi A., Kawagishi T. (2002) Effects of chemical uncouplers on microbial biomass production, metabolic activity, and community structure in an activated sludge system. *Microbes and Environments* **17**(4), 197–204.

Karim K., Gupta S. K. (2006) Effect of shock and mixed nitrophenolic loadings on the performance of UASB reactors. *Water Research* **40**(5), 935–942.

Krulwich T. A., Quirk P. G., Guffanti A. A. (1990) Uncoupler-resistant mutants of bacteria. *Microbiological Reviews* **54**(1), 52–65.

Lehninger A. L., Wadkins C. L. (1962) Oxidative phosphorylation. *Annual Review of Biochemistry* **31**, 47.

Lewis K., Naroditskaya V., Ferrante A., Fokina I. (1994) Bacterial resistance to uncouplers. *Journal of Bioenergetics and Biomembranes* **26**(6), 639–646.

Li N., Ragheb K., Lawler G., Sturgis J., Rajwa B., Melendez J. A., Robinson J. P. (2003) Mitochondrial complex I inhibitor rotenone induces apoptosis through enhancing mitochondrial reactive oxygen species production. *Journal of Biological Chemistry* **278**(10), 8516–8525.

Lin S., Jiang W. J., Tang Q., Li Y. Z. (2010) Impact of a metabolic uncoupler, 2,4-dichlorophenol on minimization of activated sludge production in membrane bioreactor. *Water Science and Technology* **62**(6), 1379–1385.

Liu Y. (2000a) Effect of chemical uncoupler on the observed growth yield in batch culture of activated sludge. *Water Research* **34**(7), 2025–2030.

Liu Y. (2000b) Effect of initial ratio of heavy metal to biomass on growth yield in batch culture of activated sludge. *Toxicological and Environmental Chemistry* **74**(1–2), 9–18.

Liu Y. (2003) Chemically reduced excess sludge production in the activated sludge process. *Chemosphere* **50**(1), 1–7.

Liu Y., Chen G.-H., Paul E. (1998) Effect of the S_0/X_0 ratio on energy uncoupling in substrate-sufficient batch culture of activated sludge. *Water Research* **32**(10), 2883–2888.

Liu, Y., Tay J. H. (2000) Interaction between catabolism and anabolism in the oxidative assimilation of dissolved organic carbon. *Biotechnology Letters* **22**(19), 1521–1525.

Liu Y., Tay J. H. (2001) Strategy for minimization of excess sludge production from the activated sludge process. *Biotechnology Advances* **19**(2), 97–107.

Low E. W., Chase H. A. (1998) The use of chemical uncouplers for reducing biomass production during biodegradation. *Water Science and Technology* **37**(4–5), 399–402.

MaCall D., Stock D., Achey P. (2001) *Introduction to Microbiology*, Wiley, Hoboken, NJ.

Mayhew M., Stephenson T. (1998) Biomass yield reduction: Is biochemical manipulation possible without affecting activated sludge process efficiency? *Water Science and Technology* **38** (8–9 pt 7), 137–144.

Mitchell P. (1961) Coupling of phosphorylation to electron and hydrogen transfer by a chemiosmotic type of mechanism. *Nature* **191**, 144–148.

Moat A. G., Foster, J. W., Spector M. P. (2002) *Microbial Physiology*, 4th ed., Wiley-Liss, New York.

Neumann J., Jagendorf A. T. (1964) Dinitrophenol as an uncoupler of photosynthetic phosphorylation. *Biochemical and Biophysical Research Communications* **16**(6), 562–567.

Ogbonda K. H., Aminigo R. E., Abu G. O. (2007) Influence of temperature and pH on biomass production and protein biosynthesis in a putative Spirulina sp. *Bioresource Technology* **98**(11), 2207–2211.

Okey R. W., Stensel H. D. (1993) Uncouplers and activated sludge: the impact on synthesis and respiration. *Toxicological and Environmental Chemistry* **40**(1–4), 235–254.

Palmen R., Driessen A. J. M., Hellingwerf K. J. (1994) Bioenergetic aspects of the translocation of macromolecules across bacterial membranes. *Biochimica et Biophysica Acta Bioenergetics* **1183**(3), 417–451.

Petty H. R. (1993) *Molecular Biology of Membrane: Structure and Function*. Plenum Press, New York.

Ray S., Peters C. A. (2008) Changes in microbiological metabolism under chemical stress. *Chemosphere* **71**(3), 474–483.

Rho S., Nam G. N., Shin J. Y., Jahng D. (2007) Effect of 3,3′,4′,5-tetrachlorosalicylanilide on reduction of excess sludge and nitrogen removal in biological wastewater treatment process. *Journal of Microbiology and Biotechnology* **17**(7), 1183–1190.

Rich L. G., Yates O. W. (1955) The effect of 2,4-dinitrophenol on activated sludge. *Applied Microbiology* **3**(2), 95–98.

Richard J. (2009) *Advances in Physical Organic Chemistry*, Academic Press, San Diego, CA.

Roach J. O'Neale and Benyon, S. (2003) *Metabolism and Nutrition*. 2nd ed., Mosby International, London.

Saini G., Wood B. D. (2008) Metabolic uncoupling of *Shewanella oneidensis* MR-1, under the influence of excess substrate and 3,3′,4′,5-tetrachlorosalicylanilide (TCS). *Biotechnology and Bioengineering* **99**(6), 1352–1360.

Schultz T. W., Cronin M. T. D. (1997) Quantitative structure–activity relationships for weak acid respiratory uncouplers to Vibrio fisheri. *Environmental Toxicology and Chemistry* **16**(2), 357–360.

Shchepina L. A., Pletjushkina O. Y., Avetisyan A. V., Bakeeva L. E., Fetisova E. K., Izyumov D. S., Saprunova V. B., Vyssokikh M. Y., Chernyak B. V., Skulachev V. P. (2002) Oligomycin, inhibitor of the Fo part of H^+-ATP-synthase, suppresses the TNF-induced apoptosis. *Oncogene* **21**, 8149–8157.

Slater E. C. (1953) Mechanism of phosphorylation in the respiratory chain. *Nature* **172**, 975–978.

Stouthamer A. H. (1973) A theoretical study on the amount of ATP required for synthesis of microbial cell material. *Antonie van Leeuwenhoek International Journal of General and Molecular Microbiology* **39**(3), 545–565.

Strand S. E., Harem G. N., Stensel H. D. (1999) Activated-sludge yield reduction using chemical uncouplers. *Water Environment Research* **71**(4), 454–458.

Tavares J. M., Duarte L. C., Amaral-Collaco M. T., Girio F. M. (1999) Phosphate limitation stress induces xylitol overproduction by Debaryomyces hansenii. *FEMS Microbiology Letters* **171**(2), 115–120.

Teixeira De Mattos, M. J., Neijssel O. M. (1997) Bioenergetic consequences of microbial adaptation to low-nutrient environments. *Journal of Biotechnology* **59**(1–2), 117–126.

Tempest D. W., Neijssel O. M. (1992) Physiological and energetic aspects of bacterial metabolite overproduction. *FEMS Microbiology Letters* **100**(1–3), 169–176.

Terada H. (1990) Uncouplers of oxidative phosphorylation. *Environmental Health Perspectives* **87**, 213–218.

Terada H., Goto S., Yamamoto K., Takeuchi I., Hamada Y., Miyake K. (1988) Structural requirements of salicylanilides for uncoupling activity in mitochondria: quantitative analysis of structure–uncoupling relationships. *Biochimica et Biophysica Acta Bioenergetics* **936**(3), 504–512.

Tissut M., Taillandier G., Ravanel P., Benoit-Guyod J. L. (1987) Effects of chlorophenols on isolated class A chloroplasts and thylakoids: a QSAR study. *Ecotoxicology and Environmental Safety* **13**(1), 32–42.

Tsubaki M. (1993) Fourier-transform infrared study of cyanide binding to the Fea3-CuB binuclear site of bovine heart cytochrome *c* oxidase: implication of the redox-linked conformational change at the binuclear site. *Biochemistry* **32**(1), 164–173.

Wilson D. F., Ting H. P., Koppelman M. S. (1971) Mechanism of action of uncouplers of oxidative phosphorylation. *Biochemistry* **10**(15), 2897–2902.

Yang X. F., Xie M. L., Liu Y. (2003) Metabolic uncouplers reduce excess sludge production in an activated sludge process. *Process Biochemistry* **38**(9), 1373–1377.

Ye F. X., Li Y. (2005) Reduction of excess sludge production by 3,3′,4′,5-tetrachlorosalicy-lanilide in an activated sludge process. *Applied Microbiology and Biotechnology* **67**(2), 269–274.

Ye F., Li Y. (2010) Oxic-settling-anoxic (OSA) process combined with 3,3′,4′,5-tetrachlor-osalicylanilide (TCS) to reduce excess sludge production in the activated sludge system. *Biochemical Engineering Journal* **49**(2), 229–234.

Ye F. X., Zhu R. F., Li Y. (2008) Effect of sludge retention time in sludge holding tank on excess sludge production in the oxic-settling-anoxic (OSA) activated sludge process. *Journal of Chemical Technology and Biotechnology* **83**(1), 109–114.

Yoshida M., Muneyuki E., Hisabori T. (2001) ATP synthase: a marvellous rotary engine of the cell. *Nature Reviews Molecular Cell Biology* **2**(9), 669–677.

Zakharov S. D., Kuzmina V. P. (1992) ATP-synthase activity of the thermophilic bacterium *Thermus thermophilus* HB-8 membranes. *BiochemistryMoscow* **57**(4), 365–371.

Zannoni D. (2004) *Respiration in Archaea and Bacteria: Diversity of Prokaryotic Electron Transport Carriers*, Springer-Verlag, Dordrecht, The Netherlands.

Zheng G. H., Chen Z. Y., Wang L., Qian Y. F., Zhou Q. (2007) Treatment of municipal wastewater with the sequence batch reactor under uncoupling metabolic conditions. *Journal of Environmental Science and Health A* **42**(13), 2059–2064.

Zheng G. H., Li M. N., Wang L., Chen Z. Y., Qian Y. F., Zhou Q. (2008) Feasibility of 2,4,6-trichlorophenol and malonic acid as metabolic uncoupler for sludge reduction in the sequence batch reactor for treating organic wastewater. *Applied Biochemistry and Biotechnology* **144**(2), 101–109.

Zubay G. L. (1998) *Biochemistry*, 4th ed., WCB Publishing, Boston.

6

REDUCTION OF EXCESS SLUDGE PRODUCTION USING OZONATION OR CHLORINATION: PERFORMANCE AND MECHANISMS OF ACTION

ETIENNE PAUL

Université de Toulouse; INSA,UPS,INP; LISBP, 135 Avenue de Rangueil, F-31077 Toulouse, France; INRA, UMR792, Ingénierie des Systèmes Biologiques et des Procédés, F-31400 Toulouse, France; CNRS, UMR5504, F-31400 Toulouse, France

QI-SHAN LIU

School of Architecture and the Built Environment, Singapore Polytechnic, Singapore

YU LIU

Division of Environmental and Water Resources Engineering, School of Civil and Environmental Engineering, Nanyang Technological University, Singapore

6.1 INTRODUCTION

Ozone has been widely used in water and wastewater treatment to remove pollutants, to kill pathogenic organisms, and to improve physical treatments such as coagulation-flocculation and biological filtration with activated carbon. Ozone is applied to sludge to limit the effect of bulking and foaming (Van Leeuwen 1988) and as a combined ozonation–biodegradation treatment to reduce excess sludge production (ESP). This combined treatment, associating an activated sludge (AS) process with an ozone contactor in its early stage, was first described by Gaudy et al. (1971) and

Biological Sludge Minimization and Biomaterials/Bioenergy Recovery Technologies, First Edition.
Edited by Etienne Paul and Yu Liu.

then by Yasui and Shibata (1994). Since this date, the process has been characterized at both laboratory and full scale combined with an activated sludge plant or anaerobic digestion (AD) (Gaudy et al. 1971; Yasui and Shibata 1994; Yasui et al. 1996; Sakai et al. 1997; Déléris et al. 1999, 2000, 2002, 2003; Déléris 2001; Huysmans et al. 2001; Salhi et al. 2003; Goel et al. 2004). Chlorine is a powerful oxidant, used widely for disinfection, biosolids stabilization, and so on. The chlorination-assisted biological process has been investigated in a lab-scale system and only for minimizing excess sludge production (Chen et al. 2001; Saby et al. 2002; Takdastan et al. 2010).

In this chapter we deal first with ozonation and then with chlorination. Considering ozonation, in the first section we present an overview of the application and performance levels of sludge ozonation systems in pilot- and full-scale plants for both the wastewater treatment line (when combined with an AS system) and the sludge treatment line (when combined with AD systems). Then we review side effects resulting from ozonation: outlet chemical oxygen demand (COD) release, extra nitrogen and phosphorus release and associated removal strategies, changes in sludge properties, and some elements of cost and energy evaluations. Then a cost assessment is given on the basis of data obtained from pilot experiments. In the fifth section, the focus is on an in-depth analysis of the mechanisms associated with mixed liquor ozonation, considering successively the basics of ozone transfer and sludge fractionation, as they are fundamental to an understanding of sludge ozonation and competition for ozone; COD solubilization and the evolution of COD biodegradability; biomass inactivation or destruction; and mechanisms associated with ozone transfer in such a complex medium containing both soluble and particulate compounds. Finally, the modeling of a combined ozonation/biological process is considered. Simulation could be used to optimize the system efficiency and improve our knowledge of ozonation. The final part of the chapter is dedicated to a review of current knowledge and results concerning chlorination-assisted biological processes.

6.2   SIGNIFICANT OPERATIONAL RESULTS FOR ESP REDUCTION WITH OZONE

In this section we first present various options for combining ozonation and biological treatments of urban wastewater. Then follows a description of organic ESP reduction performances obtained at both lab and full scale when ozonation is combined with AS or AD. Finally, mineral reduction is considered.

6.2.1   Options for Combining Ozonation and Biological Treatment

Figure 6.1 depicts a wastewater treatment plant and the various locations where ozone treatment can be used to lead to ESP reduction. Systems can be operated in the following ways:

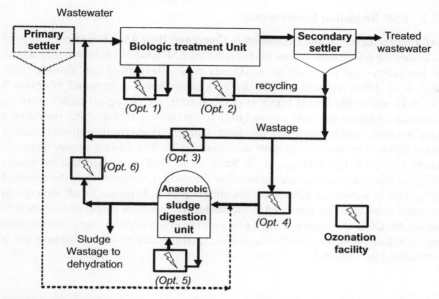

FIGURE 6.1 Proposed operational modes for a combined process associating a sludge disintegration technique such as ozonation and a biological treatment such as an AS or AD systems. [Adapted from Salhi (2003).]

1. The mixed liquor can be directly pumped from the biological reactor toward an ozonation contactor for partial oxidation and then pumped back to the biological tank for further biological degradation (option 1). Ozonation can also be applied to the settled sludge before recycling it to the biological treatment unit (options 2 and 3).

2. Ozonation can be applied to the sludge treatment route and used before digestion (option 4) or as a co-treatment, in addition to biological degradation (option 5).

3. Sludge ozonation may be applied as a posttreatment of the AD system, the resulting ozonated mixed liquor being recycled to the AS (option 6).

Depending on the system used, a primary settler may or may not be added.

Among the various options, those that give more importance to biodegradation should be preferred. Because of environmental and energy constraints, it can be interesting to combine ozonation with the anaerobic digestion unit. For example, a mesophilic–thermophilic hybrid anaerobic digestion process with ozonation of digested sludge has been proposed (Battimelli et al. 2003; Goel et al. 2004; Yasui et al. 2006; Bougrier et al. 2007; Komatsu et al. 2011a, b) which shows better energy recovery. Hence, the options that are chosen must often and described in the literature are options 1 and 4.

6.2.2 ESP Reduction Performance

Performance Levels When Ozonation Is Combined With AS   The effectiveness of the combined AS–ozonation process for reducing ESP has been demonstrated at both the laboratory- and full-scale levels (Gaudy et al. 1971; Yasui and Shibata 1994; Yasui et al. 1996; Sakai et al. 1997). The systems tested correspond to option 1 (Fig. 6.1), where the mixed liquor is pumped from the biological tank toward an ozonation contactor and then pumped back to the biological tank. After operating a plant treating wastewater from the food industry (volume of activated sludge tank $= 800\,m^3$) in association with an ozonation facility [ozone dosage approximately $0.05\,g\,O_3\,(g\,COD_{removed})^{-1}$], Sakai et al. (1997) reported that no excess sludge withdrawal was necessary to stabilize the sludge concentration in the activated sludge tank at a constant value for a five-month period. However, small amounts of inorganic substances accumulated in the sludge and a loss of suspended solids (SS) and soluble COD was observed in the effluent. The efficiency of ozone treatment with respect to ESP reduction was then assessed experimentally by various authors and is summarized in Table 6.1.

TABLE 6.1   ESP Reduction Reported in the Literature

Reference	Wastewater Type	Dosage $(kg\,O_3\,kg^{-1}\,SS)$	Dosage $(kg\,O_3\,kg^{-1}\,COD_{removed})$	Reduction of ESP (%)	Period (months)
Yasui and Shibata (1994)	Synthetic	From 0.03 to 0.05	—	100	
Yasui et al. (1996)	Pharmaceutical	>0.015	—	100	10
Sakai et al. (1997)	Urban	0034	0.04 and 0.06	70 and 100	9
Kamiya and Hirotsuji (1998)	Synthetic	0.025	—	70	
Huysmans et al. (2001)	Urban	0.019	0.025	50	
Déléris et al. (2002)	Municipal (slightly settled)	0.030	—	100	24
Déléris et al. (2003)[a]	Municipal (slightly settled)	Variable	0.1 and 0.15	70 and 100	24
Salhi et al. (2003)	Municipal (slightly settled)	<0.015	0.05 and 0.07	70 and 100	24
Cesbron et al. (2003)	Municipal (slightly settled)	<0.015	0.05 and 0.07	70 and 100	24
Sievers et al. (2004)	Municipal	0.03–0.06	—	55	
Caffaz et al. (2005)	Municipal	0.01–0.014	—	78	9
Yasui et al. (2005)	Sewage	?	—	70	24
Wolff and Hurren (2006)	Slaughterhouse	0.026	—	60–80	24
Vergine et al. (2007)	Industrial	>0.015	—	40	2
Vergine et al. (2007)	Chemical	0.056	—	45	60
Campos et al. (2009)	Seafood	0.03	—	50	

[a]Air was used to produce O_3.

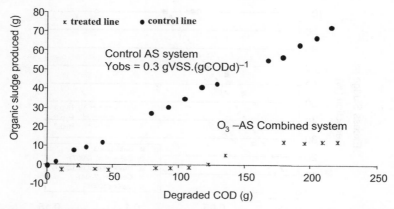

FIGURE 6.2 Comparison of the organic ESP between a conventional AS system and a combined AS–ozonation system at lab scale run at a specific ozone dosage of $0.07 \, g \, O_3 \, g^{-1}$ $COD_{removed}$. [From Salhi (2003).]

In the context of a six-year lab- and pilot-scale program of experiments, the relationship between the ozone-specific dosage and the ESP reduction was assessed (Déléris 2001; Salhi 2003; Cesbron 2004). The systems tested also corresponded to option 1 (Fig. 6.1). The wastewater, from the Toulouse (France) city network, was used to feed these systems after a simple short primary settling (15 min). The organic sludge production is presented versus the mass of degraded COD in Fig. 6.2 for a three-month experiment (representative of the entire period). For the control line (conventional activated sludge treatment alone), Y_{obs} amounted to $0.33 \pm 0.06 \, g$ volatile suspended solids (VSS) $g^{-1} \, COD_{removed}$, which is a conventional figure. In comparison, for the treated line (activated sludge treatment was combined with ozone treatment at a specific ozone dosage of $0.07 \, g \, O_3 \, g^{-1} \, COD_{removed}$) the suspended solids (SS) concentration within the reactor could be maintained almost constant even though no sludge was removed (i.e., Y_{obs} was almost zero). The SS concentration in the effluent from the combined treatment system increased slightly ($\approx +25 \, mg \, COD \, L^{-1}$) compared with the SS concentration in the effluent from the control line. However, this did not distort the ESP reduction observed by more than 5%.

Figure 6.3 shows the relationship between the reduction of ESP and the ozone dosage observed in a combined ozonation–AS treatment system. For other cases, as presented in Table 6.1, ozone dosage was expressed as the specific ozone dosage in terms of $g \, O_3 \, g^{-1} \, TSS$ (total suspended solids), which is largely dependent on the operating conditions (e.g., sludge ozonation frequency). This in turn makes comparison of the ESP reduction data reported in the literature rather difficult.

It appears from Fig. 6.3 that the specific ozone dosage applied to avoid ESP is in the same range for the various studies of lab- and full-scale plants. An ozone dosage of 0.06 to $0.07 \, g \, O_3 \, g^{-1} \, COD_{removed}$ is required to maintain the organic fraction of the volatile suspended solids (VSS) stable in the AS without sludge wastage. In addition, a linear relationship (Hyps. 1 to 3 in Fig. 6.3) between the organic ESP reduction and the specific ozone dosage is found systematically. It has been postulated by Salhi (2003)

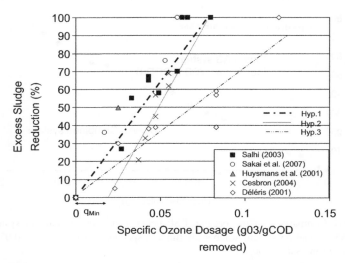

FIGURE 6.3 Relationship between the applied specific ozone dosage and the percentage of ESP reduction reported by various authors (Sakai et al. 1997; Déléris 2001; Huysmans et al. 2001; Salhi 2003; Cesbron 2004).

that the specific ozone dosage required to reach a given ESP reduction is proportional to the volumetric COD loading rate. It is, however, difficult to determine whether there is a minimal ozone dosage (q_{min}) necessary to induce an ESP reduction (Hyp. 2) or not (Hyp. 1). In Fig. 6.3, the difference observed for the results of Déléris (2001) (Hyp. 3) is attributed to the use of air instead of pure oxygen to generate ozone. Organic radicals formed during the action of ozone on sludge components would react with oxygen, increasing the oxidation of the organic matter. A system using O_3 generated with pure oxygen is thus more efficient in terms of ESP reduction. More recently, the proportionality between ESP reduction and ozone dosage has been confirmed (Dytczak et al. 2007). Cesbron (2004) obtained an ESP reduction of 70% in his lab-scale continuous ozonation–AS system (Opt. 1, Fig. 6.1) relative to the control, run in parallel, for an ozone dosage of 0.195 g O_3 g^{-1} SS$_{not\ produced}$. In the study by Dytczak and Oleszkiewicz (2008), where prolonged operation of partial sludge ozonation was carried out, the flocs seemed to adapt to ozone stress, becoming more resistant. The authors suggest that an increase in ozone dosage may be required to maintain continuously the expected level of solids destruction. This result was not observed by other authors on long term experiments (Salhi 2003; Cesbron 2004; Yasui et al. 2005).

Performance of Ozonation Combined with AD Ozonation as a sludge pretreatment prior to AD (Opt 4, Fig. 6.1) has also been used with success to enhance the anaerobic digestibility of the wasted activated sludge (Weemaes and Verstraete 1998; Scheminski et al. 2000; Weemaes et al. 2000; Goel et al. 2004; Yasui et al. 2005, 2006; Bougrier et al. 2006, 2007). A rather long acclimatization period is necessary for the anaerobic biomass, however, and the redox potential in the anaerobic phase must be kept to a low level. Weemaes et al. (2000) reported the effect of ozonation on the anaerobic digestion potential, which increased by a factor of 1.5 and 1.8 at ozone dosages of 0.04 and 0.1 g O_3 g^{-1} COD, respectively. Yasui et al. (2005) and Goel et al. (2004) described a combined ozone/anaerobic digestion process where reduction rates of 81% on the VSS and 61% on the TSS were achieved. No sludge wastage was performed; the VSS concentration in the reactor was around $26 \pm 2 \, \text{g} \, \text{L}^{-1}$ at an average VSS loading of 0.6 kg VSS (m$^3 \cdot$ d)$^{-1}$, and average specific gas recoveries of 0.36 L CH$_4$ g^{-1} VSS$_{fed}$ were obtained. At the same ESP reduction, the configuration with postozonation (Opt. 5, Fig. 6.1) required a lower ozone dosage than did the preozonation (Opt. 4, Fig. 6.1). In addition, the authors reported that mineral precipitation was observed in the sludge and that higher SS contents could easily be achieved after further dewatering of the sludge.

6.2.3   Assessing Ozone Efficiency for Mineral ESP Reduction

The question of minerals is crucial because they make a significant contribution to ESP and because they may accumulate in the sludge, modifying the sludge properties (and ozone efficiency). Mass balance on minerals should be assessed systematically when studies on ESP reduction are performed, but unfortunately, they are not seen very often. Usually, a decrease in the VSS/SS ratio is observed when ozonation is combined with biological treatment (Sakai et al. 1997; Salhi et al. 2003; Goel et al. 2004; Dytczak et al. 2007). The reasons are either lower solubilization of the mineral fraction than the organic fraction in the sludge, or mineral precipitation. However, the various studies have shown that the system stabilizes, probably because mineral leakage occurs. For example, in the combined treatment line run by Salhi et al. (2003), the VSS/SS ratio first decreased from about 0.85 to about 0.71 during the first few weeks of ozonation and then stabilized at the latter value (Fig. 6.4). This fate is confirmed in the work of Cesbron (2004), who concludes that there is a proportional solubilization of organic and mineral compounds from the sludge at steady state. These results indicate the capability of ozone to (directly or indirectly)

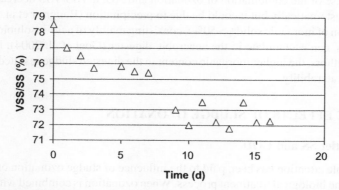

FIGURE 6.4 Variation of the sludge VSS/SS ratio for 100% ESP reduction.

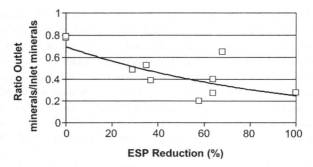

ESP Reduction (%)

FIGURE 6.5 Mass balance for suspended nonvolatile matter (total outlet, sludge wastage included, vs. total inlet) as a function of the organic ESP reduction.

solubilize a large part of the mineral fraction contained in the suspended solids destroyed. In Fig. 6.5, mass balances for solid nonvolatile matter are presented for various percentages of ESP reduction. Each point on the graph represents an average value over a period of at least three weeks. For 0% ESP reduction, 80% of the solid nonvolatile matter from the inlet is recovered as solids at the outlet. This percentage decreases sharply with increasing percentage of ESP reduction, down to about 30% for 100% ESP reduction, demonstrating an effective mineral solubilization during the combined treatment. Theoretically, it is then not possible to achieve total ESP reduction on organic and mineral sludge at the same time. However, during these experiments on the continuous ozonation combined treatment, loss of particulate matter is observed in the outlet of the activated sludge reactor. This is due to the floc-destructuring action of ozone. Nonsolubilized mineral matter can then leave the reactor with the nonsettling flocs. Particulate matter removal appears to be necessary to prevent mineral matter from accumulating in the bioreactor. If this loss does not occur, the VSS/SS would reach very low values, particularly if the system was fed with raw wastewater. Minimal sludge wastage is thus recommended. More research is required on the effect of ozonation on the mineral fraction of sludge, especially when iron is present (Cesbron 2004; Sui et al. 2011).

In the case of the combination of ozonation and AD, a VSS/TSS decrease is also observed systematically but it could be due to precipitation (Bougrier et al. 2006). A high fraction of inorganic solid ($>50\%$), consisting mainly of acid-insoluble and iron compounds, can accumulate in the anaerobic digester (Goel et al. 2004). However, for these authors, the higher inorganic content in the digested sludge resulted in better sludge dewaterability.

6.3   SIDE EFFECTS OF SLUDGE OZONATION

6.3.1   Outlet SS and COD

Considerable attention has been paid to the influence of sludge ozonation on effluent quality in the biological treatment process. When ozonation is combined with AS, the SS concentration increases slightly compared to that measured for the control line

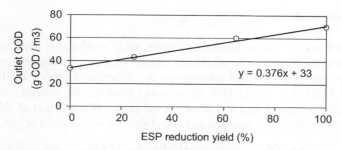

FIGURE 6.6 Variation in outlet COD (after centrifugation) for different ESP conditions. Each COD value is a mean value of three weeks of daily measurements. [From Salhi (2003).]

[$+15\,\text{mg VSS L}^{-1}$ (Cesbron 2004) and $+2$ to $15\,\text{mg VSS L}^{-1}$ (Sakai et al. 1997)]. Mainly microflocs are released. However, the additional VSS lost with the treated water amounts to less than 5% of the quantity of sludge obtained from a conventional process and does not distort the sludge reduction results reported.

The typical soluble COD contained within the treated municipal wastewater amounts to about $+40\,\text{mg COD L}^{-1}$ for a conventional AS treatment plant. Again, it increases significantly ($+15$ to $+40\,\text{mg COD L}^{-1}$) when ESP reduction is performed with ozone (Yasui and Shibata 1994; Sakai et al. 1997; Kamiya and Hirotsuji 1998; Egemen et al. 2001; Huysmans et al. 2001; Salhi et al. 2003; Camacho et al. 2005). Yasui and Shibata (1994) reported an increase in the total organic carbon (TOC) from $6\,\text{mg L}^{-1}$ to $14\,\text{mg L}^{-1}$ when the ESP reduction reaches 80%. Nevertheless, the total figure remains far below the limit value ($125\,\text{mg COD L}^{-1}$) set by the regulations in force. Salhi (2003) found the COD concentration at the outlet of the ozonation–AS system to be proportional to the sludge reduction rate and so to the specific ozone dosage transferred ($1.9\,\text{g}$ $\text{COD}_{\text{outlet}}\,\text{g}^{-1}\,\text{O}_3$). Figure 6.6 shows this relation between the extra outlet COD and the ESP reduction yield. Apparently, the amount of COD loss found in this study was higher than that observed by other authors (Sakai et al. 1997; Kamiya and Hirotsuji 1998; Egemen et al. 2001; Huysmans et al. 2001). Unlike the COD released directly during ozonation, which was found to be entirely biodegradable, this outlet COD was found to be mainly nonbiodegradable (Salhi 2003). Although it is nonbiodegradable, it may be useful to limit this COD release by using a membrane bioreactor (He et al. 2003, 2006; Oh et al. 2007; Wang et al. 2008).

To explain the apparition of a soluble nonbiodegradable COD (S_U) in the outlet of an ozonation–AS system, a delayed solubilization in the mixed liquor of the biological reactor was suggested (Salhi et al. 2003). The process responsible for the delayed solubilization was not identified, although it has been observed by other authors (Egemen et al. 2001). A possible decrease in the cohesion strength of small structures in the floc due to sludge ozonation was, however, proposed. Because of the high flow rate of water throughout the plant, this additional COD load could explain from 10 to 20% of the ESP reduction observed. Salhi et al. (2003) compared this extra soluble outlet COD to the COD removed and found an increase of $0.133\,\text{g}$ $\text{COD}_{\text{soluble}}\,\text{g}^{-1}\,\text{COD}_{\text{removed}}$ for a condition of no more sludge withdrawal.

6.3.2   N Removal

TKN Solubilization   The combined treatment, while solubilizing particulate compounds, led to the release of an additional amount of total kjeldahl nitrogen (TKN) into the system. Nitrogen and phosphorus are solubilized proportionally to the solubilized COD (ratio COD/TKN is constant) whatever the specific ozone dose transferred at the scale tested and whatever the sludge (Camacho et al. 2005). The relation between the TKN released and the sludge reduction yield is given as.

$$\text{N-TKN}_{RSP} = f_{\text{N-TKN}}(\text{ESPR})\, Y_{obs} \cdot \text{COD}_{removed} \qquad (6.1)$$

Using Eq. (6.1), for a 70% reduction in sludge production, the extra flux of nitrogen is around 15% in the case of a conventional French urban wastewater.

In a study by Zhang et al. (2009), for an ozone dosage of 50 mg O_3 (g SS)$^{-1}$, while the soluble COD increase was almost linear with the ozonation time, the increases in supernatant TN, TP, protein, and DNA were rapid in the first 15 min but then slowed down. Organic nitrogen and phosphorus compounds are the major contributors to the increase in soluble nitrogen and phosphorus concentrations (Camacho et al. 2005; Dogruel et al. 2007; Chu et al. 2008).

Nitrification   When biological nitrogen removal is achieved, both nitrification and heterotrophic COD removal occur simultaneously. As ozonation leads to a soluble COD release, nitrifiers could be outcompeted by heterotrophs for oxygen and ammonia. In addition, ozonation could inactivate nitrifiers. However, these features were not observed and it has been established (Huysmans et al. 2001; Déléris et al. 2002; Camacho et al. 2005; Paul and Debellefontaine 2007) that ozone treatment does not inactivate the autotrophic biomass if the specific ozone dosage (at the injection point) is sufficiently low. In contrast, the fraction of autotrophic biomass, quantified using respirometric tests, has been shown to increase from 5% (conventional value) to more than 10% (at an O_3 dosage of 0.04 g O_3 g^{-1} COD$_{removed}$, i.e., for a 60% ESP reduction) (Salhi 2003). It has been suggested that nitrifiers, overgrown by the faster-growing heterotrophs, may be protected inside the sludge floc and not be exposed to ozone as much as the surface-hugging heterotrophs (Böhler and Siegrist 2004). This aspect is discussed in greater depth in Section 6.5. Table 6.2 shows the nitrification yield [expressed as a ratio (in percent) of the nitrified N to the wastewater nitrifiable N]

TABLE 6.2   Nitrification Yield Obtained for a Combined Ozonation–AS System for Various Ozone Dosages (i.e., Various ESP Reductions)

ESP Reduction (%)	Additional TKN Flow (% TKN inlet)	Nitrification Yield (%)
60	15	92 ± 4
65	23	90 ± 4
100	0	94 ± 6
0	14	98 ± 2

Source: Camacho et al. (2003).

obtained in Salhi's (2003) pilot study of different ESP reduction yields. It was found that the nitrification yield was always close to 100%, and it is concluded that nitrogen removal can remain satisfactory even at high ESP reduction percentages, provided that a sufficiently large part of the treatment tank is maintained under anoxic conditions so that further denitrification can take place.

Denitrification The TKN/COD ratio obtained downstream of an ozonation unit is similar to that of a conventional French urban wastewater (0.08 to 0.11) (Camacho et al. 2005). Because the COD released is classified as easily biodegradable (S_S), this range of TKN/COD ratio is considered as sufficient for effective nitrogen removal at a conventional anoxic hydraulic retention time (HRT). In a denitrifying plant, the recycling of the ozonated sludge to the anoxic zone improves denitrification (Ahn et al. 2002; Park et al. 2004; Dytczak et al. 2007). However, ozonation saturates the mixed liquor with oxygen that will disturb the anoxic processes. A fraction of the easily biodegradable COD (S_B) released during ozonation should thus be consumed to remove the dissolved oxygen.

In the case of ozonation combined with AD, the extra nitrogen released must be removed either by a specific treatment (e.g., nitritation plus the Annamox process) or conventionally in the AS if enough oxygen and COD are provided.

P Removal P removal is often a crucial issue for wastewater treatment plants. Biological P removal is the result of both the P assimilation by all microorganisms present in sludge and of P accumulation by the phosphorus-accumulating organisms (PAOs) as described by

$$F_P = f_P p (1 - \text{PAO}) Y_{\text{obs}} \cdot \text{COD} + f_P \text{pao} \cdot \text{PAO} \cdot Y_{\text{obs}} \cdot \text{COD} \qquad (6.2)$$

where PAO represents phosphate-accumulating organisms (%), COD is the COD amount in wastewater [135 g COD (population equivalent (p.e.) $\cdot$ d^{-1}]; F_P the removal rate of phosphorus [g P (p.e. $\cdot$ d)$^{-1}$], f_Pp the P amount not in PAOs (0.02 g P g^{-1} VSS), $f_P$pao the maximum P amount accumulated in PAO (0.3 g P g^{-1} VSS), and Y_{obs} is the sludge yield factor observed (0.4 g VSS g^{-1} COD) in the case of raw wastewater treatment.

It is then clear that solubilization of particulate matter and a decrease in sludge production is not compatible with sufficient P recovery in organic sludge. For example, for 60% ESP reduction, the sludge removal efficiency would be decreased by 60%. Thus, for conventional COD and P concentrations [summed up in Eq. (6.2)], about 80% of the wastewater phosphorus (concentration: 3 g p.e.$^{-1}$) is removable by conventional AS, whereas only 30% is removable in the case where the ESP is reduced by 60%; and the P release during ozonation could even decrease this result. Including a combined physical–chemical precipitation of phosphorus in the combined system is thus necessary to cope with P removal constraints. However, methods of optimizing P removal in an ozonation–AS process with reduction of excess sludge production have been proposed by Salhi et al. (2004). According to these authors, if enhanced biological phosphorus removal is used, the PAO concentration in the sludge will increase with the reduction rate of the ESP, first due to inert fraction reduction, and second, also in proportion to the extra readily biodegradable COD flux solubilized during ozonation and consumed by PAOs. Calculations showed that a high-P concentrated sludge could thus be obtained in an ozonation–AS system, giving the opportunity to increase the P removal through the residual sludge withdrawal or to make P more available for precipitation and P recovery in a concentrated flux. Another optimization of P removal is proposed (Suzuki et al. 2006) by combining ozonation with an anaerobic-oxic-anoxic AS system having a phosphorus absorption column to achieve excess sludge reduction and phosphorus recovery. These authors ran their system for 92 d with a P removal efficiency of 85% on total phosphorus for a reduction in sludge of 34 to 100% at an ozone dose of 0.29 to 0.32 g O_3 g^{-1} TSS. Around 80% of the phosphorus was recovered.

Characteristics of the Residual Excess Sludge   During the ozonation tests, usually, the sludge volume index (SVI) strongly decreases (Kamiya and Hirotsuji 1998; Weemaes et al. 2000; Déléris et al. 2002; Böhler and Siegrist 2004; Paul and Debellefontaine 2007; Vergine et al. 2007). Sakai et al. (2003) reported an SVI

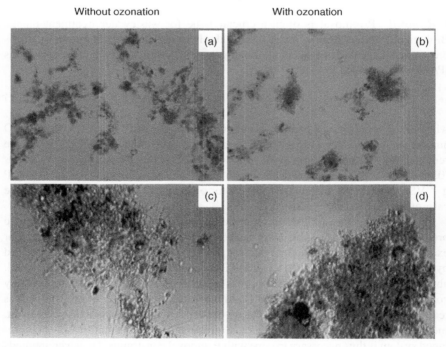

FIGURE 6.7 Comparison of the floc structure from a conventional AS (a and c) and an ozonation/AS system (b and d), showing improved compactness of the flocs (a and b) and the disappearance of filamentous bacteria (c and d). (a and b: magnifying ratio of 100, and c and d: magnifying ratio of 1000).

decrease from about 300 mL to less than 100 mL or even 50 mL, thus indicating that the sludge settled much more easily and became more compact. Micrographs of a sludge obtained during a conventional process and a sludge obtained during a treatment with ozone are compared in Fig. 6.7 (Paul and Debellefontaine 2007). They show very clearly (upper part) that the flocs were more compact when ozone was used. Figure 6.7 (lower part) shows that the use of ozone made the filamentous bacteria disappear and thus may have solved the settling problems associated with bulking. Similar trends were reported by Déléris (2001). Moreover, the negative impact of ozonation on dewaterability should be minimal in terms of the long-term operation (Dytczak et al. 2006). Bougrier et al. (2006) reported a strong increase in the capillary suction time from 151 s to 382 s for an ozone dosage of 0.1 g O_3 g^{-1} TSS. In the case of AD, the water content of the dewatered sludge cake from the train with ozonation was about 10% lower than that of the control sludge under similar dewatering conditions (Goel et al. 2004).

6.4 COST ASSESSMENT

Some studies have presented the economics of combined treatment used for ESP reduction (Yasui et al. 1996, 2005; Huysmans et al. 2001; Ahn et al. 2002; Böhler and Siegrist 2004; Caffaz et al. 2005; Paul et al. 2006; Ginestet 2007; Salsabil et al. 2010). The data given are difficult to exploit because the hypotheses used are not always well described. In this paragraph, the direct operating expense (OPEX) costs are given, based on the data obtained on pilot plants fed continuously with urban wastewater for the ozone combined processes (Paul et al. 2006; Ginestet 2007). For an SRT of 15 d, the sludge production yield was taken as 39 g TSS g^{-1} COD$_{removed}$ and the outlet COD as 50 mg L^{-1}. Sludge treatment costs were assumed to be around 160 ± 80 € [ton (t) DS]$^{-1}$. On average, sludge disposal costs (20% dryness and including transport) represent 320 ± 200 € (t DS)$^{-1}$. The total cost for sludge treatment and disposal is therefore 470 ± 280 € (t DS)$^{-1}$. It should be noted that depending on local conditions, sludge dryness, and type of disposal, the overall cost can vary from 250 to more than 1000 € (t DS)$^{-1}$. Operating costs account for the costs of the extra energy required, the reagent specifically used for the treatment, and for maintenance and labor. The energy cost was calculated using 0.065 € (kWh)$^{-1}$ for electricity, 2250 kJ kg^{-1} O_2 transferred for aeration. The ozone production yield on a fairly large scale is approximately 0.113 kg O_3 (kWh)$^{-1}$ (data from Ozone.ch), which represents an average cost for the ozone production of 580 €. (t O_3)$^{-1}$. Table 6.3 summarizes the distribution of direct OPEX and operating costs for the ozonation.

Based on these calculations, ozonation can be applied where the cost of sludge elimination is around 470 € (t DS)$^{-1}$ not produced. Ozonation appears to be competitive in combined processes. In addition, a high level of flexibility can be achieved using this technique, as the reduction yield of the ESP is a function of the ozone dosage. In Japan and some European Union countries, sludge ozonation has been applied successfully in practice (Sievers et al. 2004; Caffaz et al. 2005; Vergine et al. 2007).

TABLE 6.3   Direct Operational Expenses and Operating Cost
Distribution for a Wastewater Treatment Plant[a]

Combined Treatment	Ozone
Reduction of ESP (%)	70
Direct OPEX ($\in$ t^{-1})	367
OPEX distribution (%)	
Energy	34
Reagents	56
Labor	4
Maintenance	6

Source: Paul et al. (2006).
[a] 250,000 PE without a primary settler or anaerobic digester.

6.5   EFFECT OF OZONE ON SLUDGE

6.5.1   Synergy Between Ozonation and Biological Treatment

Considering the case of a combined process for ESP reduction, the results cited in this chapter establish, beyond any doubt, the synergistic effect between biological degradation and ozone oxidation. The results presented in Fig. 6.3 indicate that only 0.07 g O_3 was used to remove 1 g of COD, which clearly means that chemical oxidation by ozone was not the chief mechanism. However, the ratio between the amounts of O_3 used to the amount of COD treated must be monitored carefully and should be set as low as possible for economic reasons. This obviously requires advanced knowledge of the complex mechanisms involved in the process, and so far, very few studies have been devoted to understanding the reaction mechanisms and the effect of ozone on AS or ADS systems. In this section, first, the bases of ozone transfer are recalled to give better insight into the accessibility of the organic matter to ozone. Second, the mixed liquor containing the sludge is analyzed with respect to ozonation and biodegradation. A specific fractionation based on activated sludge model 1 (ASM1) (Henze et al. 1987) is useful here, to differentiate between particulate and soluble matter and between active biomass and inert particulate materials. Third, the effect of ozonation on these different fractions is considered; results on particulate COD solubilization by ozone during batch tests, on biodegradability changes of the solubilized COD, and on the dependence of microbial biomass deactivation and ozone dosage are presented. Finally, ozone transfer and sludge characteristics are considered together to improve our knowledge of the mechanisms occurring during ozonation of a complex real mixed liquor.

6.5.2   Some Fundamentals of Ozone Transfer

In gas–liquid systems, it is usually considered (Danckwerts 1970) that there is no mass transfer limitation in the gas phase when a gas with low solubility is transferred, as is the case for ozone. As this ozone transferred to the liquid is consumed primarily through fast reactions with the various dissolved organics, these reactions take place just beneath the gas–water interface—the corresponding zone is usually termed the liquid film and has a thickness of a few hundredths of a millimeter—and this results in the total absence of dissolved ozone within the bulk liquid (Danckwerts 1970). This is called the *fast kinetic regime* where the apparent rate of ozone mass transfer can exceed the maximum rate of physical gas–liquid mass transfer. This mass transfer rate enhancement is characterized by the enhancement factor, E:

$$E = \frac{N_{O3} \text{ with chemical reaction}}{k_L a C^* V} \qquad (6.3)$$

The numerator contains the actual flux of ozone, N_{O3}, transferred to the liquid, which is usually assessed by measuring the gas flow rate throughout the reactor and the concentrations of ozone at the inlet and outlet. The denominator contains the maximum flux corresponding to physical absorption, which depends on the equilibrium concentration of ozone in the liquid, C_L, and on the overall mass transfer coefficient, $k_L a$. It is important to note that the $k_L a$ value to be considered is the very value measured when transferring ozone to sewage within the reactor used. In most situations, the experimental determination will use oxygen and pure water, but correction methods, which are not developed here, exist (Cesbron 2004).

Figure 6.8 depicts the profile of dissolved ozone in this liquid film according to the value of the enhancement factor. Without any enhancement by chemical reactions, δ, the actual thickness of the film is at a maximum and the ozone concentration profile decreases linearly from the equilibrium concentration, C_L, to 0. In the presence of organic compounds leading to an enhancement of the transfer, the actual concentration profile of ozone corresponds to the dotted line and vanishes for an effective thickness, δ_{eff}, which is smaller than the total thickness and corresponds to

$$\delta_{eff} = \frac{\delta}{E} \qquad (6.4)$$

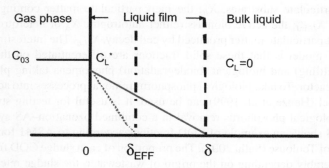

FIGURE 6.8 Schematic representation of the maximal and effective thickness of the liquid film, depending on the kinetic regime of the reaction.

Usually, the fastest-reacting compound (because of a high reactivity and/or high concentration) is preferentially attacked by ozone. It determines the E value and, consequently, the new effective film thickness, δ_{eff}, beyond which no more dissolved ozone is present. Figures commonly reported for E can reach 10, depending on the type of reactor and the conditions, leading to an effective film thickness that does not exceed a few micrometers. This phenomenon is a determining factor, first, for understanding which compound is preferentially attacked by ozone, and second, for choosing the type of gas–liquid contactor to use for ozone transfer and determining its optimal size. Usually, setups leading to a large gas–liquid contact surface, like impellors, static mixers, or venturi-like systems, should be preferred as they increase the active volume of the contactor and thus the efficiency of transfer of the ozone supplied to the system. For example, Chu et al. (2008) showed that microbubble ozonation was effective in increasing ozone utilization and improving sludge solubilization. Compared to the conventional bubble contactor, they found that more than twice the COD and total nitrogen, and eight times the total phosphorus content, were released from the sludge into the supernatant when the microbubble system was used at the same ozone dosage. Care must, however, be taken when dealing with activated sludge and/or mixed liquor because of their viscosity and their foaming capability. An in-depth analysis of ozone transfer in the case of activated sludge can be found in Cesbron's work (2004 or Cesbron et al., 2003).

6.5.3   Sludge Composition

To understand the effect of ozonation on ESP reduction, it is necessary to analyze the specific action of ozone on the various components of mixed liquor. From an overall point of view, mixed liquor contains a supernatant and a sludge that can be described as active and inactive biomass associated with organic and mineral substances organized in flocs. The sludge can be described in greater detail by considering ASM1 components (Henze et al. 1987). Notations given in Chapter 2 are used here. Two components characterize the soluble fraction: S_B is the easily biodegradable COD concentration and S_U is the refractory COD concentration. Four organic fractions are conventionally considered to characterize sludge: the slowly biodegradable particulate substrates, X_B; the inert particulate matter coming from the wastewater, $X_{U,inf}$; the active biomass (either autotrophic X_A or heterotrophic X_H); and the inert particulate matter produced by cell decay, $X_{U,E}$. The interesting point of this type of model is that these solid fractions are differentiated on the basis of physical (settling) and biological (biodegradation) phenomena taking place in the biological reactor. To take biological phosphorus removal processes into account, the ASM2 model (Henze et al. 1999) can be used. It is useful for testing strategies to improve biological phosphorus removal in a combined ozonation–AS system.

Table 6.4 shows an example of COD fractions according to ASM1 for the urban wastewater of Toulouse (Salhi 2003). The proportion of each sludge COD fraction can vary considerably depending on the origin of wastewater, the sludge retention time (SRT), and whether a primary treatment is present. These indicate that sludge fraction also varies greatly with wastewater composition and SRT (Déléris 2001; Salhi 2003).

TABLE 6.4   Proportion of the COD Fractions (Percent of Total) in Municipal Wastewater of Toulouse, France

X_H	$S_{U,inf}$	S_B	X_B	$X_{U,inf}$
19	16	11	6	48

Source: ASM1 of Henze et al. (1987).

It is important to note that the fractions $X_{U,inf}$ and $X_{U,E}$ taken together are often greater than the fraction X_H itself. As an example, Fig. 6.9 depicts the variation in the different fractions of organic sludge with SRT for a wastewater containing 20% of the total COD as $X_{U,inf}$. This confirms that the fraction of active biomass, X_H, is only a part of the total sludge. In fact, for long SRTs, the biological decay processes avoid any increase in X_H. In contrast, inert particulate material coming either from the wastewater, $X_{U,inf}$, or from the biomass through the decay processes, $X_{U,E}$, is not eliminated and will accumulate in proportion to the SRT. This accumulation should never be neglected. As an ESP reduction facility is intended to extract less sludge than does a conventional facility, it leads automatically to increased SRT. Consequently, it is concluded that an additional ozone contactor should be directed primarily at reducing these inert fractions, $X_{U,inf}$ and $X_{U,E}$, and turning them in to biodegradable COD, either soluble or at least particulate, and hydrolyzable COD. When reducing these inert fractions, attention should be paid to keeping the biological step efficient. This means that, if possible, no active biological cells, X_H, should be reduced by ozonation. This is a first fundamental point for running a treatment facility efficiently while reducing ESP. During ozonation batch experiments, the effect on active biomass and on inert materials can be differentiated by measuring the evolution of biomass activity and COD solubilization during ozonation.

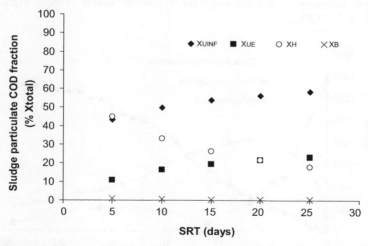

FIGURE 6.9 Calculation of sludge amounts and composition as a function of SRT for a conventional AS process according to the ASM1 (modified notation is used). [From Déléris (2001) and Salhi (2003).]

The distinction between particulate matter and soluble matter, made in the ASM models, is also essential for understanding the action of ozone on the mixed liquor and on the various COD fractions of the sludge (Cesbron et al. 2003). Because the effective film thickness, δ_{eff}, beyond which no more dissolved ozone is present, is small, a competition for ozone occurs. This aspect is analyzed in detail in the following sections.

6.5.4 Effect of Ozone on Activated Sludge: Batch Tests

In addition to the continuous tests running activated sludge pilot plants in association with ozone, a series of batch tests have been run to characterize the ozonation effect on sludge. These tests usually consist of treating samples of sludge in an ozonation contactor and analyzing the remaining compounds, notably the amount of solubilized COD and its biodegradability. The solubilized COD is quantified after centrifugation (with various accelerations) or after filtration (with various filter types and cutoffs). Biodegradability is assessed by respirometric techniques assuming a value of the growth yield or using a mass balance on the COD.

Stoechiometry Between Ozone Dose and COD Solubilization   Ozonation causes sludge COD solubilization (Kamiya and Hirotsuji 1998; Nishimura et al. 1999; Déléris et al. 2000) and if the specific dose transferred is high enough, complete COD mineralization (Déléris et al. 2000). In the latter case, the specific ozone dosage applied reaches values as high as $10 \, g \, O_3 \, g^{-1}$ VSS. Figure 6.10 describes the results obtained by showing the time course of the dissolved organic carbon, the particulate organic carbon, and the CO_2 during batch ozonation. Ozone is able to mineralize the sludge COD completely (only 5% of carbon remains unoxidized). The CO_2 production becomes significant only for a specific ozone dosage higher than $0.15 \, g \, O_3 \, g^{-1}$, COD_{VSS}.

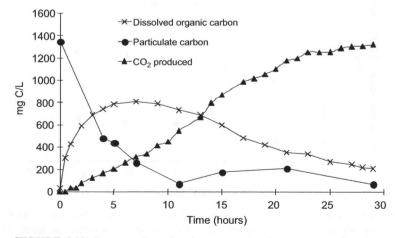

FIGURE 6.10 Concentration of carbonaceous species versus reaction time.

TABLE 6.5 Various Types and Characteristics of Activated Sludges Used during Batch Ozonation Studies[a]

Type of Sludge	Type of Wastewater	AS Plant Characteristics	Sludge Concentration (g COD L^{-1})
AS 1	Urban, raw	EBPR pilot	5.0
AS 2	Urban, settled	Highly loaded AS	3.3
AS 3	Urban, slightly settled	O$_3$/AS pilot	1.5
AS 4	Urban, slightly settled	O$_3$/AS pilot	1.5
E. coli	Synthetic glucose solution	Pure culture batch	1.0

[a] The same sludge was used by Cesbron (2004) and Salhi (2003) for a set of experiments.

A constant proportion between COD solubilization and the ozone dosage transferred has frequently been reported when the ozone dosage is not too high (Kamiya and Hirotsuji 1998; Salhi 2003; Manterola et al. 2008). Manterola et al. (2008), who used ozone dosages between 25 and 35 mg O$_3$ g^{-1} TSS, found a maximum value for this solubilization, certainly due to the start of COD mineralization. The solubilization yield, η_{O3}, calculated as the ratio of the solubilized COD to the quantity of ozone transferred, was found to be equal to 1 g DOC g^{-1} O$_3$ in the work of Kamiya and Hirotsuji (1998) and close to 2.8 g COD g^{-1} O$_3$ in a study by Salhi (2003). In the latter case, ozone dosages between 0.01 and 0.15 g O$_3$ g^{-1} COD$_{VSS}$ treated were applied to different sludges with different biochemical compositions. Sludge was sampled either on conventional AS (AS 1 and 2), or on continuously treated sludge—sludge coming from continuous ozonation–AS combined treatment pilot plants run at different ozone dosages and under steady-state conditions (AS 3 and 4)—or on a pure culture of *Escherichia coli*. The characteristics of these ASs are given in Table 6.5, and Fig. 6.11 shows the time course of the solubilized COD for the four sludges and the *E. coli* culture. It is obvious

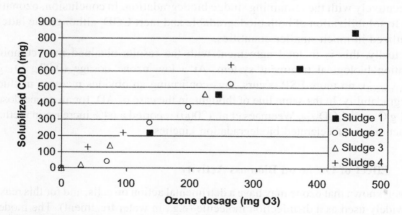

FIGURE 6.11 Solubilized COD versus ozone dosage for four sludges with different compositions. [From Salhi (2003).]

that η_{O3} remains identical whatever the sludge composition, although it is slightly lower for *E. coli* (in that case, equal to 1.5 g COD g^{-1} O$_3$). The linearity between the ozone dosage and the solubilized COD demonstrates that ozone availability limits the solubilization reaction.

COD Biodegradability   One key point for efficient use of the sludge ozonation strategy to reduce ESP is based on the transformation of the inert particulate COD into biodegradable COD. The change in biodegradability is assessed primarily using batch biological degradation tests [ultimate biochemical oxygen demand (BOD), biological methane potential (BMP), or use of a respirometer to indicate the short-term biodegradability]. It can also be determined by performing a COD mass balance on a continuous treatment system. Usually, after sludge ozonation, a strong increase in COD biodegradability is observed by all the authors who have quantified it (Scheminski et al. 2000; Saktaywin et al. 2005; Salhi 2003). However, the extent of biodegradability varies from one author to another. In the work of Saktaywin et al. (2005), working only on solubilized COD, 60% of the soluble COD generated due to ozonation was found to be biodegradable, while the remaining soluble COD was still refractory. During short-term biodegradability tests performed on the COD solubilized by ozone, Salhi (2003) found a ratio of biodegraded COD to the initially solubilized COD equal to 1, indicating that the entire solubilized COD can be considered as biodegradable and classified as readily biodegradable or hydrolyzable, according to the ASM1 model classification (Henze et al. 1987). Very similar results were obtained for the other samples of sludge (described in Table 6.5), and in addition, complete biodegradability of the solubilized COD was confirmed through ultimate BOD tests for some of the samples. However, on a continuous lab-scale pilot, to close the COD mass balance taking into account the physical (soluble or particulate) form of the COD, Salhi (2003) demonstrated that an extra nonbiodegradable COD had to be solubilized, in a delayed fashion, directly in the continuous biological reactor consecutively with the remaining sludge biodegradation. In conclusion, ozonation leads to solubilization of both biodegradable and inert COD, although the latter is solubilized in much smaller quantities.

Actually, this is in total agreement with the results obtained in a combined ozonation–biological treatment system. At a low ozone dosage (0.07 g O$_3$ g^{-1} COD$_{removed}$), no more ESP occurs, thus confirming an obvious increase in sludge biodegradability. In the same line of thought, in the case of AD, for an ozone dosage of 0.1 g O$_3$ g^{-1} COD$_{VSS}$, Weemaes et al. (2000) reported a 64% increase in methane production and accelerated biodegradation kinetics.

6.5.5   Effect of Ozone on Biomass Activity

It is well known that ozone may have a detrimental action on cells, and for this reason, it is widely used as a disinfection molecule (e.g., in water treatment). The mode of action of ozone on cells is complex and not fully understood. An effect of ozone on the cell membrane was suggested very early (Christensen and Giese 1954), and many

TABLE 6.6 Cell Inactivation by Ozone for Organic Sludge[a]

Reference	Specific Ozone Dosage (g O_3 g^{-1} SS)	Cell Inactivation
Yasui and Shibata (1994)	< 0.05	10%
Nishimura et al. (1999)	0.03	No loss of dehydrogenase activity
	0.05	80% (for nitrifiers)
Kobayashi et al. (2001)	< 0.01	No deactivation
Salhi (2003)	0.1	90%
Saktaywin et al. (2005)	0.03–0.04	70%
Lee et al. (2005)	0.05	97%
Chu et al. (2008)	0.02 (bubble reactor)	50%
	0.02 (microbubble reactor)	80%
Yan et al. (2009)	> 0.02	Alteration in DGGE profile

[a] Correction factor between COD and VSS taken as 1.4.

other studies have been performed to better understand the mechanisms or the kinetics of ozone action on cells (Hoigné and Bader 1983; Finch and Smith 1989; Finch et al. 1992). It has been shown that the cell deactivation follows the Chick–Watson model:

$$\frac{dN}{dt} = -kN \cdot [\text{oxidant}] \tag{6.5}$$

where N is number of active cells and k is an inactivation constant. However, various authors have pointed out the requirement for a minimum ozone dose to start the reduction of cell activity, this critical ozone dose being necessary to oxidize other, more reactive compounds, such as humic acids (Finch et al. 1992).

Few studies have been reported on the effect of ozonation on cells embedded in flocs and in the case of real mixed liquor. Table 6.6 summarizes results on cell inactivation at various specific ozone dosages from various authors. To understand these results, one should always consider the specific ozone dose transferred to sludge, the sludge characteristics, and the quality of the supernatant of the mixed liquor, as ozone transfer and ozone action depend strongly on these aspects (Cesbron et al. 2003; Cesbron 2004; Chu et al. 2008).

Salhi (2003) reported an in-depth analysis of cell deactivation in ozonation batch experiments with *E. coli* and AS 1 to 4, whose characteristics are presented in Table 6.5, and on other sludges whose characteristics are not described here. Heterotrophic and autotrophic activities were determined by measuring the maximum oxygen uptake rate (OUR_{max}). PAO activity was also determined following the capacity for P release. These activity measurements were conducted in two steps: just after sampling the sludges from their reactor of origin, and just after treating these sludges with doses of ozone ranging between 0.001 and 0.2 g O_3 transferred g^{-1} COD_{VSS}. It can be seen in Fig. 6.11 that the cell survival rate, defined as the ratio between the residual OUR_{max} of the sludge (after ozonation) and the initial OUR_{max} of the sludge (before ozonation), is plotted versus the ozone dosage for the four AS. In this log-log plot, a conventional linear relationship was found between the two variables, as previously reported (Finch and Smith 1989), and for all sludge samples, biomass inactivation began to occur only when the ozone dosage was set above a threshold value close to 0.01 g O_3 transferred g^{-1} COD in the sludge sample. It has to be pointed out that the ozone dosage ($\times 10$) must be increased strongly to reduce the cell activity significantly, and this is not realistic economically.

This threshold value of 0.01 g O_3 transferred g^{-1} COD is much higher than the ozone dose actually injected into the ozonation contactor during the combined continuous treatment process run by Salhi (2003). In consequence, he concluded that no cell deactivation due to ozonation occurred in his continuous ozonation–AS system run during his Ph.D. work. Consequently, if the ozone-specific dosage (in terms of g O_3 g^{-1} $SS_{treated}$) at the injection point is sufficiently low, cell deactivation by ozone is very limited in the ozone–AS combined treatment and is not the dominant mechanism for excess sludge reduction. Actually, ozone probably reacts preferentially with the inert particulate material coming either from the wastewater, $X_{U,inf}$, or from the biomass through the decay processes, $X_{U,E}$. To explain this observation, we recall the ozone transfer theory and that ozone is in limited amounts compared to the total COD. Due to a high E value induced by high reactivity and high COD concentration, the effective film thickness, δ_{eff}, is very small compared to the size of the flocs containing the viable biomass. It is assumed that the organic matter $X_{U,inf}$ and $X_{U,E}$ (which represented more than 50% of total soluble COD under the actual operating conditions of the various AS pilot plants) in some way protected the viable cells, X_H, against ozonation. Thus, ozone was specifically directed to the inert organic and mineral material present in the sludge. The fact that the inactivation rate found in activated sludge was 10 times lower than that in the pure *E. coli* culture (Fig. 6.12) confirms this assumption.

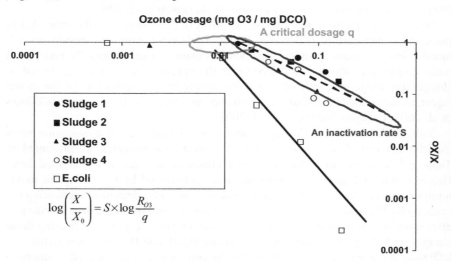

FIGURE 6.12 Activity loss (as the ratio of residual to initial OUR_{max}) resulting from batch ozonation for four types of sludge and a pure culture of *E. coli*. Dependence on the ozone dosage is shown.

6.5.6 Competition for Ozone in Mixed Liquor

The various factors affecting the performance of ozonation on activated sludge are the pH value, the nature and concentrations of the various oxidizable organics, and the ozone dose. However, the competition between a target refractory organic compound and other biodegradable organic compounds, the presence of soluble oxidant scavengers, and the efficiency of ozone mass transfer are also key factors. Hoigné and Bader (1976) stress the importance of the competition between particulate organic matter (e.g., microorganisms) and dissolved species to react with OH$^\bullet$ radicals produced by the decomposition of ozone during water treatment. Because these OH$^\bullet$ radicals react very rapidly with most categories of dissolved species, they are likely to be completely scavenged before they encounter a dispersed target particle. Inhibition of the indirect reaction of ozone by some radical scavengers, such as lactic acid and SO_4^{2-} released from the microbial cell into the soluble part is also mentioned by Yan et al. (2009). This can also occur with the various particulate organic fractions of an AS. In such a mixed liquor, a huge number of particulate species can react rapidly with hydroxyl radicals—or with molecular ozone—so that hardly any ozone will remain available for destroying the targeted inert particulate matter. Consequently, an optimized ozone treatment system should attempt to reduce this possible major drawback. It is important to consider that the relative importance of the ozone attack toward each fraction or compound of the sludge can be different from one reactor to another because of different enhancement factors, E, which have an influence on the selectivity, even when the various reactors have been correctly designed for transferring identical quantities of ozone. To illustrate competition processes in the case of mixed liquor, a study by Cesbron (2004) is discussed next.

Ozone Transfer and Reactivity with Sludge   Cesbron (2004) performed batch ozonation tests with the same four types of sludges as those used by Salhi (2003). The characteristics of these sludges are presented in Table 6.5. The ozone transferred into the liquid is plotted against the ozonation time in Fig. 6.13. In all cases, the amount of

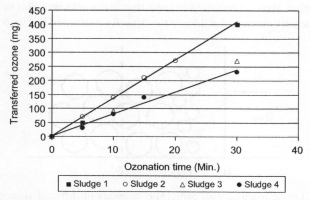

FIGURE 6.13 Amount of ozone transferred into the liquid phase versus the batch ozonation time for the various sludges tested. [From Cesbron et al. (2004).]

ozone transferred appears to be proportional to the contact time. The maximal physical absorption rate, $k_L a C_L^*$, was determined previously and found to be constant throughout a given experiment, so the enhancement factor E [Eq. (6.3)] can simply be deduced from the slope of the straight line in Fig. 6.13. The E values are always higher than 2, confirming that ozone is consumed through fast reactions, which take place only in the liquid film near the water–gas interface. The same E value—about 3.5—was obtained for sludges 1 and 2 taken from treatment facilities where no ozone was used. A lower (but again constant) E value—about 2.3—was obtained for sludges 3 and 4 taken, this time, from combined ozone–activated sludge pilot-scale plants. This suggests that the reactions involved are slower in the second case, certainly because the compounds leading to the highest E values no longer accumulate in the continuously ozonated sludge. Thus, affinity for ozone controls the chemical reactions whatever the sludge COD fractions. However, even for the sludges having the lowest reactivity, cell activity does not decrease and the same solubilization yield is observed. The highly reactive molecules come mainly from the inert organic suspended material, as no cell deactivation occurs. This is again proof that the amount of COD available from the refractory fractions, $X_{U,\text{inf}}$ and $X_{U,E}$, is large compared to the amount of ozone injected, A_{O3}.

Ozone Transfer in Systems Containing Particulate Matter   The maximum thickness of the film, δ, is expressed by Eq. (6.6), where the diffusivity of ozone is $D_{O3} = 1.74 \times 10^{-9}\,\mathrm{m^2\,s^{-1}}$ and the film transfer coefficient is $k_L \approx 1 \times 10^{-4}\,\mathrm{m\,s^{-1}}$ in the ozone contactor used. This leads to $\delta = 15$ to $20\,\mu\mathrm{m}$. In consideration of the actual enhancement factor (E), the effective thickness of the film (δ_{eff}) is always less than $10\,\mu\mathrm{m}$. As the reaction with ozone occurs only in the liquid film, it appears necessary to consider the specificities of reactions with particulate material having a characteristic size somewhat greater than the effective film thickness, in addition to the specificities of reactions with dissolved organic matter:

$$\delta = \frac{D_{O3}}{k_L} \tag{6.6}$$

In the case of ozonation of activated sludge, this particulate material may enhance the gas absorption, thus contributing to reduction in the effective film thickness, δ_{eff}: The smaller the particles are, the thinner the film. As illustrated in Fig. 6.14, reacting

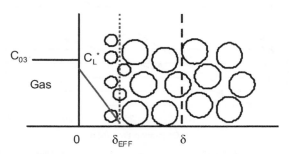

FIGURE 6.14 Ozone reacting with particulate materials of different sizes. The effective thickness of the transfer film is shown in relation to the actual particle size.

particles migrate to the limit of the effective film, where they react with ozone. They produce solubilized species associated with small colloids, which are partially oxidized by ozone near the gas–liquid interface, but which migrate primarily toward the bulk liquid for further biological degradation. In consequence, gas absorption will be very high if small flocs are in high concentration, which could be achieved by destructuring the flocs prior to their ozonation. In addition, soluble compounds (both organic and mineral) can decrease the efficiency of particulate matter ozonation. The negative effect on ozonation efficiency of compounds produced during anaerobic treatments or of $FeCl_3$ used for dephosphatation has been studied by Cesbron (2004).

6.6 MODELING OZONATION EFFECT

Models are useful to help our understanding of the mechanisms of ozonation and the behavior of the combined ozonation–biodegradation system or to help in process design. The first model for a combined process of ozone oxidation–AS treatment was presented by Yasui and Shibata (1994) from a study on a bench-scale reactor fed continuously with a synthetic broth made primarily of peptone and yeast extract. This model, based on mass balance, considers an active and an inactive biomass, X_H and X_U, respectively:

$$V \frac{dX_H}{dt} = Y \cdot \mathrm{VLR_{rem}} - bVX_H - Q_dX_H - Q_rX_H + yQ_r(X_H + X_U) \qquad (6.7)$$

$$V \frac{dX_U}{dt} = -Q_dX_U - Q_rX_U + rQ_r(X_H + X_U) \qquad (6.8)$$

In Eq. (6.7), the variation in active biomass concentration is mainly a balance between biomass net production, due to growth and decay, and the net biomass generated after ozonation. The effect of ozonation on sludge is represented by the term y, a global parameter with the signification of a net growth yield. It is the net difference between biomass inactivation by ozone and growth on the substrate generated by the chemical treatment. An additional mass balance is performed on inactive biomass X_U.

In Eq. (6.8) the effect of ozonation on inert biomass is represented by a second parameter, r, which is the mass of inactive biomass produced per total mass of ozone-treated sludge.

Under steady-state conditions, combining Eqs. (6.7) and (6.8) leads to

$$b \frac{X_A}{X} + D + (1 - z)R = \frac{Y \cdot \mathrm{VLR_{rem}}}{X} \qquad (6.9)$$

in which reduction in excess sludge production is defined as a function of parameters y and r and of the treatment frequency (daily mass of sludge treated per mass of sludge in the reactor) (Yasui and Shibata 1994). The term $1-z$ represents the biological mineralization ratio between ozonated sludge and treated sludge [i.e., $1-(y+r)$]. Then Yasui and Shibata (1994) calculated an excess sludge reduction efficiency (η_{ESP}) under different ozonation conditions by comparing sludge production with and without ozonation:

$$\eta_{ESP} = 1 - \frac{Y \cdot OLR - b/(X_H/X) - (1-z)R}{Y \cdot OLR - b} \tag{6.10}$$

At a given organic loading rate, this equation indicates how η_{ESP} depends on $1-z$ and R, that is, on the ozone dosage and the recirculation ratio between the ozonation and the activated sludge reactor. This model is interesting for visualizing the ozone consumption in a combined process, but the use of global parameters does not provide an understanding of why ozone efficiency may change with SRT or with the wastewater characteristics.

Salhi (2003) proposed a combination of the ASM1 model (Henze et al. 1987) with an ozonation model (termed O_3M). The main advantages of this were (1) to use the different fractions of AS that are linked to the wastewater COD fractionation and to biological processes such as growth, decay, and hydrolysis, and (2) to establish an ozonation model based on experimental results characterizing the various effects of ozone on sludge mineralization, solubilization, X_H and X_A deactivation, and ozonation-generated COD biodegradability. In batch experiments by Salhi (2003), the effect of ozone on activated sludge was quantified by looking into the ozone transfer rate, COD solubilization, and biotreatability versus the ozone dosage. Results led to the development of a simple model for sludge ozonation with consideration of the ASM1 COD fractions in sludge. This model rests on the following hypotheses:

- For a specific ozone dosage lower than the threshold value of 0.01 g O_3 transferred g^{-1} COD, heterotrophic biomass (X_H) was not deactivated, and as no decrease was observed in the Y_H value, it can be concluded that ozone attacks only the nonviable fractions ($X_{U,inf}$, $X_{U,E}$, and X_B) of the sludge.
- Because each of the sludges studied had different COD fractionations (in the ASM1 sense) and because a constant solubilization yield was found for these sludges, COD solubilization due to ozone appeared to be independent of the type of inert COD fractions present in the sludge. Therefore, a proportional attack of nonviable sludge COD fractions was proposed [term 1 of Eq. (6.11)] to describe the ozone-solubilizing effect on a treated sludge. In addition, no COD compound could resist the ozone attack.
- Within the SRT applied, a delayed solubilization of soluble inert COD was observed in the biological reactor, classified as S_U production resulting from ozone attack on $X_{U,inf}$, and $X_{U,E}$ [term 2 of Eq. (6.11)].

Equation (6.11) gives the fluxes of particulate matter that will be solubilized due to ozonation:

$$Q_{xj} = \eta_{O3}Q_{O3}\frac{X_j}{X_{U,inf} + X_B + X_{U,E}} + \eta'_{O3}Q_{O3}\frac{X_j}{X_{U,inf} + X_B + X_{U,E}} \tag{6.11}$$

where Q_{XJ} is the COD solubilization rate of the X_J fraction (g COD d^{-1}), Q_{O3} the ozone dosage (g O$_3$ d^{-1}); X_J the nonviable sludge COD fractions $X_{U,\text{inf}}$ or X_B or $X_{U,E}$, η_{O3} the ratio of S_S production from X_J to the ozone amount: 2.8 g COD g^{-1} O$_3$, η'_{O3} the ratio of S_U production from X_J to the ozone amount: 1.9 g COD g^{-1} O$_3$. This "ozonation model" was thus combined with a conventional ASM1 model (Henze et al. 1987) describing the AS. Equation (6.12) gives the ESP$_{\text{ozone}}$ in an ozonation–AS combined system:

$$\text{ESP}_{\text{ozone}} = f_{UP}Q_{\text{COD}} + Y_H \frac{1}{1 + [b'/[\theta_{B,\text{ref}}/(1 - \text{ESPR})]][1 - Y_H(1 - f')]} \left[1 + b'\frac{\theta_{B,\text{ref}}}{1 - \text{ESPR}}f'\right]$$
$$\cdot [(1 - f_{UP})Q_{\text{COD}} + \eta_{O3}Q_{O3}] - (\eta_{O3} + \eta'_{O3})Q_{O3}$$

$$(6.12)$$

In Fig. 6.15, simulation results are compared with some experimental results obtained using the combined process in a bench-scale pilot plant. It can be observed that the model correctly predicts the ESP reduction depending on the ozone dosage. The authors also characterize the capacity of the model to predict the VSS concentration in the aerated tank, the outlet soluble COD, and nitrogen removal.

Other approaches have recently been described in the literature to take the specific action of ozone on the COD fraction of sludge into account. For example, three models were proposed to test the action of ozone on active biomass or on all the particulate solids (Frigon and Isazadeh 2011). Model 1 assumes that ozone affects only active biomass by promoting cryptic growth, model 2 assumes that ozone affects all the solid fractions (X_H, $X_{U,E}$, $X_{U,\text{inf}}$) equally, and model 3 assumes that biomass is inactivated at a specific rate higher than the specific rate of transformation of the other solid fractions by ozone. These models are extensions of IWA ASM3, and validation was performed by comparing the results from simulation with data obtained from a

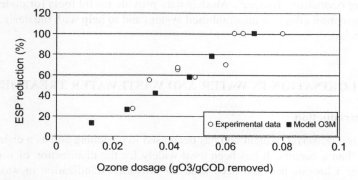

FIGURE 6.15 Comparison of experimental excess sludge reduction and excess sludge reduction simulated using the OM3 ozonation model developed by Salhi (2003). Excess sludge reduction is expressed as a percentage of the ESP of a control line. Ozone dosage is expressed as a ratio between the ozone transferred and the ozonated sludge COD removed in the biological system.

pilot plant. Contrary to what was found by Salhi (2003), Frigon and Isazadeh (2011) found that the best fit of the data of a pilot-scale system was obtained by a model 3, where active biomass was inactivated at a higher rate than the rest of the solid fractions. In our opinion, this could be reached only at a high ozone-specific dosage (high contact time).

6.7 REMARKS ON SLUDGE OZONATION

Considering studies available from the literature, ozonation–biodegradation appears as an efficient, flexible system to reduce the ESP. In the case of AS, an ozone dosage around 0.05 to 0.07 g O_3 g^{-1} COD$_{removed}$ applied at around 0.03 g O_3 g^{-1} SS is necessary to avoid sludge wastage completely. However, to avoid mineral accumulation, it is advisable to maintain a low level of sludge leakage. Different systems have been tested at full scale, and some are currently running cost-effectively in wastewater treatment plants that have high sludge disposal costs, operational problems such as sludge foaming and bulking, or constraints on outlet refractory COD. Combined with AD, ozonation can decrease the sludge wastage amount and increase methane production. The ozone dosage should be determined with more accuracy in that case.

The sludge ozonation treatment phase is compatible with the biological system: An increase in effluent COD is observed, but COD and nitrogen removal efficiencies are maintained, and provided that the ESP reduction yield is not too high, phosphorus can still be eliminated from the system together with the remaining residual sludge. Sludge dewatering does not seem to be strongly modified.

Understanding the mechanisms of the action of ozone on sludge is the key factor for a rational design of the ozonation contactors and of the ozonation–biodegradation system. Ozone transfer and selectivity are key parameters in optimizing ozonation efficiency. Models may provide useful tools for understanding the ozonation effect on the combined system and to help with the design of the entire process.

6.8 CHLORINATION IN WATER AND WASTEWATER TREATMENT

6.8.1 Introduction

Chlorine is a powerful oxidant and has been used in bleaching and as a disinfectant for more than a century. It has been used widely for the disinfection of water and wastewater. Chlorine has also been used for biosolids stabilization in wastewater treatment plants to reduce sludge putrescibility and pathogen concentration as well as to improve sludge dewaterability (Wang et al. 2007). At standard temperature and pressure, chlorine is a yellow-green gas that has a distinctive strong smell, the smell of bleach. The dissolved chlorine oxidizes organic material, including pathogenic organisms and viruses. Various theories have been put forward to explain the germicidal effects of chlorine. These include oxidizing the germ cells, altering cell permeability, altering cell protoplasm, inhibiting enzyme activity, and damaging the cell DNA and RNA (Korich et al. 1990). Chlorine appears to react strongly with lipids in the cell membrane, and membranes having high lipid concentrations appear to be more susceptible to destruction (Black & Veatch Corporation 2010).

When chlorine is added to water, it reacts to form a pH-dependent equilibrium mixture of chlorine, hypochlorous acid, and hydrochloric acid (Hammer 2008):

$$Cl_2 + H_2O \rightarrow HOCl + HCl \tag{6.13}$$

Depending on the pH, hypochlorous acid partly dissociates to hydrogen and hypochlorite ions:

$$HClO \rightarrow H^+ + ClO^- \tag{6.14}$$

In an acidic solution, the major species are Cl_2 and HOCl, whereas in an alkaline solution, effectively only ClO^- is present. The effectiveness of the disinfection using chlorine is determined by the pH of the water. Hypochlorous acid (HOCl, electrically neutral) and hypochlorite ions (OCl^-, electrically negative) will form free chlorine when bound together. Hypochlorous acid is more reactive and has a stronger oxidizing ability than hypochlorite. The cell wall of pathogenic microorganisms is negatively charged by nature. As such, it can be penetrated by the neutral hypochlorous acid rather than by the negatively charged hypochlorite ion. As a result, hypochlorous acid can penetrate slime layers, cell walls, and protective layers of microorganisms and effectively kill them. The microorganisms will either die or suffer from reproductive failure. In the presence of ammonia and organic nitrogen in the water, chloramines and organic chloramines will also be formed. These are also effective germicides and viricides (Black & Veatch Corporation 2010).

6.8.2 Chlorination-Assisted Biological Process for Sludge Reduction

Chlorine is a strong oxidizing agent, as discussed above. When sludge is in contact with chlorine, most of the sludge microorganisms will be killed and oxidized to organic substances. These organic substances can be biodegraded in the biological process of the aeration tank when they are returned to the tank. In fact, chlorination has been used for sludge solubilization and cell lysis (Wang et al. 2007; Paola et al. 2010). A chlorination-assisted biological process was investigated in a lab-scale system for minimizing excess sludge production (Chen et al. 2001; Saby et al. 2002; Takdastan et al. 2010). This chlorination-assisted biological process is similar to the ozonation-activated sludge process: that is, a portion of excess sludge was subjected to a chlorine dose and the chlorinated mixed liquor was then returned to the aeration tank for its further biodegradation. Figure 6.16 is a process diagram of the chlorination-assisted biological process for sludge reduction. It shows that the equipment needed for this process is minimal, and this is one of the main attractions of the process. The clarifier

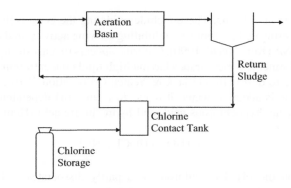

FIGURE 6.16 Process diagram of chlorination-assisted biological process for sludge reduction.

may not be needed if a membrane bioreactor is used in the process. The portion for the chlorination can be equal to the amount of sludge wastage.

The chlorination-assisted biological process for sludge reduction has the following advantages (Liu 2003; Paola et al. 2010):

- Chlorine is cheaper than other oxidants.
- Equipment for chlorination is cheaper and the operation is simpler than ozonation.

The operating cost of chlorination is only 10% that of ozonation in terms of disinfection practice (Tchobanoglous et al. 2003; Wang et al. 2009). It is clear that the chlorination-assisted biological process has advantages over the ozonation-activated sludge system in terms of operational cost. It should be recalled that chlorine is a weak oxidant compared to ozone. The dosage of chlorine used in the chlorination-activated sludge process is about 7 to 13 times higher than that of ozone applied in the ozonation-activated sludge process (Liu 2003). On the other hand, a chlorination-assisted biological process for sludge reduction has the following disadvantages (Saby et al. 2002; Liu 2003, Paola et al. 2010):

- Formation of by-products of trihalomethanes
- Increase in soluble COD in the effluent
- Worsening of sludge settleability

Although the chlorination-assisted biological process is more cost-effective than the ozonation-activated sludge system, chlorination generates potentially harmful by-products that would pose a serious challenge to the full-scale application of this technique. These disinfection by-products may increase the risk of certain cancers (Karanfil et al. 2008). Previous research has shown that when raw water is made to react with chlorine, the yield of trihalomethanes (THMs) increases according to the amount of chlorine input (Park 2001), while long-term chlorine demand and the formation of THMs could follow second-order kinetics (Gallard and von Gunten 2002). Saby et al. (2002) found that a concentration not higher than 200 bbp of THMs was detected during the entire period of operation of a bioreactor. Such a low THM concentration was probably due to the volatization of THMs during the chlorine treatment. However, it is necessary to investigate the potential of THM formation and its gas emission.

Chlorination treatment of the excess sludge resulted in the increase of soluble chemical oxygen demand in the effluent and poor sludge settleability (Saby et al. 2002; Wei et al. 2003; Takdastan et al. 2010). These will surely create potential problems when the chlorination process is used for sludge reduction. However, to minimize these potential problems, it is recommended that a separate membrane unit be used instead of a conventional sedimentation tank (Saby et al. 2002). So far, the use of chlorination has been limited to lab-scale systems; no full-scale application has been reported in the literature. Studies of a full-scale application in a plant will surely be required to demonstrate the feasibility of this technique.

6.8.3 Effect of Chlorine Dosage on Sludge Reduction

Dosing of chlorine to a portion of return sludge has a significant impact on sludge production. The study by Saby et al. (2002) showed that excess sludge treated with 66 mg Cl_2 g^{-1} MLSS showed a 67% sludge reduction compared with a reference system without chlorination, as shown in Fig. 6.17. Although the system could not reach 100% sludge reduction as obtained by the ozonation treatment, it is expected

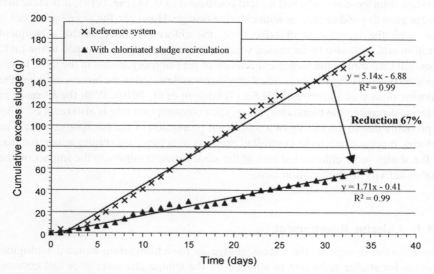

FIGURE 6.17 Sludge production rates in a continuous system without and with chlorination treatment of the excess sludge. [From Saby et al. (2002).]

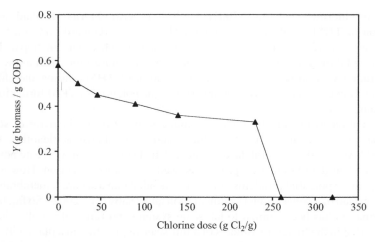

FIGURE 6.18 Effect of chlorine dosage on sludge production. [From Takdastan et al. (2010).]

that by increasing the chlorine dose, a more complete minimization of excess sludge may be achieved. Thus, zero sludge growth could be achieved in such a system.

An increase in the chlorine dosage decreases the sludge production rate: that is, the yield coefficient. It was reported by Takdastan et al. (2010) that a 90-mg chlorine dose in 1 g of MLSS of the excess resulted in a yield coefficient of 0.41 g biomass g^{-1} COD in a sequencing batch reactor operated at a solid retention time of 10 days, while a 230-mg chlorine dose only had a yield coefficient of 0.33 (Fig. 6.18). It is clear that sludge growth yield decreases with chlorine dosage. However, the negative impact is that, with the increase in chlorine dose, the chlorine residue in the subsequent aeration tank will also be increased when chlorinated sludge is returned to the tank. This will then inhibit the biological activity of the microorganisms in the tank. It was reported that 0.01 mg L^{-1} of residual chlorine was detected in the bioreactor when the chlorine dose was 140 mg g^{-1} MLSS (Takdastan et al. 2010). With the increase in chlorine dosage to the bioreactor, the oxygen consumption rate is also reduced. This is probably due to the killing of a significant proportion of the microorganisms. The chlorine dosage needs to be controlled properly to achieve maximum mineralization of the sludge to be chlorinated and, at the same time, to minimize the impact on the sludge activity in the aeration tank.

6.8.4 Chlorine Requirement

The chlorine dosage to the excess sludge in the chlorination-assisted biological process for sludge reduction is affected by the sludge characteristics and concentration, contact time, pH, and temperature. The requirement of the residual chlorine level in the aeration tank must also be considered when determining the chlorine

TABLE 6.7 Sludge Reduction Potential by Chlorination and Ozonation

Chlorine/Ozone Dosage	Sludge Reduction (%)	References
Lab-scale activated sludge membrane bioreactor		
66 mg Cl_2 g^{-1} MLSS	67	Saby et al. (2002)
Lab-scale SBR		
90 mg Cl_2 g^{-1} MLSS	32	Takdastan et al. (2010)
230 mg Cl_2 g^{-1} MLSS	45	
320 mg Cl_2 g^{-1} MLSS	100	
Full-scale plant for pharmaceutical wastewater		
Higher than 15 mg O_3 g^{-1} TSS	100	Yasui et al. (1996)
Full-scale plant for municipal wastewater		
34 mg O_3 g^{-1} TSS	100	Sakai et al. (1997)
Full-scale plant for slaughterhouse wastewater		
26 mg O_3 g^{-1} TSS	60–80	Wolff and Hurren (2006)
Lab-scale SBR with intermittent ozonation		
10 mg O_3 g^{-1} MLSS	29	Takdastan et al. (2009a, b)
18 mg O_3 g^{-1} MLSS	55	
22 mg O_3 g^{-1} MLSS	100	

dosage. It has been demonstrated that with 66 mg Cl_2 g^{-1} mixed liquor suspended solids (MLSS) of chorine dosage, 67% sludge reduction is achieved (Saby et al. 2002). However, the study also found that there was an accumulation of small suspended particles less than 1 μm in size and a decrease in the MLSS/TS ratio from 0.95 to 0.80. It is speculated that this was due to the incomplete disruption of sludge flocs; that is, the chlorine dose of 66 mg Cl_2 g^{-1} MLSS used in the study was not adequate to mineralize the sludge effectively. The study by Takdastan et al. (2010) showed that 100% of sludge reduction (i.e., no excess sludge) was generated from the bioreactor when 320 mg Cl_2 g^{-1} MLSS of chorine was used. Table 6.7 comparies chlorine and ozone dosage with sludge reduction.

Chlorine dosage varies and is affected by many factors, as mentioned earlier. It is recommended that a chlorine dose above 133 mg Cl_2 g^{-1} MLSS be used for the chlorination of excess sludge. However, a high chlorine dose generates more chlorine residue, which will disrupt the operation of the treatment process when it enters the system with the returning chlorinated sludge (Saby et al. 2002). More studies are needed to determine the appropriate chlorine dosage and the impact on sludge mineralization of various factors, such as sludge characteristics, sludge concentration, and pH.

6.9 NOMENCLATURE

Parameter	Description	Unit
B	Decay rate	d^{-1}
b'	Decay constant of active biomass (death–regeneration concept)	d^{-1}
BOD	Biological oxygen demand	$g\,O_2\,m^{-3}$
C_{O3}	Concentration of ozone in the gas	$g\,O_3\,m^{-3}$
C_L	Equilibrium concentration of ozone in the liquid	$g\,O_3\,m^{-3}$
C_L^*	Saturation concentration of ozone in the liquid	$g\,O_3\,m^{-3}$
COD	Chemical oxygen demand	$gO_2\,m^{-3}$
COD_{VSS}	Chemical oxygen demand for the VSS of sludge	$g\,O_2\,m^{-3}$
D	Sludge drawing rate	$L\,L^{-1}\,d^{-1}$
DOC	Dissolved organic carbon	$g\,C\,m^{-3}$
D_{O3}	Diffusivity of ozone	$m^2\,s^{-1}$
E	Enhancement factor (dimensionless)	
ESP_{ozone}	Excess sludge production for a combined ozonation/AS system	$g\,COD\,d^{-1}$
ESPR	Excess sludge production reduction	$g\,COD\,g^{-1}\,COD$
$f_{N\text{-}TKN}$	Fraction of N in sludge	$g\,N\,g^{-1}\,COD$
f'	Inert fraction of dead biomass (death–regeneration concept)	$g\,COD\,g^{-1}\,COD$
f_{UP}	Fraction of inert COD in the wastewater	$g\,COD\,g^{-1}\,COD$
HRT	Hydraulic retention time	d
k	Cell inactivation constant	s^{-1}
$k_L a$	Overall oxygen mass transfer coefficient	s^{-1}
N	Active cell number	-
N_{O3}	Flux of ozone transferred	$g\,O_3\,m^{-3}\,s^{-1}$
OLR	Organic loading rate	$kg\,BOD\,kg^{-1}\,SS\,d^{-1}$
OUR_{max}	Maximum oxygen uptake rate	$g\,O_2\,m^{-3}\,s^{-1}$
Q_d	Sludge drawing rate	$L\,d^{-1}$
Q_r	Volumetric flow between the aeration tank and the ozone contactor	$L\,d^{-1}$
Q_{DCO}	COD mass flow	$g\,COD\,d^{-1}$
Q_{O3}	Ozone mass flow	$g\,O_3\,d^{-1}$
Q_{XJ}	COD solubilization rate of the X_J fraction	$g\,COD\,d^{-1}$
q_{min}	Minimal ozone dosage to obtain a ESP reduction	$g\,O_3\,g^{-1}\,COD_{removed}$
r	Residual ratio of ozonated sludge to biomass in aeration tank	$g\,SS\,g^{-1}\,SS$
R	Ratio of recircultation rate to the aeration tank volume	$L\,L^{-1}\,d^{-1}$

$S_{U,inf}$	Soluble nonbiodegradable	g COD m^{-3}
SRT	Sludge retention time	d
SS	Suspended solids concentration	g m^{-3}
S_B	Soluble readily biodegradable COD concentration	g COD m^{-3}
S_U	Soluble unbiodegradable COD produced	g COD m^{-3}
SVI	Sludge volume index	mL
TKN	Total Kjeldahl nitrogen	g N m^{-3}
TKN$_{RSP}$	Additional TKN due to ESP reduction	g d^{-1}
TSS	Total suspended solids	g m^{-3}
VLR	Volumetric loading rate	kg BOD m^{-3} d^{-1}
VSS	Volatile suspended solids concentration	g m^{-3}
X_B	Hydrolyzable biodegradable COD concentration	g COD m^{-3}
X_H	Heterotrophic biomass	g COD m^{-3}
X_J	Nonviable sludge COD fractions, $X_{U,inf}$ or X_B or $X_{U,E}$	g COD m^{-3}
X_A	Autotrophic nitrifying biomass	g COD m^{-3}
X_U	Particulate unbiodegradable COD concentration	g COD m^{-3}
$X_{U,E}$	Particulate unbiodegradable COD concentration from cell decay	g COD m^{-3}
$X_{U,inf}$	Particulate unbiodegradable COD concentration in wastewater	g COD m^{-3}
Y	Generation ratio of ozonated sludge to biomass in aeration tank	g SS g^{-1} SS
Y	Growth yield (model: Yashui and Shibata 1994)	g SS g^{-1} BOD
Y_H	Maximal growth yield	g X$_H$ g^{-1} COD$_{removed}$
Y_{obs}	Observed sludge production yield	g VSS g^{-1} COD$_{removed}$
$1-z$	Ozonated fraction of the sludge that will be biologically degraded in the AS (model: Yasui and Shibata 1994)	g SS g^{-1} SS
δ	Total thickness of the liquid film	m
δ_{eff}	Active thickness of the liquid film	m
θ_{Bref}	Reference SRT of the control AS line	d^{-1}
η_{O3}	Ratio of S_S production from X_J to ozone amount	g COD$_{solubilized}$ g^{-1} O$_{3transferred}$
η'_{O3}	Ratio of S_U production from X_J to ozone amount	g COD$_{solubilized}$ g^{-1} O$_{3transferred}$
η_{VSS}	VSS degradation yield	%
η_{ESP}	ESP reduction yield compared to a reference for a conventional AS	%

REFERENCES

Ahn K. H., Yeom I. T., Park K. Y., Maeng S. K., Lee Y., Song K. G., Choi S. (2002) Reduction of sludge by ozone treatment and production of carbon source for denitrification. *Water Science and Technology* **46**(11–12), 121–125.

Battimelli, A., Millet C., Delgenes J.P., Moletta R. (2003) Anaerobic digestion of waste activated sludge combined with ozone post-treatment and recycling. *Water science and technology* **48**(4), 61–68.

Black & Veatch Corporation. (2010) *White's Handbook of Chlorination and Alternative Disinfectants*, 5th ed., Wiley, Hoboken, N.J.

Böhler M., Siegrist H. (2004) Partial ozonation of activated sludge to reduce excess sludge, improve denitrification and control scumming and bulking. *Water Science and Technology* **49**(10), 41–49.

Bougrier C., Albasi C., Delgenès J. P., Carrère H. (2006) Effect of ultrasonic, thermal and ozone pre-treatments on waste activated sludge solubilisation and anaerobic biodegradability. *Chemical Engineering and Processing* **45**(8), 711.

Bougrier C., Battimelli A., Delgenès J. P., Carrère H. (2007) Combined ozone pretreatment and anaerobic digestion for the reduction of biological sludge production in wastewater treatment. *Ozone Science and Engineering* **29**(3), 201–206.

Caffaz S., Santianni D., Cerchiara M., Lubello C., Stecchi R. (2005) Reduction of excess biological sludge with ozone: experimental investigation in a full-scale plant. In: IOA 17th World Ozone Congress, Strasbourg, France.

Camacho P., Ginestet P., Audic J. M. (2003) Pilot plant demonstration of reduction technology during activated sludge treatment of wastewater, Los Angeles, October 11–15.

Camacho P., Ginestet P., Audic J. M. (2005) Understanding the mechanisms of thermal disintegrating treatment in the reduction of sludge production. *Water Science and Technology* **52**(10–11), 235–245.

Campos J. L., Otero L., Franco A., Mosquera-Corral A., Roca E. (2009) Ozonation strategies to reduce sludge production of a seafood industry WWTP. *Bioresource Technology* **100**, 1069–1073.

Cesbron D. (2004) Caractérisation et analyse des compétitions lors de l'action de l'ozone sur une boue: implications pour un procédé de réduction de production de boue combinant traitement biologique et oxydation. INSA Toulouse, France.

Cesbron D., Déléris S., Debellefontaine H., Roustan M., Paul E. (2003) Study of competition for ozone between soluble and particulate matter during activated sludge ozonation. *Chemical Engineering Research and Design* **81**(A9), 1165–1170.

Chen G. H., Saby S., Djafer M., Mo H. K. (2001) New approaches to minimize excess sludge in activated sludge systems. *Water Science and Technology* **44**(10), 203–208.

Christensen E., Giese A. C. (1954) Changes in absorption spectra of nucleic acids and their derivatives following exposure to ozone and ultraviolet radiation. *Archives of Biochemistry and Biophysies* **51**, 208–216.

Chu L. B., Xing X. H., Yu A. F., Sun X. L., Jurcik B. (2008) Enhanced treatment of practical textile wastewater by microbubble ozonation. *Process Safety and Environmental Protection* **86**(5), 389.

Danckwerts P. V. (1970) *Gas–Liquid Reactions*, McGraw-Hill, New York.

Déléris S. (2001) Réduction de la production de boues par couplage d'un procédé chimique et d'une boue activée. INSA, Toulouse, France.

Déléris S., Paul E., Debellefontaine H., Geaugey V. (1999) Sludge reduction in wastewater treatment plants. Mass balances for assessing the efficiency of a combined treatment system. In: Activated Sludge and Ozonation, Montpellier, France, October 5–7, pp. 9–20.

Déléris S., Paul E., Audic J. M., Roustan M., Debellefontaine H. (2000) Effect of ozonation on activated sludge solubilization and mineralization. *Ozone Science and Engineering* **22**(5), 473–486.

Déléris S., Geaugey V., Camacho P., Debellefontaine H., Paul E. (2002) Minimization of sludge production in biological processes: an alternative solution for the problem of sludge disposal. *Water Science and Technology* **46**(10), 63–70.

Déléris S., Larose A., Geaugey V. T. L. (2003) Innovative strategies for the reduction of sludge production in activated sludge plant: Biolysis® O and Biolysis® E., International Conference on Wastewater Sludge as a Resource (BIOSOLIDS 2003) Trondheim, Norway, June 23–25, pp. 55–61.

Dogruel S., Sievers M., Germirli-Babuna F. (2007) Effect of ozonation on biodegradability characteristics of surplus activated sludge. *Ozone Science and Engineering* **29**(3), 191–199.

Dytczak M. A., Oleszkiewicz J. A. (2008) Performance change during long-term ozonation aimed at augmenting denitrification and decreasing waste activated sludge. *Chemosphere* **73**(9), 1529–1532.

Dytczak M. A., Londry K., Siegrist H., Oleszkiewicz J. A. (2006) Extracellular polymers in partly ozonated return activated sludge: impact on flocculation and dewaterability. *Water Science and Technology* **54**(9), 155–164.

Dytczak M. A., Londry K. L., Siegrist H., Oleszkiewicz J.A. (2007) Ozonation reduces sludge production and improves denitrification. *Water Research* **41**(3), 543–550.

Egemen E., Corpening J., Nirmalakhandan N. (2001) Evaluation of an ozonation system for reduced waste sludge generation. *Water Science and Technology* **44**(2–3), 445–452.

Finch G. R., Smith D. W. (1989) Ozone dose–response of *Escherichia coli* in activated-sludge effluent. *Water Research* **23**(8), 1017–1025.

Finch G. R., Yuen W. C., Uibel B. J. (1992) Inactivation of *Escherichia coli* using ozone and ozone–hydrogen peroxide. *Environmental Technology* **13**(6), 571–578.

Frigon D., Isazadeh S. (2011) Evaluation of a new model for the reduction of excess sludge production by ozonation of return activated sludge: What solids COD fraction is affected? *Water Science and Technology* **63**(1), 156–163.

Gallard H., von Gunten U. (2002) Chlorination of natural organic matter: kinetics of chlorination and of THM formation. *Water Research* **36**(1), 65–74.

Gaudy A. F., Yang P. Y., Obayashi A. W. (1971) Studies on the total oxydation of activated sludge with and without hydrolytic treatment. *Journal of the Water Pollutin Control Federation* **43**, 40–54.

Ginestet P. (2007) In: Research E. W. (ed.), *Comparative Evaluation of Sludge Reduction Routes*. IWA Publishing, London.

Goel R., Komatsu K., Yasui H., Harada H. (2004) Process performance and change in sludge characteristics during anaerobic digestion of sewage sludge with ozonation. *Water Science and Technology* **49**(10), 105–113.

Hammer M. J. (2008) *Water and Wastewater Technology*, Prentice Hall, Upper Saddle River, NJ.

He S. B., Wang B. T., Wang L., Jiang Y. F., Zhang L. Q. (2003) A novel approach to treat combined domestic wastewater and excess sludge in MBR. *Chinese Journal of Environmental Sciences* **15**(5), 674–679.

He S. B., Xue G., Wang B. Z. (2006) Activated sludge ozonation to reduce sludge production in membrane bioreactor (MBR). *Journal of Hazardous Materials* **135**(1–3), 406–411.

Henze M., Grady C. P. L., Gujer W., Marais G. V. R., Matsuo T. (1987) A general-model for single-sludge waste-water treatment systems. *Water Research* **21**(5), 505–515.

Henze M., Gujer W., Mino T., Matsuo T., Wentzel M. C., Marais G. V. R., van Loosdrecht M. C. M. (1999) Activated Sludge Model No. 2d, ASM2d. *Water Science and Technology* **39**(1), 165–182.

Hoigné J., Bader H. (1976) Role of hydroxyl radical reactions in ozonation processes in aqueous solutions. *Water Research* **10**(5), 377–386.

Hoigné J., Bader H. (1983) Rate constants of reactions of ozone with organic and inorganic-compounds in water: 2. Dissociating organic-compounds. *Water Research* **17**(2), 185–194.

Huysmans A., Weemaes M., Fonseca P. A., Verstraete W. (2001) Ozonation of activated sludge in the recycle stream. *Journal of Chemical Technology and Biotechnology* **76**(3), 321–324.

Kamiya T., Hirotsuji J. (1998) New combined system of biological process and intermittent ozonation for advanced wastewater treatment. *Water Science and Technology* **38**(8–9), 145–153.

Karanfil T., Krasner S. W., Westerhoff P., Xie Y. F. (2008) Recent Advances in Disinfection By-product Formation, Occurrence, Control, Health Effects, and Regulations. Disinfection By-Products in Drinking Water: Occurrence, Formation, Health Effects, and Control **995**, 2–19.

Kobayashi T., Arakawa K., Katu Y., Tanaka T. (2001) Study on sludge reduction and other factors by use of an ozonation process in activated sludge treatment. Proceedings of 15th Ozone World Congress, London 2001, International Ozone Association 321–329.

Komatsu K., Yasui H., Goel R. Li Y.Y., Noike T. (2011a) Novel anaerobic digestion process with sludge ozonation for economically feasible power production from biogas. *Water science and technology* **63**(7), 1467–1475.

Komatsu K., Yasui H., Goel R. Li Y.Y., Noike T. (2011b) Feasible Power Production from Municipal Sludge Using an Improved Anaerobic Digestion System. *Ozone-science & engineering* **33**(2), 164–170.

Korich D. G., Mead J. R., Madore M. S., Sinclair N. A., Sterling C. R. (1990) Effects of ozone, chlorine dioxide, chlorine, and monochloramine on *Cryptosporidium parvum* oocyst viability. *Applied Environmental Microbiology* **56**(5), 1423–1428.

Lee J.W., Cha H.Y., Park K.Y., Song K.G., Ahn K.H. (2005) Operational strategies for an activated sludge process in conjunction with ozone oxidation for zero excess sludge production during winter season. *Water research* **39**(7), 1199–1204.

Liu Y. (2003) Chemically reduced excess sludge production in the activated sludge process. *Chemosphere* **50**(1), 1–7.

Manterola G., Uriarte I., Sancho L. (2008) The effect of operational parameters of the process of sludge ozonation on the solubilisation of organic and nitrogenous compounds. *Water research* **42**(12), 3191–3197.

Nishimura F., Katoh G., Fujiwara T. (1999) *Improvement and reduction of activated sludge by ozonation and first application to wastewater treatment.* In: 15th World Congress IOA, London.

Oh Y.K., Lee K.R., Ko K.B., Yeom I.T. (2007) Effects of chemical sludge disintegration on the performances of wastewater treatment by membrane bioreactor. *Water Research* **41**(12), 2665–2671.

Paola F., Gianni A., Giuliano Z. (2010) *Sludge Reduction Technologies in Wastewater Treatment Plants*, IWA Publishing, London.

Park K. Y., Lee J. W., Ahn K. H., Maeng S. K., Hwang J. H., Song K. G. (2004) Ozone disintegration of excess biomass and application to nitrogen removal. *Water Environment Research* **76**(2), 162–167.

Park Y. G. (2001) Impact of ozonation on biodegradation of trihalomethanes in biological filtration system. *Journal of Industrial and Engineering Chemistry* **7**(6), 349–357.

Paul E., Debellefontaine H. (2007) Reduction of excess sludge produced by biological treatment processes: effect of ozonation on biomass and on sludge. *Ozone Science and Engineering* **29**(6), 415–427.

Paul E., Camacho P., Spérandio M., Ginestet P. (2006) Technical and economical evaluation of a thermal, and two oxidative techniques for the reduction of excess sludge production. *Process Safety and Environmental Protection* **84**(B4), 247–252.

Saby S., Djafer M., Chen G. H. (2002) Feasibility of using a chlorination step to reduce excess sludge in activated sludge process. *Water Research* **36**(3), 656–666.

Sakai Y., Fukase T., Yasui H., Shibata M. (1997) An activated sludge process without excess sludge production. *Water Science and Technology* **36**(11), 163–170.

Sakai Y., Kato N., Saito T., Hashizume H., Sasaki S., Ishikawa S., Watanabe T. (2003) Sewage treatment by activated magnetic sludge process without excess sludge production. *Abstracts of Papers of the American Chemical Society* **225**, 229-IEC.

Saktaywin W., Tsuno H., Nagare H., Soyama T., Weerapakkaroon J. (2005) Advanced sewage treatment process with excess sludge reduction and phosphorus recovery. *Water Research* **39**(5), 902–910.

Salhi M. (2003) Procédés couplés boues activées-ozonation pour la réduction de la production de boues: étude, modélisation et intégration dans la filière de traitement de l'eau. INSA, Toulouse, France.

Salhi M., Déléris S., Debellefontaine H., Ginestet P., Paul E. (2003) More insights into the understanding of reduction of excess sludge production by ozone. *Wastewater Sludge as a Resource*, pp. 39–46.

Salhi M., Berthe L., Spérandio M., Paul E. (2004) Ways of optimization of P removal in an ozonation-activated sludge process with excess sludge production reduction. In: Proceedings of the IWA Biennial, Marrakech, Morocco.

Salsabil M. R., Laurent J., Casellas M., Dagot C. (2010) Techno-economic evaluation of thermal treatment, ozonation and sonication for the reduction of wastewater biomass volume before aerobic or anaerobic digestion. *Journal of Hazardous Materials* **174**(1–3), 323–333.

Scheminski A., Krull R., Hempel D. C. (2000) Oxidative treatment of digested sewage sludge with ozone. *Water Science and Technology* **42**(9), 151–158.

Sievers M., Ried A., Koll R. (2004) Sludge treatment by ozonation: evaluation of full-scale results. *Water Science and Technology* **49**(4), 247–253.

Sui P.Z., Nishimura F., Nagare H., Hidaka T., Nakagawa Y., Tsuno H. (2011) Behavior of inorganic elements during sludge ozonation and their effects on sludge solubilization. *Water Research* **45**(5), 2029–2037.

Suzuki Y., Kondo T., Nakagawa V., Tsuneda S., Hirata A., Shimizu Y., Inamori Y. (2006) Evaluation of sludge reduction and phosphorus recovery efficiencies in a new advanced wastewater treatment system using denitrifying polyphosphate accumulating organisms. *Water Science and Technology* **53**(6), 107–113.

Takdastan A., Mehrdadi N., Azimi A. A., Torabian A., Bidhendi G. N. 2009a. Investigation of the excess sludge reduction in SBR by oxidizing some sludge by ozone. *Iranian Journal of Chemistry and Chemical Engineering International English Edition* **28**(4), 95–104.

Takdastan A., Mehrdadi N., Torabian A., Azimi A. A., Bidhendi G. N. 2009b. Investigation of excess biological sludge reduction in sequencing Bach reactor. *Asian Journal of Chemistry* **21**(3), 2419–2427.

Takdastan A., Azimi A. A., Jaafarzadeh N. (2010) Biological excess sludge reduction in municipal wastewater treatment by chlorine. *Asian Journal of Chemistry* **22**(3), 1665–1674.

Tchobanoglous G., Burton F. L., Stensel H. D. (2003) In: ME, Inc. (ed.), *Wastewater Engineering: Treatment and Reuse*, 4th ed., McGraw-Hill, New York.

Van Leeuven J. 1988. Improved sewaage treatment with ozonated activated sludge. *Journal of the Institute of Water Environment Management*, pp. 493–499.

Vergine P., Menin, G., Canziani, R., Ficara, E., Fabiyi, M., Novak, R., Sandon, A., Bianchi, A., Bergna, G. (2007) Partial ozonation of activated sludge to reduce excess sludge production: evaluation of effects on biomass activity in a full scale demonstration test. In: International Water Association Specialist Conference, Moncton, New Brunscvick, Canada.

Wang L. K., Shammas N. K., Hung Y-T. (2007) In: Engineering HoE (ed.), *Biosolids Treatment Processes*, Humana Press, Totowa, NJ.

Wang L. K., Pereira N. C., Hung Y. T., Shammas N. K. (2009) In: Engineering HoE (ed.), *Biological Treatment Processes*. Humana Press, Totowa, NJ.

Wang Z., Wang L., Wang B. Z., Jiang Y. F., Liu S. (2008) Bench-scale study on zero excess activated sludge production process coupled with ozonation unit in membrane bioreactor. *Journal of Environmental Science and Health*, **43**(11), 1325–1332.

Weemaes M. P. J., Verstraete W. H. 1998. Evaluation of current wet sludge disintegration techniques. *Journal of Chemical Technology and Biotechnology* **73**(2), 83–92.

Weemaes M., Grootaerd H., Simoens F., Huysmans A., Verstraete W. (2000) Ozonation of sewage sludge prior to anaerobic digestion. *Water Science and Technology* **42**(9), 175–178.

Wei Y. S., Van Houten R. T., Borger A. R., Eikelboom D. H., Fan Y. B. (2003) Minimization of excess sludge production for biological wastewater treatment. *Water Research* **37**(18), 4453–4467.

Wolff S., Hurren D. (2006) Reduction of excess sludge by up to 80% with ozone injection: practical experience. In: 11th European Biosolids and Organic Resources Conference, Wakefield, UK.

Yan S.T., Chu L.B., Xing X.H., Yua A.F., Sun X.L. Jurcikc B. (2009) Analysis of the mechanism of sludge ozonation by a combination of biological and chemical approaches. *Water research* **43**(1), 195–203.

Yasui H., Shibata M. 1994. An innovative approach to reduce excess sludge production in the activated sludge process. *Water Science and Technology* **30**(9), 11–20.

Yasui H., Nakamura K., Sakuma S., Iwasaki M., Sakai Y. (1996). A full-scale operation of a novel activated sludge process without excess sludge production. *Water Science and Technology* **34**(3–4), 395–404.

Yasui H., Komatsu K., Goel R., Li Y. Y., Noike T. (2005) Full-scale application of anaerobic digestion process with partial ozonation of digested sludge. *Water Science and Technology* **52**(1–2), 245–252.

Yasui H., Matsuhashi R., Noike T., Harada H. (2006) Anaerobic digestion with partial ozonation minimises greenhouse gas emission from sludge treatment and disposal. *Water Science and Technology* **53**(3), 255–263.

Zhang G.M., Yang J., Zhang J. (2009) Sludge ozonation: Disintegration, supernatant changes and mechanisms. *Bioresource Technology* **100**(3), 1505–1509.

7

HIGH-DISSOLVED-OXYGEN BIOLOGICAL PROCESS FOR SLUDGE REDUCTION

ZHI-WU WANG

Bioscience Division, Oak Ridge National Laboratory, Oak Ridge, Tennessee

7.1 INTRODUCTION

Biological wastewater treatment involves the transformation of dissolved and suspended organic matter to biomass, microbial by-products, and gases (Wei et al. 2003). More than 90% of municipal wastewater treatment plants utilize the activated sludge process as a core technology for domestic and industrial wastewater treatment in the world (Liu 2003). This is because activated sludge systems can treat up to 10 times more wastewater per unit volume of reactor than can fixed-film processes, without involving high operational costs (Chen et al. 2001; Liu and Tay 2001; Liu 2003; Wei et al. 2003). However, one of a the drawbacks of a conventional activated sludge process is its high sludge production. Daily production of excess sludge from a conventional activated sludge process is approximately 15 to $100 \, L \, kg^{-1}$ BOD_5 removed, in which over 95% is water (Liu and Tay 2001). The production of excess sludge from an activated sludge process has become one of the most serious problems encountered in aerobic wastewater treatment. The treatment and disposal of sludge from wastewater treatment plants is estimated to cost about 60% of the total operational cost of the wastewater treatment plant (Canales et al. 1994; Springer et al. 1996; Chen et al. 2001; Wei et al. 2003). Various methods available for sludge disposal, such as incineration, landfill, and sea disposal, are found to have a negative impact on the environment (Ramakrishna and Viraraghavan 2005). Hence, one of the ideal ways to

Biological Sludge Minimization and Biomaterials/Bioenergy Recovery Technologies, First Edition.
Edited by Etienne Paul and Yu Liu.
© 2012 John Wiley & Sons, Inc. Published 2012 by John Wiley & Sons, Inc.

solve the sludge problem is to reduce sludge production in the wastewater treatment process rather than in post-treatment of the sludge generated (Liu and Tay 2001). Therefore, it is necessary to develop new strategies to minimize the excess sludge production.

Low sludge yield has commonly been observed in pure oxygen-aerated activated sludge processes (Liu 2003). Side-by-side comparison of the pure oxygen- and air-aerated full-scale activated sludge systems treating the same wastewater for a relatively long period of time in the late 1960s revealed that the excess sludge produced per pound of biomass removed was reduced by more than 50% when using pure oxygen instead of air to provide dissolved oxygen over a wide food/microorganism (F/M) range of 0.3 to 0.9 (McWhirter 1978). Boon and Burgess (1974) also found that at a similar sludge age, the sludge growth yield observed in the pure oxygen-aerated system was only 60% of that in the air-aerated system. Similarly, the results from purified oxygenation-activated sludge processes show that the growth yield can be lowered by up to 54% compared with a conventional air-activated sludge system, even at high sludge loading rates (Liu and Tay 2001). These broad reports imply that a high dissolved-oxygen concentration could have the potential to promote sludge reduction (Kumke and Sutton 1973; Liu 2003). A study by Travers and Lovett (1984) showed that the sludge yield tended to decrease as the dissolved oxygen concentration was increased. An even more detailed study on the effect of dissolved oxygen on excess sludge production was conducted by Abbassi et al. (2000), showing that the excess sludge production decreased from 0.28 to 0.2 mg MLSS mg^{-1} BOD as the dissolved oxygen concentration increased from 1.8 to 6.0 mg O_2 L^{-1} in a laboratory-scale conventional activated sludge reactor. Similarly, according to Hu et al. (2009), compared with the control system, an increase in aeration by 23% led to reduced discharge of excess sludge by 34.6%. In an experiment by Roques et al. (1984), dissolved oxygen was brought directly into the liquid phase without the exchange at the gas–liquid interface, and it was found that sludge production can be reduced considerably by varying the dissolved oxygen concentration. Mahmood and Elliott (2006) added that while consuming approximately 25% more oxygen, the sludge production process produced 36% less sludge than did the conventional activated sludge system. As a matter of fact, such a high dissolved-oxygen reduced microbial yield is observed not only for an activated sludge system, but is also found with pure cultures. For example, Landwall and Holme (1977) reported a rapid decrease in the growth yield of *Escherichia coli*-b in the presence of a high concentration of dissolved oxygen. Nagai et al. (1971) compared the metabolism of *Azotobacter* in oxygen- and glucose-limited condition and found that the bacterial growth yield ranged from 0.2 to 0.25 mg bacteria mg^{-1} glucose in the oxygen-limited condition which was considerably higher than the growth yield, ranging from 0.03 to 0.18 mg bacteria mg^{-1} glucose observed when oxygen was in excess, suggesting that the dissolved oxygen interferes in the metabolism of the growing *Azotobacter*.

Existing evidence supports a basic idea that use of a high level of dissolved oxygen is able to promote sludge reduction. In addition, maintaining a high dissolved oxygen concentration also benefits a biological wastewater treatment system in aspects of filamentous growth repression, high biomass retention, better sludge settling and thickening, as well as higher oxygen transfer efficiency and thus more stable operation (Benefield and Randall 1980; Pérez-Elvira et al. 2006). A successful high-purity oxygen process has been demonstrated in full-scale application (Pérez-Elvira et al. 2006). It can be anticipated that the high dissolved-oxygen biological process could have great industrial potential in reducing excess sludge production in the future.

7.2 MECHANISM OF HIGH-DISSOLVED-OXYGEN REDUCED SLUDGE PRODUCTION

In contrast to the widely reported positive effect of high dissolved oxygen on sludge minimization, the mechanism of reduced sludge production at a high dissolved-oxygen concentration is not yet thoroughly clear, and different opinions can be found in the literature. They can be largely categorized into three aspects in terms of changes made to the specific loading rate, microbial population, and metabolism pathway by high dissolved oxygen in wastewater treatment process.

7.2.1 High-Dissolved-Oxygen Decreased Specific Loading Rate

It is generally believed that activated sludge production, in principle, is closely associated with the specific organic loading rate that is imposed on a bioreactor (e.g., low sludge production usually comes with a low organic loading rate on a unit activated sludge basis). As postulated by McWhirter (1978) and Ramakrishna and Viraraghavan (2005), a high dissolved oxygen concentration would produce a higher level of activated biomass. This is evidenced by a study of the effect of dissolved oxygen on sludge viability; higher adenosine triphosphate (ATP) viabilities were observed at higher dissolved oxygen levels of 2 to 15 mg DO L^{-1} (Williamson and Nelson 1981). As the result, the specific loading rate based on active biomass would be lowered at higher dissolved oxygen concentrations. The lowered true sludge loading rate, in turn, results in a relatively lower sludge production rate at the same apparent measured value of the volumetric loading rate (Liu and Tay 2001). This gives a simple interpretation of one of the mechanisms underlying the sludge reduction at high dissolved oxygen levels.

Technically, an increase in the oxygen concentration in the bulk liquid also promotes a deeper penetration of oxygen, which subsequently leads to an enlargement of the aerobic volume inside the bioflocs (Fig. 7.1). As a result, a greater fraction of the active biomass will get involved in and make a higher degree of endogenous respiration than at a comparably lower dissolved oxygen concentration at the same organic substrate loading. Consequently, more biomass in the bioflocs matrix can be hydrolyzed and degraded aerobically. Results by Chapman et al. (1976) confirmed the reduction in sludge production in the high dissolved-oxygen system with regard to the significantly increased penetration of the oxygen into the bioflocs and the increase in the sludge viability. A model proposed by Abbassi et al. (2000) may better explain this deeper diffusion of oxygen, which resulted in enlargement of the aerobic

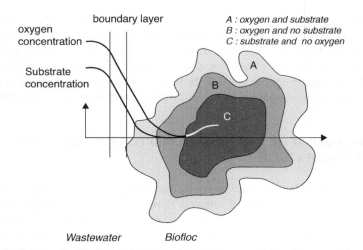

FIGURE 7.1 Model describing the increased oxygen penetration into bioflocs at a high dissolved-oxygen concentration. [From Abbassi et al. (2000).]

volume inside the bioflocs (Fig. 7.1). As presented, even though the degradation of the bulk substrate takes place primarily in region A, where both substrate and oxygen are supplied, when the bioflocs is exposed to a high oxygen concentration, oxygen starts to become available in region B (Fig. 7.1). In this part of the bioflocs, the content of dead cells can be oxidized and the amount of excess sludge is thus reduced, even though in the core of the bioflocs, an anaerobic region C may remain and the organisms in this part do not participate in the degradation process. This is a good example to illustrate that a high dissolved oxygen level is able to produce a higher level of active biomass and thus a lower true F/M than would be measured in a low dissolved-oxygen system. The lower true F/M, in turn, results in a relatively lower specific loading rate and thus reduced sludge production. However, as Liu (2003) pointed out, such an explanation may not fully reveal the mechanism behind the high-dissolved-oxygen reduced activated sludge production, so other underlying mechanisms are probably taking place at a higher than usual dissolved oxygen concentration.

7.2.2 High-Dissolved-Oxygen Uncoupled Microbial Metabolism Pathway

Liu and Tay (2001) predicted that the dissolved oxygen may have some impact on the energy metabolism of activated sludge, which further determines carbon flux flowing between anabolism and catabolism, based on the fact that the cell surface hydrophobicity, microbial activity, and extracellular polymer production are all linked to the dissolved oxygen level in bioreactor (Roques et al. 1984; Mishima and Nakamura 1991; Palmgren et al. 1998; Pena et al. 2000). In this case, the reduced sludge production at a high dissolved-oxygen concentration could be a consequence of high dissolved-oxygen-induced metabolic uncoupling in activated sludge.

However, a detailed study in this regard is still lacking (Liu and Tay 2001). According to del Giorgio and Cole (1998), when microbial growth is unconstrained, as in batch cultures, there is often a high degree of coupling between catabolism and anabolism. However, when growth is constrained by the supply of organic substrate or inorganic nutrients, different degrees of uncoupling could invariably be observed. For example, washed suspensions of bacteria oxidize substrates, such as glucose at a high rate under conditions at which cell synthesis is severely impeded (Tempest 1978). This uncoupling is manifested especially at high oxygen and organic substrate consumption rates through metabolite overproduction and excretion, excess heat production, and energy-spilling pathways (Russell and Cook 1995). All these processes could eventually result in reduced microbial growth efficiency.

In general, catabolism appears to proceed at the maximum rate at which the organisms are capable under the cultivation conditions, irrespective of whether or not the energy so produced can be used for biosynthesis (Russell 1991). Under conditions of severe constraints to growth, it has been suggested that maintaining the highest possible flow of energy would be advantageous (Russell 1991; Russell and Cook 1995). One of the potential advantages of a high energy flux in the cell may be to maintain the energization of the cell membrane and the function of active transport systems, both of which are essential for resumption of growth whenever growth conditions get better (Dawes 1985; Morita 1997). Phillips and Johnson (1961) and Nagai et al. (1971) reported that an oxygen-wasting system functions when dissolved oxygen exceeds a critical level. From the analysis of enzymes responsible for growth in a glucose-limited chemostat culture, Nagai et al. (1971) showed that the oxygen-wasting system became predominant at high oxygen concentrations, and the yield from glucose decreased appreciably with the increase in dissolved oxygen concentrations. In addition, according to Zhulin et al. (1997), in the presence of high oxygen concentrations, bacteria employ multiple strategies to protect against reactive oxygen derivatives that are generated by the partial reduction of oxygen. They may regulate the expression of genes involved in aerobic metabolism and in the enzymatic defense against reactive oxygen species (Nystrom et al. 1996). Bacteria may also use noncoupled respiration and a mild uncoupling mechanism to accelerate the respiratory consumption of oxygen and thereby lower the concentration of intracellular oxygen as part of the respiratory protection concept (Skulachev 1996). Dalton and Postage (1969) assumed that in the N_2-reducing bacteria, rapid consumption of oxygen by a highly active oxidase maintains low intracellular oxygen concentration, compatible with nitrogenase function, which is arrested at higher oxygen concentration. The most demonstrative and direct verification of the respiratory protection concept was carried out in experiments on *Azotobacteria vinelandii*. This bacterium shows an unusually high rate of oxygen consumption accompanied by dissipation of a large portion of energy, which results in fast heating of the growth medium. Similarly, according to O'beirne and Hamer (2000), when *E. coli* strains are grown aerobically to high cell densities on glucose, two fundamental problems occur. The first is overflow metabolism, which occurs at a high specific growth rate under conditions of excess oxygen (Xu et al. 1999), where the overabundant supply of energy results in acetate excretion (Holms 1996). The second occurs as a result of either oxygen limitation or oxygen starvation, where glucose metabolism occurs via the mixed acid fermentation, with acetate again being one of the products. Under both circumstances, acetate formation detracts from the conversion of glucose carbon into either biomass or product carbon, and the yield coefficients concerning this are markedly depressed.

In line with this metabolism-uncoupling hypothesis, the overproduction of extracellular polysaccharides has been reported widely, with microorganisms growing in a high dissolved-oxygen environment (Lee et al. 1997; Kim et al. 2005). For example, a sufficient supply of oxygen was suggested to be necessary for extracellular polysaccharides production (Lee et al. 1997), and the extracellular polysaccharide yield was found to increase with dissolved oxygen as well (Kim et al. 2005). In contrast, Shin et al. (2001) reported that the oxygen limitation generally caused a decrease in the carbohydrate concentration in the extracellular polysaccharides. A higher aeration rate was also reported to be necessary for enhancing the extracellular polysaccharide production (Lee et al. 2001). As noted by Lawford and Rousseau (1991), to achieve a high production of curdlan, a high-molecular-weight polymer of glucose, a high dissolved oxygen concentration has to be employed.

Technically, a high dissolved oxygen concentration means a high specific respiration rate of the activated sludge, thus a fast catabolism of substrates, which translates to a quick specific ATP generation. However, the quick ATP generation may not give a high ATP yield over substrate consumption, which is closely related to microbial growth yield. Instead, heterotrophic organisms generally face a trade-off between rate and yield of ATP production, as do the rate and yield of their growth (Pfeiffer et al. 2001). It is well-known that heterotrophic organisms can obtain their energy by the degradation of organic substrates into products with lower free energy. The free-energy difference can in part be conserved by production of ATP and in part be used to drive the degradation reaction. As noted by Pfeiffer et al. (2001), if the maximal ATP yield is obtained through conservation of the entire free-energy difference as ATP, the reaction will be at thermodynamic equilibrium, and therefore the rates of substrate degradation and ATP production vanish. However, if some of the free-energy difference is used to drive the reaction, the rate of ATP production will thus increase with the decreasing yield until a maximum rate is reached. For such a fundamental thermodynamic reason, there is always an inverted relationship between the yield and the rate of ATP production in heterotrophic organisms (Stucki 1980; Angulobrown et al. 1995; Waddell et al. 1999). Since the ATP production rate is rapidly saturated at high levels of dissolved oxygen, this will in turn play down the ATP and thus the bacterial growth yield (Postma et al. 1989; Vandijken et al. 1993; Voet and Voet 1995).

7.2.3 High-Dissolved-Oxygen Shifted Microbial Population

Diverse microbial populations have been observed in wastewater treatment bioreactors operating under different dissolved oxygen conditions. Microscope observation indicates that small rod-shaped and spherical clusters were dominant in a high-dissolved-oxygen reactor (above 3 mg O_2 L^{-1} on average), but filamentous bacteria and long rod-shaped bacteria coexisted in the low-dissolved-oxygen reactor (0.4 to

$0.8 \, mg \, O_2 \, L^{-1}$) (Guo et al. 2009). In fact, it has been demonstrated sufficiently that low levels of dissolved oxygen in aeration basins favor the growth of filamentous organisms that cause sludge bulking, one of the most serious operational problems encountered in activated sludge processes (Richard et al. 1985; Nowak et al. 1986). On the contrary, the development of filamentous organisms was repressed in those high-dissolved-oxygen activated sludge processes (McWhirter 1978; Bitton 1994; Abbassi et al. 2000). In addition, experiments also showed that a low-dissolved-oxygen concentration (e.g., less than $1.1 \, mg \, O_2 \, L^{-1}$), had a strong negative effect on sludge settleability, which again is associated with the proliferation of filamentous bacteria, supporting the importance of high dissolved oxygen in the suppression of filamentous growth (Martins et al. 2003). For this reason, the high-dissolved-oxygen process has been believed to come with the added advantage of better sludge settling and thickening compared with the conventional aeration process (Benefield and Randall 1980).

The mechanism behind the reported microbial population shift with dissolved oxygen level might link to the disparate energy efficiency and growth rate of various microbial species under different dissolved oxygen conditions. As aforementioned, the microbial energy efficiency and growth rate usually do not go hand in hand with each other. Microbial species with a higher level of energy efficiency often grow at a lower rate, and vice versa (Stucki 1980; Angulobrown et al. 1995; Waddell et al. 1999). Pfeiffer et al. (2001) simulated the competition of several different strains for the same food source. The outcome of the competition was found to be determined by the one with the highest growth rate but not the highest growth yield. Such a high growth rate can be translated to a high rate of ATP production that is driven by the high rate of respiration achievable under high-dissolved-oxygen conditions. This implies that a cell population using a pathway with low growth yield but a high respiration rate can invade and replace another cell population using a pathway with a high growth yield and a low respiration rate. Only in the case of a pure culture will the population size depend on the growth yield but not the rate of ATP production, which is opposite to the scenario in a mixed culture full of interspecies competition for the limited substrate, such as those in wastewater treatment reactors (Pfeiffer et al. 2001).

7.3 LIMITS OF HIGH-DISSOLVED-OXYGEN PROCESS FOR REDUCED SLUDGE PRODUCTION

A high dissolved-oxygen level undoubtedly plays a positive role in sludge reduction through various types of mechanisms. However, like many other parameters, dissolved oxygen concentration should have its effective range. According to study by Ji et al. (2006), as illustrated in Fig. 7.2, along with the increase in dissolved oxygen level, the sludge growth yield observed kept decreasing until a threshold at $1.25 \, mg$ $O_2 \, L^{-1}$, above which the sludge yield remained at a constant value around $0.14 \, g$ sludge g^{-1} COD. Even though there is still room for the dissolved oxygen level to be elevated, the sludge growth yield may not be reduced further (Fig. 7.2). In line with

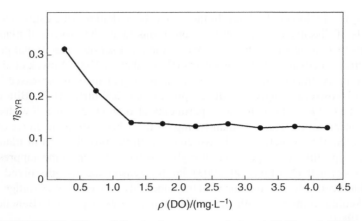

FIGURE 7.2 Effect of dissolved oxygen on sludge yield (Ji et al. 2006).

this study, Rickard and Gaudy (1968) also found no effect on respiration rate or sludge yield in a mechanically mixed activated sludge system when dissolved oxygen was increased from 1.4 to 7.1 mg O_2 L^{-1}. This may explain the results by Thabaraj and Gaudy (1969) obtained from a study of the effect of dissolved oxygen on shock loading response. In the dissolved oxygen range 1.3 to 7.4 mg O_2 L^{-1}, no difference in cell yield was observed. Some researchers thought that a dissolved-oxygen concentration above 2 mg L^{-1} would not further benefit sludge reduction in an activated sludge process (Kalinske 1976; Parker and Merrill 1976). A similar conclusion was reached by Benefield et al. (1977).

A significant fraction of the heterotrophic population in activated sludge could use nitrate as the terminal electron acceptor when dissolved oxygen is sufficiently low (Copp and Dold 1998). This mechanism is known as *anoxic respiration* or *denitrification*. Copp and Dold (1998) observed that the growth yield of activated sludge under anoxic conditions was 38% lower than that under aerobic conditions. Similarly, Muller et al. (2004) also reported that the biomass yield under anoxic condition was reduced to approximately 81% of that under aerobic conditions. These suggest that less sludge production can be expected when anoxic denitrification occurs in a biological system (Copp and Dold 1998; Hao et al. 2001; Koch et al. 2001; Peng et al. 2001; Muller et al. 2004).

REFERENCES

Abbassi B., Dullstein S., Rabiger N. (2000) Minimization of excess sludge production by increase of oxygen concentration in activated sludge flocs: experimental and theoretical approach. *Water Research* **34**, 139–146.

Angulobrown F., Santillan M., Callejaquevedo E. (1995) Thermodynamic optimality in some biochemical reactions. *Nuovo Cimento Della Societa Italiana di Fisica D* **17**, 87–90.

Benefield L. D., Randall C. W. (1980) *Biological Process Design for Wastewater Treatment*, Prentice-Hall, Englewood Cliffs, NJ.

Benefield L. D., Randall C. W., King P. H. (1977) Effect of high purity oxygen on activated sludge process. *Journal of the Water Pollution Control Federation* **49**, 269–279.

Bitton G. (1994) *Wastewater Microbiology*, Wiley-Liss, New York.

Boon A. G., Burgess D. R. (1974) Treatment of crude sewage in two high-rate activated sludge plants operated in series. *Water Pollution Control* **74**, 382.

Canales A., Pareilleux A., Rols J. L., Goma G., Huyard A. (1994) Decreased sludge production strategy for domestic wastewater treatment. *Water Science and Technology* **30**, 97–106.

Chapman TD., Matsch LC., Zander EH. (1976) Effect of high dissolved-oxygen concentration in activated-sludge systems. *Journal of the Water Pollution Control Federation* **48**, 2486–2510.

Chen G. H., Yip W. K., Mo H. K., Liu Y. (2001) Effect of sludge fasting/feasting on growth of activated sludge cultures. *Water Research* **35**, 1029–1037.

Copp J. B., Dold P. L. (1998) Comparing sludge production under aerobic and anoxic conditions. *Water Science and Technology* **38**, 285–294.

Dalton H., Postage J. P. (1969) Effect of oxygen on growth of *Azotobacter ehroococcum* in batch and continuous cultures. *Journal of General Microbiology* **54**, 463–473.

Dawes E. (1985) Starvation, survival and energy reserves. In: M. Fletcher, G. D. Foodgate (eds.), *Bacteria in Their Natural Environment*, Academic Press, New York, pp. 43–79.

del Giorgio P. A., Cole J. J. (1998) Bacterial growth efficiency in natural aquatic systems. *Annual Review of Ecology and Systematics* **29**, 503–541.

Guo J., Peng Y., Wang S., Zheng Y., Huang H., Wang Z. (2009) Long-term effect of dissolved oxygen on partial nitrification performance and microbial community structure. *Bioresource Technology* **100**, 2796–2802.

Hao X., Heijnen J. J., Qian Y., van Loosdrecht M. C. M. (2001) Contribution of P-bacteria in biological nutrient removal processes to overall effects on the environment. *Water Science and Technology* **44**, 67–76.

Holms H. (1996) Flux analysis and control of the central metabolic pathways in *Escherichia coli*. *FEMS Microbiology Reviews* **19**, 85–116.

Hu X. B., Chai H. X., Han W. Y., Ji F. Y., Long T. R. (2009) Performance of a sludge reduction system on removal of nitrogen and phosphorus controlled by low dissolved oxygen. *Journal of Civil, Architectural and Environmental Engineering* **31**, 112–116.

Ji F Y., Zuo N., Yang S. B., Hu Y. Q. (2006) Advanced sludge reduction and phosphorus removal process. *Journal of Central South University of Technology* **13**, 313–317.

Kalinske A. A. (1976) Comparison of air and oxygen activated-sludge systems. *Journal of the Water Pollution Control Federation* **48**, 2472–2485.

Kim H. H., Na J. G., Chang Y. K., Lee S. J. (2005) Effects of dissolved oxygen control on cell growth and exopolysaccharides production in batch culture of *Agaricus blazei*. *Korean Journal of Chemical Engineering* **22**, 80–84.

Koch G., Kuhni M., Siegrist H. (2001) Calibration and validation of an ASM3-based steady-state model for activated sludge systems: I. Prediction of nitrogen removal. and sludge production. *Water Research* **35**, 2235–2245.

Kumke G. W., Sutton J. A. (1973) Advancements in the use of high purity oxygen in the activated sludge process. *Hwahak Konghak* **11**, 220–231.

Landwall P., Holme T. (1977) Influence of glucose and dissolved-oxygen concentrations on yields of *Escherichia coli* B in dialysis culture. *Journal of General Microbiology* **103**, 353–358.

Lawford H. G., Rousseau J. D. (1991) Bioreactor design considerations in the production of high-quality microbial exopolysaccharide. *Applied Biochemistry and Biotechnology* **28–29**, 667–684.

Lee H., Park S., Lee J., Lee H. (2001) Effect of aeration rates on production of extracellular polysaccharide, EPS-R, by marine bacterium *Hahella chejuensis*. *Biotechnology and Bioprocess Engineering* **6**, 359–362.

Lee I. Y., Seo W. T., Kim G. J., Kim M. K., Ahn S. G., Kwon G. S., Park Y. H. (1997) Optimization of fermentation conditions for production of exopolysaccharide by *Bacillus polymyxa*. *Bioprocess Engineering* **16**, 71–75.

Liu Y. (2003) Chemically reduced excess sludge production in the activated sludge process. *Chemosphere* **50**, 1–7.

Liu Y., Tay J. H. (2001) Strategy for minimization of excess sludge production from the activated sludge process. *Biotechnology Advances* **19**, 97–107.

Mahmood T., Elliott A. (2006) Activated sludge process modification for sludge yield reduction using pulp and paper wastewater. *Journal of Environmental Engineering ASCE* **132**, 1019–1027.

Martins A. M. P., Heijnen J. J., van Loosdrecht M. C. M. (2003) Effect of dissolved oxygen concentration on sludge settleability. *Applied Microbiology and Biotechnology* **62**, 586–593.

McWhirter J. R. (1978) Oxygen and activated sludge process. In: McWhirter J. R. (ed.), *The Use of High-Purity Oxygen in the Activated Sludge Process*, CRC Press, Boca Raton, FL, pp. 57–60.

Mishima K., Nakamura M. (1991) Self-immobilization of aerobic activated-sludge: a pilot-study of the aerobic upflow sludge blanket process in municipal sewage-treatment. *Water Science and Technology* **23**, 981–990.

Morita R. (1997) *Bacteria in Oligotrophic Environments*, Chapman & Hall, New York.

Muller A. W., Wentzel M. C., Ekama G. A. (2004) Experimental determination of the heterotroph anoxic yield in anoxic–aerobic activated sludge systems treating municipal wastewater. *Water SA* **30**, 555–560.

Nagai S., Nishizawa Y., Onodera M., Aiba S. (1971) Effect of dissolved oxygen on growth yield and aldolase activity in chemostat culture of *Azotobacter-vinelandii*. *Journal of General Microbiology* **66**, 197–203.

Nowak G., Brown G., Yee A. (1986) Effects of feed pattern and dissolved oxygen on growth of filamentous bacteria. *Journal of the Water Pollution Control Federation* **58**, 978–984.

Nystrom T., Larsson C., Gustafsson L. (1996) Bacterial defense against aging: role of the *Escherichia coli* ArcA regulator in gene expression, readjusted energy flux and survival during stasis. *EMBO Journal* **15**, 3219–3228.

O'beirne D., Hamer G. (2000) Oxygen availability and the growth of *Escherichia coli* W3110: a problem exacerbated by scale-up. *Bioprocess Engineering* **23**, 487–494.

Palmgren R., Jorand F., Nielsen P. H., Block J. C. (1998) Influence of oxygen limitation on the cell surface properties of bacteria from activated sludge. *Water Science and Technology* **37**, 349–352.

Parker D. S., Merrill M. S. (1976) Oxygen and air activated-sludge: another view. *Journal of the Water Pollution Control Federation* **48**, 2511–2528.

Pena C., Trujillo-Roldan M. A., Galindo E. (2000) Influence of dissolved oxygen tension and agitation speed on alginate production and its molecular weight in cultures of *Azotobacter vinelandii. Enzyme and Microbial Technology* **27**, 390–398.

Peng D. C., Bernet N., Delgenes J. P., Moletta R. (2001) Simultaneous organic carbon and nitrogen removal in an SBR controlled at low dissolved oxygen concentration. *Journal of Chemical Technology and Biotechnology* **76**, 553–558.

Pérez-Elvira S., Nieto Diez P., Fdz-Polanco F. (2006) Sludge minimisation technologies. *Reviews in Environmental Science and Biotechnology* **5**, 375–398.

Pfeiffer T., Schuster S., Bonhoeffer S. (2001) Cooperation and competition in the evolution of ATP-producing pathways. *Science* **292**, 504–507.

Phillips D. H., Johnson M. J. (1961) Aeration in fermentations. *Journal of Biochemical and Microbiological Technology and Engineering* **3**, 277–309.

Postma E., Verduyn C., Scheffers W. A., Vandijken J. P. (1989) Enzymic analysis of the crabtree effect in glucose-limited chemostat cultures of *Saccharomyces-cerevisiae. Applied and Environmental Microbiology* **55**, 468–477.

Ramakrishna D. M., Viraraghavan T. (2005) Strategies for sludge minimization in activated sludge process: a review. *Fresenius Environmental Bulletin* **14**, 2–12.

Richard M., Hao O., Jenkins D. (1985) Growth kinetics of sphaerotilus species and their significance in activated sludge bulking. *Journal of the Water Pollution Control Federation* **57**, 68–81.

Rickard M. D., Gaudy A. F. (1968) Effect of oxygen tension on O_2-uptake and sludge yield in completely mixed heterogeneous populations. Proceedings of the 23th Industrial Waste Conference, Purdue University, West Lafayette, IN.

Roques H., Capdeville B., Seropian J. C., Grigoropoulou H. (1984) Oxygenation by hydrogen-peroxide of the fixed biomass used in biological water treatment. *Water Research* **18**, 103–110.

Russell J. B. (1991) A reassessment of bacterial growth efficiency: the heat production and membrane potential of *Streptococcus bovis* in batch and continuous culture. *Archives of Microbiology* **155**, 559–565.

Russell J. B., Cook G. M. (1995) Energetics of bacterial growth: balance of anabolic and catabolic reactions. *Microbiological Reviews* **59**, 48–62.

Shin H. S., Kang S. T., Nam S. Y. (2001) Effect of carbohydrate and protein in the EPS on sludge settling characteristics. *Water Science and Technology* **43**, 193–196.

Skulachev V. P. (1996) Role of uncoupled and non-coupled oxidations in maintenance of safely low levels of oxygen and its one-electron reductants. *Quarterly Reviews of Biophysics* **29**, 169–202.

Springer A. M., DietrichVelazquez G., Higby C. M., Digiacomo D. (1996) Feasibility study of sludge lysis and recycle in the activated-sludge process. *TAPPI Journal* **79**, 162–170.

Stucki J. W. (1980) The optimal efficiency and the economic degrees of coupling of oxidative phosphorylation. *European Journal of Biochemistry* **109**, 269–283.

Tempest D. W. (1978) Biochemical significance of microbial growth yields: reassessment. *Trends in Biochemical Sciences* **3**, 180–184.

Thabaraj G. J., Gaudy A. F. (1969) Effect of DO concentration on metabolic response of completely mixed activated sludge. Proceedings of the 24th Industrial Waste Conference, Purdue University, West Lafayette, IN.

Travers S. M., Lovett D. A. (1984) Activated-sludge treatment of abattoir wastewater: 2. Influence of dissolved-oxygen concentration. *Water Research* **18**, 435–439.

Vandijken J. P., Weusthuis R. A., Pronk J. T. (1993) Kinetics of growth and sugar consumption in yeasts. *Antonie Van Leeuwenhoek International Journal of General and Molecular Microbiology* **63**, 343–352.

Voet D., Voet J. G. (1995) *Biochemistry*, 2nd ed., Wiley, New York.

Waddell T. G., Repovic P., Melendez-Hevia E., Heinrich R., Montero F. (1999) Optimization of glycolysis: new discussions. *Biochemical Education* **27**, 12–13.

Wei Y. S., Van Houten R. T., Borger A. R., Eikelboom D. H., Fan Y. B. (2003) Minimization of excess sludge production for biological wastewater treatment. *Water Research* **37**, 4453–4467.

Williamson K. J., Nelson P.O. (1981) Influence of dissolved-oxygen on activated-sludge viability. *Journal of the Water Pollution Control Federation* **53**, 1533–1540.

Xu B., Jahic M., Enfors S. O. (1999) Modeling of overflow metabolism in batch and fed-batch cultures of *Escherichia coli*. *Biotechnology Progress* **15**, 81–90.

Zhulin I. B., Johnson M. S., Taylor B. L. (1997) How do bacteria avoid high oxygen concentrations? *Bioscience Reports* **17**, 335–342.

8

MINIMIZING EXCESS SLUDGE PRODUCTION THROUGH MEMBRANE BIOREACTORS AND INTEGRATED PROCESSES

PHILIP CHUEN-YUNG WONG

Division of Environmental and Water Resources Engineering, School of Civil and Environmental Engineering, Nanyang Technological University, Singapore

8.1 INTRODUCTION

Energy considerations have spurred a reevaluation of wastewater treatment processes. Not only is treatment efficiency and effluent quality important, the energy required for treatment is equally so. The largest operating cost in wastewater treatment is that associated with sludge disposal (Low and Chase 1999), followed by the provision of oxygen in aerobic processes (Yoon et al. 2004b). As such, any strategy that seeks to reduce energy consumption substantially must involve reducing sludge output and oxygen input.

A reduction in oxygen use can be realized through the inclusion of nutrient removal schemes, such as predenitrification or biological phosphorus removal. It is also possible to replace aerobic processes with anaerobic processes if nutrient removal is of secondary importance. Irrespective of the biological processes employed and the reactor configuration, sludge is always produced and must be disposed of properly. The handing of excess sludge typically follows anaerobic digestion, dewatering, sludge drying, and finally, either landfilling or incineration. Depending on the specific constraints, one or more of these steps may be omitted.

Biological Sludge Minimization and Biomaterials/Bioenergy Recovery Technologies, First Edition.
Edited by Etienne Paul and Yu Liu.
© 2012 John Wiley & Sons, Inc. Published 2012 by John Wiley & Sons, Inc.

Each sludge management process involves substantial investment cost and has its own drawbacks. For example, a digester of considerable size is required for solids digestion due to the inherently low hydrolysis rate (Pavlostathis and Gossett 1986; Vavilin et al. 1996). Dewatering, sludge drying, and incineration all require significant amounts of energy. Landfilling requires investment in landfill sites and earthmoving equipment, and is increasingly difficult to implement, due to land scarcity and potential problems with leachate.

Although a digester or a landfill can be operated such that energy in the form of biogas can be tapped and thus partially offset the cost of sludge management, it is of greater advantage if sludge production can be reduced at the generation site. This brings about an immediate savings in sludge disposal. Downstream processes can also be scaled down.

The direct manner in which sludge production can be reduced is to lower the sludge wasting rate, thereby raising the sludge age and the cell concentration in the bioreactor. A high sludge concentration results in a viscous suspension, making solids separation by gravity difficult. This is exacerbated by the selection of filamentous microorganisms prevalent at long solids residence times (Massé et al. 2006). As a result, excess sludge reduction by adjusting the sludge wasting rate can only be carried out to the extent to which the clarifier can still function efficiently. It is for the same reason that sludge reduction is often not the deciding factor when selecting a minimum sludge age in conventional treatment plants. Instead, settleability issues necessitate that an upper limit be placed.

Membrane bioreactors (MBRs) eliminate settling concerns through replacement of the clarifier by membrane modules. The micro- or ultrafiltration membranes do not allow suspended solids to escape, and hence completely decouple the hydraulic and solid residence times. This dramatically increases the range of operating sludge ages possible. Reactors can be operated at very long solid residence times, or even without wasting. These long cell ages brought about a new set of interesting observations and opportunities. For example, there is an apparent decrease in yield due to lysis-cryptic growth, maintenance metabolism, and predation (Hamer 1985). These occurrences can be exploited further via integrated processes that enhance cell lyses, or by having an additional step for predation. In this chapter, some of these approaches are presented, with a focus on aerobic membrane bioreactors.

8.2 MASS BALANCES

It is instructive to review mass balances on active cells (X_a), inert organic particulates (X_i), biodegradable particulates (S_p), and soluble substrates (S) in MBRs. The aim is to employ a simple model with just enough complexity to elucidate the underlying processes and to provide an estimated trend of sludge production as a function of various parameters. The influent (flow rate, Q^0) contains biodegradable particulates (S_p^0) and soluble organics (S^0), inert organic solids (X_i^0), and inorganic solids (X_{in}^0). It is assumed that the membrane does not retain colloids and macromolecules so that the permeate chemical oxygen demand (COD) is equal to the reactor soluble COD.

The respective mass balances are

$$V\frac{dX_a}{dt} = -Q^w X_a + \left(\frac{Y\hat{q}S}{K_S + S} - b\right)X_a V \tag{8.1}$$

$$V\frac{dX_i}{dt} = Q^0 X_i^0 - Q^w X_i + (1 - f_d)bX_a V \tag{8.2}$$

$$V\frac{dS_p}{dt} = Q^0 S_p^0 - Q^w S_p - k_{hyd}S_p V \tag{8.3}$$

$$V\frac{dS}{dt} = Q^0(S^0 - S) + k_{hyd}S_p V - \frac{\hat{q}S}{K_S + S}X_a V \tag{8.4}$$

where Y is the true yield, $\hat{q}$ the maximum specific rate of substrate utilization, b the endogenous respiration rate, f_d the fraction of active cells that are biodegradable, and k_{hyd} the first-order hydrolysis rate constant. The reactor volume and waste flow rate are denoted V and Q^w, respectively.

At steady state, Eqs. (8.1) and (8.2) can be rearranged to give

$$\frac{Q^w}{V} = \frac{Y\hat{q}S}{K_S + S} - b \tag{8.5}$$

and

$$\frac{Q^w X_i}{V} = \frac{Q^0 X_i^0}{V} + (1 - f_d)bX_a \tag{8.6}$$

respectively. Recognizing that V/Q^w and V/Q^0 are the sludge age (θ_x) and hydraulic retention time (θ), Eqs. (8.5) and (8.6) are rewritten as

$$S = \frac{K_S(1 + b\theta_x)}{\theta_x(Y\hat{q} - b) - 1} \tag{8.7}$$

and

$$X_i = \theta_x\left[\frac{X_i^0}{\theta} + (1 - f_d)bX_a\right] \tag{8.8}$$

respectively.

Removing the time dependency and making S_p and X_a the subjects, Eqs. (8.3) and (8.4) become

$$S_p = \frac{Q^0 S_p^0}{Q^w + k_{hyd}V} \tag{8.9}$$

and

$$X_a = \frac{(K_S + S)\left[Q^0(S^0 - S) + k_{\text{hyd}}S_p V\right]}{\hat{q}SV} \tag{8.10}$$

respectively. Dividing the numerator and denominator of Eq. (8.10) by S, followed by substituting K_S/S obtained from Eq. (8.7) and S_p from Eq. (8.9), gives the active cell concentration:

$$X_a = \frac{\theta_x}{\theta}\left\{\frac{Y}{1 + b\theta_x}\left[S^0 + \frac{S_p^0 k_{\text{hyd}}\theta_x}{1 + k_{\text{hyd}}\theta_x} - S\right]\right\} \tag{8.11}$$

The corresponding inert particulate concentration is obtained by substituting Eq. (8.11) into Eq. (8.8):

$$X_i = \frac{\theta_x}{\theta}\left\{X_i^0 + \frac{Y(1 - f_d)b\theta_x}{1 + b\theta_x}\left[S^0 + \frac{S_p^0 k_{\text{hyd}}\theta_x}{1 + k_{\text{hyd}}\theta_x} - S\right]\right\} \tag{8.12}$$

Therefore, the total volatile solids, $X_v\ (= X_i + S_p/c_p + X_a)$, is

$$X_v = \frac{\theta_x}{\theta}\left\{X_i^0 + \frac{1}{1 + k_{\text{hyd}}\theta_x}\frac{S_p^0}{c_p} + \frac{Y[1 + (1 - f_d)b\theta_x]}{1 + b\theta_x}\left[S^0 + \frac{S_p^0 k_{\text{hyd}}\theta_x}{1 + k_{\text{hyd}}\theta_x} - S\right]\right\} \tag{8.13}$$

where c_p is the chemical oxygen demand (COD)-to-mass ratio of the nonactive organic particulates, typically around 2. The second term within the braces originate from Eq. (8.9) and represents the particulate contribution from the influent. The total suspended solids concentration is given by

$$X = \frac{\theta_x}{\theta}\left\{X_i^0 + X_{\text{in}}^0 + \frac{1}{1 + k_{\text{hyd}}\theta_x}\frac{S_p^0}{c_p} + \frac{Y[1 + (1 - f_d)b\theta_x]}{0.85(1 + b\theta_x)}\left[S^0 + \frac{S_p^0 k_{\text{hyd}}\theta_x}{1 + k_{\text{hyd}}\theta_x} - S\right]\right\} \tag{8.14}$$

where a volatile-to-total solids ratio of 0.85 is used.

The volatile and total sludge production rates are then

$$P_{X_v} = Q^w X_v = Q^0\left\{X_i^0 + \frac{1}{1 + k_{\text{hyd}}\theta_x}\frac{S_p^0}{c_p} + \frac{Y[1 + (1 - f_d)b\theta_x]}{1 + b\theta_x}\left[S^0 + \frac{S_p^0 k_{\text{hyd}}\theta_x}{1 + k_{\text{hyd}}\theta_x} - S\right]\right\} \tag{8.15}$$

and

$$P_X = Q^w X = Q^0 \left\{ X_i^0 + X_{\text{in}}^0 + \frac{1}{1 + k_{\text{hyd}}\theta_x} \frac{S_p^0}{c_p} + \frac{Y[1 + (1 - f_d)b\theta_x]}{0.85(1 + b\theta_x)} \left[S^0 + \frac{S_p^0 k_{\text{hyd}}\theta_x}{1 + k_{\text{hyd}}\theta_x} - S \right] \right\}$$

(8.16)

respectively.

The true yield of anaerobic consortia (acid formers and methanogens) is around four times lower than that of the aerobic counterparts. As such, a low sludge production is characteristic of anaerobic processes. However, local conditions might not favor anaerobic treatment, for a variety of reasons. If aerobic processes must be applied, one strategy of reducing the true yield of the aerobic community is to employ chemical uncouplers (Low et al. 2000).

More generally, the straightforward way to minimize excess sludge is to reduce the wasting rate. This results in an increase in sludge age, and hence the MLSS (mixed liquor suspended solids). In a conventional activated sludge process (CAS), where cell separation is carried out by gravity, θ_x is typically not more than 20 d. This is necessary not only to limit an excessively high MLSS level but also to prevent the selection of difficult-to-settle filamentous microorganism. Settling related issues, including bulking and foaming, are immaterial in an MBR from a cell separation perspective. This greatly expands the range of θ_x that can be applied. From a sludge disposal standpoint, a high solids concentration in the wasting line is beneficial, as the costs of dewatering, drying, and incineration are reduced.

The Observed yield, $Y_{\text{obs}} \left[= P_{X_v}/Q^0(S^0 + S_p^0 - S) \right]$, decreases with θ_x, as can be deduced from the equations. If X_i^0 and S_p^0 are small and can be neglected, the trend is more easily described:

$$Y_{\text{obs}} = \frac{Y[1 + (1 - f_d)b\theta_x]}{1 + b\theta_x}$$

(8.17)

Y_{obs} decreases monotonically and approaches $(1 - f_d)Y$ when $\theta_x \gg 1/b(1 - f_d)$ ($=25$ d using typical values of $b = 0.2\,\text{d}^{-1}$ and $f_d = 0.8$; Rittmann and McCarty 2001). The various solids concentrations are reduced to the following at a large solids residence time (SRT):

$$X_a = \frac{Y}{b\theta} \left[S^0 + S_p^0 - S \right]$$

(8.18)

$$X_i = X_v = \frac{\theta_x}{\theta} \left\{ X_i^0 + Y(1 - f_d) \left[S^0 + S_p^0 - S \right] \right\}$$

(8.19)

$$X = \frac{\theta_x}{\theta} \left\{ X_i^0 + X_{\text{in}}^0 + \frac{Y(1 - f_d)}{0.85} \left[S^0 + S_p^0 - S \right] \right\}$$

(8.20)

Thus, simple mass balances predict that when $\theta_x \gg 25$ d, the active cell concentration approaches a constant, whereas the inert solids concentration increases linearly with θ_x and dominates the volatile solids content. Similar trends are predicted by more sophisticated models, such as those based on the IWA (International Water Association) activated sludge models (ASM; Henze et al. 2000), albeit with differing accuracies, particularly at large SRTs (Spérandio and Espinosa 2008; Lubello et al. 2009; Fenu et al. 2010).

Although the increasing trend in X is observed in practice, it has also been noted that the MLSS and MLVSS (mixed liquor volatile suspended solids) have a reduced rate of increase at very large θ_x (Muller et al. 1995; Rosenberger et al. 2002; Pollice et al. 2004, 2008). Moreover, the observed yields tend to decline (Huang et al. 2001). These are due to a combination of factors, including maintenance metabolism (Rosenberger et al. 2002; Witzig et al. 2002), predation (Teck et al. 2009), hydrolysis and biodegradation of inert solids (Pollice et al. 2004, 2008), dissolution of inorganic solids (Laera et al. 2005), and settling of inorganic solids within the bioreactor (Rosenberger et al. 2002).

8.3 INTEGRATED PROCESSES BASED ON LYSIS-CRYPTIC GROWTH

Sludge minimization solely through an increase in SRT can cause difficulties in MBR operation because of excessive solids accumulation. A high MLSS value is associated with high sludge viscosity (Laera et al. 2007; Trussell et al. 2007; Pollice et al. 2008) and oxygen transfer resistance (Muller et al. 1995; Yoon et al. 2004b; Henkel et al. 2009a,b). Membrane clogging and fouling are also exacerbated (Pollice et al. 2004; Chang and Kim 2005; Trussell et al. 2007; Wu et al. 2011; Wu and Lee 2011). Elevated SRTs may also affect nutrient removal negatively (Ersu et al. 2010). As such, a complete excess sludge reduction strategy would typically incorporate sludge disintegration and solubilization to enhance the decay rate or the biodegradability of solids. This gives rise to sludge disintegration methods that disrupt the solids structure, solubilizing the solids before channeling the treated products back to the reactor for further digestion. These processes provide additional control of sludge concentration.

An effective disintegration and solubilization process can substantially reduce the SRT without increasing the quantity of sludge discharged from an MBR. Conversely, the wasting rate can be reduced considerably without a corresponding increase in mixed liquor concentration. The process involves lysing a portion of the bioreactor suspended solids in a sidestream vessel and returning the partially solubilized products to the reactor. This can be carried out in batch or continuous mode. The mass flow to be disintegrated hinges largely on the influence that cycling of disintegrated products has on effluent quality and the economics of the process.

Disintegration and solubilization techniques are varied and include physical processes such as ultrasound and mechanical cell disruption, chemical processes such as alkali treatment and ozonation, and thermal heating (Ødegaard 2004). Some of these techniques can be combined for better effect. Although the underlying mechanisms of the methods differ, the flow of carbon and electrons from whole cells to solubilized organics can be conceptualized as depicted in Fig. 8.1. The distinction

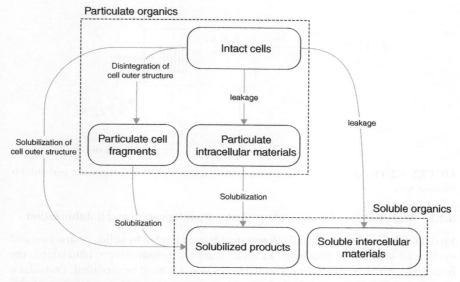

FIGURE 8.1 Schematic depicting the disintegration and solubilization of intact cells.

between particulates and solutes is defined operationally (e.g., filtration using a 1.2- or 0.45-μm filter), allowing disintegration and solubilization to be undertaken irrespective of the actual underlying mechanism. For example, sonication first weakens the intermolecular forces of the outer cell structure of an intact cell, creating particulate cell fragments. This is considered disintegration. The fragments can be further broken into colloidal materials in the solubilization step. In contrast, chemical treatment undermines the outer cell structure by direct reaction, forming soluble products. The unevenly weakened structure then disintegrates into particulates. In both cases, a compromised cell wall and membrane allow intracellular materials to be released and be available for further physical or chemical attacks.

For completeness, intracellular particulates such as storage polymers (polyhydroxyalkanoates, glycogen) are included in Fig. 8.1. Their importance depends on the bioprocess adopted (biological phosphorus removal, presence of feast–famine cycles, etc.) and the specific reactor from which sludge is removed for treatment. For example, in biological phosphorus removal, sludge is withdrawn from the aerobic reactor where polyhydroxyalkanoates are biologically oxidized, and polyphosphates are synthesized. The concentration of the former would be low and may be neglected, but an elevated phosphorus concentration is expected from solubilization of the latter (Saktaywin et al. 2005).

Depending on the process selected, the major route(s) from whole cells to soluble organics, and the kinetics associated with each route differ. As a result, the disintegration and solubilization efficiency is expected to be markedly different, which ultimately affects the quantity and composition of disintegrated products. These are discussed in ensuing sections.

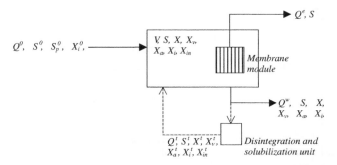

FIGURE 8.2 Process flow of a membrane bioreactor with a disintegration and solubilization unit.

8.3.1 Mass Balance Incorporating Sludge Disintegration and Solubilization

Mixed liquor concentration and effluent quality are affected by solids destruction and cycling of solubilized products. To understand the quantitative relationships, the basic mass balance equations presented in Section 8.2 must be modified. Consider a generic process flow consisting of a one-stage bioreactor with a sidestream disintegration and solubilization (DS) unit, as shown in Fig. 8.2. For simplicity, both vessels are treated as completely mixed and continuous-flow reactors. In addition, it is assumed that no cell growth takes place in the DS unit.

Taking the bioreactor as the control volume, the mass balance equation on active cells is

$$V\frac{dX_a}{dt} = Q^t(X_a^t - X_a) - Q^w X_a + \left(\frac{Y\hat{q}S}{K_S + S} - b\right)X_a V \qquad (8.21)$$

where the flow rate to the DS unit is denoted Q^t. It is assumed that the same flow returns to the bioreactor. Active cells from the DS unit are denoted X_a^t.

At steady state, Eq. (8.21) becomes

$$\frac{Q^t\left(X_a - X_a^t\right) + Q^w X_a}{X_a V} = \frac{Y\hat{q}S}{K_S + S} - b \qquad (8.22)$$

which allows the SRT of a MBR with a DS unit to be defined:

$$\theta_x^t \equiv \frac{VX_a}{Q^t(X_a - X_a^t) + Q^w X_a} \qquad (8.23)$$

Therefore, the substrate concentration has the same form as Eq. (8.7), but with θ_x^t in place of θ_x:

$$S = \frac{K_S(1 + b\theta_x^t)}{\theta_x^t(Y\hat{q} - b) - 1} \qquad (8.24)$$

A minimum θ_x^t can be defined:

$$\theta_{x,min}^t \equiv \frac{V}{Q^t + Q^w} \tag{8.25}$$

which corresponds to the case in which disintegration and solubilization are very effective $(X_a^t \ll X_a)$. An upper bound in θ_x^t can be conceptualized similarly:

$$\theta_{x,\,max}^t \equiv \frac{V}{Q^w} \tag{8.26}$$

This corresponds to an ineffective process $(X_a^t \approx X_a)$ and is equal to the SRT without sludge disintegration. Equations (8.24) to (8.26) indicate that the reactor substrate concentration must increase if sludge disintegration is carried out and if Q^w is unchanged. However, such an increase can be marginal if θ_x^t is not pushed too low through prudent control of Q^t. Suitably reducing Q^w as Q^t is increased would reduce sludge production without compromising effluent quality.

The direct application of Eq. (8.23) is problematic, as X_a is not known. If the fraction of active cells out of all volatile solids (X_v) is similar for both bioreactor sludge and that from the DS unit (i.e., $X_a^t/X_v^t \approx X_a/X_v$), X_a in Eq. (8.23) can be replaced by X_v, which is easily measured as MLVSS. However, since active cells are likely to be impaired or deactivated while simultaneously being solubilized, it is possible that $X_a^t/X_v^t \leq X_a/X_v$. The approach would then yield an overestimated SRT:

$$\theta_{x,max2}^t = \frac{VX_v}{Q^t(X_v - X_v^t) + Q^wX_v} \geq \theta_x^t \tag{8.27}$$

Nevertheless, Eq. (8.27) provides a convenient estimate of θ_x^t and is a more realistic upper limit than Eq. (8.26), especially when no wasting is carried out.

Mass balance on inert solids gives the following:

$$V\frac{dX_i}{dt} = Q^0X_i^0 + Q^t(X_i^t - X_i) - Q^wX_i + (1 - f_d)bX_aV \tag{8.28}$$

which at steady state becomes

$$\frac{Q^t(X_i - X_i^t) + Q^wX_i}{VX_i} = \frac{Q^0X_i^0}{VX_i} + \frac{(1 - f_d)bX_a}{X_i} \tag{8.29}$$

If the mass ratio of active to inert cells is similar in the reactor and in the DS sludge $(X_a^t/X_i^t \approx X_a/X_i)$, X_a can be replaced with X_i in Eq. (8.23) and substituted into Eq. (8.29) to give

$$X_i \approx \theta_x^t \left[\frac{X_i^0}{\theta} + (1 - f_d)bX_a\right] \tag{8.30}$$

Before writing the mass balance on the soluble substrate, the additional contributions from the solubilized particulates (S^t) and the nonactive biodegradable solids (S_p^t) exiting the DS unit need to be clarified. S^t and S_p^t are given by

$$S^t = c_v(X_v - X_v^t) + S \tag{8.31}$$

and

$$S_p^t = c_p(X_v^t - X_a^t - X_i^t) \tag{8.32}$$

respectively. A different COD-to-mass ratio (c_v) is used in Eq. (8.31) to represent solubilized organics of both microbial and nonmicrobial origin. Since the former is in much larger amounts, c_v is expected to be close to 1.42. It is assumed that no substrate mineralization occurs in the DS unit—an appropriate approximation in most cases except where significant oxidation is allowed to take place, in which case S^t given by Eq. (8.31) would be an overestimate.

The mass balance of nonactive biodegradable solids in the bioreactor, $S_p \left[= c_p(X_v - X_a - X_i)\right]$, is

$$V\frac{dS_p}{dt} = Q^0 S_p^0 + Q^t(S_p^t - S_p) - Q^w S_p - k_{\text{hyd}} S_p V \tag{8.33}$$

At steady state, Eq. (8.33) gives

$$S_p = \frac{Q^0 S_p^0 + Q^t S_p^t}{Q^t + Q^w + k_{\text{hyd}} V} \tag{8.34}$$

which upon hydrolysis, contributes to the available soluble organics in the bioreactor. Therefore, the mass balance of S is

$$V\frac{dS}{dt} = Q^0(S^0 - S) + Q^t(S^t - S) + k_{\text{hyd}} S_p V - \frac{\hat{q}S}{K_S + S}X_a V \tag{8.35}$$

At steady state, Eq. (8.35) can be rearranged to give

$$X_a = \frac{K_S + S}{\hat{q}S\theta}\left[S^0 + \frac{Q^t(S^t - S) + k_{\text{hyd}} S_p V}{Q^0} - S\right] \tag{8.36}$$

Dividing the numerator and denominator by S, followed by substituting K_S/S from Eq. (8.24), S_p from Eq. (8.34), and then invoking Eq. (8.25), Eq. (8.36) becomes

$$X_a = \frac{\theta_x^t}{\theta}\frac{Y}{(1 + b\theta_x^t)}\left[S^o + \frac{S_p^0 k_{\text{hyd}} \theta_{x,\text{min}}^t}{1 + k_{\text{hyd}} \theta_{x,\text{min}}^t} + \frac{Q^t}{Q^0}\left(S^t - S + \frac{S_p^t k_{\text{hyd}} \theta_{x,\text{min}}^t}{1 + k_{\text{hyd}} \theta_{x,\text{min}}^t}\right) - S\right] \tag{8.37}$$

The second term in brackets is related to the hydrolysis of organic particulates in the influent, whereas the third term contains components related to the solubilized and organic particulates exiting the DS unit.

Substituting Eq. (8.37) into Eq. (8.30) gives the estimated inert solids concentration,

$$X_i \approx \frac{\theta_x^t}{\theta} \left\{ X_i^0 + \frac{Y(1-f_d)b\theta_x^t}{(1+b\theta_x^t)} \left[S^0 + \frac{S_p^0 k_{hyd}\theta_{x,min}^t}{1+k_{hyd}\theta_{x,min}^t} + \frac{Q^t}{Q^0}\left(S^t - S + \frac{S_p^t k_{hyd}\theta_{x,min}^t}{1+k_{hyd}\theta_{x,min}^t} \right) - S \right] \right\} \tag{8.38}$$

The volatile and total solids concentrations are

$$X_v \approx \frac{\theta_x^t}{\theta} \left\{ \begin{array}{l} X_i^0 + \dfrac{1}{\theta_x^t/\theta_{x,min}^t + k_{hyd}\theta_x^t} \dfrac{1}{c_p}\left(S_p^0 + \dfrac{Q^t}{Q^0}S_p^t \right) \\[2ex] + \dfrac{Y\left[1+(1-f_d)b\theta_x^t\right]}{1+b\theta_x^t}\left[S^0 + \dfrac{S_p^0 k_{hyd}\theta_{x,min}^t}{1+k_{hyd}\theta_{x,min}^t} + \dfrac{Q^t}{Q^0}\left(S^t - S + \dfrac{S_p^t k_{hyd}\theta_{x,min}^t}{1+k_{hyd}\theta_{x,min}^t} \right) - S \right] \end{array} \right\} \tag{8.39}$$

and

$$X \approx \frac{\theta_x^t}{\theta} \left\{ \begin{array}{l} X_i^0 + X_{in}^0 + \dfrac{1}{\theta_x^t/\theta_{x,min}^t + k_{hyd}\theta_x^t} \dfrac{1}{c_p}\left(S_p^0 + \dfrac{Q^t}{Q^0}S_p^t \right) \\[2ex] + \dfrac{Y\left[1+(1-f_d)b\theta_x^t\right]}{0.85(1+b\theta_x^t)}\left[S^0 + \dfrac{S_p^0 k_{hyd}\theta_{x,min}^t}{1+k_{hyd}\theta_{x,min}^t} + \dfrac{Q^t}{Q^0}\left(S^t - S + \dfrac{S_p^t k_{hyd}\theta_{x,min}^t}{1+k_{hyd}\theta_{x,min}^t} \right) - S \right] \end{array} \right\} \tag{8.40}$$

respectively. The second and third terms in braces in Eqs. (8.39) and (8.40), respectively, originate from Eq. (8.34), representing particulate contribution from the influent. Sludge production may then be estimated accordingly.

One should be mindful of the assumptions made in developing the preceding equations, and make modifications depending on the actual configuration and process. In the derivations of the solids concentrations, it was implied that inert and inorganic particulates are conservative. Recent research indicates that solids such as endogenous residue, traditionally considered to be inert, may be degraded, albeit at low rates (Ramdani et al. 2010). Soluble microbial products were also not considered. Additionally, no distinction was made between cells and biodegradable particulates in the influent; hence the same hydrolysis rate was employed for both.

To include the performance of disintegration and solubilization in the preceding development, a representation of solubilization efficiency is necessary. This can be either from the percentage reduction in MLVSS (or MLSS) or the increase in soluble

TABLE 8.1 Summary of MBRs Integrated With Disintegration–Solubilization Units Employing Various Lysis–Cryptic Growth Techniques

Process	Substrate (mg L^{-1})	Membrane	Disintegration and Technique Solubilization	$\theta'_{x,\min}$ (d)	$\theta'_{x,\max}$ (d)	$\theta'_{x,\max}$ (d)	X_v (g L^{-1})	Y_{obs} (g VSS g^{-1} COD)	Effluent quality (mg L^{-1}) and Remarks	Ref.
Anoxic–aerobic MBR Recirculation ratio = 3, HRT$_{anox}$ = 3 h, HRT$_{aer}$ = 6 h, Q^0 = 200 L d^{-1}	Real sewage COD ≈ 230, SS ≈ 66, TN ≈ 53, TP ≈ 5, ALK as CaCO$_3$ ≈ 216	Immersed flat sheet PVDF, 0.22 μm, Flux = 17 LMH (constant flux operation; 10 min suction, 2 min pause)	Thermal-alkaline (NaOH). Mixed liquor from aerobic reactor treated at a rate of (a) 0 (control) (b) 0.015Q^0 at 80°C, pH 11 for 3 h, α_s = 0.2. Treated sludge returned to anoxic reactor.	(a) 76 (b) 23	(a) 76 (b) 64	(a) 76 (b) 113	(a) 5.6 (b) 5.4	(a) 0.145 (b) 0.094	Similar effluent quality for both units: COD ≈ 8, TN ≈ 19, TP ≈ 3. No observable difference in sludge viscosities and membrane fouling rates	Do et al. (2009)
Recirculation ratio = 2, HRT$_{anox}$ = 3.2 h, HRT$_{aer}$ = 5 h, Q^0 = 30 L d^{-1} TP ≈ 4	Sewage source not reported COD ≈ 224, SS ≈ 41, NH$_4^+$-N ≈ 30, TN ≈ 38	Immersed flat sheet, 0.4 μm, Flux = 15 LMH (constant flux operation; 10 min suction, 2 min pause)	Ozonation. Mixed liquor from aerobic reactor batch-treated at a rate of (a) 0 (control) (b) 0.0039Q^0 (= 0.95 g MLSS d^{-1}) Dosage = 100 mg O$_3$ g^{-1} MLSS (90% utilization). Contact time and α not reported. Estimated α_x = 0.53 using Eq. (8.46). Treated sludge returned to anoxic reactor.	(a) 120 (b) 89	(a) 120 (b) 165	(a) 120 (b) ∞	(a) 6.9 (b) 6.1	(a) 0.12 (b) 0	(a) COD ≈ 9, NH$_4^+$-N ≈ 0.3, TN ≈ 12, TP ≈ 2, P_X ≈ 1.04 g d^{-1} (b) COD ≈ 12, NH$_4^+$-N ≈ 1.4, TN ≈ 11, TP ≈ 2, P_X ~ 0. Similar membrane performance for both units; TMP < 10 kPa for 40 d	Song et al. (2003)
Aerobic MBR HRT = 6 h,	Synthetic, COD ≈ 342, SS ≈ 178,	Immersed hollow-fiber, PE, 0.05 μm	Ozonation. Mixed liquor treated at a rate of	(a) ∞ (b) 50	(a) ∞ (b) 94	(a) ∞ (b) ∞	(a) 1.8–9.0 (b) 1.8–6.4	(a) 0.025 (b) 0.016	(a) COD ≈ 32 (b) COD ≈ 38	He et al. (2006)

Table (rotated 90°; continued):

Reactor / feed & operation	Sludge reduction technique							Reference
V = 16.5 L, NH$_4^+$-N ≈ 41, TN ≈ 54, TP ≈ 3; DO = 2 mg L^{-1}; HRT = 7 h; Immersed flat sheet (unknown polyalkene), 0.22 μm; Flux = 20 LMH (constant flux operation; 10 min suction, 2 min pause)	(a) 0 (control) (b) 0.005Q^0 (c) 0.010Q^0 Dosage = 160 mg O$_3$ g^{-1} MLSS, contact time = 2 h, α$_t$ = 0.02, α$_t$ = 0.53; Alkaline (NaOH) and ozonation; Mixed liquor treated at a rate of	(c) 25	(c) 47	(c) ∞	(c) 1.8–3.7 Values from day 0–120	(c) ~ 0 Values after day 60, when P_X is constant	(c) COD ≈ 41 Estimated from COD removal from day 60–120	Oh et al. (2007)
Real sewage. COD ≈ 292, SS ≈ 182, TN ≈ 48; V = 28 L, TN ≈ 48, DO = 3–5 mg L^{-1}, TP ≈ 9, ALK as CaCO$_3$ ≈ 165	(a) 0 (control)	(a) ∞	(a) ∞	(a) ∞	(a) 8.9–11.9	(a) 0.13	(a) COD ≈ 13	
	(b) 0.015Q^0 at pH 11 for 3 h, followed by ozonation. Dosage = 20 mg O$_3$ g^{-1} MLSS (90–95% utilization), contact time = 0.44–0.59 h, α$_t$ = 0.19	(b) 19	(b) 97	(b) ∞	(b) 8.1 Values from day 0–120	(b) ~ 0 Values from day 0–120	(b) COD ≈ 13 Values from day 0–120. Fouling in control MBR associated with high MLSS. Solubilization reduces MLSS and appears to mitigate fouling.	
Synthetic; COD ≈ 4036; HRT = 96 h; 20°C; V = 8.5 L; Immersed hollow-fiber, PVDF, 0.1 μm; Flux = 1.3 LMH (constant flux operation; 2 min suction, 4 min pause)	(a) Control; Sonication	(a) ∞	(a) ∞	(a) ∞	(a) 5.7–10.7	(a) 0.18	(a) COD ≈ 46	Yoon et al. (2004a)
	(b) 1 L mixed liquor batch-treated daily (equivalent to 0.47 Q^0) for 1 h at 600 W, 20 kHz; specific energy input = 295 kJ g^{-1}; ultrasonic density = 0.6 W mL^{-1}; α not reported.	(b) 8.5	(b) Unable to estimate	(b) ∞	(b) 5.2–6.6 Values from day 0–28	(b) 0.05 Values from day 0–28	(b) COD ≈ 76 Estimates from day 0–28	

organics relative to the initial solids concentration. Designating the former and latter by α_x and α_s, respectively, they are

$$\alpha_x = \frac{X_v - X_v^t}{X_v} \qquad (8.41)$$

and

$$\alpha_s = \frac{S^t - S}{c_v X_v} \qquad (8.42)$$

Conceptually, these two equations are equivalent, and both lead to

$$S^t = \alpha c_v X_v + S \qquad (8.43)$$

and

$$S_p^t = (1 - \alpha) S_p \qquad (8.44)$$

where α is either α_x or α_s. In practice, α_s is typically smaller than α_x due to more stringent laboratory procedures in defining soluble components (e.g., filtering through 0.2 or 0.45 μm membranes). Additionally, processes that oxidize soluble organics while undertaking solubilization would reduce α_s, complicating its interpretation.

The upper limit of the effective sludge age [Eq. (8.27)] can be rewritten as

$$\theta_{x,\text{max2}}^t = \frac{VX_v}{Q^t(\alpha X_v) + Q^w X_v} = \frac{V}{\alpha Q^t + Q^w} \qquad (8.45)$$

using the general α. Equation (8.45) thus relates the reduction in sludge age with solubilization efficiency.

In the next three sections, common lysis-cryptic growth techniques for which efforts have been made to integrate with MBRs are presented. They include thermal and thermal-alkaline methods, ozonation, and sonication. Where appropriate, data from the cited literature are reanalyzed in accordance with the framework developed in this section. For easy reference, a summary of the work cited is presented in Table 8.1.

8.3.2 Thermal and Thermal-Alkaline Treatment

Heating is a simple method that promotes lyses of temperature-sensitive cells. This can be attractive if a source of waste heat is readily available. The efficacy of heating and the compositional changes of sludge during thermal treatment were studied specifically by Yan et al. (2008). Sludge from a conventional sewage treatment plant was heated at 60°C for 24 h. The initial 6200 mg L^{-1} MLSS decreased by 20, 28,

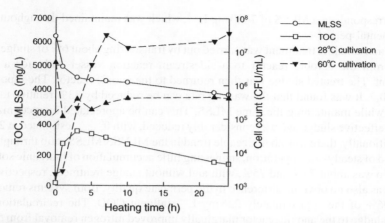

FIGURE 8.3 Changes in concentrations of solids and soluble organics during heat treatment at 60°C. Also depicted are cell counts of heat-treated bacteria grown at 28 and 60°C. [Data from Yan et al. (2008).]

and 29% after 1, 3, and 5 h, respectively, before reaching a final concentration of 3800 mg L^{-1} after 24 h (Fig. 8.3)—a 39% reduction or an α_x of 0.39. The trend in MLSS indicates that treatment beyond 3 h did not improve solubilization substantially. This could be due to an accumulation of cell fragments that resist solubilization and/or the continued growth of certain groups of microorganism.

Cells sampled at periodic intervals were cultivated at 28 and 60°C to track the population of viable thermoduric microorganisms. The population (in colony-forming units per milliliter) cultivated at 28°C decreased by 98% after a 1-h heating period, followed by a small apparent increase before stabilizing after 3 h of heating (Fig. 8.3). This represents a 94% reduction in the initial active mesophilic population. The lysate and solubilized solids were utilized concurrently by another group of thermoduric (and thermophilic) bacteria that were better adapted to the higher temperature. The production and consumption of these soluble organics resulted in a rise and fall in soluble total organic carbon (TOC; Fig. 8.3).

The dominance of thermophilic microorganisms was evidenced by a four-order-of-magnitude increase in the population of cells cultivated at 60°C during the first 7 h of heating. To limit the multiplication of these cells, heating time should be controlled between 1 and 3 h, or additional methods employed to inhibit cell growth. Energy and space considerations also call for short thermal treatment times.

When combined with alkaline treatment, heat can prevent cell growth and enhance solubilization. One technique involves heating the sludge at 80°C at pH 11. This process was investigated by Do et al. (2009) in a nitrogen-removing MBR treating real sewage. The predenitrifying configuration consists of a 25-L anoxic reactor and a 50-L aerobic reactor. Sludge was cycled at a recirculation ratio of 3 between the aerobic and anoxic reactors via a 12.5-L intermediate oxygen stripping tank. Two setups, with and without thermal-alkaline treatment, were compared. For the control, the sludge age calculated from the reported wasting rate was about 76 d.

This corresponds to a MLSS of 7400 mg L^{-1}, which was maintained throughout the experimental period.

Thermal-alkaline treatment was carried out by transferring about 6% of sludge (by mass) from the aerobic reactor to a sidestream reaction vessel daily for a 3-h treatment. The treated sludge was then returned to the anoxic reactor. The reported α_s was 0.2. It was found that the wasting rate can be reduced by 33% relative to the control while maintaining the same MLSS. This can be appreciated by recognizing that the effective sludge age was considerably reduced, with $\theta^t_{x,\, max2}$ estimated at 28 d.

Additionally, there was no noticeable trend in the MLVSS/MLSS ratio throughout the 120 d of steady-state operation, suggesting little accumulation of inorganic solids. The ratio was about 73% and 75%, with and without sludge treatment, respectively. There was also no obvious difference in the permeate quality. Both systems removed about 96% of the approximately 226 mg L^{-1} influent COD. The recirculation of treated sludge to the anoxic reactor marginally improved nitrogen removal from 59% to 61%, due primarily to the increase in effective influent C/N ratio from 4.2 to 4.8. Thermal-alkaline sludge treatment did not increase fouling rate. Both sets of immersed PVDF microfiltration (MF) membranes, operated in 10-min suction, 2-min pause cycles, showed similar rates of transmembrane pressure (TMP) increase from 1.3 to about 6 kPa in 180 d while maintaining the flux at 17 LMH.

8.3.3 Ozonation

The mechanisms of ozonation for sludge reduction and disinfection are similar. Ozone has a high redox potential, allowing it to oxidize bacterial cell wall and membrane, leading to cell lysis. Following this simultaneous disintegration and solubilization of the cell outer structure, the intracellular materials become accessible for further oxidative attack. These may be carried out by ozone itself, or indirectly via hydroxyl radicals decomposed from ozone (Staehelin and Hoigne 1985).

The oxidizing power of ozone notwithstanding, most of the organic solids are merely solubilized, or may only be partially oxidized, instead of being mineralized. For example, He et al. (2006) observed a 30% COD reduction in the soluble portion of 5260 mg L^{-1} of mixed liquor when ozonated for 1 h at a dosing rate of 240 mg h^{-1}. When the same dose was applied to whole sludge, soluble COD increased from 32 mg L^{-1} to about 175 mg L^{-1}. The demonstration of solubilization overwhelming oxidation notwithstanding, partial oxidation is sufficiently significant to yield a low α_s of 0.02. In another batch test, an initial 2750 mg L^{-1} MLVSS was reduced by 56% in 2 h (i.e., an α_x of 0.56). This is in line with the findings of Saktaywin et al. (2005), who related α_x (measured via changes in MLSS, in COD units) with the specific ozone consumption (SOC, mg O_3 g^{-1} MLSS). SOC is the amount of ozone utilized and is independent of reactor specific parameters. Reanalyzing their data by nonlinear regression, an empirical fit is obtained:

$$\alpha_x = 0.76 \tanh(0.0095 \times SOC) \tag{8.46}$$

which holds irrespective of the ozone concentration in the ozone contactor and the initial sludge concentration. The experimental range of the former was 20 to

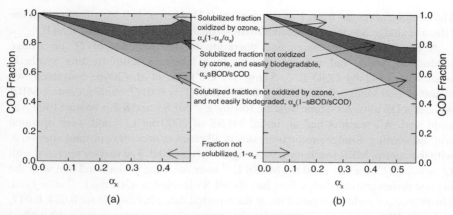

FIGURE 8.4 Area plot fractionating total COD following ozonation at various solubilization efficiency for (a) 50 and (b) 90 mg L^{-1} residual ozone. [Derived using data from Saktaywin et al. (2005).]

90 mg L^{-1}, and the latter 1200 to 4000 mg MLSS L^{-1}. The 95% confidence intervals of the two coefficients are (0.72, 0.81) and (0.0083, 0.0108).

Equation (8.46) suggests that about 24% of particulate sludge COD resists solubilization. Of those solubilized, the ozone-oxidizable fraction $1 - \alpha_s/\alpha_x$ increases with the residual ozone concentration, but is reduced when α_x increases, due to the release of chemically resistant components such as lipids. The biodegradable fraction of the solubilized organics (represented by the soluble BOD/COD ratio) not oxidized by ozone decreases with α_x. These parameters and trends, derived from Saktaywin et al. (2005), are depicted in Fig. 8.4 for 50 and 90 mg L^{-1} residual ozone concentrations.

In their comprehensive study, Saktaywin et al. (2005) also assessed the loss in activities of ozonated sludge and related it to α_x. The former was defined by the oxygen uptake rate of ozonated sludge (OUR^t) normalized by that of nonozonated sludge (OUR). Regression analysis of their data yields the empirical equation

$$\frac{OUR^t}{OUR} = 1 - \frac{1.08\alpha_x}{0.124 + \alpha_x} \tag{8.47}$$

which is valid in the experimented range $0 < \alpha_x < 0.36$. The form of Eq. (8.47) is identical to that provided by Saktaywin et al. (2005), although the coefficients differ as the authors included data on the ratio of phosphorus released as a measure of activity loss in their derivation. OUR^t/OUR can be considered a proxy for X_a^t/X_a, whereas $X_v^t/X_v = 1 - \alpha_x$, from Eq. (8.41). Taken together, a relation between the fractional active solids following ozonation and that of nonozonated sludge can be deduced:

$$\frac{X_a^t}{X_v^t} = \frac{1}{1 - \alpha_x}\left(1 - \frac{1.08\alpha_x}{0.124 + \alpha_x}\right)\frac{X_a}{X_v} \tag{8.48}$$

The coefficient ranges from 1 when α_x is 0 to 0.31 when α_x is 0.36, affirming that the effective sludge age in an integrated MBR-ozonation process is smaller than $\theta^t_{x, max2}$.

A consideration in design and operation is the influence of Q^t on sludge production, yield, and effluent quality. In a lab-scale setup treating synthetic wastewater (342 mg COD L^{-1}, 54 mg TN L^{-1}), He et al. (2006) compared two disintegration sludge flows, $Q^t = 0.005Q^0$ and $Q^t = 0.01Q^0$ with a control MBR without a DS unit. An ozone dose of 160 mg g^{-1} MLSS and a 2-h contact time was employed. All reactors had an initial MLSS of 2000 mg L^{-1} and were operated without wasting. Sludge production rates in all reactors becomes constant after 60 d, with the control MBR reaching 10,000 mg L^{-1} after 120 d. The reactor operated with $Q^t = 0.005Q^0$ reached 7500 mg MLSS L^{-1} over the same period, and that with the highest disintegrating sludge flow had its MLSS leveled at 4300 mg L^{-1} after 60 d. The respective yields computed using the reported data after day 60 are 0.024, 0.017, and ~ 0 g VSS g^{-1} COD. Compared to the control, the permeate quality at the highest Q^t was only slightly inferior, both in terms of COD (91 vs. 88% removal) and NH_4^+ (93% vs. 91%), affirming that at the exact balance between cell growth and disintegration, effluent quality need not be severely compromised.

Zero sludge production was also demonstrated in a predenitrifiying MBR (Song et al. 2003) in which the ozonated sludge was returned to the anoxic reactor. The Q^t applied was $0.0039Q^0$ and the average SOC was 90 mg O_3 g^{-1} MLSS. Ozonation was sufficient in maintaining a constant MLVSS of about 6100 mg L^{-1}. In contrast, a wasting rate of 1.04 g MLSS d^{-1} is necessary to maintain a MLVSS of 6900 mg L^{-1} in a control MBR without sludge ozonation. Effluent qualities from both MBRs were similar. Probably because of the similar sludge concentration, no apparent performance difference in the immersed flat sheet MF membranes in the two setups was observed. Hence, it was concluded that ozone treatment did not show any propensity to enhance fouling rates.

Despite the solubilizing efficacy of ozone, the cost of ozone production is high (Chu et al. 2009), and this may limit its adoption. Apart from improving on ozone mass transfer into sludge, which entails better designs of ozone contactors, ozonation can be combined with alkaline (NaOH) treatment for the purpose of reducing ozone dosage. This is possible, as NaOH is itself a solubilizing agent. It also has the additional advantage of being able to moderate pH decrease due to ozonation and nitrification.

Sequential alkaline-ozone solubilization was investigated in a MBR, in which the disintegrating sludge flow $(Q^t = 0.015Q^0)$ was first subjected to 3 h of alkaline (pH 11) treatment followed by 0.44 to 0.59 h of ozonation (Oh et al. 2007). The ozone dose was 20 mg g^{-1} MLSS with 90 to 95% utilization. The performance of combined treatment is shown in Fig. 8.5. The average α_s following NaOH and ozone treatment is 0.14 and 0.19, respectively. The corresponding α_x, which was not measured, should be even higher. Nevertheless, the final α_s was already larger than the α_x for ozone treatment alone—a value of 0.13, which can be estimated using Eq. (8.46). It can be further deduced, by setting $\alpha_x = 0.19$, that at least a 30% reduction in ozone dosage is possible in sequential alkaline-ozone solubilization.

In the control MBR operated without wasting, MLSS steadily increased from 12,000 to 17,000 mg L^{-1} from day 0 to day 120 (Fig. 8.6). Thereafter, the rate of

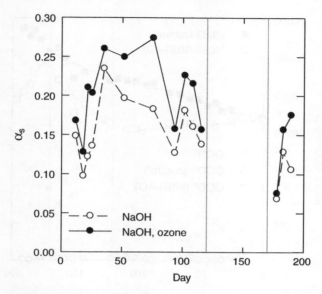

FIGURE 8.5 Changes in α_s following alkaline and ozone solubilization. Sludge treatment was paused between days 120 and 170. [Data from Oh et al. (2007).]

increase increases due to the higher influent COD (COD^0). With sequential alkaline-ozone solubilization, the MBR (MBR-AO) maintained a MLSS value between 9800 and $11,000\,mg\,L^{-1}$. In fact, there appears to be a marginal rate of decrease ($\sim 14\,mg\,d^{-1}$), suggesting that the Q^t selected might be slightly on the high side. Between days 120 and 170, sludge disintegration was paused, to which the system responded immediately with an increase in MLSS. This also indicates that sludge activity was not impaired by the chemical treatments. On day 170, sludge treatment was restarted, and a prompt reduction in MLSS ensued. Throughout the experiment, the effluent COD (COD^e) in both the control and the MBR-AO were similar. Membrane performances in the two MBRs were also similar except after day 150, when the TMP in the control MBR begins to show a much higher rate of increase. This is due primarily to the MLSS approaching a high $20,000\,mg\,L^{-1}$ (Fig. 8.6). Therefore, although solubilization may elevate the concentration of potentially fouling colloids and soluble organics, the net effect is a reduction in fouling rate by virtue of a reduction in solids concentration.

8.3.4 Sonication

Sonication involves the use of acoustic energy for cell disintegration. In an ultra-sonication device, sounds waves are generated typically by a piezoelectric transducer that converts electrical signals to vibrations. These vibrations are amplified by the booster and horn. The latter, which is in direct contact with the suspension, is the source of the propagating sound energy. In the acoustic field, regions of low pressure

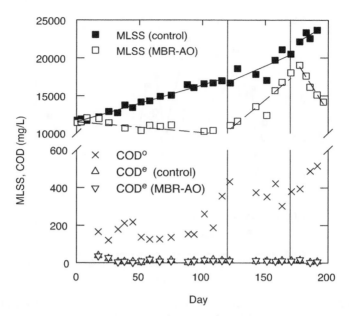

FIGURE 8.6 Time series of sludge concentrations and effluent CODs with and without alkaline-ozonation treatment. Disintegration and solubilization in the MBR-AO was paused between days 120 and 170. [Data from Oh et al. (2007).]

(rarefactions) favor the generation of microbubbles, which contain gas originally dissolved in the solution. These gas bubbles grow in size and are simultaneously influenced by the propagating pressure wave. Once a critical dimension is reached, the bubbles collapse, a phenomenon termed *acoustic cavitation.*

The high local pressure generated when a bubble collapses, and the interactions of the innumerable collapsing bubbles, give rise to very high local shear sufficient to break up flocs and disintegrate cells. The associated high local temperatures also play a part by disrupting the lipid membrane and denaturing cellular components (Khanal et al. 2007). Sonication can also produce free radicals such as $OH\bullet$, especially at high frequencies ($> 100\,kHz$, Tiehm et al. 2001). Since the typical frequency employed in sludge disintegration is 20 to 25 kHz (ultrasound range), disintegration and solubilization is contributed primarily by mechanical shear acting in synergy with elevated temperatures (Chu et al. 2001).

The extent of disintegration and solubilization is a function of factors such as the specific energy input (energy per mass of total suspended solids, $kJ\ g^{-1}\ TSS$), ultrasonic power density (power supplied per volume, $W\ mL^{-1}$), sludge concentration, and sonication time. Ultrasonic power density has the greatest influence on disintegration (Khanal et al. 2007; Akin 2008). The specific energy input which accounts implicitly for sonication time is also very influential. These relations are exemplified in Fig. 8.7 (Chu et al. 2001), where the floc size of waste activated sludge

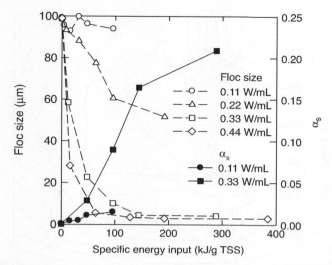

FIGURE 8.7 Floc size and solubilization efficiency for various specific energy input and ultrasonic density. Initial total solids concentration was 8240 mg L^{-1}. The temperature was not controlled. [Data from Chu et al. (2001).]

(initial concentration $= 8240$ mg L^{-1}) is plotted against the specific energy input. Using Chu et al.'s data, α_s was computed and plotted on the same graph. These data show that a minimum ultrasonic density is necessary for floc disruption and solubilization. Zhang et al. (2009) observed negligible solubilization when the power density is less than 0.5 W mL^{-1}. Additionally, when it exceeds 1.6 W mL^{-1}, there is modest additional benefit. The difference in the critical minimums in these studies is probably setup-specific.

When a sufficiently high ultrasonic density is applied, such as 0.33 and 0.44 W mL^{-1} in Fig. 8.7, disintegration and solubilization proceed rapidly, as indicated by the large gradients. However, even at high ultrasonic density and specific energy input, the extent of solubilization is low compared to chemical methods. Salsabil et al. (2009) obtained less than 10% solubilization at a high specific energy input of 110 kJ g^{-1} TSS and an ultrasonic density of 1.2 W mL^{-1}. The plateauing of α_s at some specific energy further suggests the futility of increasing sonication time. To obtain a high α_s value at maximal energy efficiency, a high power density, low sonication duration, and a high sludge concentration should be applied (Gonze et al. 2003; Khanal et al. 2007; Zhang et al. 2009).

Other factors that affect sonication efficiency include the device type and their location(s) within the vessel, and reactor design. These factors make comparisons between studies and scale-up difficult. Attenuation of sound signals with distance depends on the solids concentration and ultrasonic power. One example is shown in Fig. 8.8 using the data of Grönroos et al. (2005). Acoustic signals in a large reactor ($\sim$10 L) containing 2.3% MLSS were measured, varying the ultrasonic power and distance from the horn. Below 300 W, the signal attenuation was negligible. As power

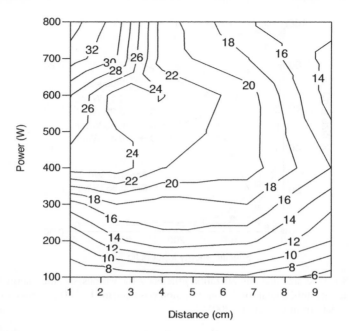

FIGURE 8.8 Contour plot of acoustic signal (in volts) as a function of ultrasonic power and distance from the sonotrode. [Derived using data from Grönroos et al. (2005).]

increases, the spatial rate of attenuation increases. As a result, the intensity of acoustic cavitation and hence sludge disintegration is location dependent. In a large-scale setup, active mixing might be required instead of relying solely on acoustic streaming.

Most research on sonication has been in the context of pretreatment to improve aerobic or anaerobic digestibility (Tiehm et al. 2001; Grönroos et al. 2005; Khanal et al. 2007; Salsabil et al. 2009). A number of studies combine sonication with sequencing batch reactors for excess sludge minimization (Zhang et al. 2007, 2009; He et al. 2011). Integration with an aerobic MBR was attempted by Yoon et al. (2004a). A 8.5-L lab-scale reactor was fed with synthetic wastewater (COD = 4036 mg/L) composed on yeast extract, tryptone, and glucose. 1 L of sludge was sonicated daily for 1 h (equivalent to $Q^t = 0.47Q^0$), using a 600-W sonicator at a frequency of 20 kHz. This integrated MBR (MBR-US) was compared with a control MBR.

The evolution of the MLVSS and the effluent COD in both reactors are shown in Fig. 8.9 for the period without sludge wasting. A reanalysis of Yoon et al.'s MLVSS and MLSS data to determine the average change in sludge concentration (hence production) was made using simple regression. For the control MBR, MLSS production was 1830 mg d^{-1}, compared to 507 mg d^{-1} for MBR-US (VSS/TSS ratios in both reactors were consistently around 0.81to 0.82). The mean COD^e of the

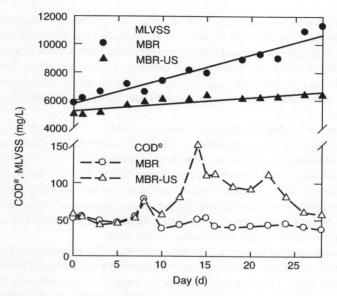

FIGURE 8.9 Temporal variations in MLVSS and effluent COD in the control MBR and MBR-US. The average influent COD was 4036 mg L^{-1}. [Data from Yoon et al. (2004a).]

control was 46 mg L^{-1}, with an average absolute deviation (AAD) of 7 mg L^{-1}. That from MBR-US was 79 mg L^{-1}, with a much higher fluctuation (AAD = 24 mg L^{-1}). The fluctuation could be attributed to the batch treatment of sludge, which upon return to the reactor constitutes a shock load if disintegration was performed inconsistently. From these estimates, observed yields of 0.18 and 0.05 mg VSS mg^{-1} COD were computed for the control and MBR-US, respectively.

The solubilization efficiency was not reported, but may be speculated to be low, thereby necessitating the large amount of sludge sonicated daily and the high energy input. Our estimate of the specific energy applied was 295 kJ g^{-1} TSS (ultrasonic density = 0.6 W mL^{-1}), based on an average MLSS of 7320 mg L^{-1} in the MBR-US.

The low operational flux (1.3 LMH) maintained by the immersed membranes did not permit an investigation of fouling. However, others have observed that in dead-end filtrations (-0.45-μm membrane) of sonicated sludge, the filtration resistance can be a few orders of magnitude higher compared to untreated sludge (Gonze et al. 2003), suggesting the heighten risk of pore plugging on MF membranes.

8.4 PREDATION

The ecological community in bioreactors comprises not only bacterial cells but predatory organisms as well. They include bacteriophage, predatory prokaryotes (Jurkevitch, 2007), protozoans (e.g., flagellates, ciliates), and metazoans (e.g., rotifers, nematodes, oligochaete). Bacteriophage and predatory prokaryotes, which thrive within bacterial cells, are the least understood. Not much is known about their impact on sludge production and reactor performance. Estimates of mortality due to these parasitoids either vary widely or are uncertain (Jurkevitch 2007). It is possible that their impact is minimal, due to their high prey selectively, leading to the dominance of resistant bacterial strains over time. However, it remains speculative at this point.

The influence of phagotrophic organisms on wastewater treatment is known with somewhat greater certainty (Ratsak et al. 1996). These predators actively control the population of bacterial cells, which from the perspective of the latter constitute part of their external decay (van Loosdrecht and Henze 1999). The premise behind excess sludge reduction via predation is founded on the notion of ecological inefficiency— the loss of energy during transfer from the prey to the predator, which ultimately leads to a lower biomass production. As a result, bioreactors in which the growths of predators are favored should see a lower sludge yield.

This was recognized by Lee and Welander (1996), who experimented with a two-stage process comprising of a chemostat first stage and a carrier-based biofilm reactor in the second stage. The chemostat selects for dispersed cells, whereas the biofilm reactor favors the growth of protozoans and metazoans. The much reduced overall sludge yield motivated Ghyoot and Verstraete (2000) to investigate a similar scheme but with a MBR in the second stage. This scheme was compared to a parallel setup that employed a second-stage CAS.

Several influent concentrations (400 to 1000 mg COD L^{-1}), HRTs (first stage: 8 to 34 h; second stage: 17 to 74 h) and SRTs (10 to 122 d) were tested. In all cases, in both configurations, COD removal of at least 83% was achieved in the first stage. Acting as a polishing step, the second stage removed additional COD with an efficiency higher ($> 90\%$) than that of the first stage for the CAS, but (in most cases) lower for the MBR. Ghyoot and Verstraete (2000) attributed the higher COD^e from the MBR to the retention of organics by the immersed hollow fiber MF ($0.2\,\mu m$) membranes. This could have been originated from the grazing of bacterial cells, which reduced the active bacterial population and increased the nonactive hydrolyzable solids concentration. The hydrolyzed products were apparently slowly biodegradable, thus leading to an elevated COD. Higher concentrations of nitrate and phosphate were also observed in the MBR effluent, probably due to the grazing of populations such as nitrifiers (Moussa et al. 2005). Compared to CAS, the density of protozoans and metazoans was found to be higher in the MBR, which also resulted in a 20 to 30% lower sludge yield for the MBR configuration. Ghyoot and Verstraete's data also suggest that this percentage difference increases with SRT and could be much bigger at large SRTs.

The two perceptible trends are that predation appears to increase with sludge age and that MBRs provide better predator selection pressures than CAS. Predation rate depends on the predator characteristics (size and clearance rate being some of the underlying factors; Ratsak et al. 1996), and the predator population. As predators are slow growers (Ni et al. 2010), appropriately reducing wasting rate should prevent their washout. From this perspective, the large SRT at which MBR can operate should favor predators. Even if the MBR is operating at a SRT similar to CAS, predator population may be higher as observed by Ghyoot and Verstraete (2000). This could be related in part to the solids separation process. For example, nonsettleable free-swimming ciliates are washed out in CAS (Ratsak et al. 1996) but not in MBRs. However, the prevalence of protozoans and metazoans in MBRs was not observed universally. Witzig et al. (2002) and Wei et al. (2003) reported few sightings in single-stage MBRs, suggesting indirectly that process staging may be helpful, or might even be essential in creating the conditions conducive for predators.

Wei et al. (2003) also observed the lack of native oligochaete in the MBR. Despite inoculation with worms, the average worm density was low ($10\,mg^{-1}$ VSS), about seven times lower than that in a corresponding CAS reactor. Attempt to increase the MBR worm density by decreasing the wasting rate was unsuccessful. Although oligochaete have been determined to reduce sludge at a rate ranging from 0.1 to $0.8\,g\,g^{-1}$ worm·d (Liang et al. 2006b), the low numbers in the MBRs were insufficient to decrease sludge production measurably. In contrast, the presence of worms in CAS has been correlated with sludge reduction to various extents (Wei et al. 2003; Liang et al. 2006a).

The difficulty in maintaining a high oligochaeta density in MBRs may be overcome by having a dedicated oligochaeta reactor treating excess sludge, with the possibility of returning the treated sludge to the main reactor. This scheme has been studied in oxidation ditch processes (Guo et al. 2007; Wei et al. 2009) with mixed results. Nonetheless, there appears to be potential for integrating oligochaeta reactors with MBRs, an area that is still underexplored.

Besides ecological factors, the quantity of predators may to some degree be influenced by the physical environment. Menniti and Morgenroth (2010) compared low- and high-shear single-staged aerobic MBRs immersed with flat sheet MF membranes. As the fluid shears were induced by aeration, the confounding effects of dissolved oxygen and pH cannot be separated. Nevertheless, oligochaetes were observed only in low-shear MBRs, although both MBRs contain protozoans and other metazoans. There was also limited evidence indicating a positive correlation between EPS (extracellular polymeric substances) and SMP (soluble microbial products) productions, with the presence of oligochaetes. As both EPS and SMP were implicated in membrane fouling (Chang et al. 2002; Le-Clech et al. 2006; Jiang et al. 2010), the benefit of excess sludge reduction has to be weighed against fouling-related costs.

8.5 SUMMARY AND CONCLUDING REMARKS

Sludge disposal is the single largest cost component in sewage treatment. The rising energy cost has provided the impetus to examine methods of minimizing excess sludge production. MBRs allow operation at an elevated sludge age, which directly reduces the quantity of excess sludge to be processed. However, this creates another set of issues associated primarily with membrane fouling and clogging at elevated MLSS. A practical approach is to integrate MBRs with lysis-cryptic growth processes. A portion of reactor solids is channeled to a sidestream disintegration–solubilization reactor in the "lysis" stage and the solubilized content returned to the MBR as "growth" substrates. This allows the system wasting rate to be reduced or eliminated while maintaining a constant MLSS. Mass balance indicates that the substrate and solids concentration depends on a modified SRT, which is primarily a function of the solubilization efficiency and disintegrating sludge flow. As such, the character of disintegration and solubilization, and the way it is being performed, has an effect on effluent quality and the reactor solids concentration.

This chapter concentrates on lysis-cryptic growth processes that have featured in MBRs: thermal-alkaline, ozonation, and sonication. Other processes, such as the use of chemical uncouplers, have been employed in CAS and should see more applications and research in MBRs in the near future. Ozonation appears to offer the best performance with an easily attainable solubilization efficiency of 0.5. With a suitable disintegrating sludge flow, zero sludge production was established with little impact on effluent quality. The downside is the cost of ozone generation, which can be minimized by reducing the ozone required through sludge pretreatment with sodium hydroxide. Improvements in mass transfer efficiency can also reduce ozone dosage.

Sodium hydroxide by itself is also a solubilizing agent. Reasonably good performance was obtained when used at elevated temperatures. In MBR integrated with thermal-alkaline solubilization, a much reduced excess sludge production without deterioration in effluent quality was demonstrated. Sonication has a lower efficacy in relative terms. Although yield in the integrated ultrasonication MBR was low, energy requirement seems to be on the high side. Additionally, the scale-up of a sonication process can be fairly involved and may require specialized design of the ultrasonication vessel. Nevertheless, successful resolutions of these difficulties would see sonication as a practicable alternative.

Irrespective of the disintegration-solubilization technique, the direct impact on membrane performance was marginal and cannot be distinguished from the counterparts without sludge disintegration. However, by reducing sludge concentration, solubilization could indirectly mitigate membrane fouling.

Sludge production can also be minimized via predation. The difficulty is the creation of suitable environments for the predators. In staged MBR, a substantial reduction in yield has been observed. However, better control of predator selection and population remains a challenge. The successful exploitation of predation could potentially be more cost-effective than lysis-cryptic growth techniques.

REFERENCES

Akin B. (2008) Waste activated sludge disintegration in an ultrasonic batch reactor. *Clean— Soil, Air, Water* **36**(4), 360–365.

Chang I.-S., Kim S.-N. (2005) Wastewater treatment using membrane filtration: effect of biosolids concentration on cake resistance. *Process Biochemistry* **40**(3–4), 1307–1314.

Chang I.-S., Le-Clech P., Jefferson B., Judd S. (2002) Membrane fouling in membrane bioreactors for wastewater treatment. *Journal of Environmental Engineering* **128**(11), 1018–1029.

Chu C. P., Chang B.-V., Liao G. S., Jean D. S., Lee D. J. (2001) Observations on changes in ultrasonically treated waste-activated sludge. *Water Research* **35**(4), 1038–1046.

Chu L., Yan S., Xing X.-H., Sun X., Jurcik B. (2009) Progress and perspectives of sludge ozonation as a powerful pretreatment method for minimization of excess sludge production. *Water Research* **43**(7), 1811–1822.

Do K.-U., Banu J. R., Chung I.-J., Yeom I.-T. (2009) Effect of thermochemical sludge pretreatment on sludge reduction and on performances of anoxic–aerobic membrane bioreactor treating low strength domestic wastewater. *Journal of Chemical Technology and Biotechnology* **84**(9), 1350–1355.

Ersu C. B., Ong S. K., Arslankaya E., Lee Y.-W. (2010) Impact of solids residence time on biological nutrient removal performance of membrane bioreactor. *Water Research* **44**(10), 3192–3202.

Fenu A., Guglielmi G., Jimenez J., Spèrandio M., Saroj D., Lesjean B., et al. (2010) Activated sludge model (ASM) based modelling of membrane bioreactor (MBR) processes: a critical review with special regard to MBR specificities. *Water Research* **44**(15), 4272–4294.

Ghyoot W., Verstraete W. (2000) Reduced sludge production in a two-stage membrane-assisted bioreactor. *Water Research* **34**(1), 205–215.

Gonze E., Pillot S., Valette E., Gonthier Y., Bernis A. (2003) Ultrasonic treatment of an aerobic activated sludge in a batch reactor. *Chemical Engineering and Processing* **42**(12), 965–975.

Grönroos A., Kyllönen H., Korpijärvi K., Pirkonen P., Paavola T., Jokela J., et al. (2005) Ultrasound assisted method to increase soluble chemical oxygen demand (SCOD) of sewage sludge for digestion. *Ultrasonics Sonochemistry* **12**(1–2), 115–120.

Guo X.-S., Liu J.-X., Wei, Y.-S., Li L. (2007) Sludge reduction with Tubificidae and the impact on the performance of the wastewater treatment process. *Journal of Environmental Sciences* **19**(3), 257–263.

Hamer G. (1985) Lysis and "cryptic" growth in wastewater and sludge treatment processes. *Acta Biotechnologica* **5**(2), 117–127.

He J., Wan T., Zhang G., Yang J. (2011) Ultrasonic reduction of excess sludge from activated sludge system: Energy efficiency improvement via operation optimization. *Ultrasonics Sonochemistry* **18**(1), 99–103.

He S.-B., Xue G., Wang B.-Z. (2006) Activated sludge ozonation to reduce sludge production in membrane bioreactor (MBR). *Journal of Hazardous Materials* **135**(1–3), 406–411.

Henkel J., Cornel P., Wagner M. (2009a) Free water content and sludge retention time: impact on oxygen transfer in activated sludge. *Environmental Science and Technology* **43**(22), 8561–8565.

Henkel J., Lemac M., Wagner M., Cornel P. (2009b) Oxygen transfer in membrane bioreactors treating synthetic greywater. *Water Research* **43**(6), 1711–1719.

Henze M., Gujer W., Mino T., van Loosdrecht M. C. M. (2000) *Activated Sludge Models ASM1, ASM2, ASM2d and ASM3*, IWA Scientific and Technical Report 9, IWA Publishing, London.

Huang X., Gui P., Qian Y. (2001) Effect of sludge retention time on microbial behaviour in a submerged membrane bioreactor. *Process Biochemistry* **36**(10), 1001–1006.

Jiang T., Kennedy M. D., Schepper V. D., Nam S.-N., Nopens I., Vanrolleghem P. A., et al. (2010) Characterization of soluble microbial products and their fouling impacts in membrane bioreactors. *Environmental Science and Technology* **44**(17), 6642–6648.

Jurkevitch E. (2007) *Predatory Prokaryotes*, Springer-Verlag, New York.

Khanal S. K., Grewell D., Sung S., van Leeuwen J. (2007) Ultrasound applications in wastewater sludge pretreatment: a review. *Critical Reviews in Environmental Science and Technology* **37**(4), 277–313.

Laera G., Pollice A., Saturno D., Giordano C., Lopez A. (2005) Zero net growth in a membrane bioreactor with complete sludge retention. *Water Research* **39**(20), 5241–5249.

Laera G., Giordano C., Pollice A., Saturno D., Mininni G. (2007) Membrane bioreactor sludge rheology at different solid retention times. *Water Research* **41**(18), 4197–4203.

Le-Clech P., Chen V., Fane T. A. G. (2006) Fouling in membrane bioreactors used in wastewater treatment. *Journal of Membrane Science* **284**(1–2), 17–53.

Lee N. M., Welander T. (1996) Use of protozoa and metazoa for decreasing sludge production in aerobic wastewater treatment. *Biotechnology Letters* **18**(4), 429–434.

Liang P., Huang X., Qian Y. (2006a) Excess sludge reduction in activated sludge process through predation of *Aeolosoma hemprichi*. *Biochemical Engineering Journal* **28**(2), 117–122.

Liang P., Huang X., Qian Y., Wei Y., Ding G. (2006b) Determination and comparison of sludge reduction rates caused by microfaunas' predation. *Bioresource Technology* **97**(6), 854–861.

Low E. W. Chase H. A. (1999) Reducing production of excess biomass during wastewater treatment. *Water Research* **33**(5), 1119–1132.

Low E. W., Chase H. A., Milner M. G., Curtis T. P. (2000) Uncoupling of metabolism to reduce biomass production in the activated sludge process. *Water Research* **34**(12), 3204–3212.

Lubello C., Caffaz S., Gori R., Munz G. (2009) A modified activated sludge model to estimate solids production at low and high solids retention time. *Water Research* **43**(18), 4539–4548.

Massé A., Spérandio M., Cabassud C. (2006) Comparison of sludge characteristics and performance of a submerged membrane bioreactor and an activated sludge process at high solids retention time. *Water Research* **40**(12), 2405–2415.

Menniti A., Morgenroth E. (2010) The influence of aeration intensity on predation and EPS production in membrane bioreactors. *Water Research* **44**(8), 2541–2553.

Moussa M. S., Hooijmans C. M., Lubberding H. J., Gijzen H. J., van Loosdrecht M. C. M. (2005) Modelling nitrification, heterotrophic growth and predation in activated sludge. *Water Research* **39**(20), 5080–5098.

Muller E. B., Stouthamer A. H., Van Verseveld H. W., Eikelboom D. H. (1995) Aerobic domestic waste water treatment in a pilot plant with complete sludge retention by cross-flow filtration. *Water Research* **29**(4), 1179–1189.

Ni B., Rittmann B. E., Yu H. (2010) Modeling predation processes in activated sludge. *Biotechnology and Bioengineering* **105**(6), 1021–1030.

Ødegaard H. (2004) Sludge minimization technologies: an overview. *Water Science and Technology* **49**(10), 31–40.

Oh Y.-K., Lee K.-R., Ko K.-B., Yeom I.-T. (2007) Effects of chemical sludge disintegration on the performances of wastewater treatment by membrane bioreactor. *Water Research* **41**(12), 2665–2671.

Pavlostathis S. G., Gossett J. M. (1986) A kinetic model for anaerobic digestion of biological sludge. *Biotechnology and Bioengineering* **28**(10), 1519–1530.

Pollice A., Laera G., Blonda M. (2004) Biomass growth and activity in a membrane bioreactor with complete sludge retention. *Water Research* **38**(7), 1799–1808.

Pollice A., Laera G., Saturno D., Giordano C. (2008) Effects of sludge retention time on the performance of a membrane bioreactor treating municipal sewage. *Journal of Membrane Science* **317**(1–2), 65–70.

Ramdani A., Dold P., Déléris S., Lamarre D., Gadbois A., Comeau Y. (2010) Biodegradation of the endogenous residue of activated sludge. *Water Research* **44**(7), 2179–2188.

Ratsak C. H., Maarsen K. A., Kooijman S. A. L. M. (1996) Effects of protozoa on carbon mineralization in activated sludge. *Water Research* **30**(1), 1–12.

Rittmann B. McCarty P. (2001) *Environmental Biotechnology: Principles and Applications*, McGraw-Hill, New York.

Rosenberger S., Krüger U., Witzig R., Manz W., Szewzyk U., Kraume M. (2002) Performance of a bioreactor with submerged membranes for aerobic treatment of municipal waste water. *Water Research* **36**(2), 413–420.

Saktaywin W., Tsuno H., Nagare H., Soyama T., Weerapakkaroon J. (2005) Advanced sewage treatment process with excess sludge reduction and phosphorus recovery. *Water Research* **39**(5), 902–910.

Salsabil M. R., Prorot A., Casellas M., Dagot C. (2009) Pre-treatment of activated sludge: effect of sonication on aerobic and anaerobic digestibility. *Chemical Engineering Journal* **148**(2–3), 327–335.

Song K.-G., Choung Y.-K., Ahn K.-H., Cho J., Yun H. (2003) Performance of membrane bioreactor system with sludge ozonation process for minimization of excess sludge production. *Desalination* **157**(1–3), 353–359.

Spérandio M., Espinosa M. C. (2008) Modelling an aerobic submerged membrane bioreactor with ASM models on a large range of sludge retention time. *Desalination* **231**(1–3), 82–90.

Staehelin J., Hoigne J. (1985) Decomposition of ozone in water in the presence of organic solutes acting as promoters and inhibitors of radical chain reactions. *Environmental Science and Technology* **19**(12), 1206–1213.

Teck H. C., Loong K. S., Sun D. D., Leckie J. O. (2009) Influence of a prolonged solid retention time environment on nitrification/denitrification and sludge production in a submerged membrane bioreactor. *Desalination* **245**(1–3), 28–43.

Tiehm A., Nickel K., Zellhorn M., Neis U. (2001) Ultrasonic waste activated sludge disintegration for improving anaerobic stabilization. *Water Research* **35**(8), 2003–2009.

Trussell R. S., Merlo R. P., Hermanowicz S. W., Jenkins D. (2007) Influence of mixed liquor properties and aeration intensity on membrane fouling in a submerged membrane bioreactor at high mixed liquor suspended solids concentrations. *Water Research* **41**(5), 947–958.

van Loosdrecht M. C. M. Henze M. (1999) Maintenance, endogeneous respiration, lysis, decay and predation. *Water Science and Technology* **39**(1), 107–117.

Vavilin V. A., Rytov S. V., Lokshina L. Y. (1996) A description of hydrolysis kinetics in anaerobic degradation of particulate organic matter. *Bioresource Technology* **56**(2–3), 229–237.

Wei Y., van Houten R. T., Borger A. R., Eikelboom D. H., Fan Y. (2003) Comparison performances of membrane bioreactor and conventional activated sludge processes on sludge reduction induced by oligochaete. *Environmental Science and Technology* **37**(14), 3171–3180.

Wei Y., Wang Y., Guo X., Liu J. (2009) Sludge reduction potential of the activated sludge process by integrating an oligochaete reactor. *Journal of Hazardous Materials* **163**(1), 87–91.

Witzig R., Manz W., Rosenberger S., Krüger U., Kraume M., Szewzyk U. (2002) Microbiological aspects of a bioreactor with submerged membranes for aerobic treatment of municipal wastewater. *Water Research* **36**(2), 394–402.

Wu B., Yi S., Fane A. G. (2011) Microbial behaviors involved in cake fouling in membrane bioreactors under different solids retention times. *Bioresource Technology* **102**(3), 2511–2516.

Wu S. C., Lee C. M. (2011) Correlation between fouling propensity of soluble extracellular polymeric substances and sludge metabolic activity altered by different starvation conditions. *Bioresource Technology* **102**(9), 5375–5380.

Yan S., Miyanaga K., Xing X.-H., Tanji Y. (2008) Succession of bacterial community and enzymatic activities of activated sludge by heat-treatment for reduction of excess sludge. *Biochemical Engineering Journal* **39**(3), 598–603.

Yoon S.-H., Kim H.-S., Lee S. (2004a) Incorporation of ultrasonic cell disintegration into a membrane bioreactor for zero sludge production. *Process Biochemistry* **39**(12), 1923–1929.

Yoon S.-H., Kim H.-S., Yeom I.-T. (2004b) The optimum operational condition of membrane bioreactor (MBR): cost estimation of aeration and sludge treatment. *Water Research* **38**(1), 37–46.

Zhang G., Zhang P., Yang J., Chen Y. (2007) Ultrasonic reduction of excess sludge from the activated sludge system. *Journal of Hazardous Materials* **145**(3), 515–519.

Zhang G., He J., Zhang P., Zhang J. (2009) Ultrasonic reduction of excess sludge from activated sludge system: II. Urban sewage treatment. *Journal of Hazardous Materials* **164**(2–3), 1105–1109.

9

MICROBIAL FUEL CELL TECHNOLOGY FOR SUSTAINABLE TREATMENT OF ORGANIC WASTES AND ELECTRICAL ENERGY RECOVERY

SHI-JIE YOU, NAN-QI REN, AND QING-LIANG ZHAO

State Key Laboratory of Urban Water Resource and Environment, School of Municipal and Environmental Engineering, Harbin Institute of Technology, Harbin, China

9.1 INTRODUCTION

Activated sludge and biofilm processes together with their modified forms have been in wide use as efficient biotechnologies for removing organic pollutants from various types of wastewaters (Henze et al. 2008). However, for several reasons, these methods may face new bottlenecks and challenges alongside the progressively developed concepts toward more energy-efficient, cost-effective, and sustainable treatment of wastewater. First, proliferation of aerobic microorganisms needs continuous supplement of oxygen as an electron donor, which indeed represents a great amount of energy consumption. Second, the emission of gaseous carbon dioxide to the atmosphere resulting from microbial metabolism can make a considerable contribution to the increased amount of greenhouse gases. Finally, excessive sludge produced from microbial growth must be disposed of properly in technologically and economically feasible ways, and this accounts for 25 to 65% of the overall cost for the operation of a wastewater treatment plant (Liu and Tay 2001). In addition to the end-of-pipe manner for sludge minimization, such

Biological Sludge Minimization and Biomaterials/Bioenergy Recovery Technologies, First Edition.
Edited by Etienne Paul and Yu Liu.
© 2012 John Wiley & Sons, Inc. Published 2012 by John Wiley & Sons, Inc.

as alkaline-thermal treatment, ozonation, chlorination, and metabolic uncoupling (Liu 2003), several novel methods have been developed recently, some of which are expected to be a possible alternative to the conventional solutions.

Microbial fuel cells (MFCs), in which electrochemically active microorganisms serve as biocatalysts for oxidation of organic compounds to generate current, may provide a completely new approach to organic waste disposal while recovering energy in the form of electricity (Logan and Regan 2006a). Combining the structural and functional superiority of biological processes (e.g., anaerobic digestion) and chemical fuel cells (e.g., H_2/O_2 fuel cell), MFCs may offer several particular advantages in waste handling, in terms of high efficiency due to one-step conversion, ambient temperature and pressure, and the ability to utilize a broad range of feedstock, as well as negligible production yield of excessive sludge and secondary by-products (Rabaey and Verstraete 2005). These factors are giving rise to a promising potential and opportunity for a more sustainable and environmentally friendly approach to simultaneous waste treatment and energy recovery.

Bioelectricity produced from a fuel cell–like system was first reported in 1911 by Potter (Potter 1911), who found electrical current yield by a bacterium in a yeast culture, although the current was extremely low. It was not until the end of twentieth century that MFCs began to draw growing attention, because they agree well with the current trend toward green and sustainable development of environmental and energy industries. This has inspired many researchers to dedicate considerable effort not only toward a better understanding of the mechanisms involved in MFCs, but also toward seeking an effective way in which to enhance power production in a variety of ways. By means of enriching highly active bacteria, applying effective electrode materials, and optimizing reactor design and operation, the maximum power produced from a lab-scale MFC can achieve an increase from less than $10^{-1}\,\mathrm{mW\,m^{-2}}$ to more than $4 \times 10^3\,\mathrm{mW\,m^{-2}}$ (Logan and Regan 2006b). Meanwhile, MFCs have been shown to be able to achieve the synthesis of chemical products and environmental remediation in a sustainable manner.

Despite substantial advances made in improving MFC performance compared with the first MFCs reported by Potter, it is worth noting that power density remains extremely low toward large-scale applications at the current status. Due to poor reactivity, high solution resistance, and slow mass transfer, MFCs can only produce a maximum power density of 10^{-2} to $10^{-1}\,\mathrm{mW\,cm^{-2}}$, which is three to five orders of magnitude lower than that of an H_2/O_2 fuel cell (on the order 10^2 to $10^3\,\mathrm{mW\,cm^{-2}}$) and other types of fuel cells. Design and operation of a high-efficiency MFC are highly dependent on a thorough understanding of different biological and electrochemical reactions, interfacial interactions, and ionic transport and transformation processes. Therefore, in this chapter we review the state of the art of MFC technology for sustainable treatment of wastewater and electricity recovery, with a focus on (1) the fundamentals, performance assessment, and design of MFCs; (2) anode performance, including electrode materials, biological electron transfer, and electron donors; (3) cathode performance, including electron acceptors and air cathode design; (4) separators; (5) operational problems associated with separators and buffers; and (6) various applications of MFCs in addition to power generation.

9.2 FUNDAMENTALS, EVALUATION, AND DESIGN OF MFCs

9.2.1 Principles

An MFC can be defined as a device that converts chemical energy stored in the chemical bonds of organic matters into electrical energy by means of microbial metabolism. Similar to a H_2/O_2 fuel cell, a typical MFC essentially has a two-compartment structure with a negative electrode (anaerobic anode) and a positive electrode (oxidative cathode), separated by a cationic exchange membrane (CEM). Figure 9.1 illustrates the working principle of an MFC. For example, in complete oxidation of fermentative glucose (electron donor, 5 mM, pH 7.0), electrochemically active microorganisms enriched on the anode surface are capable of oxidizing glucose to release energy for growth. In the absence of any other electron acceptors having a high positive potential compared to fermented by-products under anaerobic conditions, the electrons produced are transferred from microbial cells to the electrode as a final electron acceptor [Eq. (9.1)]. In most cases, glucose is converted to small-molecular volatile organic acids (e.g., acetate and butyrate) via fermentation rather than being oxidized directly to CO_2 via a respiration pathway. If the anode (e.g., copper wire) is connected to a high-potential cathode where the reduction of oxidative species (e.g., oxygen) occurs, electrons are driven to flow to the cathode by the potential difference, participating in the reduction reaction of the oxidant through combining equivalent protons across the CEM [Eq. (9.2)].

$$\text{Anode:} \quad C_6H_{12}O_6 + 6H_2O \rightarrow 6CO_2 + 24H^+ + 24e^-, \qquad E = -0.41 \text{ V} \quad (9.1)$$

$$\text{Cathode:} \quad O_2 + 4H^+ + 4e^- \rightarrow H_2O, \qquad E = +0.804 \text{ V} \quad (9.2)$$

$$\text{Overall reaction:} \quad C_6H_{12}O_6 + 6H_2O \rightarrow 6CO_2 + 6H_2O, \quad \Delta G^0 = -2843 \text{ kJ mol}^{-1} \quad (9.3)$$

In addition to transporting protons, the membrane also mitigates oxygen diffusion to maintain the anaerobic condition of the anode. Owing to favorable thermodynamics ($\Delta G^0 = -2843 \text{ kJ mol}^{-1}$) for the overall reaction, the current generation can be sustained at the external circuit as long as dynamic equilibrium is established.

9.2.2 Performance Evaluation

The performance of an MFC is generally evaluated by power normalized by the geometrical area of the anode (rate-limiting electrode), which gives power density in units of milliwatts per square meter (mW m^{-2}). Sometimes, the power from an MFC with a packed-bed anode can also be normalized by the wet liquid volume of the anode zone, giving a volumetric power density (W m^{-3}).

In an MFC, the theoretical potential difference for the two half-reactions in Eqs. (9.1) and (9.2) is 1.214 V, which is also referred to as the *thermodynamic equilibrium potential*. When the external load is incorporated into the circuit, the MFC will generate current at the external circuit; meanwhile, polarization occurs. The consequence of polarization is to render the resulting potential diverged from the theoretical potential: that is, overpotential resulting from (1) Nernst loss, (2) electrochemical activation loss related to catalytic reactions at both electrodes, (3) ohmic loss due to electrolyte conductivity, and (4) diffusion loss caused by limitation of mass transfer of reactants onto the reactive site of the electrode. The sum of these overpotentials determines the order of magnitude of power density generated by an MFC.

In addition to power density, coulombic efficiency (CE) is another important parameter used to assess the total number of coulombs recovered from organic matter. In general, CE is defined as a relative ratio of the total experimental coulombs (C_{EX}) accumulated at a given time interval to the theoretical coulombs (C_{TH}) calculated by Faraday's law:

$$C_{EX} = \int_0^t I \, d\tau = \sum_{i=0}^{t} I_i \, \Delta\tau_i \tag{9.4}$$

$$C_{TH} = \frac{(COD_{in} - COD_{out})V_A}{M_{O_2}} bF \tag{9.5}$$

where t is the experimental time, I_i the current in the ith time interval τ_i, COD the chemical oxygen demand, V_A the volume of the anode, M_{O_2} the molecular mass of oxygen ($32 \, g \, mol^{-1}$), b the number of the moles of electrons per mole of substrate ($4 \, mol \, mol^{-1}$), and F the Faraday constant ($96{,}485 \, C \, mol^{-1}$).

9.2.3   MFC Configurations

Similar to an H_2/O_2 fuel cell, a conventional MFC has one anode compartment and one cathode compartment separated by a CEM (Fig. 9.1). Such *batch-fed* MFCs have often been employed in fundamental studies of the isolation of electricity-producing bacteria, identification of microbial communities, and exploration of new materials and their electrochemical behavior. It has been known that the internal resistance (R) of an electrochemical cell–type reactor is the function of resistivity of the electrolyte (ρ), electrode spacing (l), and electrode area (A): $R = \rho l/A$. Thus, many innovative designs of MFCs have been reported toward decreasing its internal resistance for high-efficiency, cost-effective recovery of electricity from wastewater.

One technical breakthrough is to replace the active-aeration cathode compartment by a passive air-breathing waterproof gas diffusion electrode (GDE), and this has led to the development of single-chamber membrane-less MFCs, which have the advantages of reduced energy input for active aeration, easy operation, and adjustment of electrode spacing and area (Liu and Logan 2004). Due to these inherent advantages, this type of MFC has been widely accepted as a model reactor in many lab-scale experiments for testing microbial activity, innovative materials, and so on.

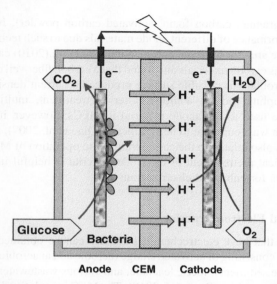

FIGURE 9.1 Schematic representation of a typical MFC for electricity production.

Another development in MFCs is the transformation from a small-scale batch-fed reactor to flow-through *continuous* electricity generation and wastewater treatment (He et al. 2005). The packed-bed reactor allows for the use of large-surface-area graphite granule materials as the three-dimensional electrode, which largely increases the treatment capacity and stability of the system. Also, the tubular design enables a close electrode spacing, leading to power production at a sufficiently low internal resistance. These provide the principal guidance for scale-up of an MFC reactor for practical applications. Nevertheless, it should be realized that technical and economical challenges remain, due to an increased overpotential with an increase in reactor size. Hence, the design and use of pilot- and large-scale MFCs are still under extensive investigation.

9.3 PERFORMANCE OF ANODES

9.3.1 Electrode Materials

In an MFC, electrochemically active microorganisms responsible for substrate degradation and electron transfer to the external circuit are attached primarily to the anodic electrode. Thus, the anode materials need to have a good electrically conductive capacity for efficient delivery of electrons, high resistance to electro-chemical corrosion in aqueous salt solution, and a rough and porous surface to facilitate microbial attachment. So far, a large number of materials have been tested as the MFC anode, including noncorrosive metallic stainless steel and carbon-based materials (e.g., carbon plate, carbon paper, carbon felt, carbon cloth, carbon fiber brush, graphite granule, carbon foam, activated carbon powder). It is difficult to compare the performance of different anode materials due to such technical obstacles as effective active area for bacterial colonization. Liu et al. (2010) carried out a CV analysis of various carbon materials and found that a carbon fiber veil or carbon paper with a large microbially accessible surface produced a current density 40% higher than that of graphite rod. In addition, after pretreatment, multiwalled carbon nanotubes can be used as the anode material in MFCs; however, improvement in power production was found not to be significant (Qiao et al. 2007). Selection of an anode material is also related to the configuration and operation of MFCs. Chemical and physiochemical pretreatment of electrode material is helpful in improving its surface properties for enhanced electron transfer.

9.3.2   Microbial Electron Transfer

Microorganisms that have electrochemical activity can be obtained from a broad range of sources, consisting of activated sludge (aerobic and anaerobic) in wastewater treatment, marine sediments, feces, leachate, and various wastewaters (e.g., domestic, swine, food processing) (Pant et al. 2010). The MFC inoculation is accomplished once the anode is colonized by electrophilic microorganisms. Regardless of energy conversion during anoxic metabolisms for heterotrophic microorganisms, microbial electron transfer is a measure of primary importance of how fast electrochemically active microorganisms transfer electrons onto the electrode in MFCs. A critical question is: In what way are electrons transferred from an aqueous medium to a solid electrode? To address this question, a number of fundamental studies have been carried out to uncover the mechanisms governing electron transfer in MFCs, and several identifiable mechanisms have been proposed. On the basis of the benchmark proposed by Schröder (2007), microbial electron transfer can commonly be categorized into direct and indirect ways. No matter which mechanism predominates, the electron transfer needs electrochemical active matter to have interfacial contact with the electrode, and possesses a redox potential close to that of the starting substrate and considerably lower than that of the cathodic electron acceptor.

Direct Ways   Applies to electron transfer by (1) electronically conductive outer membrane cytochromes via physical contact between microbial cell and electrode (Fig. 9.2a), *or* (2) electronically conductive filamentous pili (nanowires) (Fig. 9.2b). In the former mechanism, since the electrochemically active bacteria prevail only in the first monolayer of biofilm developed at the electrode surface, the maximal cell density in the monolayer dominates the rate at which electrons are transferred. Several bacterial strains, including *Shewanella putrefaciens, Rhodoferax ferrireducens*, and *Geobacter sulfurreducens*, have been demonstrated capable of transferring electrons in this manner, producing current in MFCs (Logan and Regan 2006b). However, this way seems inefficienct, due to the fact that the majority of bacteria identified, except *R. ferrireducens,* can only feed on small-molecular substrates such as acetate and alcohols. Peng et al. (2010) found that the electrode potential regulated the accumulation of cytochromes OmcA and MtrC at the cell membrane–electrode interface, but

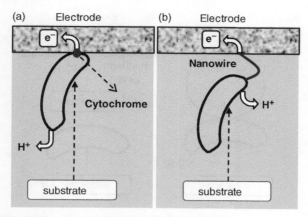

FIGURE 9.2 Simplified view of direct electron transfer via (a) a cell cytochrome and (b) nanowires.

the reactivity of the cytochromes was observed to be much less than that of diffusive electron shuttle flavins, which are probably responsible for current output.

There is strong evidence indicating that nanowire is a highly conductive material that is produced by *Shewanella* (Gorby et al. 2006) and *Geobacter* species (Reguera et al. 2005). The conductivity of nanowire can be identified qualitatively by scanning tunneling microscopy (STM) technology. In this case, electron transfer is achieved through connecting membrane-bound cytochromes at the end of nanowires to the electrode surface (Fig. 9.2b). Compared to monolayer biofilm for electron transfer via membrane cytochromes, nanowires allow the formation of multilayer active biofilm in series/parallel way, thus resulting in a higher electron transfer rate and power production. The finding of nanowires also uncovers the possible mechanisms of interactions through transferring electrons between different microbial cells (Gorby et al. 2006).

Indirect Ways Refers to the way in which electron transfer occurs through redox mediators or shuttles without the need of direct contact between the bacteria and the electrode. The electron mediator functions as a reversible electron acceptor between the bacterial cell and the electrode by altering its redox state (Fig. 9.3a). Park and Zeikus (2000) noted that the incorporation of an electron mediator such as neutral red dye, Fe(III), or Mn(IV) onto a graphite electrode was able to improve substantially the electron transfer efficiency from $NADH^+$ to the electrode, thereby increasing the power yield 1000-fold. In addition to the mediators mentioned above, a variety of mediator materials based on phenazine, phenothiazine, phenoxazine, and quinine are also available for MFC uses (Schröder 2007). Another feasible indirect way is to oxidize primary metabolites, such as H_2 and formate produced from anaerobic fermentation, as electron carriers to accomplish electron transfer. By immersing an electrode coated with a electrocatalyst such as platinum and electronically conductive polymers into an aqueous culture, the small-molecular metabolites generated

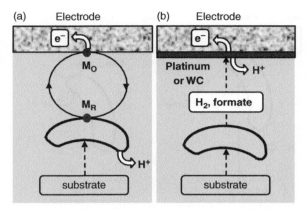

FIGURE 9.3 Simplified view of indirect electron transfer via (a) a redox mediator and (b) fermentative primary metabolites.

from fermentation are oxidized at the catalyst surface as a result of current output. In this case, the electrochemical reactions take place at the three-phase boundary (solid catalyst/gaseous H_2/aqueous H^+) of the electrode surface. The essence of this is the implementation of a chemical fuel cell to utilize H_2 and formate in situ (Fig. 9.2b). Platinum was shown to be effective for H_2 oxidation, while the oxidation of formate had to rely on tungsten carbide (Rosenbaum et al. 2006). This method can not only achieve a substantially increased power density (as great as $6000\,mW\,m^{-2}$), but can also synthesize hydrogen peroxide at the cathode from glucose dark fermentation (You et al. 2010).

In summary, electron transfer proceeding in indirect ways is commonly reported to be more efficient and produces a higher power density than that via direct ways in MFCs. Despite great progress in electron transfer mechanisms based on pure-culture experiments, there remains a region with many unclear problems to better understand which mechanism may predominate and how to manipulate the electron transfer process artificially in an effective manner, particularly in a mixed-culture system.

9.3.3   Electron Donors

In contrast to chemical fuel cells, which operate upon oxidation of only a minority of simple electron donors such as H_2, methanol, and ethanol on precious noble metals (Pt and Au) (Steele and Heinzel 2001), MFCs can feed on a much wider range of macromolecule organic substances, even complex organic wastes and biomass. In lab-scale experiments, acetate and glucose represent the most available electron donors for MFC tests. By using fixed substrates for the anode, substrate-independent performances (e.g., electron transfer, electrode reactions, electrolyte behavior, cathodic reduction) can be well defined. Additionally, a large variety of organic compounds can be adopted as a substrate for power production in MFCs (Pant et al. 2010). The statistical data clearly reveal that the power density and CE recovered from pure cultures are much higher than those converted from real wastewaters. Unlike pure cultures, there exist limitations for real wastewaters with respect to the concentration of biodegradable materials, ionic conductivity and buffer capacity, and the adverse impact on reactivity and the microbial community of electrophilic organisms induced by chemical impurities and aboriginal microbial communities in wastewater. The MFC performances reported for different organic substrates vary widely, with power density changing from a few ($<$ 10) mW m^{-2} to thousands of mW m^{-2} and CE ranging from less than 10% to more than 80%, respectively. A comparison of MFC performances with different substrates is consciously avoided here, because the design and operation of the MFCs used in these studies differed from each other significantly.

Recent research showed that activated sludge could also be used as an electron donor to sustain electricity production in MFCs. Scott and Murano (2007) reported that manure sludge could be treated stably in a two-chamber MFC, as indicated by 95% reduction of carbohydrates during three months of operation. Jiang et al. (2009) found that by feeding a two-chamber MFC with sludge produced from biotreatment, the total chemical oxygen demand can be decomposed by nearly 50%. It is well known that only soluble components are biodegradable, so activated sludge requires being properly hydrolyzed before it can be the fuel for MFCs. The methods available for sludge pretreatment may include alkaline-thermal treatment, ozonation, and ultrasound-based sonication. Pretreatment can solubilize the insoluble organic compounds in the sludge by alerting the fraction of aromatic proteins and some microbial by-products (e.g., fluorescent matter) that supplies the electricity-producing microorganisms with soluble electron donors continuously, thus allowing the MFCs to last for much longer. These findings are expected to provide a completely new proof-of-concept method to handle sludge waste while recovering electricity from the sludge.

Another breakthrough worthwhile noting is the utilization of biomass materials for electricity in MFCs. Biomass, which is known to store solar energy in chemical bonds through natural biocycling, is being regarded as a feedstock of great sustainability for its large-scale production and, cost-effective and renewable nature. Ren et al. (2007) reported electricity generation from cellulose serving as a sole electron donor in a two-chamber MFC based on a co-culture of the cellulolytic fermenter *Clostridium cellulolyticum* and electricity-producing bacterium *Geobacter sulfurreducens*. By feeding the MFC with 1000 mg L^{-1} carboxymethylcellulose, the maximum power density reached 143 mW m^{-2}, corresponding to a CE of 47% and chemical oxygen demand (COD) removal of 38%. Wang et al. (2009) used an air-cathode MFC to produce electricity from waste corn stover and obtained a maximum power density of 331 mW m^{-2} from the bioaugmented mixed culture.

9.4 CATHODE PERFORMANCES

When striving toward optimization of an MFC, cathode performance is another important concern. The cathode design can substantially affect the cathodic reactivity and sustainability of the entire system. The cathode configuration should be well matched by the MFC architecture. For example, the aqueous electron acceptor requires a two-compartment MFC equipped with a membrane, whereas both the two- and single-compartment architecture can accept gaseous oxygen. In this section we discuss the electron acceptors used and access their properties in MFCs, the electrochemical fundamentals of the air-breath cathode, and the challenges and opportunities faced by an air-cathode MFC.

9.4.1   Electron Acceptors

In MFCs, the electron acceptor plays the role of a terminal sink for electrons diverted from the anodic oxidation. Because the electrons are transferred thermodynamically toward high redox potential, all the oxidizing species can, in theory, possibly be used as the cathodic electron acceptor. During the early period of MFC research, aqueous potassium ferricyanide [$K_3Fe(CN)_6$] was frequently used as the electron acceptor in two-compartment MFCs by virtue of its good mass transfer and reactivity (Schröder et al. 2003). Based on these considerations, a variety of new aqueous or gaseous oxidizing chemicals have successively been explored and tested for power generation from MFCs in ongoing studies. Table 9.1 summarizes and compares various types of representative electron acceptors and their overall performance in terms of thermo-dynamic and kinetic reactions, and sustainability. By using chemicals that have a redox couple of great oxidative potential, MFCs yielded remarkably improved cathode performance as a result of the cathode potential exceeding $+1.0\,V$ [e.g., $+1.53\,V$ for acidic permanganate (You et al. 2006), $+0.91\,V$ for acidic dichromate (Wang et al. 2008), and $+1.59\,V$ for persulfate (Li et al. 2009)]. Clearly visible is the fact that the cathode potential values are actually much higher than those reported in previous studies. Nonetheless, it may be problematic to use these chemicals in MFCs, for several reasons.

First, the highest cathode potential can only be obtained under low pH conditions for MnO_4^-/MnO_2 (pH < 4) and $Cr_2O_7^{2-}/Cr^{3+}$ couple (pH < 4), causing reverse diffusion of protons across the membrane from the cathode to the anode side, driven by concentration difference. Second, the oxidants require periodic compensation for depletion, which may be of less technological and economical sustainability in large-scale uses unless these chemicals can be reproduced. Nitrate (NO_3^-) can also serve as an electron acceptor as a result of the terminal production of nitrite, even gaseous N_2 (Clauwaert et al. 2007b). Through recirculating the anodic-treated effluent contain-ing ammonium–nitrogen to the cathode compartment, ammonium–nitrogen is oxidized to NO_3^- by aerobic ammonia-oxidizing bacteria, followed by nitrogen removal by a denitrifer (Virdis et al. 2008). In this novel manner, biological denitrification is linked to carbon removal in one MFC system. Due to such a process catalyzed by a specific community of microorganisms in the absence of any chemical catalyst, the cathode-reducing NO_3^- is called *biocathode*. As discussed below, a biocathode is able to catalyze oxygen reduction in addition to nitrate reduction. Of all the electron acceptors listed above, gaseous oxygen–air has clearly been shown to be the optimal choice for sustainable power generation, and extensive research has been carried out to improve the electrocatalyzing reduction of oxygen in

TABLE 9.1 Summary of the Cathodic Electron Acceptors and Their Performances in MFCs

Redox Couple	Half-Reaction[a]	E^o (V)[b]	E (V)[c]	OCP (V)[d]	Conditions		Catalyst	Sustain-ability	References
					pH	Conc. (mM)[e]			
Fe^{3+}/Fe^{2+}	$Fe^{3+} + e^- \rightarrow Fe^{2+}$	+0.77	+0.58	0.8	2.0	2.38	No	No	Ter Heijne al. (2007)
	$[Fe(CN)_6]^{3-} + e^- \rightarrow [Fe(CN)_6]^{3-}$	+0.36	—	0.895	7.0	50	No	No	Schröder et al. (2003)
MnO_4^-/MnO_2	$MnO_4^- + H^+ + e^- \rightarrow MnO_2 + H_2O$	+1.70	+1.284	1.532	3.5	10	No	No	You et al. (2006)
MnO_2/Mn^{2+}	$MnO_2 (s) + 4H^+ + 2e^- \rightarrow Mn^{2+} + 2H_2O$	+1.28	+0.36	0.809	7.2	—	Bacteria	Yes	Rhodas et al. (2005)
$Cr_2O_7^{2-}/Cr^{3+}$	$Cr_2O_7^{2-} + 14H^+ + 6e^- \rightarrow 2Cr^{3+} + 7H_2O$	+1.33	—	0.91	2.0	3.85	No	No	Wang et al. (2008)
$S_2O_8^{2-}/SO_4^{2-}$	$S_2O_8^{2-} + 2H^+ + 2e^- \rightarrow 2HSO_4^-$	+2.12	+1.21	1.592	1.0	10	No	No	Li et al. (2009)
NO_3^-/NO_2^-	$NO_3^- + 2H^+ + 2e^- \rightarrow NO_2^- + H_2O$	+0.42	+0.045	0.36	7.0	—	Bacteria	Yes	Clauwaert et al. (2007a)
H_2O_2/H_2O	$H_2O_2 + 2H^+ + 2e^- \rightarrow 2H_2O$	+1.27	—	0.62	6.9	—	No	No	Tartakovsky and Guiot (2006)
O_2/H_2O	$O_2 + 4H^+ + 4e^- \rightarrow 2H_2O$	+0.804[f]	+0.425	0.7	7.0	0.21 atm[g]	Yes	Yes	Liu and Logan (2004); Zhao et al. (2006)
O_2/H_2O_2	$O_2 + 2H^+ + 2e^- \rightarrow H_2O_2$	+0.29[f]	+0.20	0.5	7.0	0.21 atm[g]	Yes	Yes	Rozendal et al. (2009)

[a] The reactions are assumed to take place at a temperature of 298 K and a pressure of 1.0 atm.
[b] Standard cathode potential vs. SHE at pH 0 and a reactant concentration of 1 M.
[c] Real cathode potential.
[d] Open-circuit potential.
[e] Reactant concentration.
[f] pH 7.0.
[g] Partial pressure of oxygen (21%) in air.

MFCs. It is well known that oxygen is normally reduced at a slow rate at the electrode surface; thus, catalysts with a large surface area and high reactivity are needed. For this reason, particular emphasis should be placed on intensive understanding of oxygen electrochemistry to explore effective strategies in optimizing the cathode performance of an MFC.

9.4.2   Electrochemical Fundamentals of the Oxygen Reduction Reaction

The electrochemical reduction of oxygen is a heterogeneous catalytic reaction occurring at the electrode surface in several steps, including the adsorption of reactants and the catalytic reaction and desorption of products. The kinetics and mechanisms of electrochemical reduction of oxygen are function of the electro-catalyst and electrolyte. Generally, the oxygen reduction reaction (ORR) takes place through two pathways in an aqueous electrolyte [normal conditions; E^0 vs. standard hydrogen electrode (SHE)] (Kinoshita 1992).

1. *Direct four-electron route*

$$\text{Acid conditions:}\quad O_2 + 4H^+ + 4e^- \rightarrow 2H_2O \qquad E^0 = +1.229 \text{ V} \quad (9.6)$$

$$\text{Alkaline conditions:}\quad O_2 + 2H_2O + 4e^- \rightarrow 4OH^- \qquad E^0 = +0.401 \text{ V} \quad (9.7)$$

2. *Indirect two-electron route*

$$\text{Acid conditions:}\quad O_2 + 2H^+ + 2e^- \rightarrow H_2O_2 \qquad E^0 = +0.67 \text{ V} \quad (9.8)$$

$$H_2O_2 + 2H^+ + 2e^- \rightarrow 2H_2O \qquad E^0 = +1.77 \text{ V} \qquad (9.9)$$

$$2H_2O_2 \rightarrow 2H_2O + O_2 \qquad (9.10)$$

$$\text{Alkaline conditions:}\quad O_2 + H_2O + 2e^- \rightarrow HO_2^- + OH^- \qquad E^0 = -0.065 \text{ V}$$
$$(9.11)$$

$$HO_2^- + H_2O + 2e^- \rightarrow 3OH^- \qquad E^0 = +0.867 \text{ V} \qquad (9.12)$$

$$2HO_2^- \rightarrow 2OH^- + O_2 \qquad (9.13)$$

So, ORR is an extremely complex process that may involve a large number of reaction intermediates and rate-limiting steps through either four- or two-electron series–parallel pathways (Fig. 9.4), depending on the electrocatalyst used. Route (1) should be predominant at the surface of a noble metallic catalyst (e.g., Pt, Pd) and some N_4-coordinating macrocyclics containing transition metals (e.g., Fe, Co); while it appears most likely that route (2) dominates the ORR on graphite and the majority of carbon, gold, and transition metal oxides. Generally speaking, ORR via a two-electron pathway is observed more commonly than that via a four-electron pathway.

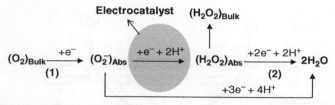

FIGURE 9.4 Typical model describing ORR in aqueous acid electrolyte. When O_2 diffuses from bulk solution to the catalyst surface, an electron is added to the O_2 to form adsorbed electronegative O_2^-, followed by successive reduction by addition of three electrons to produce water or one electron to generate absorbed H_2O_2. The two-electron route proceeds with desorption of H_2O_2 into bulk solution or decomposition to water.

It is possible to qualitatively differentiate the two pathways for a specific catalyst in acid or alkaline conditions using a rotating ring-disk electrode.

9.4.3 Air-Cathode Structure and Function

Since oxygen (air) has been fully acknowledged as the most suitable electron acceptor for MFC applications, it should be of great significance to create the optimal conditions for the ORR to proceed effectively. At the beginning of MFC research, the air-cathode was established simply by immersing a graphite rod or plate in electrolyte and aerating it actively by air. However, several limitations caused the cathode to work so inefficiently that only a low power density was obtained. Afterward, learning from experience gained in oxygen-reduction cathode design for H_2/O_2 fuel cells, the gas diffusion electrode (GDE) was introduced into MFCs, first by Liu and Logan (2004) and later by Cheng et al. (2006a). An MFC with a passive air-breathing cathode was accompanied by substantially increased power density.

As shown in Fig. 9.5, the GDE used for MFC cathodes consists basically of a gas diffusion layer (GDL), a back layer (BL), a substrate layer (SL), and an electrocatalytically active layer (EAL).

GDL   GDL, which is commonly made from 60% polytetrafluoroethylene (PTFE) suspension, functions to supply gaseous air to the catalyst layer and to prevent the aqueous solution from leakage or weeping. Previous studies showed that applying four layers of GDL was most effective for power production with the maximal power density and CE values in a single-chamber MFC (Cheng et al. 2006a).

BL   BL plays the role of supporting layer and current collector, and is prepared by mixing a PTFE emulsion and fine carbon powders uniformly. The BL, located between the GDL and the substrate layer, needs to be highly permeable to gas and electrical conductivity.

SL   The SL, serving as the base layer, is required to have good mechanical strength, chemical stability, and electrical conductivity. This means that the SL can be made from inert porous carbon paper, carbon cloth, or stainless steel mesh.

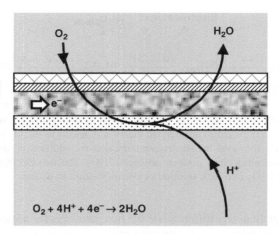

FIGURE 9.5 Schematic composition of a typical GDE used in MFCs. The four layers, indicated by different symbols, are (from top to bottom) the gas diffusion layer, the back layer, the substrate layer, and the electrocatalytically active layer, containing catalyst and binder.

EAL   The layer that adheres to the other side of the SL is the electrochemically active layer, which contains an electrocatalyst for ORR. This layer is often known as a three-phase boundary (TPB), where solid catalyst, gaseous oxygen, and aqueous protons combine to form water. Binder solution should be used to attach the catalyst to the electrode surface by PTFE emulsion or Nafion solution (5%), depending on the hydrophobicity and hydrophilicity required. A Nafion solution performs better, due to its ability to improve the interfacial contact of the TPB. The electrocatalyst constitutes the core of the GDE because it is the sole determiner of the reactivity, selectivity, and stability of the ORR process.

Admittedly, the use of a GDE greatly facilitates the ORR in an MFC, but several limitations will continue to exist. Principally, three issues may contribute to the air-cathode to make them the limiting factors in MFC performance. First, the direct contact between the TPB and the electrolyte causes the TPB to work under flooding conditions, which hinders oxygen transport by blocking the pores in the EAL, covers up active sites in the EAL, and plugs the oxygen diffusion channels in the DL, making the MFC performance degradable, unpredictable, and unreliable. Second, the slow kinetics in the ORR necessitates the development of high-efficiency sustainable catalysts as discussed below. Finally, water loss through the cathode by vaporization will be a serious problem in a scaled-up system.

9.4.4 Electrocatalyst

The most widely used catalyst for ORR is platinum (Pt); however, its high cost and sensitivity to poisoning place considerable restrictions on its universal acceptability. In addition to Pt, some organic N_4 macrocycle complexes containing transition metals (e.g., Co, Fe) can also be used as available catalysts. The catalytic reactivity

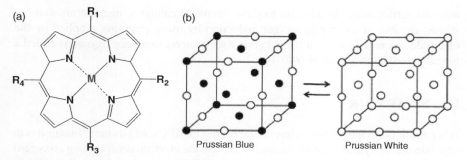

FIGURE 9.6 (a) Framework of N_4 macrocycles containing transition metals (M = Fe, Co), and (b) Prussian blue/Prussian white shuttle for oxygen reduction (●) Fe(III); (○) Fe(II).

is the function of both the core metal coordinated by nitrogen and the functional groups located at R_1 to R_4 (Fig. 9.6a). These Pt-free compounds, some of which carry comparably high electrocatalytic activity to the Pt catalyst for oxygen reduction as tested in chemical fuel cells, can be a promising candidate in MFCs. For example, substituting a methoxyphenyl group for R_1 to R_4 (M = Co) gives a classical ORR catalyst (i.e., CoTMPP), which has been demonstrated to yield cathode performance comparable to that of Pt in MFCs (Zhao et al. 2005; Cheng et al. 2006b). To increase the active surface area of the TPB and the effectiveness of catalyst utilization, the catalyst needs to be highly dispersed onto electrically conductive carriers on a nanometer scale, and the applicable materials can be fine carbon powders (Vulcan X72) or multiwalled carbon nanotubes (MWCNTs).

Several studies also reported on metal oxides [e.g., MnO_2 (Zhang et al. 2009)] or metal-free materials containing active carbon, graphite powder, or MWCNTs pretreated by chemical or thermal methods for MFC cathode modification. However, it should be realized that the reactivity and selectivity of one specific catalyst cannot be measured solely by polarization and power data reported individually. As mentioned earlier, only noble metals and a minority of dual-core metallic N_4-based macrocycles are capable of catalyzing oxygen reduction through direct four-electron pathways. In other words, in common cases, with the exception of these catalysts, a two-electron (H_2O_2) or indirect four-electron route can proceed, both of which are side reactions responsible for cathode performance degradation. Surprisingly, however, it seems a common practice to make an assumption that oxygen is reduced to water other than H_2O_2, regardless of what catalyst is being used. In fact, this postulation may, to some extent, mislead MFC researchers into designing a catalyst in an unreasonable way. Recently, Fu et al. (2011) reported a new type of Prussian blue (PB)/polyaniline-composed cathode for oxygen reduction in MFCs through redox transformation between N-coordinating Fe(III) and C-coordinating Fe(II) located on a face-centered cubic lattice (Fig. 9.6b). This novel catalyst (i.e., electron shuttle) substantially improves the kinetics of oxygen reduction and reoxidation of Fe(II) (Prussian white) back to Fe(III) (PB), and achieved a maximum power density very close to that of aqueous ferricyanide. In addition to these chemical catalysts, bacteria are demonstrated capable of catalyzing oxygen reduction by using electrons supplied by the electrode. As noted earlier, a cathode that uses bacteria to reduce oxygen is called a biocathode (Clauwaert et al. 2007b).

9.5 SEPARATOR

A separator plays the role of an interfacial barrier in MFCs, and its main function is to separate the anolyte and catholyte, and to prevent the electron acceptor (e.g., oxygen) from diffusion from the cathode to the anode. Unlike chemical fuel cells, where a perfluorosulfonic membrane serves as a solid polymer electrolyte, the membrane does not appear to be a compulsory component in MFCs because the solution itself, functioning as an electrolyte, has the ability to conduct cations. For this reason, the incorporation of a separator in an MFC leads to an increase in the overall internal resistance and a decrease in the power efficiency.

The most widely used separator is perfluorosulfonic acid membrane (Fig. 9.7a), consisting primarily of Nafion (Dupont, Inc.) and Ultrex CMI 7000 (Membranes, Inc.). All cationic-exchange membranes (CEMs) have two features in common: (1) the polymer chains contain mainly a hydrophobic PTFE backbone, which forms segments several units in length; and (2) the perfluorinated vinyl polyether, a few ether links long, joins these segments into a flexible branch pendant to the main perfluoro chain and carries a terminal hydrophilic acidic group (e.g., sulfonate) to supply cation-exchange capability. CEMs are highly conductive to cationic species H^+, Na^+, K^+, NH_4^+, Ca^{2+}, and Mg^{2+}, and are also permeable to some small organic and gaseous molecules. Owing to low-concentration protons in the anode of MFCs, cation exchange membranes (PEMs) often behave poorly in conducting protons, and thus an anion exchange membrane (AEM) was tested as an alternative to CEMs. In contrast to CEMs, AEMs are made up of a hydrophobic fluorocarbon backbone connected by a terminal alkaline quaternary ammonium group (Fig. 9.7b). They have the ability to transport anionic species such as OH^-, Cl^-, HCO_3^-, CO_3^{2-}, $H_2PO_4^-$, and HPO_4^{2-} with high selectivity. Although protons can be migrated more efficiently with phosphate or carbonate as carriers by AEMs, high-concentration buffer chemicals are still required to maintain pH within a neutral range.

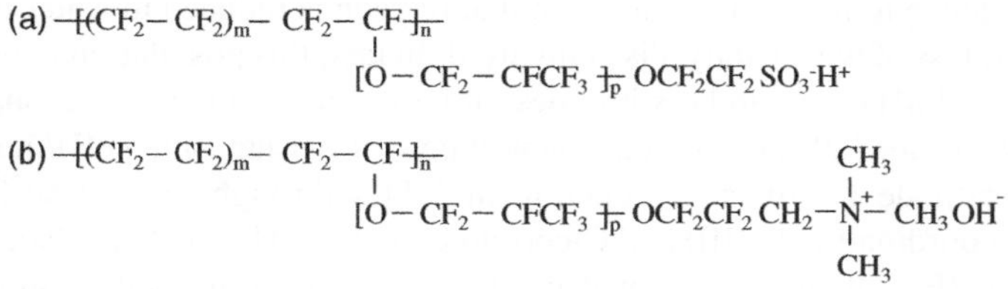

(a) $-\mathrm{[(CF_2-CF_2)_m-CF_2-CF]_n}-$
$$[O-CF_2-CFCF_3]_p\ OCF_2CF_2\ SO_3^-H^+$$

(b) $-\mathrm{[(CF_2-CF_2)_m-CF_2-CF]_n}-$
$$[O-CF_2-CFCF_3]_p\ OCF_2CF_2\ CH_2-\overset{\overset{\displaystyle CH_3}{|}}{\underset{\underset{\displaystyle CH_3}{|}}{N^+}}-CH_3OH^-$$

FIGURE 9.7 Structural formulas for (a) PEM and (b) AEM, where $m = 5$ to 13, $n = 1000$, and $p = 1, 2, 3$.

TABLE 9.2   Summary of Separators and Evaluation of Their Properties in MFCs

Separator	Primary Function	Problems	Cost	Reference
PEM[a]	Transport cation	pH gradient, high resistance	High	Kim et al. (2007)
AEM[b]	Transport anion	Higher resistance	High	Kim et al. (2007)
BM[c]	Transport cation and anion	pH gradient, high cross-membrane overpotential	Very high	Ter Heijne et al. (2007)
MFM[d]	Transport proton	High oxygen and substrate permeation, high resistance	Moderate	Biffinger et al. (2007)
UFM[e]	Transport proton	High resistance	Moderate	Kim et al. (2007)
GF[f]	Prevent oxygen diffusion	Substrate permeation	Low	Ghangrekar and Shinde (2007)
J-cloth	Prevent oxygen diffusion	Biodegradable, high oxygen and substrate permeation	Low	Fan et al. (2007)

[a] Cation-exchange membrane.
[b] Anion-exchange membrane.
[c] Bipolar membrane.
[d] Microfiltration membrane.
[e] Ultrafiltration membrane.
[f] Glass fiber.

Apart from PEMs and AEMs, some other separators including bipolar membranes, microfiltration membranes, ultrafiltration membranes, glass fibers and J-cloth, can be used in MFCs, and their primary functions and problems are assessed and compared in Table 9.2. Taken together, all the separators are needed to conduct protons and at the same time to mitigate back diffusion of oxygen and organic substrate to their negative sides. This is a very helpful strategy to enable a high CE and energy efficiency during electricity generation. On the other hand, because the separators are permeable to organic substrate and molecular oxygen in addition to ionic species, overall loss of efficiency cannot be avoided. Moreover, as earlier an mentioned MFC with a separator is commonly observed to have much greater internal resistance than the without, which accounts for its higher ohmic overpotential and lower power density. This is attributed to the additional resistance to salt solution for proton transfer when a separator is introduced. Finally, a significant concern associated with the use of separator is the pH gradient of the electrolyte, which may heavily discount the duration and stability of an MFC, an issue that is discussed in detail below.

9.6   pH GRADIENT AND BUFFER

In comparison with an H_2/O_2 fuel cell, where a membrane electrode assembly is fabricated by sandwiching Pt-containing GDEs and solid polymer electrolyte with

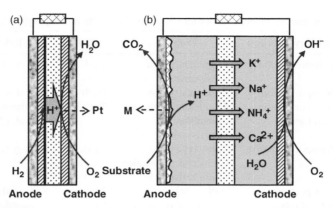

FIGURE 9.8 Schematic view of ionic migration for charge neutralization in (a) an H_2/O_2 fuel cell and (b) an MFC.

excellent proton conductivity (Fig. 9.8a), an MFC needs to work under pH-neutral aqueous culture for microorganism growth. Such a feature affects the way in which the membrane transports cationic species from the anode to the cathode, making an MFC differ from any other type of chemical fuel cell. For this reason, one significant impediment to making advances in scaling up an MFC system is the lack of buffer capacity and conductivity for real wastewater (Rozendal et al. 2006a; You et al. 2009). As a consequence, the actual behavior of the membrane should be quite different from that given in Fig. 9.1. Taking PEM as an example, the protons produced from substrate oxidation by electrochemically active microorganisms are in approximately 10^4-fold lower concentration than other cationic species existing in the anolyte, such as Na^+, K^+, NH_4^+, Ca^{2+} and Mg^{2+}. Due to permeability to a variety of cations apart from protons for PEM, these cations in higher concentration will inevitably take precedence over protons to be migrated by CEM into catholyte at a much faster rate to achieve electroneutralization. As a result, this gives rise to a substantial loss of pH balance between the anode and cathode compartments (Fig. 9.8b). The alteration in membrane behavior also results in a great difference in the manner in which oxygen is electrochemically reduced at the cathode for an H_2/O_2 fuel cell and an MFC. In an H_2/O_2 fuel cell, protons can be fully conducted toward the Pt catalyst and participate in oxygen reduction to form water at the cathode. Whereas the cathode lacks available protons in an MFC, oxygen has to combine with water to form OH^- (Fig. 9.8b). The increased pH in the catholyte leads to a considerable degradation of the thermodynamic and kinetic performance of the ORR.

For this reason, stable and efficient operation of an MFC system is bound to require that the electrolytes hold sufficient buffer capacity that the pH value can be preserved within a nearly neutral range. To achieve this goal, it once was, and now is again common practice to use a buffer chemical consisting of hydrogen phosphate and dihydrogen phosphate (50 to $100\,mmol\,L^{-1}$) in the electrolyte. In view of wastewater treatment, however, it seems impractical for engineered use because

50 to 100 mmol L^{-1} phosphate means that total phosphate in the effluent reaches an extraordinarily high level of 1.95 to 3.90 g P L^{-1}. To prevent eutrophication, the phosphate must be reduced below the adopted criterion of 0.5 mg P L^{-1} prior to being discharged into the receiving water body. This represents an enormous additional investment to deal with such a problem, and it seems unclear whether the costs of phosphate removal could be balanced by power generated from an MFC (You et al. 2009).

Possible solutions to the problems related to pH gradient may include (1) removing membrane to eliminate pH gradient; (2) using an AEM other than a PEM to transport phosphate-carrying protons; (3) applying alternative environmentally friendly buffer materials, such as carbonates, to phosphate; and (4) exploring effective approaches to recovering buffer chemicals. Although there have been reports showing that methods (1) to (3) are effective for improving the MFC performance, the increase in maximum power density remains very limited. Recovering buffer may become a promising choice for wastewater treatment and sustainable power generation, but at the current stage, it appears quite difficult to find an efficient manner to separate such high-concentration phosphate from pure water. Taken together, the bottlenecks in relevance to the pH gradient and buffer use will continue to be a crucial issue in this area for a long time.

9.7 APPLICATIONS OF MFC-BASED TECHNOLOGY

Apart from electricity generation originating from microbial oxidation of organic compounds, MFCs can be utilized in diverse ways, including biosensors, in hydrogen recovery, in hydrogen peroxide synthesis, in desalination, and in bioelectrochemical remediation. The use of MFC technology can be transformed from original sole power production to other purposes, such as the synthesis of valuable chemicals and environmental remediation of pollutants in a more energy-efficient, sustainable way. These alterations suggest a promising potential to stretch the applicability of MFCs for various goals.

9.7.1 Biosensors

The most common way to assess the organic strength of wastewater is through a biological oxygen demand (BOD) test, which is normally conducted by measuring the oxygen consumption of aerobic microorganisms in diluted samples (20°C) within 5 or 7 d. However, this method appears very time consuming and labor intensive. Taking into account the proportional correlation between the substrate concentration and coulombs accumulated over a defined time interval, MFCs can possibly be used in sensor targeting the BOD in wastewater. By feeding organic substrate to the anode while recording the response of current or voltage, the BOD can be determined in real time. Chang et al. (2004) reported on a two-chamber

MFC-type biosensor for continuous monitoring of BOD variation during an experimental period of five years. They found that the current responded linearly to BOD at concentrations below $100\,mg\,L^{-1}$, within which BOD values can be determined. Kumlanghan et al. (2007) developed an MFC biosensor for fast estimation of easily biodegradable compounds at a responce time of 3 to 5 minutes with good reproducibility. However, these results were obtained from the use of artificial wastewater (glucose) rather than real wastewater. In reality, the presence of various impurities, such as sulfate, nitrate, nitrite, and metallic elements, some of which take part in electrochemical reactions during current production, may lead to overestimation of the relationship between the current and BOD values. In comparison with conventional sensor-based methods such as dissolved oxygen electrode, photodiode, and fluorescence technique, in MFC serving as a BOD sensor can provide several inherent advantages for fast online measurement of organic matter in wastewater. Thus, MFCs are widely expected to sense as a novel alternative to conventional methods of assessing wastewater strength. Even so, the commercial use of this technology necessitates more intensive investigations of real wastewater, combined with further improvements toward better accuracy, sensitivity, reproducibility, and stability.

9.7.2 Hydrogen Production

An MFC reactor can be modified to produce hydrogen gas assisted by electrons created by anodic oxidation of organic substrates by anophilic bacteria. In general, the anode potential approaches about $-0.3\,V$ vs. SHE (e.g., acetate oxidation), while H_2 is evolved spontaneously on the oxygen-free cathode at a redox potential exceeding $-0.414\,V$ in a pH-neutral solution (298 K). This means that a voltage of at least $0.114\,V$ should be provided additionally to realize H_2 formation at the cathode (Fig. 9.9a). In general, to overcome overpotential, a higher voltage ($> 0.25\,V$) is needed (Liu et al. 2005; Rozendal et al. 2006b). Since H_2 production is the result of combined microbial oxidation and electrolysis, this process is called *microbial electrolysis cell* (MEC). A voltage supply of $0.25\,V$ for an MEC is undoubtedly much lower than that of $> 1.6\,V$ for H_2 generation by water electrolysis. Additionally, an MEC will theoretically be able to produce H_2 from the oxidation of any type of biodegradable organic matter, such as both organic waste and renewable biomass material. An illustrative example of breakthrough has been given by Cheng and Logan (2007), who for the first time successfully realized high-efficiency H_2 recovery from domestic wastewater in an MEC. This makes the H_2-producing MEC hold the most promising potential to be scaled up for practical uses.

9.7.3 Desalination

Working from the principle of electrodialysis for desalination, Cao et al. (2009) first reported a modified three-chamber MFC separated by a CEM and an AEM (Fig. 9.9b), giving what they called a *microbial desalination cell* (MDC), which

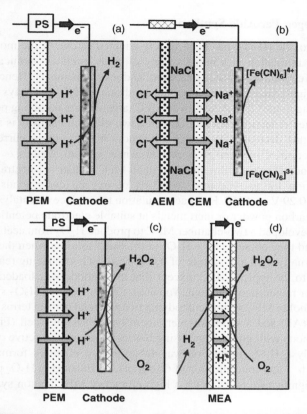

FIGURE 9.9 Schematic diagram of (a) a microbial electrolysis cell (MEC) for H_2 production, (b) an AEM/CEM MFC for desalination, (c) an MEC for H_2O_2 synthesis, and (d) H_2O_2 formation in SPE–MFC with biofermented H_2 as a hydrogen carrier. PS, power supply.

was very effective for splitting NaCl in synthetic sea water. Unlike a traditional electrolysis cell, an MDC was able to accomplish desalination driven by microbial oxidation of organic matters at the anode rather than by applying external power to the cell. By using acetate for anophilic bacteria and ferricyanide [$K_3Fe(CN)_6$] for the catholyte, NaCl was demonstrated to be removed from its original 35 g L^{-1} to final concentration lower than 4 g L^{-1} (removed by 90%) in the middle compartment, which was accompanied by a tremendous increase in ohmic impedance from 25 to 950 Ω, observed for MDCs at the end of the reaction cycle. Meanwhile, MDCs also produced electricity with a maximum power density of 2000 mW m^{-2}. As is clearly seen from these results, MDCs opened a completely new approach to effective desalination of seawater in the most sustainable and economic way. In the ongoing studies, MDCs need to be tested further with air rather than a $K_3Fe(CN)_6$ cathode for desalination, and more efforts are required to solve the pH-gradient problem so as to improve the duration and stability of the system.

9.7.4 Hydrogen Peroxide Synthesis

Hydrogen peroxide (H_2O_2) has been widely adopted as one of the most important chemicals for utilization in a broad variety of areas, such as chemical processes, medical disinfection, wastewater treatment, and green chemistry. Hence, exploring methods for high-efficiency, low-cost, safe synthesis of H_2O_2 is always a significant area. According to the ORR theory, in an MFC targeted at maximizing power output, cathodic oxygen reduction proceeding with a two-electron pathway is an unwanted side reaction that decreases the power efficiency. Whereas the occurrence of two-electron reduction of oxygen gives rise to a new way to synthesize H_2O_2 using organic compounds as a starting material in an MFC. Under pH-neutral conditions, the half-reaction for two-electron reduction of oxygen corresponds to a redox potential of $+0.29$ V vs. SHE. H_2O_2 accumulation takes place on catalyst containing either active carbon powder or inert metals at suitable electrode potential. Rozendal et al. (2009) developed a two-chamber MFC to produce H_2O_2 from acetate oxidation (Fig. 9.9c), and they obtained 83% H_2O_2 in the NaCl solution when the system was powered externally by a low voltage of 0.5 V. This H_2O_2-producing reactor appears quite similar to the typical MFC, except that the cathode was loaded with active carbon powder rather than platinum. You et al. (2010) reported H_2O_2 synthesis in a primary-metabolite MFC system embodying two essential parts in terms of anaerobic fermentation (AF) and a solid polymer electrolyte (SPE) fuel cell (Fig. 9.9d). By feeding the anode with glucose and using thermally pretreated active carbon as the cathodic catalyst, H_2O_2 production was achieved at a maximal formation rate of $35 \, \text{mmol m}^{-2} \, \text{h}^{-1}$ and concentration of $60 \, \text{mmol L}^{-1}$. Enhancing H_2O_2 production is of essential significance to establish a high-efficiency MFC/Fenton system.

9.7.5 Environmental Remediation

Electrochemical methods are regarded as a powerful and green alternative to conventional chemical and physiochemical processes, especially for degradation of those nonbiodegradable pollutants. However, one limiting factor is the high operational cost due to the requirement of external electrical power input into the system. MFCs are able to produce electrons from anodic oxidation spontaneously, and then provide the cathode with electrons for electrochemical remediation of various pollutants. This process can be called a *bioelectrochemical treatment*. As discussed below, the representative treatment based on this manner (but not limited to these) can include biodenitrification, the Fenton system, and the remediation of heavy metals.

Denitrification A two–compartment MFC was suggested capable of cathodic denitrification by microorganisms using electrons produced from anodic oxidation, as shown in Fig. 9.10a. The electrode potential and nitrate concentration applied to a biocathode are the two most significant parameters dominating the rate at which denitrification proceeds (Clauwaert et al. 2007a). The MFC can be further modified via the change in the designing and operating mode for simultaneous removal of

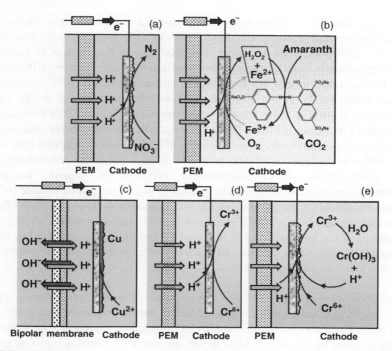

FIGURE 9.10 Schematic diagram of (a) a biodenitrification cathode; (b) an MFC/Fenton system for amaranth decomposition; (c) copper recovery in bipolar membrane MFC; (d) direct Cr(VI) reduction at the electrode; and (e) biological Cr(VI) reduction.

carbon and nitrogen in one system (Virdis et al. 2008). Compared to a conventional biodenitrification process where external electron donors should be provided, an MFC is obviously advantageous because (1) it completely eliminates the need to supply both an electron donor (e.g., methanol) and a power input for liquid recirculation; and (2) electricity is recovered during pollutant remediation, although the maximum power for nitrate-feeding biologically catalyzing cathode is not as high as that for noble metal-catalyzing oxygen cathode.

Bioelectrochemical Fenton System   One promising application of H_2O_2-producing MFCs is the microbial oxidation-driven in situ electrochemical Fenton system [H_2O_2/Fe(II)] for indirect degradation of nonbiodegradable or persistent materials. When the cathode produces H_2O_2, followed by the addition of Fe(II) ions and pollutants, the reactions will take place in sequence as

$$O_2 + 2H^+ + 2e^- \rightarrow H_2O_2 \tag{9.14}$$

$$Fe^{3+} + e^- \rightarrow Fe^{2+} \tag{9.15}$$

$$Fe^{2+} + H_2O_2 \rightarrow Fe^{3+} + {}^\bullet OH + OH^- \tag{9.16}$$

Incorporating Fe^{2+} solution into H_2O_2 produced from two-electron ORR gives a Fenton reaction that produces a hydroxyl radical ($^\bullet$OH) having a redox potential as great as $+2.80$ V vs. SHE. In theory, hydroxyl radical has the ability to oxidize organic compounds nonselectively to their finalized mineralization. Fe(III) generated from Fenton reaction can be transformed electrochemically into its originally reduced form, Fe(II), at the electrode, followed by participating in the Fenton process once again (Fig. 9.10b). By using this approach, Fu et al. (2010) successfully constructed a two-chamber MFC/Fenton system, whereby the azo dye amaranth can be decomposed continuously at an efficiency of 82.59% after a reaction time of 1 h, along with a maximum power density of 28.3 W m^{-3} produced concurrently. This MFC configuration allows simultaneous treatment of organic wastewater and remediation of nonbiodegradable pollutants in one integrated reactor by individually manipulating the parameters for two subsystems. However, more efficient design and operation of an MFC/Fenton reactor requires better understanding of the interactions at the interface of different species and electrode, and the key factors affecting $^\bullet$OH-generating kinetics and reactivity when pollutants are introduced into the catholyte.

Removal/Recovery of Heavy Metals   Several types of wastewater contain oxidative heavy metals that must to be eliminated before being discharged into a receiving water body. These metals can take part in electrochemical reduction at the cathode of an MFC assisted by anodic microbial oxidation, as a result of being transformed into chemically inactive forms for removal or recovery purposes. Two illustrative examples document this possibility well. As shown in Fig. 9.10c, an MFC equipped with a bipolar membrane can achieve Cu^{2+} reduction and subsequent Cu deposition at the surface of the cathode (Ter Heijne et al. 2010). A bipolar membrane is essential because it electrolyzes water to H^+ and OH^- and then transports OH^- to the anode side and H^+ to the cathode side, respectively. This results in a relatively low pH of the catholyte, so that the soluble copper tends to deposit onto the electrode rather than combining with OH^- to develop $Cu(OH)_2$ precipitation in the solution. Another representative case is the reduction of Cr(VI) that can occur through a direct electrochemical (Fig. 9.10d) or an indirect biological pathway (Fig. 9.10e). For the direct electrochemical way, Cr(VI) is reduced by electrons to Cr(III) at the cathode surface (Wang et al. 2008, Li et al. 2008); for the indirect way, Cr(VI) is reduced by a specific bacterial community, followed by being removed as $Cr(OH)_3$ precipitation (Tandukar et al. 2009). As analyzed by a 16S rRNA gene based on a clone library, the biomass responsible for Cr(VI) reduction appeared most likely to be dominated by phylotypes closely related to putative Cr(VI) reducers of *Trichococcus pasteurii* and *Pseudomonas aeruginosa*.

9.8   CONCLUSIONS AND REMARKS

MFC is currently the focus of considerable interest and is viewed as a novel strategy for developing sustainable treatment of waste materials, and research efforts in this area have increased substantially. This multidisciplinary area lies at the interface of microbiology, electrochemistry, materials science and technology, and chemical engineering, and has a wide range of applications, such as green power production from complex macromolecular organic biofuels, as a biosensor for monitoring organic components in wastewater, in chemical synthesis of H_2 and H_2O_2, and in environmental remediation. In the field of fundamental research, several new scientific findings have been derived from the MFC system, including the isolation and identification of new electricity-producing bacteria, the way that electrochemically active microorganisms interact with electrodes and with other microbial communities, operating problems associated with the use of membranes and pH gradients in a bioelectrochemical system, as well as several innovative principles of cathode reactions.

Notwithstanding this, it should also be realized that the power density produced from an MFC remains extraordinarily small, and to date, all the tests have been conducted on the lab scale, before field and practical applications have been undertaken, so scaled-up studies and ongoing on-site experimental experiences are highly desired. Several inherent technical bottlenecks that may coexist in MFCs will present the main challenges to the development of scaling-up methodologies for practical and commercial applications. These problems should be solvable by in the future improving the design and operation of the reactor, enriching highly active electricity-producing bacteria, exploring effective electrode and membrane materials, and developing specific highly active catalysts.

REFERENCES

Biffinger J. C., Ray R., Little B., Ringeisen B. R. (2007) Diversifying biological fuel cell designs by use of nanoporous filters. *Environmental Science and Technology* **41**, 1444–1449.

Cao X. X., Huang X., Liang P., Xiao K., Zhou Y. J., Zhang X. Y., Logan B. E. (2009) A new method for water desalination using microbial desalination cells. *Environmental Science and Technology* **43**, 7148–7152.

Chang I. S., Jang J. K., Gil G. C., Kim M., Kim H. J., Cho B. W., Kim B. H. (2004) Continuous determination of biochemical oxygen demand using microbial fuel cell type biosensor. *Biosensors and Bioelectronics* **19**, 607–613.

Cheng S. A., Logan B. E. (2007) Sustainable and efficient biohydrogen production via electrohydrogenesis. Proceedings of the National Academy of Sciences USA 104, 18871–18873.

Cheng S. A., Liu H., Logan B. E. (2006a) Increased performance of single-chamber microbial fuel cell using an improved cathode structure. *Electrochemistry Communications* **8**, 489–494.

Cheng S. A., Liu H., Logan B. E. (2006b) Power densities using different cathode catalysts (Pt and CoTMPP) and polymer binders (Nafion and PTFE) in single chamber microbial fuel cells. *Environmental Science and Technology* **40**, 364–369.

Clauwaert P., Rabaey K., Aelterman P., Schamphelaire I. D., Pham T. H., Boeckx P., Boon N., Verstraete W. (2007a) Biological denitrification in microbial fuel cells. *Environmental Science and Technology* **41**, 3354–3360.

Clauwaert P., van der Ha D., Boon N., Verbeken K., Verhaege M., Rabaey K., Verstraete W. (2007b) Open air biocathode enables effective electricity generation with microbial fuel cells. *Environmental Science and Technology* **41**, 7564–7569.

Fan Y. Z., Hu H. Q., Liu H. (2007) Enhanced coulombic efficiency and power density of air-cathode microbial fuel cells with an improved cell configuration. *Journal of Power Sources* **171**, 348–354.

Fu L., You S. J., Zhang G. Q., Yang F. L., Fang X. H. (2011) PB/PANI-modified electrode used as a novel oxygen reduction cathode in microbial fuel cell. *Biosensors and Bioelectronics* **26**, 1975–1979.

Fu L., You S. J., Zhang G. Q., Yang F. L., Fang X. H. (2010) Degradation of azo dyes using in-situ Fenton reaction incorporated into H_2O_2-producing microbial fuel cell. *Chemical Engineering Journal* **160**, 164–169.

Ghangrekar M. M., Shinde V. B. (2007) Performance of membrane-less microbial fuel cell treating wastewater and effect of electrode distance and area on electricity production. *Bioresource Technology* **98**, 2879–2885.

Gorby Y. A., Yanina S., McLean J. S., et al. (2006) Electrically conductive bacterial nanowires produced by *Shewanella oneidensis* strain MR-1 and other microorganisms. Proceedings of the National Academy of Sciences USA 130, 11358–11363.

He Z., Minteer S. D., Angenent L. T. (2005) Electricity generation from artificial wastewater using an upflow microbial fuel cell. *Environmental Science and Technology* **39**, 5262–5267.

Henze M., van Loosdrecht M. C. M., Ekama G. A., Brdjanovic D. (2008) Biological wastewater treatment: principles, modeling and design. International Water Association, London, UK.

Jiang J. Q., Zhao Q. L., Zhang J. N., Zhang G. D., Lee D. J. (2009) Electricity generation from bio-treatment of sewage sludge with microbial fuel cell. *Bioresource Technology* **100**, 5808–5812.

Kim J. R., Cheng S. A., Oh S. E., Logan B. E. (2007) Power generation using different cation, anion, ultrafiltration membranes in microbial fuel cells. *Environmental Science and Technology* **41**, 1004–1009.

Kinoshita K. (1992) *Electrochemical Oxygen Technology*, Wiley, New York.

Kumlanghan A., Liu J., Thavarungkul P., Kanatharana P., Mattiasson B. (2007) Microbial fuel cell-based biosensor for fast analysis of biodegradable organic matter. *Biosensors and Bioelectronics* **22**, 2939–2944.

Li J., Fu Q., Liao Q., Zhu X., Ye D. D., Tian X. (2009) Persulfate: a self-activated cathodic electron acceptor for microbial fuel cells. *Journal of Power Sources* **194**, 269–274.

Li Z., Zhang X., Lei L. (2008) Electricity production during the treatment of real electroplating wastewater containing Cr(VI) using microbial fuel cell. *Process Biochemistry* **43**, 1352–1358.

Liu Y. (2003) Chemically reduced excess sludge production in the activated sludge process. *Chemosphere* **50**, 1–7.

Liu H., Logan B. E. (2004) Electricity generation using an air-cathode single chamber microbial fuel cell in the presence and absence of a proton exchange membrane. *Environmental Science and Technology* **38**, 4040–4046.

Liu Y., Tay J. H. (2001) Strategy for minimization of excess sludge production from activated sludge process. *Biotechnology Advances* **19**, 97–107.

Liu H., Grot S., Logan B. E. (2005) Electrochemically assisted microbial production of hydrogen from acetate. *Environmental Science and Technology* **39**, 4317–4320.

Liu Y., Harnisch F., Fricke K., Schröder U., Climent V., Feliu J. M. (2010) The study of electrochemically active microbial biofilms on different carbon-based anode materials in microbial fuel cells. *Biosensors and Bioelectronics* **25**, 2167–2171.

Logan B. E., Regan J. M. (2006a) Microbial fuel cells: challenges and applications. *Environmental Science and Technology* **40**, 5172–5180.

Logan B. E., Regan J. M. (2006b) Electricity-producing bacterial communities in microbial fuel cells. *Trends in Microbiology* **14**, 512–518.

Pant D., van Bogaert G., Diels L., Vanbroekhoven K. (2010) A review of the substrates used in microbial fuel cells. (MFCs) for sustainable energy production. *Bioresource Technology* **101**, 1533–1543.

Park D. H., Zeikus J. G. (2000) Electricity generation in microbial fuel cell using neutral red as electronophore. *Applied Environmental Microbiology* **66**, 1292–1297.

Peng L., You S. J., Wang J. Y. (2010) Electrode potential regulates cytochrome accumulation on *Shewanella oneidensis* cell surface and the consequence to bioelectrocatalytic current generation. *Biosensors and Bioelectronics* **25**, 2530–2533.

Potter M. C. (1911) Electrical effects accompanying the decomposition of organic compounds. *Proceedings of the Royal Society of London Series B* **84**, 260–276.

Qiao Y., Li C. M., Bao S. J., Bao Q. L. (2007) Carbon nanotube/polyaniline composite as anode material for microbial fuel cells. *Journal of Power Sources* **170**, 79–84.

Rabaey K., Verstraete W. (2005) Microbial fuel cells: novel biotechnology for energy generation. *Trends in Biotechnology* **23**, 291–298.

Reguera G., McCarthy K. D., Mehta T., Nicoll J. S., Tuominen M. T., Lovley D. R. (2005) Extracellular electron transfer via microbial nanowires. *Nature* **435**, 1098–1101.

Ren Z. Y., Ward T. E., Regan J. M. (2007) Electricity production from cellulose in a microbial fuel cell using a defined binary culture. *Environmental Science and Technology* **41**, 4781–4786.

Rhodas A., Beyenal H., Lewandowski Z. (2005) Microbial fuel cell using anaerobic respiration as an anodic reaction and biomineralized manganese as a cathodic reactant. *Environmental Science and Technology* **39**, 4666–4671.

Rosenbaum M., Zhao F., Schröder U., Scholz F. (2006) Interfacing electrocatalysis and biocatalysis with tungsten carbide: a high-performance, noble-metal-free microbial fuel cell. *Angewandte Chemie* **118**, 1–4.

Rozendal R. A., Hamelers H. V. M., Buisman C. J. N. (2006a) Effects of membrane cation transport on pH and microbial fuel cell performance. *Environmental Science and Technology* **40**, 5206–5211.

Rozendal R. A., Hamelers H. V. M., Euverink G. J. W., Metz S. J., Buisman C. J. N. (2006b) Principle and perspectives of hydrogen production through biocatalyzed electrolysis. *International Journal of Hydrogen Energy* **31**, 1632–1640.

Rozendal R. A., Leone E., Keller J., Rabaey K. (2009) Efficient hydrogen peroxide generation from organic matter in a bioelectrochemical system. *Electrochemistry Communications* **11**, 1752–1755.

Schröder U. (2007) Anodic electron transfer mechanisms in microbial fuel cells and their energy efficiency. *Physical Chemistry Chemical Physics* **9**, 2619–2629.

Schröder U., Niessen J., Scholz F. (2003) A generation of microbial fuel cells with current outputs boosted by more than one order of magnitude. *Angewandte Chemie International Edition* **42**, 2880–2883.

Scott K., Murano C. (2007) A study of a microbial fuel cell battery using manure sludge waste. *Journal of Chemical Technology and Biotechnology* **82**, 809–817.

Steele B. C. H., Heinzel A. (2001) Materials for fuel-cell technologies. *Nature* **414**, 345–352.

Tandukar M., Huber S. J., Onodera T., Pavlostathis S. G. (2009) Biological chromium(VI) reduction in the cathode of a microbial fuel cell. *Environmental Science and Technology* **43**, 8159–8165.

Tartakovsky B., Guiot S. R. (2006) A comparison of air and hydrogen peroxide oxygenated microbial fuel cell reactors. *Biotechnology Progress* **22**, 241–246.

Ter Heijne A., Hamelers H. V. M., Buisman C. J. N. (2007) Microbial fuel cell operation with continuous biological ferrous iron oxidation of the catholyte. *Environmental Science and Technology* **41**, 4130–4134.

Ter Heijne A., Liu F., van der Weijden R., Weijma J., Buisman C. J. N., Hamelers H. V. M. (2010) Copper recovery combined with electricity production in a microbial fuel cell. *Environmental Science and Technology* **44**, 4376–4381.

Virdis B., Rabaey K., Yuan Z. G., Keller J. (2008) Microbial fuel cell for simultaneous removal of carbon and nitrogen. *Water Research* **42**, 3013–3024.

Wang G., Huang L. P., Zhang Y. F. (2008) Cathodic reduction of hexavalent chromium [Cr(VI)] coupled with electricity generation in microbial fuel cells. *Biotechnology Letters* **30**, 1959–1966.

Wang X., Feng Y. J., Wang H. M., Qu Y. P., Yu Y. L., Ren N. Q., Li N., Wang E., Lee H., Logan B. E. (2009) Bioaugmentation for electricity generation from corn stover biomass using microbial fuel cell. *Environmental Science and Technology* **43**, 6088–6093.

You S. J., Zhao Q. L., Zhang J. N., Jiang J. Q., Zhao S. Q. (2006) A microbial fuel cell using permanganate as a cathodic electron acceptor. *Journal of Power Sources* **162**, 1409–1415.

You S. J., Ren N. Q., Zhao Q. L., Kiely P. D., Wang J. Y., Yang F. L., Fu L., Peng L. (2009) Improving phosphate buffer-free cathode performance of microbial fuel cell based on biological nitrification. *Biosensors and Bioelectronics* **24**, 3698–3701.

You S. J., Wang J. Y., Ren N. Q., Wang X. H., Zhang J. N. (2010) Sustainable conversion of glucose into hydrogen peroxide in solid polymer electrolyte microbial fuel cell. *ChemSusChem* **3**, 334–338.

Zhang L. X., Liu C. S., Zhuang L., Li W. S., Zhou S. G., Zhang J. T. (2009) Manganese dioxide as an alternative cathodic catalyst to platinum in microbial fuel cell. *Biosensors and Bioelectronics* **24**, 2825–2829.

Zhao F., Harnisch F., Schröder U., Scholz F., Bogdanoff P., Herrmann I. (2005) Application of pyrolysed iron(II) phthalocyanine and CoTMPP based oxygen reduction catalysts as cathode materials in microbial fuel cells. *Electrochemistry Communications* **7**, 1405–1410.

Zhao F., Harnisch F., Schröder U., Scholz F., Bogdanoff P., Herrmann I. (2006) Challenges and constraints of using oxygen cathodes in microbial fuel cells. *Environmental Science and Technology* **40**, 5193–5199.

10

ANAEROBIC DIGESTION OF SEWAGE SLUDGE

KUAN-YEOW SHOW

Department of Environmental Engineering, Faculty of Engineering and Green Technology, University Tunku Abdul Rahman, Jalan University, Bandar Barat, Perak, Malaysia

DUU-JONG LEE

Department of Chemical Engineering, National Taiwan University of Science and Technology, Taipei, Taiwan

JOO-HWA TAY

Department of Environmental Science and Engineering, Fudan University, Shanghai, China

10.1 INTRODUCTION

Sewage sludge is an unavoidable by-product of wastewater treatment. Raw sludge is not only rich in organic carbon and pathogens but also in heavy metals and other environmental pollutants. Therefore, the sludge must be stabilized to enable environmentally safe disposal or utilization. Currently anaerobic digestion is the most commonly used process for the stabilization of sewage sludge. Although anaerobic digestion of sludge was first used more than a century ago, it has only been during the last two decades that due consideration has been given to the process. The use of an anaerobic process for sludge digestion has evolved from the earliest septic tanks to complex digestion systems involving modern technologies. There are many positive features of anaerobic treatment; for example, methane can be generated to be utilized as fuel, digestion has a low energy requirement, the pathogenic microorganisms in sludge are effectively killed, attention to operations

Biological Sludge Minimization and Biomaterials/Bioenergy Recovery Technologies, First Edition.
Edited by Etienne Paul and Yu Liu.
© 2012 John Wiley & Sons, Inc. Published 2012 by John Wiley & Sons, Inc.

is minimized, seasonal treatment is optimized, and the digested sludge is stable and may be disposed of harmlessly.

However, despite its proven significance and potential development, the process has not generally been used as widely as it might deserve, due primarily to a lack of fundamental understanding and the operational limitations of the process. A main drawback of anaerobic digestion is its slow biological degradation rate, which results in long fermentation times and large fermenter volumes. A retention time of more than 20 days and the construction of huge digesters are usually required for efficient anaerobic degradation. Moreover, due to the low concentration of soluble organic matter contained in sludge, only 30 to 50% of the total chemical oxygen demand (COD) or volatile solids (VS) can be degraded over very long digestion times (Chiu et al. 1997). The process of rapid industrialization and urbanization has dramatically increased the volume of sludge quantity generated. Hence, there is an urgent need to shorten the digestion period and enhance the degradation efficiency of anaerobic digestion.

Advances in science along with recent research studies have helped to better understand the complex biochemistry and microbiology of anaerobic process, and this helps to stimulate further interest and application of the process in sludge digestion. In this chapter we describe key fundamentals of anaerobic digestion, including biochemistry and microbiology, environmental requirements, control and design considerations of digesters, evaluation of process designs, and advantages and limitations of anaerobic digestion. Perspectives and applications of anaerobic digestion are also illustrated.

10.2   PRINCIPLES OF ANAEROBIC DIGESTION

Advances in science along with recent research studies have helped to better understand the complex biochemistry and microbiology of anaerobic process. The anaerobic fermentation process converts organic materials biologically to methane and carbon dioxide in an environment devoid of oxygen. A historical overview of the process recognizes that anaerobic microorganisms were first discovered by Pasteur in 1861 while studying fermentive reactions. The process was not utilized for waste treatment until late in the nineteenth century. Since then, anaerobic digestion has been recognized as a useful process for waste treatment from the earliest household septic tanks to modern waste treatment systems.

The mechanisms of anaerobic processes are much more complicated than that of aerobic processes, due to the many pathways available for an anaerobic community. The biochemistry and microbiology responsible for the reactions are not fully understood, but during the last 30 years a broad outline of the processes has been reported by various researchers. Anaerobic digestion of complex organic substances is usually considered to be a two-stage process consisting of acid formation (liquefaction) and gas formation (gasification) in an environment devoid of oxygen as depicted in Fig. 10.1. The process is performed by two physiologically distinct bacterial populations: the *acid formers* and the *methane formers*.

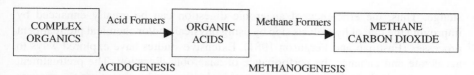

FIGURE 10.1 Two-stage acidogenesis–methanogenesis anaerobic digestion.

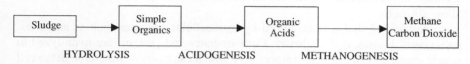

FIGURE 10.2 Three-stage hydrolysis–acidogenesis–methanogenesis anaerobic sludge digestion.

Many researchers prefer to consider anaerobic digestion of complex organic substances such as sludge to be a three-stage process consisting of hydrolysis, acidogenesis, and methanogenesis (Fig. 10.2). Anaerobic digestion of sludge must initially be hydrolyzed to soluble organics of lower molecular weight. The first stage is the hydrolysis of long-chain complex organics such as carbohydrates, proteins, and fats to simpler molecules. Complex organics are catalyzed by extracellular enzymes such as amylases, proteinases, lipases, and nucleases. Carbohydrates and proteins are hydrolyzed to simple sugars and amino acids, respectively. Fats are hydrolyzed to glycerol and long-chain fatty acids. These lower-molecular-weight organic compounds are then used by the acid formers to produce simple volatile fatty acids.

In the second stage, organic materials are converted into simple volatile fatty acids by the group of facultative and obligate anaerobes commonly termed acid formers. The products of this second-stage acidogenic conversion comprise predominantly organic fatty acids and a small portion of biological cells. Although no waste stabilization is brought about during this stage of treatment, it is normally considered as an intermediate reaction to prepare the organic matter in a form amenable for the third stage of treatment. It is in the methanogenesis stage of treatment that actual waste stabilization occurs. The organic acids produced by the acid formers are converted by the unique group of microorganisms identified as methane formers into gaseous end products consisting of carbon dioxide, methane, and cells.

10.2.1 Hydrolysis and Acidogenesis

Hydrolysis is a rather slow stage and has been identified as the rate-limiting step that limits the speed of the entire process and leads to poor degradation results. Even after some decades of optimization, a retention time of more than 20 d and the construction of huge digesters are usually necessary for efficient degradation in an anaerobic process. Acceleration and better performance of the anaerobic process could be achieved by finding an alternative to the slow and rate-determining hydrolysis of the sludge. Thus, the efficiency of anaerobic digestion can be greatly enhanced by improving the rate of hydrolysis step by using physical and/or chemical pretreatment processes (Eastman and Ferguson 1981). Extensive studies have explored ways to accelerate and enhance the performance of anaerobic digestion. The pretreatment process may include thermal pretreatment, high-pressure homogenization, enzyme treatment, chemical solubilization by alkali, acid, or base addition, mechanical disintegration, and ultrasound treatment. Among these processes, ultrasonication exhibits a greater potential of not being hazardous to the environment and is economically competitive (Mao et al. 2004; Show et al. 2006, 2007; Mao and Show 2007a,b).

Hydrolysis of sludge is catalyzed by extracellular enzymes such as amylases, proteinases, lipases, and nucleases. Carbohydrates and proteins are hydrolyzed to simple sugars and amino acids, respectively, which can easily diffuse through the cell wall into the bacteria. Fats are hydrolyzed to glycerol and long-chain fatty acids. While glycerol can move across the cell wall, the fatty acid molecules are too large to be assimilated by the bacterial cell. The acids dissolve in the lipopolysaccharide on the bacteria surface and are pulled into the cell while being metabolized by β-oxidation. The end products resulting from hydrolysis are generally used as carbon and energy sources by acid formers which carry out the first-stage fermentation.

The bacteria responsible for the hydrolysis and initial fermentation are a very complicated mixture of various bacterial genera. Most of these bacteria are obligate anaerobes, but some facultative anaerobes that can metabolize either aerobically or anaerobically may be present. The obligate bacteria are strict anaerobes sensitive to oxygen, and *Clostridium* is the major group of this species, which produce spores in order to survive under aerobic conditions. *Flavobacterium, Alcaligenes, Achromobacter*, and various enteric bacteria are common facultative microorganisms that have been identified in wastewater treatment systems. It was originally thought that acid formation was performed primarily by facultative bacteria. Studies have shown that the obligate anaerobes are the primary organisms involved in this process.

The oxidized end products from the first-stage conversion are primarily volatile acids such as acetic, propionic acids, and to a lesser extent, butyric, valeric, and caproic acids can also be found as shown in Table 10.1. These are called *fatty acids* since compounds of this type are readily available from naturally occurring fats and oils. It has been reported that acetic and propionic acids are the precursors of about

TABLE 10.1 Basic Volatile Fatty Acid Intermediates

Common Name	IUPAC Name	Structural Formula	Salt Name
Formic acid	Methanoic	$HCOOH$	Formate
Acetic acid	Ethanoic	CH_3COOH	Acetate
Propionic acid	Propanoic	CH_3CH_2COOH	Propionate
Butyric acid	Butanoic	$CH_3 (CH_2)_2COOH$	Butyrate
Valeric acid	Pentanoic	$CH_3 (CH_2)_3COOH$	Valerate
Caproic acid	Hexanoic	$CH_3 (CH_2)_4COOH$	Caproate

85% of the methane produced from the digestion of complex organic wastes. Relative concentrations of the various intermediates are influenced by both the environmental conditions and the specific growth rate imposed on the substrate.

Some of the acidogenic bacteria possess a distinctive enzyme system enabling them to oxidize reduced coenzymes without passing the electrons to an organic acceptor and releasing hydrogen to the medium. The collective activity carried out by these hydrogen-producing bacteria is called *hydrogenogenesis*, and the responsible bacteria may be thought of as a subset of the acid-producing bacteria. It has been shown that hydrogen production and utilization can influence the fermentation process. The acidogenic bacteria are relatively fast growing and have typical doubling times of approximately 30 min at 35°C (McCarty 1964; Zhang et al. 2008; Lee et al. 2011).

10.2.2 Methane Formation

The methane-producing bacteria are subdivided into acetoclastic methane bacteria (acetophilic) and methane bacteria (hydrogenophilic). These methanogenic bacteria are strictly anaerobic and thus vulnerable to even small amounts of oxygen. Naturally, they are only found in completely anaerobic environments such as the bottom of lakes, rumen of cattle, and the wet wood of trees. The methanogenic bacteria are very difficult to isolate in pure culture. Although many studies have been conducted, relatively little is known about their biochemistry. One of the most significant features of the methanogenesis is that very few substrates can act as energy sources for the methanogens. The discovery that methanogenic bacteria are unable to metabolize alcohols other than methanol, or organic acids other than acetate or formate, indicates that there must be at least three groups of bacteria responsible for the decomposition of organic material into the final gaseous products.

The bioconversion of organics into methane proceeds through a series of complex biochemical changes, and little is known about the individual steps involved. One identified source of methane in anaerobic decomposition is acetate cleavage into methane and carbon dioxide through decarboxylation. The reaction proposed by McCarty (1964) is

$$CH_3COOH \rightarrow CH_4 + CO_2 \qquad (10.1)$$

Acetic acid is one of the most important volatile acids formed from the decomposition of organics and is the main source of methane in anaerobic digestion. Most of the remaining methane is formed from the reduction of carbon dioxide, using hydrogen as the energy source by the carbon dioxide–reducing methanogens through the reaction

$$CO_2 + 8H \rightarrow CH_4 + 2H_2O \qquad (10.2)$$

Carbon dioxide is reduced by hydrogen, which is removed from the organic matter by enzymes. The carbon dioxide hence functions as a hydrogen or electron acceptor.

There is always an excess of carbon dioxide in the system, and thus the availability of carbon dioxide is never a limiting factor for the methanogenesis.

Early taxonomic studies included methanogens in the family Methanobacteriaceae, which is divided into three genera on the basis of cell morphology. They are generally grouped by *Methanobacterium* in rods, *Methanosarcina* in curves, and *Methanococcus* in spheres. More new genera have been added to the family, including *Methanobrevibacter*, *Methanomicrobium*, *Methanogenium*, and *Methanospirillum*. It had been demonstrated that 65 to 70% of methane production from a complex substrate is through acetate cleavage accomplished by *Methanosarcina* and *Methanothrix*, while reduction of carbon dioxide by hydrogen-oxidizing methanogens is responsible for the rest, and that *Methanosarcina* predominated at high acetate concentration, whereas *Methanothrix* predominated at lower acetate levels (Barker 1956; McCarty 1964).

A sound anaerobic decomposition of waste requires a balance among the acidogenic and methanogenic bacteria. The methanogens and acidogens form a syntrophic relationship in which each bacteria group constitutes a significant link in a complex chain of bioconversion. The establishment and maintenance of this balance is usually indicated by the control test of volatile acid concentration. An increase in the acid concentration indicates that the activity of slow-growing methane formers lags behind fast-growing acid formers. An excess of volatile acids develops rapidly, leading to a decrease in system pH and possible upsetting of the fermentation process. Such upsets are often caused by shock loadings of organic solids to the system, or the system buffering capacity is suddenly reduced. As the growth rate of methane formers is extremely low compared with that of acid formers, it appears that the entire anaerobic decomposition process is dependent on the vitality of methane formers. This has led to the conclusion that the metabolism of methane formers is rate-limiting in the anaerobic treatment process (Barker 1956).

10.3 ENVIRONMENTAL REQUIREMENTS AND CONTROL

Anaerobic waste treatment is a sensitive biological process such that a variety of environmental conditions must be maintained for efficient treatment. The environmental requirements include careful control of optimum system pH, temperature, nutrients, and tolerable toxic substances.

10.3.1 pH

Anaerobic treatment proceeds well at a system pH varying from 6.6 to 7.6, with an optimum range of 7.0 to 7.2. The efficiency drops off rapidly at a pH below 6.2. Acidic conditions occur when the methane formers are overburdened, due to a rapid increase in volatile fatty acids concentrations. The acidic conditions are usually caused by organic overloading or hydraulic stress by washing out excessive amounts of the slow-growing methane formers (Liu et al. 2002; Wong et al, 2008).

Maintaining an optimum system pH is especially crucial during the sensitive startup period. A pH below 6.5 can increase the length of startup considerably. The anaerobic systems are able to tolerate higher fluctuation of pH only when steady-state conditions are reached, and also able to recover rapidly from short-term departures of pH from optimum. To maintain the system in the desired pH range, addition of adequate buffer is essential. Desirable levels of alkalinity are usually around 2500 to 5000 as $CaCO_3$ mg L^{-1}, depending on the organic loading conditions. Lime is often added to the systems to maintain a proper pH. However, it must be used with caution to prevent calcium ion toxicity (Show et al. 2004a,b; Wang et al. 2004).

10.3.2 Alkalinity

Sufficient alkalinity is essential for proper pH control. Alkalinity is derived from the breakdown of organics and is present primarily in the form of bicarbonates, which are in equilibrium with the carbon dioxide in the gas at a given pH. This relationship among alkalinity, the carbon dioxide in the gas, and pH is shown by the reactions

$$CO_2 + H_2O \rightarrow H_2CO_3 \tag{10.3}$$

$$H_2CO_3 \rightarrow H^+ + HCO_3^- \tag{10.4}$$

The hydrogen ion concentration $[H^+]$ and pH of the system may be calculated from the following equilibrium equation for the ionization of H_2CO_3:

$$[H^+] = k_1 \frac{[H_2CO_3]}{[HCO_3^-]} \tag{10.5}$$

At values of pH between 6.6 and 7.4 and at a carbon dioxide content in the gas of 30 to 40% by volume, the bicarbonate alkalinity will range between 1000 and 5000 mg L^{-1} as $CaCO_3$. The concentration of bicarbonate alkalinity should be approximately 3000 mg L^{-1} as $CaCO_3$. The bicarbonate alkalinity is approximately equal to the total alkalinity of the anaerobic system. A portion of the alkalinity appears as "volatile acid salts" alkalinity, which results from the reaction of volatile acids with the bicarbonate present, yielding carbon dioxide. At low volatile acid concentrations, the bicarbonate alkalinity represents approximately the total alkalinity; however, as the volatile acids concentration increases, the bicarbonate alkalinity is much lower than the total alkalinity. About 83.3% of the volatile acid concentration contributes to the alkalinity as volatile acids salts alkalinity, and the following equation may be used to estimate the concentration of bicarbonate alkalinity:

$$BA = TA - (0.85)(0.833) TVA \tag{10.6}$$

where BA is bicarbonate alkalinity (mg L^{-1} as $CaCO_3$), TA is total alkalinity (mg L^{-1} as $CaCO_3$), and TVA is total volatile acids (mg L^{-1} as acetic acid). The factor 0.85

accounts for the fact that 85% of the volatile acid salts alkalinity is measured by titration to pH = 4.0 (McCarty 1964; Cook 1987).

10.3.3 Temperature

Temperature has a significant effect on the rate of reaction in anaerobic systems. The systems perform better at elevated temperatures in the thermophilic range 45 to 65°C. Although waste decomposition proceeds more rapidly at thermophilic temperatures, the costs associated with maintaining such temperatures may offset the benefits of higher reaction rates. Therefore, most anaerobic treatment systems are designed to operate in the mesophilic range 20 to 45°C. It has been shown that most optimum temperatures are around 33 to 40°C.

Anaerobic treatment can be performed at a temperature below 20°C in the psychrophilic range. However, operation of the system in this low-temperature range is disadvantageous, owing to the extremely reduced rates of reaction and the resulting longer solids retention times. Sudden temperature changes are often detrimental to anaerobic systems. It has been reported that changes of only a few degrees in temperature can cause an imbalance between the major bacteria populations, leading to process failure (Cook 1987).

10.3.4 Nutrients

The anaerobic process is dependent on bacterial activities. For microorganisms to grow, they must be provided with sufficient quantities of macronutrients (nitrogen and phosphorus) and micronutrients (trace nutrients) to support the synthesis of new biomass for active biomass growth. Unlike municipal wastewater, industrial wastes are often more specific in composition, and various nutrients must be added for optimum treatment. With knowledge of the yield coefficient, the necessary nutrient concentrations in the substrate can be calculated.

The amount of nitrogen and phosphorus needed for anaerobic growth can be estimated by first assuming a common empirical formula for bacterial cell material as $C_5H_7O_2N$. This indicates that nitrogen constitutes about 12% of the dry cell mass. The phosphorus content of bacteria is approximately one-seventh to one-fifth of the nitrogen requirement. By next assuming that 10% of the COD that undergoes biodegradation is converted to new bacterial cells (growth yield of $0.1 \, \text{kg VSS kg}^{-1}$ COD removed), it is a simple matter to calculate the nitrogen and phosphorus requirements.

By convention, the quantities of N and P required for growth are expressed in proportion to the COD, with the amount of N normalized to 7. In this fashion, the nutrients required in the examples would be described by a COD/N/P ratio of 580 : 7 : 1. If nutrient supplementation is required, nitrogen is most commonly added as urea, aqueous ammonia, or ammonium chloride. Phosphorus can be supplemented as phosphoric acid or as a phosphate salt. Since the growth yield for anaerobic bacteria varies somewhat with process operating conditions, some flexibility must be adopted in setting nutrient levels. The COD/N ratio is a function of the specific biomass loading or food/microorganism ratio (F/M, $kg\,COD\,kg^{-1}\,VSS\,d^{-1}$). The highest nitrogen requirement (COD/N of 350 : 7) is associated with highly loaded biomass. Another approach that can be followed for nitrogen requires that the reactor effluent be monitored for NH_4-N. As long as 5 to $10\,mg\,L^{-1}$ of residual NH_4-N is detected, nitrogen should not be limiting. However, with some wastewaters, the requirement for 100% higher levels of residual ammonium-N have been identified.

In addition to nitrogen and phosphorus, several other substances have been identified as micronutrients for methanogens. The most important of these are calcium, magnesium, iron, cobalt, nickel, and sulfide, all of which are required in $mg\,L^{-1}$ levels. Generally, these elements are present in sufficient quantities in wastewaters. However, it is advisable to analyze the reactor effluent and verify that it contains residual levels of these elements in the soluble form. During anaerobic treatment, significant quantities of the metals can be precipitated as carbonates or sulfides, making them unavailable for bacterial uptake. Pulsing addition of trace metals to disturb the solubility equilibria temporarily had been proposed.

To sustain healthy microbial populations in the systems, the COD/N/P ratio is often quoted as a useful process parameter. Speece and McCarty (1964) have shown that the minimum theoretical COD/N/P ratio may be assumed to be 350 : 7 : 1 for anaerobic systems. Van den Berg and Lentz (1977) have quoted 420 : 7 : 1 as an acceptable maximum ratio for systems loaded in the range 0.8 to $1.2\,kg\,COD\,kg^{-1}$ $VSS\,d^{-1}$. Values of around 1000 : 7 : 1 have been reported for organic loading below $0.5\,kg\,COD\,kg^{-1}\,VSS\,d^{-1}$ (Benjamin et al. 1981).

10.3.5 Toxicity

There are many substances that may be toxic or inhibitory to the anaerobic treatment. Toxicity in biological treatment is normally considered as a relative phenomenon since the extent of inhibition is in relation to the concentration of the toxic material. At low concentrations, some inhibiting materials have a stimulative effect on the process. As the concentration is increased above the optimum level, the bacterial activity begins to decrease.

Microorganisms are often able to adapt to some degree to inhibitory concentrations of most substances. The extent of adaptation is relative, and in some cases, the biological activity after adaptation may revert to the original levels, as in the absence of the toxicity. It seems that an important property of the bacteria is their ability to acclimatize to toxic substances. In general, methanogenic bacteria are more susceptible to toxicity than other groups of bacteria in anaerobic process. The sensitivity to toxicant of the anaerobes can be reduced by acclimation and by maintaining a longer solid retention time (Owen et al. 1979).

Apart from various organic substances which can inhibit anaerobic systems, there are more common toxic materials that cause process failure or upset in anaerobic treatment. These include volatile acids, ammonia, heavy metals, alkali and alkaline-earth salts, and sulfide.

Volatile fatty acids (VFAs) are perhaps the most common inhibitors of anaerobic system since they are generated as intermediates in the decomposition of organics.

The mechanism is somewhat obscure, but it is believed that nonionized volatile acids (NVAs) play a role. The toxic level for free NVAs has been quoted in the range 1000 to 2000 mg L^{-1} as acetic acid. The toxic level for long-chain fatty acids seems to be of the same magnitude. But inhibition has been reported at an NVA level of 30 to 60 mg L^{-1} as acetic acid (McCarty 1961).

It has been shown that the extent of NFA inhibition is influenced by the system pH. It had been reported that when the pH was held consistently near neutrality, neither acetic nor butyric acid had any significant toxic effects on hydrogen-utilizing methanogens at concentrations up to 10,000 mg L^{-1}. Similar results for acetic acid in sewage sludge digestion had been reported. It appears that at neutral pH, only propionic acid is likely to exhibit toxic effects in an anaerobic process when its concentration is as high as 1000 mg L^{-1}. NVAs have a more deleterious effect as the pH decreases. Weak acids are poorly dissociated at low pH and can penetrate bacterial cells readily in nonionized forms, thereby changing the internal cell pH. This explains the phenomenon that NFAs exhibit toxicity at low pH values but do not have an inhibitory effect at neutral pH. As far as operation of anaerobic reactors is concerned, little inhibition by NFAs will occur if the system pH is maintained near neutrality.

Ammonia is a common toxic substance resulting from the degradation of wastes containing proteins or urea. Ammonia may be present either in the form of ammonium ion (NH_4^+) or as dissolved ammonia gas (NH_3). It is believed that free undissociated ammonia is most toxic, with inhibition reported at 0.1 to 0.2 kg N m^{-3}. If concentration of free ammonia exceeds 150 mg L^{-1}, severe toxicity will occur, whereas concentration of ammonia ion must exceed 3000 mg L^{-1} to exert the same effect. Total ammonia and ammonium concentrations as high as 5 to 8 kg N m^{-3} can be tolerated if the reactor pH is within normal operation limits. When the ammonia–nitrogen exceeds 3000 mg L^{-1}, the ammonium ion itself will become toxic regardless of system pH, and process failure can be expected (Owen 1979).

Heavy metals have been blamed for many anaerobic system failures, particularly for sludge digesters. Soluble heavy metals such as copper, zinc, and nickel salts can be toxic even at very low concentrations. Hexavelant chromium is relatively less toxic because it can be reduced to insoluble trivalent form. Iron and aluminum salts are also less toxic, due to their low solubility.

It has been demonstrated that the toxicity of heavy metals is directly related to the solubility product of their sulfide salts (Mosey and Hughes 1975). The presence of sulfide will enable precipitation of soluble heavy metal ions to insoluble and inert sulfide salts. The tolerable levels for heavy metals in anaerobic systems are directly related to the sulfide concentration. Although sulfides by themselves are toxic materials, they form insoluble salts with heavy metals. Such salts are quite inert and have no detrimental effect on microorganisms. In fact, one of the most effective ways for the control of heavy metal toxicity is by adding sodium sulfide, which will be reduced to sulfide under anaerobic conditions.

Alkali and alkaline-earth salts concentrations, such as those of sodium, potassium, calcium, or magnesium, may be very high in industrial wastes. These are often the cause of process failure in anaerobic treatment. It has been found that alkali and alkaline-earth salt toxicity is normally associated with the cation rather than the anion portion of the salt (Kugelman and McCarty 1964).

The combined effects of these cations are somehow complex, as some of the cations act antagonistically and reduce the toxicity of other cations, while others act synergistically, which increases the toxicity of other cations. Calcium and magnesium are normally poor antagonists but may become stimulatory if another antagonist is already present. Sodium and potassium are the best antagonists and are most effective if present at the stimulatory concentrations. It has been recommended that antagonists are best added as the chloride salts.

Sulfides in anaerobic treatment result from the introduction of sulfides with the wastewater or from the biological reduction of sulfates and other sulfur-containing inorganic compounds in the digester, as well as from anaerobic decomposition of proteins. The toxicity of sulfide is closely associated with the free hydrogen sulfide concentration, which is pH dependent (Lawrence and McCarty 1965). Sulfide toxicity has been reported at different concentrations, depending on process operation and type of reactor. For general operation, influent sulfate-sulfur levels below 0.3 to $0.6 \, \text{kg S m}^{-3}$ may be regarded as noninhibitory. Free hydrogen sulfide seems to inhibit at lower levels around $0.1 \, \text{kg m}^{-3}$. Various methods have been used successfully to reduce sulfide toxicity. These include the addition of iron salts to the feed, which precipitates the sulfide as insoluble metal sulfides, gas stripping of H_2S from the digester gas, and pure oxygen stripping.

10.4 DESIGN CONSIDERATIONS FOR ANAEROBIC SLUDGE DIGESTION

The purpose of anaerobic digestion is to achieve destruction of a portion of the volatile solids in the sludge to enhance the dewaterability of the digested sludge and to minimize the putrescibility of the sludge. Volatile solids degradation is time dependent. Therefore, the design criteria for anaerobic digestion systems are based on the hydraulic detention time required to achieve a specific reduction in the volatile solids content of the digested sludge. The hydraulic detention time and mean cell residence time are the same for an anaerobic digestion system with no recycle. The design parameters that must be considered and controlled include hydraulic detention time, uniform solids loading, temperature, and mixing.

10.4.1 Hydraulic Detention Time

The generation times (i.e., the time required to double the number of bacteria or to double the microbial population) of methane-forming bacteria are relatively long compared to those reported for aerobic and facultative bacteria. The generation times for methane-forming bacteria range from less than 2 d to more than 20 d at a temperature of 35°C. Therefore, typical detention times for anaerobic sludge digestion are about 15 to 20 d. However, hydraulic detention times as low as 7 d may be used at facilities where a high level of operational control of the process is maintained (McCarty 1964).

The hydraulic retention time affects the rate and extent of methane production, which in turn is affected by environmental conditions within the digestion tank, the operating temperature maintained, and the solids concentration and volatile solids content of the feed sludge. Typically, sludges introduced into a municipal anaerobic digestion system contain equal amounts on a weight basis of primary solids and excess activated sludge. At a trickling filter plant where the sloughed trickling filter sludge is returned to the primary clarifier, sludge from only the primary clarifier is fed to the anaerobic digestion tank. The volatile solids content controls the rate and amount of gas production. However, the concentration of total solids affects the ability to mix the sludge effectively to eliminate pockets of raw sludge and pockets of sludge at different temperatures. The conversion of volatile solids to gaseous products is controlled by the hydraulic detention time. Therefore, the design detention time is a function of the final disposition of the digested sludge (i.e., land application or incineration) (Liu et al. 2002).

10.4.2 Solids Loading

The hydraulic detention time controls the degree of stabilization of volatile solids. High solids loadings would reduce the required digester volume for a given detention time; however, the actual volatile solids loadings achievable are controlled in most treatment facilities by the efficiency of the sedimentation basins in removing solids and in concentrating the sludge, which is pumped to the digester. Therefore, the concentration of solids in the feed sludge actually controls the loading to, and the size of, the anaerobic digester. The ability to thicken the sludge becomes an important design and operating consideration and may be a major limitation to digester loadings. Pretreatment of sludge may involve blending of primary sludge with thickened excess activated sludge or thickening the blended primary and biological sludges to maintain the organic loading to the digester. The design solids loading to anaerobic digestion systems should be between 3.2 and 7.2 kg of volatile solids per cubic meter per day. A concentration of 50% volatile solids in the digested sludge usually is considered satisfactory. The ultimate disposal of the digested sludge determines the degree of digestion required (Metcalf & Eddy, Inc., 2003).

The hydraulic detention time affects the extent of destruction of the volatile solids in the anaerobic digestion process and the size of digestion tank required. In turn, the size of the digestion tank and the concentration of solids in the feed sludge dictate the solids loading that it is possible to have and still maintain the required minimum hydraulic detention time. For example, in order to operate an anaerobic digestion system at a volatile solids loading of $3.2 \, \text{kg m}^{-3} \text{d}^{-1}$ and a detention time of 10 days, the concentration in the feed sludge must be about 3.2% based on volatile solids. This concentration translates to a solids concentration of approximately 4.5% total solids (assuming 72% volatile solids). To achieve this loading, the combined primary and biological sludges would have to be thickened to at least 2% and the solids concentration of primary sludge would have to approach 7%. If the design hydraulic detention time is 15 days, the solids concentration would have to be increased to 4.6% based on volatile solids (6.4% total solids) to maintain a solids loading of $3.2 \, \text{kg m}^{-3} \text{d}^{-1}$. Separate continuously operated gravity- or dissolved-air flotation thickeners would be required to concentrate excess activated sludges at most treatment plants to ensure continuous volatile solids loading as high as possible (Cook 1987; Metcalf & Eddy, Inc. 2003).

10.4.3 Temperature

It is essential that the operating temperature be maintained as constant as possible. Sharp and frequent fluctuations in temperature affect the performance of the methane-forming bacteria to a greater extent than the operating temperature, within the mesophilic and thermophilic ranges. Gas production is higher at mesophilic temperatures of 35°C and 55°C. However, at temperatures near 45°C, the gas production is lower, indicating that the methane-forming bacteria are inhibited in this intermediate temperature range (Liu et al. 2002). One important advantage of thermophilic digestion is greater destruction of pathogenic organisms than is reported for sludges digested at mesophilic temperatures. The increased cost of providing the additional heat required to maintain the thermophilic conditions is not offset by increased gas production or more complete digestion.

10.4.4 Mixing

The principal advantages of mixing anaerobic digestion tanks, other than eliminating the scum, are: (1) the elimination of thermal stratification and maintenance of a uniform temperature throughout the tank by maintaining chemical and physical uniformity throughout the digesting sludge; (2) maintenance of intimate contact between the active biomass and the feed sludge by mixing the raw feed sludge and the digesting sludge; (3) rapid dispersion of metabolic end products produced during digestion and any toxic materials entering the system in the feed sludge, thereby minimizing inhibitory and toxic effects on the microbial activity; and (4) prevention of the formation of surface scum layers and the deposition of silt, grit, and other heavy inert solids on the bottom of the tank and in the corners of the digestion tank.

The major disadvantage of mixing a digestion tank completely, in addition to the cost of mixing, is the need for a facility that will enhance the separation of the digested solids from the liquid phase, depending on the final disposal of the digested sludge. The initial attempts at mixing anaerobic digesters were directed at breaking the scum or keeping the scum moist so that the gas could escape. Methods of mixing that have been employed include pumping sludge from one digester to another, pumping supernatant to keep the scum moist, use of a vertical screw pump, recirculating gas, and mixing with a mechanical device (Metcalf & Eddy, Inc. 2003).

10.5 COMPONENT DESIGN OF ANAEROBIC DIGESTER SYSTEMS

10.5.1 Tank Configurations

There are two types of commonly used anaerobic digesters: standard rate and high rate. In the standard-rate digestion process, the contents of the digester are usually unheated and unmixed. Since the sludge content is not mixed, it separates into layers of scum, supernatant, and active and stabilized solids. The gas is collected at the floating gas dome. The retention times of standard-rate digesters are over 30 d. Because of the long retention times, the process is inefficient. In a high-rate digester, the contents of the digester are heated and mixed either mechanically or by the recycling of biogas. This creates an active zone of digestion and the reaction speeds up significantly. The required detention time is typically 15 d or less (Metcalf & Eddy, Inc. 2003).

A combination of these two basic processes is known as the two-stage process. The sludge in the first tank is heated to a temperature of about 35°C and is thoroughly mixed. The digestion process is essentially completed in the first tank within about 15 d of detention time. The sludge then flows into a second tank, which serves primarily for sludge settling and storage. The digester supernatant is pumped back to the influent stream of the treatment plant. Digested sludge is withdrawn from the second tank for subsequent processing.

Floating covers generally are used for anaerobic digestion tanks, although digestion tanks with fixed covers also have been designed. The floating covers are preferred because the cover rises and falls with the depth of sludge in the tank, thus maintaining a relatively constant and positive pressure in the tank. With a positive pressure in the tank, oxygen in the air is not likely to leak into the tank. In some designs the floating cover is designed to store excess digester gas also.

Anaerobic digestion tanks are either cylindrical or egg-shaped. The shape of the anaerobic digestion tank affects the type of external mixing required. Circular anaerobic digestion tanks are relatively shallow, with diameters larger than the depth. Shallow cylindrical digestion tanks require external mixing to ensure uniform temperature and distribution of raw and digesting sludge in the tank. The walls are usually reinforced concrete or post-tensioned concrete. The bottoms of the tanks slope toward the center, forming a cone in which digested sludge solids can concentrate. Some digestion tanks are designed with waffle bottoms in which the tank floor is subdivided into 12 pie-shaped hoppers, each sloping toward a separate draw-off port along the outside wall of the digestion tank. This design allows for steeper floor slopes, reduces the distance the settled solids must transverse, and minimizes the amount of grit accumulated in the tank. Construction costs are higher for this type of bottom because of the complex excavation, formwork, and piping required. However, savings are realized because of the reduced costs of cleaning the tanks.

The egg-shaped digestion tank design in which the depth of the tank is much larger than the diameter has been used in Germany for more than 50 years. This design has been gaining popularity all over the world. The purpose of forming an egg-shaped tank is the elimination of the need to clean the digester sides, which form a cone so steep at the bottom that grit cannot accumulate. However, the construction of egg-shaped tanks requires complex formwork and special construction techniques; therefore, the construction costs are higher than those of more conventional tanks.

In an egg-shaped digester the sludge surface at the top is small and the gas produced causes mixing as the gas rises to the surface of the sludge contents. The mixing caused by rising gas is augmented by pumped circulation of sludge from the bottom of the egg-shaped digester through the heat exchanger to the top of the tank. Gas spargers may be located along the inside walls of the tank. The gas discharged through these spargers is effective in keeping the walls clean and in detaching any materials adhering to the walls, or to increase mixing. The need for external mixing and problems with excessive grit and scum accumulation are minimal. The scum contained at the surface is kept fluid with a mixer and removed through a special scum removal port (Metcalf & Eddy, Inc. 2003).

10.5.2 Temperature Control

External heat exchange units are used to heat raw sludge and to maintain the temperature of the sludge undergoing digestion. Pumping the digesting sludge from the digestion tank through the external heat exchange unit permits seeding the raw sludge with digesting sludge; however, this external mixing does not markedly affect the circulation pattern in the digester and does not replace the need for effective mixing of the digesting sludge.

Some of the equipment used to mix the digesting sludge is designed with internal exchangers. An internal heat exchanger has been incorporated in the draft tube of a digestion system mixed by recirculated gas. Water jackets are placed around the periphery of draft tubes through which the sludge is pumped mechanically or by gas recirculation. Steam injection directly into the sludge has been used to heat sludge. However, the addition of steam only adds more water to the sludge and dilutes the concentration of the digested sludge. In addition, a greater volume of supernatant is generated (Metcalf & Eddy, Inc. 2003).

10.5.3 Sludge Heating

The temperature of the feed sludge must be increased to the temperature of the digestion tank, and the temperature of the digesting sludge must be maintained at the operating temperatures. The amount of heat required to raise the temperature of the incoming sludge is

$$q_s = Q_m C_p (T_2 - T_1) \tag{10.7}$$

where Q_m is the mass flow rate of sludge (kg h^{-1}), q_s the heat required to raise the temperature of the incoming sludge from T_1 to T_2 (kJ h^{-1}), C_p the specific heat of the sludge (approximately 2.32 kJ kg^{-1} sludge °C^{-1}), T_1 the temperature of the feed sludge (°C), and T_2 the temperature desired within the digestion tank (°C).

The concentration of solids in the sludge markedly affects the heat requirements (kJ kg^{-1} solids °C^{-1}). As the solids content increases, the amount of sludge solids remain constant, but the amount of water associated with the sludge is reduced; therefore, the heating requirements per pound of solids decrease. For example, sludge at 2% solids may have a heating requirement of approximately 140 kJ kg^{-1} sludge °C^{-1}; however, the heating requirements are reduced to about 35 kJ kg^{-1} sludge °C^{-1} when the sludge is concentrated to 8% solids (Cook 1987).

The heat requirements must be adjusted to make up for heat losses to the air and to the soil surrounding the digestion tank. These heat losses depend on the shape of the digestion tank, the materials of construction, and the temperature gradient from the temperature of the digesting sludge and the outside air and/or soil temperature. The heat losses can be reduced by insulating the digestion tank cover and walls exposed to the ambient air. Common insulating materials used include a dead air space, lightweight insulating concrete, glass wool, insulation board, and urethane foam. The insulation material is often covered to protect the insulation and for aesthetic purposes. Common facing materials include brick, metal siding, precast concrete panels, and plaster.

10.5.4 Auxiliary Mixing

A certain amount of mixing occurs naturally in an anaerobic digestion tank. The rising gas bubbles mix the sludge, and the recirculation of heated sludges causes some thermal convection currents. However, auxiliary mixing is essential to maximize the advantages of complete mixing and to ensure stable performance and control of the anaerobic digestion process.

Various systems for mixing anaerobic digesters include external pumped recirculation, recirculation of compressed digester gas, and mechanical mixing. The first application of gas recirculation was employed to break the scum layer. Pumped circulation is relatively simple and effective at keeping the scum layer moist so that gas produced during digestion can escape. However, the large flow rates required for complete mixing of the volume of the digestion tank limit the use of pumped circulation as the only method of mixing. Minimum power requirements for pumped circulation are 5.3 to 7.9 kW 1000 m^{-3} and may be much higher if friction losses are excessive. Cost-effective use of pumped circulation is in combination with other mixing systems. Pumped circulation is used to circulate the digesting sludge through the external heat exchangers, where the digesting sludge is blended with the feed sludge and heated prior to return to the digestion tank (Metcalf & Eddy, Inc. 2003).

If a gas recirculation system is used to break the scum layer, a compressor can be mounted on the cover of the digestion tank to pump gas from the head space in the anaerobic digester through a series of vertical pipes that were located at a distance of about one-half the tank radius. The gas is released at a point about 3.05 to 3.66 m below the liquid surface. However, this gas recirculation system has been modified to provide more complete mixing of the digesting sludge rather than just breaking the scum layer. Specific design conditions for the Pearth system vary with the different applications. The location of the gas recirculation pipes away from the center of the tank prevents disturbances within the cone of the tank and permits the classification of bottom materials, thereby minimizing the amount of raw sludge that is withdrawn and resulting in a more concentrated sludge for transfer to a second-stage digester or to sludge dewatering and disposal facilities (Metcalf & Eddy, Inc. 2003).

The quantity of gas required to mix a digester tank varies with the volume of sludge undergoing digestion, the concentration of sludge in the digester, the volatile solids content of the digesting sludge, and the diameter of the tank. In the Pearth process the number of gas discharge points and the gas discharge rate are a function of the diameter of the tank. For example, three or four discharge points discharging an average of between 5 and 9 L min^{-1} per 1 m^3 of digester capacity are used for 6- to 10-m-diameter digestion tanks. However, for digestion tanks that are 30 to 35 m in diameter, six to eight discharge points are typical and the average gas discharge rate is between 0.66 and 1.0 L min^{-1} m^{-3} of digester capacity. The actual power requirements range from about 1290 J s^{-1} per 1000 m^3 for 30- to 35-m-diameter tanks to 10 kW per 1000 m^3 of digester capacity for smaller tanks (6 to 10 m in diameter). These power requirements correspond to nameplate power ratings of 2 to 20 kW per 1000 m^3 digester capacity, respectively (Metcalf & Eddy, Inc. 2003).

In other systems, compressed gas is released through diffusers located at the bottom of the cone in the digestion tank, or the recirculated gas is introduced into a draft tube. Introduction of the recirculated compressed gas at the bottom of the tank sets up circulation of the sludge as the gas rises in the center of the tank. The entire volume of the tank is mixed and is used for digestion; however, no solids separation or concentration can take place in the digestion tank. The rate of gas recirculation required for mixing the digester varies with the diameter of the tank. The required gas discharge rate is 3.33 L min^{-1} m^{-3} of digester capacity for a 6-m-diameter tank, with a required power of 1 kW (6.6 kW per 1000 m^3 digester capacity). The required gas discharge decreases as the diameter and volume of the tank decrease. For a 35-m-diameter digestion tank the power required is 7.5 kW (2.4 kW per 1000 m^3 digester capacity). The operating data indicate that the gas discharge rate is approximately 93 L min^{-1} per meter of digester diameter (Metcalf & Eddy, Inc. 2003).

Recirculated compressed gas is introduced through spargers into a draft tube. The gas released in the draft tube acts like a gas lift pump in the digester, and sludge is carried upward through the draft tube to the surface of the digesting sludge, where the sludge is directed radially toward the tank periphery. The rising gas bubbles cause sludge near the bottom of the tank to be drawn into the draft tube. This recirculation pattern causes mixing of the entire tank volume. Operating data indicate that the power requirements for this type of gas recirculation system are between 2.63 and 3.16 kW per 1000 m^3 digester capacity (Metcalf & Eddy, Inc. 2003).

A comparison of the operating data for these three gas recirculation systems used to mix anaerobic digestion tanks indicates that for large-diameter tanks (35 m) the power requirements are lowest for the Pearth process (1.29 kW per 1000 m^3) and almost twice this requirement (2.6 kW per 1000 m^3) for the other two systems. However, for smaller-diameter tanks (6 to 10 m) the system with gas recirculation through a draft tube requires the least amount of power (3.16 kW per 1000 m^3). The power requirements for a 6-m-diameter tank with the Pearth system installed is approximately 9.88 kW per 1000 m^3, while the gas recirculation system with diffusers at the bottom of the tank requires approximately 65.8 kW per 1000 m^3 (Metcalf & Eddy, Inc. 2003).

Various mechanical methods of mixing the digesting sludge have been employed. Mixing can be maintained by a number of mechanical draft tube mixers located to provide maximum mixing. Sludge may also be recirculated by an external pump that draws sludge from the central portion of the digester, which discharges the sludge tangentially through nozzles near the surface to break the scum, and near the bottom of the tank. Surface mixers have also been used to mix the sludge in anaerobic digestion tanks. The circulation pattern is from the bottom of the central portion of the tank and radially along the surface to the periphery. One disadvantage of the use of rotary machines to mix digesting sludge is potential problems with rags and other stringy materials in the sludge wrapping around the drive shaft, which could cause eccentric torques on the shaft, resulting in uneven wearing of the bearings. An accumulation of rags, hair, and other stringy material on the impeller (propeller) of axial-type mixers would also reduce the efficiency of the mixers.

The ability of mixing devices to circulate the contents of a digestion system completely is not without limits. The relative content of fixed and volatile solids in the feed sludge affects mixing. Mixing by gas recirculation may be hindered, as the total solids content of the digesting sludge exceeds 5%. Feed sludges should not be concentrated to more than 8% total solids if the volatile solids content is less than 70%; that is, the fixed solids exceed 30%. However, in most municipal wastewater treatment plants, mixing capabilities do not control the solids loading as much as the ability to concentrate the feed sludge in the sedimentation and thickening processes (Metcalf & Eddy, Inc. 2003).

10.6   REACTOR CONFIGURATIONS

The principal objective of any anaerobic digester system is to allow the retention of slow-growing microorganisms for a sufficient time for successful waste stabilization. Based on this principle, the fundamental design considerations for anaerobic digesters include the provision of the following requirements: (1) biomass accumulation by means of settling, adhesion to biofilm, entrapment within the system, or recirculation for longer solids retention time; (2) good contact between biomass and wastewater, by overcoming problems of diffusion of substrates and products from the liquid to biofilm or granules; and (3) maintenance of an environment suitable for bacterial growth.

10.6.1   Conventional Anaerobic Digesters

The simplest version of the conventional anaerobic process is the single-stage standard rate anaerobic digester which has been used widely in the past to treat domestic waste. The process does not employ mixing, and the digester contents are allowed to stratify into layers of stabilized solids, active biomass, supernatant, and scum. It is highly inefficient, for it utilizes only 50% of the total waste volume and requires a very long solids retention time (SRT), usually greater than 30 days (Owen 1982). The digester is generally heated to increase the rate of biological reaction, thereby decreasing the retention time. Major disadvantageous of a single-stage process are large tank volume requirement, low applied organic loading rates, and the formation of thick scum layer.

To improve on the standard-rate digester, the high-rate digester, which incorporates external mixing in the process, was developed. This additional mixing improved the process tremendously by reducing the SRT required to between 6 and 30 d while increasing the organic loading rate approximately five fold. Completely mixed digesters are particularly suitable for wastewaters containing high concentrations of particulates or extremely high concentrations of soluble biodegradable organic materials. In both cases, the reactor contents will contain high concentrations of suspended solids that originate from either the raw wastewater or from anaerobic biological growth during digestion. Since a completely mixed reactor does not contain a fixed support medium, the potential for plugging and dead volume accumulation is less than in fixed-film anaerobic processes. However, particulate material can easily settle and accumulate in a conventional digester if the internal mixing is inadequate. Over lengthy periods of operation, solids accumulation can reduce digester performance as the reactor hydraulics become characterized by significant dead volume and flow short-circuiting.

The relatively low biomass concentrations and short operating SRTs maintained in completely mixed digesters render the process susceptible to toxic and shock loadings. If an input of a toxicant is of short duration, the long hydraulic retention time of a completely mixed digester may provide some protection against process upset by diluting the toxicant to a no-effect level. To avoid process instabilities and upsets, thorough process monitoring should be carried out on a frequent basis. In a completely mixed digester, the only process control available to stabilize the reactor after a shock is a reduction of the loading to the process. This assumes, of course, that the process environmental parameters, such as temperature, pH, and nutrient supplementation, are also maintained within acceptable ranges.

The organic loading rates to conventional digester systems are usually expressed in terms of volatile solids (VS) since the predominant application of the process is to high particulate wastes. Loading rates of 0.5 to 6.0 kg VS $m^{-3} d^{-1}$ are typical. For comparison to other anaerobic treatment processes, the organic loading rates applied in conventional digesters correspond roughly to COD loading rates of 1 to 10 kg COD $m^{-3} d^{-1}$ (Owen 1982).

The simple single-stage process has latter evolved into a two-stage high-rate digester as depicted in Fig. 10.3. In the high-rate system, two digesters are operated in

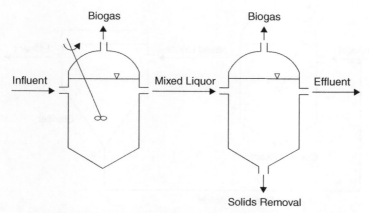

FIGURE 10.3 Schematic two-stage anaerobic digester.

series, separating the functions of fermentation and solid–liquid separation. The contents of the first unit are mixed by gas recirculation, draft-tube mixer, or sludge pumping, and are also heated to increase the rate of fermentation. The mixed treated waste and microorganisms are pumped into the second tank, where the solids are allowed to settle and subsequently are removed. These tanks are typically about 25 m in diameter and about 15 m deep. The retention time required for the first unit is normally between 10 and 15 d. The mixing provided significant influences on the process efficiency. It maintains a uniform temperature and pH in the reactor and helps to disperse biological flocs, thereby providing better contact between waste and microorganisms. More important, the mixing helps to prevent the formation of a scum layer in the reactor. The two-stage arrangement is mainly designed to "thicken" the waste in the second tank and aid in the collection of digester gas. Nevertheless, this system frequently fails to separate the waste completely, making this arrangement inefficient and impractical (Metcalf & Eddy, Inc. 2003).

10.6.2 Anaerobic Contact Processes

Anaerobic contact processes were developed to overcome the problems associated with conventional reactors. Commonly regarded as the first significant advance on the conventional anaerobic digesters, anaerobic contact process design is similar to the aerobic activated sludge process, because it includes a set of reactors in series, often with recycle. The anaerobic contact reactor is able to retain biomass systematically within the anaerobic reactor. Influent waste is passed through a contact reactor containing a high concentration of active biomass. A clarifier is incorporated downstream of the contact reactor and is used to remove the active biomass from the effluent stream for recycling back to the contact unit (Fig. 10.4). The biomass would not be washed out with the effluent, but is returned and maintained in the

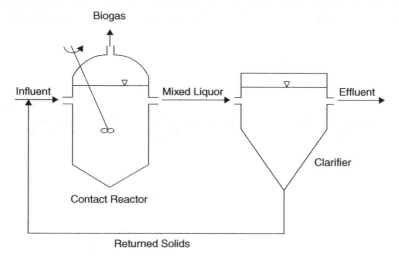

FIGURE 10.4 Schematic diagram of anaerobic contact process.

system. As with the aerobic activated sludge process, recycled solids result in higher microbial growth and improve the ability of the system to tolerate organic loading as well as temperature variations. The resulting increase in the solids/hydraulic retention time (SRT/HRT) ratio enables higher reactor performance. With a good solids settling property, the process can be operated successfully with an average HRT as low as 12 h.

Anaerobic contact process performance depends to a large extent on the settleability of the biological solids. The major practical problem encountered in the contact process is the effective separation and concentration of biological solids in the clarifier prior to their return to the contact chamber. Modifications have been made on the anaerobic contact process, and in general, effective solid–liquid separation can be accomplished by degasification followed by gravity sedimentation. Several other methods have been employed, including settling of polymer-enhanced flocculation, centrifugation, floatation, vacuum degasification, thermal shock, and low-level turbulence caused by a packing material.

The anaerobic contact configuration can be utilized to overcome some of the disadvantages of the conventional digester process by separating and recycling effluent suspended solids back to the mixed anaerobic reactor. Since the process biomass content can then be controlled independent of the wastewater flow, the system SRT can also be controlled separate from the HRT. This enables the process designer to maintain the SRT required for biomass growth while increasing the applied loading rate and reducing the HRT for capital cost economy. The biomass separation system used in the anaerobic contact process will retain both active microorganisms and undigested influent suspended solids, thus promoting more extensive biodegradation of wastewater particulates. The anaerobic contact process retains most of the advantages of a conventional digester with the extra benefits of increased SRTs and smaller reactor volumes. However, the advantages of an anaerobic contact process are completely dependent on the production of an anaerobic biomass with satisfactory properties for adequate solid–liquid separation.

Anaerobic contact reactor VSS concentrations of 4000 to 6000 mg L^{-1} are typical of the process. A settling tank with a liquid upflow velocity of less than 1 m h^{-1} is a common device used for solids separation. Membrane filtration of the reactor effluent has also been utilized as a more positive method of biosolids control. Anaerobic contact systems that utilize gravity settling for solids separation are heavily dependent on the settling properties of the anaerobic floc. Since active anaerobic flocs are usually associated with trapped or attached biogas, solids settleability can often be problematic (Metcalf & Eddy, Inc. 2003).

A number of approaches have been developed to enhance sludge settleability, including gas stripping, stirred or vacuum degasification, inclined plate or lamella settlers, and the addition of coagulants and flocculants to promote floc formation. One alternative design approach involves short-term cooling of the settler influent to temporarily reduce the rate of biogas production in anaerobic flocs. In a system that is sensitive to sludge settleability characteristics, it is important to minimize transient inputs of toxic and organic shock loads that can impair floc settleability.

The anaerobic contact process can be applied over a wide range of wastewater concentrations. Although the lower economically practical limit of wastewater concentration is probably in the range 1000 to 2000 mg $COD L^{-1}$, there is no well-established upper concentration limit. At very high wastewater concentrations, the completely mixed anaerobic reactor is the best alternative for efficient digestion while minimizing internal reactor hydraulic inefficiencies. Wastewaters of up to 100,000 mg $COD L^{-1}$ can theoretically be treated in an anaerobic contact process as long as the anaerobic floc produced has satisfactory settling properties (Owen 1982). In practice, the floc settleability can be impaired by the presence of high concentrations of dissolved solids. If the untreated wastewater contains significant concentrations of poorly biodegradable suspended solids, a biomass recycle system can lead to the accumulation of inert solids in the reactor. Over long periods the accumulation of inert material can cause the displacement of active anaerobic biomass from the process.

The treatment efficiency of an anaerobic contact process is usually much greater than that of a completely mixed digester. Total COD reductions of 90 to 95% are possible for highly biodegradable wastewaters with COD concentrations of 2 to $10 g L^{-1}$. Typical organic loading rates in anaerobic contact systems are between 0.5 and $10 kg COD m^{-3} d^{-1}$, with HRTs of 0.5 to 5 d (Metcalf & Eddy, Inc. 2003).

10.6.3   Other Types of Configurations

In addition to the commonly used conventional anaerobic digesters and the anaerobic contact processes, other configurations are used in a lesser extent. These systems include upflow anaerobic sludge blanket (UASB) reactors, the expanded- and fluidized-bed processes, and anaerobic packed-bed reactors. In a UASB reactor, the wastewater flows upward through a blanket of concentrated biological solids at the upper portion of the reactor, where a three-phase separator device is installed for the separation of biogas from sludge granules and treated effluent.

The waste is introduced at the bottom of the reactor, where upon contact with the sludge bed, it is degraded to CH_4 and CO_2. Gas formation and evolution supply sufficient mixing in the bed. Some solids are buoyed up by rising gas bubbles, but a quiescent settling zone is provided for their separation and return to the lower portions of the reactor. This internal recycling of solids removes the need for external solids recycle.

The design of the gas separator and solids settling zone is important to the success of the reactor and, if incorrect, significant solids losses may occur, which could result in failure. The clarifier is normally incorporated into the top of the reactor to conserve space. New designs sometimes include flexi-rings or other media in the upper portion of the reactor to trap solids and encourage fixed-film growth. This results in a hybrid sludge blanket–fixed film reactor.

Successful operation of the UASB process seems to be dependent on good process control and a feed that imparts satisfactory sludge settling characteristics. Loading rates for UASB reactors range on a COD basis from 0.5 to $40 kg m^{-3} d^{-1}$. The high density of solids in the sludge zone is responsible for retaining the biomass well in excess of minimum SRT for methanogens (Show et al. 2004a).

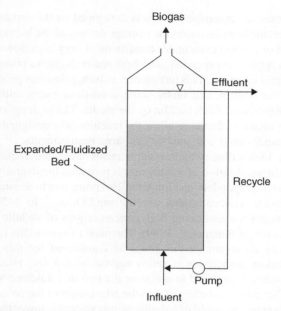

FIGURE 10.5 Schematic diagram of a fluidized/expanded-bed reactor.

A major limitation of the UASB process is based essentially on problems associated with the development of dense and settleable granular sludge that will not easily be washed out. Difficulty in restarting inactive UASB reactors, sensitivity to hydraulic and organic shock loadings or to changing wastewater characteristics, and inability to handle insoluble wastes have also limited their use. With the expanded- and fluidized-bed processes (Fig. 10.5), attempts have been made to improve anaerobic reactor mass-transfer characteristics by the utilization of small media particles with very high surface-to-volume ratios. Spherical silica sand of 0.2 to 0.5 mm diameter and specific gravity of 2.65 is the most common medium used in full-scale anaerobic fluidized-bed systems. With such small-diameter media, the interstitial void spaces in a settled bed would normally become plugged very rapidly. However, by applying high liquid-upflow velocities, the media can be expanded to produce a substantial increase in bed voidage.

The difference between expanded and fluidized beds relates simply to the upflow velocity used and the degree of media expansion maintained. In expanded-bed systems, sufficient flow is applied to increase the settled bed volume by 15 to 30%. At this point, individual particles are supported partly by the fluid flow and partly through contact with adjacent particles. The higher upflow velocities utilized in the fluidized bed produce 25 to 300% bed expansions. In the fluidized state, the media particles are supported entirely by the flowing liquid and are therefore able to move freely in the bed. The energy required for effluent recycle for bed expansion or fluidization is one of the most significant disadvantages of these systems (Heijnen et al. 1989).

In both processes, an anaerobic biofilm is developed on the surface of the media particles. The inert medium increases the average density of the biomass particle and prevents washout of the bed even under conditions of very high flow rate. The large upflow velocities applied in expanded- and fluidized-bedsystems promote turbulence at the biofilm–liquid interface. This turbulence, in turn, promotes good mass transfer into and out of the biofilm, and under some conditions exerts sufficient shear to prevent the development of thick biofilm on the media. The high upflow velocities in expanded- and fluidized-bedsystems allow the reactors to be designed with relatively large height/diameter ratios and smaller land area requirements.

Because very high effluent recirculation ratios are often required for media fluidization, maximum dilution of wastewater is provided incidentally at the reactor inlet. This enables the expanded- and fluidized-bed processes to accommodate a wide variety of wastewater concentrations ($< 1000 \, \text{mg COD L}^{-1}$ to $> 20,000 \, \text{mg COD L}^{-1}$) without concern for generating high concentrations of volatile acids near the bottom of the reactor (Heijnen et al. 1989). The need to expand the reactor contents represents a major disadvantage that must be considered for this process. High effluent recirculation, sometimes at ratios approaching a few hundred times the influent waste stream, is required to maintain the bed in a fluidized state. This may incur high pumping costs, and often offsets the advantages of the process. It has been reported that the net energy yield of a fluidized-bed system is lower than that of other reactors considering the high capital cost of the flow distribution system and the pumping equipment.

Anaerobic packed-bed reactors or "anaerobic filters" are similar to the upflow bioreactor, yet they contain an additional internal medium that supports bacterial growth. The reactors usually consist of a submerged bed of the packing medium through which the waste is passed either in upflow or downflow mode, as shown in Fig. 10.6. Random loose-fill packings such as plastic pall rings, and ordered, modular block media formed from plastic sheets have both been used in full-scale applications. The advantage of the synthetic packings lies in their large open structures and high void volumes. The large voidage maximizes the reaction volume available and provides space for the accumulation of nonattached biomass. The media surface allows the development of an attached biofilm.

The specific surface-to-volume ratios of the most commonly used packed-bed packings are relatively low (about $100 \, \text{m}^2 \, \text{m}^{-3}$). Research evidence suggests that media-specific surface areas of up to $220 \, \text{m}^2 \, \text{m}^{-3}$ do not produce a significant improvement in reactor performance (Tay et al. 1996a,b, 1997; Show and Tay 1999). In a process with packed media and a tortuous liquid flow path, excess biomass accumulation can become an operational difficulty if it causes flow short-circuiting and dead volume accumulation (Tay and Show 1998). Media plugging in randomly packed anaerobic reactors has been reported at pilot scale and at full scale. Mixing induced by biogas evolution helps to prevent media blockage, but an efficient flow distribution system must also underlie the packed bed.

The recent trend in upflow packed-bed reactor design is toward the use of a hybrid process in which the lower 50 to 75% of the media in anaerobic filters could produce a hybrid sludge blanket/anaerobic filter. The resulting hybrid design has the

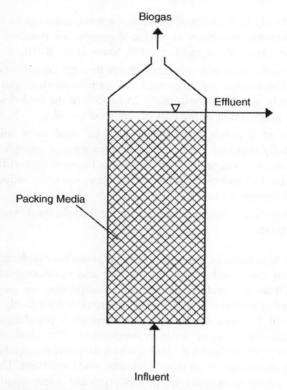

FIGURE 10.6 Schematic diagram of a packed-bed reactor.

potential to substantially reducing the media plugging and the associated hydraulic and mass-transfer problems found in packed-bed reactors while realizing the advantages of both fixed-film and upflow sludge blanket treatment.

10.7 ADVANTAGES AND LIMITATIONS OF ANAEROBIC SLUDGE DIGESTION

The principal advantages of anaerobic sludge digestion compared to other methods of sludge stabilization include:

1. Production of methane gas, which is a usable source of energy. The process is a net energy producer at most treatment facilities that employ anaerobic sludge digestion used. The energy produced is in excess of that required to maintain the temperature of the digesting sludge and to meet the energy requirements for mixing. The surplus energy may be used to heat buildings, to drive the engines for the aeration blowers, or to generate electricity that can be used to drive the sewage pumps. In addition to contributing to sustainable development with

energy recovery in the form of methane, carbon credits can be claimed by the use of anaerobic processes in sludge digestion for reducing emissions of greenhouse gases (Show and Lee 2008; Show et al. 2010).

2. Reduction in the mass and volume of sludge through the conversion of organic matter in the volatile solids to methane, carbon dioxide, and water. Solids destruction is usually approximately 25 to 45% of the feed sludge solids and can result in reduction in the cost of sludge disposal.

3. Production of a solids residue that may be used as a soil conditioner. Anaerobically digested sludge contains nitrogen and phosphorus and other nutrients, as well as organic material that can improve the fertility and texture of soils. The odor associated with raw sludge is markedly reduced to a musty odor by anaerobic digestion.

4. Inactivation of pathogens associated with the feed sludge during the anaerobic digestion process.

The principal limitations of anaerobic sludge digestion are high capital costs, and the large covered tanks and pumps for feeding and circulating sludge that are required, as well as the heat exchangers and compressor for gas mixing. The slow growth rates of methane-producing bacteria require a relatively long retention time, in excess of 10 days, to develop and maintain a population of methane-producing bacteria for adequate waste decomposition. The sensitive and delicate nature of methanogens also limits the rate at which the process can adapt to changing organic loadings, temperatures, or other environmental conditions. This has resulted in a long startup period in an anaerobic process, typically a few months. The quality characteristics of the supernatant resulting from anaerobic sludge digestion are poor. The supernatants contain suspended solids, dissolved and particulate organic materials (oxygen-consuming compounds), nitrogen, and phosphorus. This return flow adds to the solids, oxygen demand, and nutrient loads to the treatment system.

10.8   SUMMARY AND NEW HORIZONS

Microbial-mediated anaerobic digestion has attracted considerable scientific and technical attention throughout the world, largely because of the promise and intrigue associated with their ubiquity, but of more significance from an environmental and waste management perspective, their ability to compete favorably and thrive as integral participants in the nutrient and energy cycles of a variety of natural and simulated environmental settings. Indeed, the early rather restricted and frequently isolated investigations of microbiologists/physiologists and wastewater treatment chemists/operators have broadened into a productive harmony between an exceedingly diverse amalgamation of interdisciplinary scientific and engineering inquiry, with unprecedented communication of basic principles, applications, and opportunities for future development. The ever-expanding literature, replete with contributions from all sectors, provides ample evidence of this status and overall vitality.

Notwithstanding the many significant and impressive advances in anaerobic microbial process fundamentals and applications over the past few decades, there are areas that require additional attention and development. Perceived as foremost among these are the following:

- Further elucidation of principal and controlling mechanisms in the anaerobic conversion of complex and relatively recalcitrant sludges, including the microbiology and biochemistry of biotic hydrolytic, fermentative, oxidative, respiratory, acetoclastic, and methanogenic reactions, as well as the abiotic counterparts, either alone or in combination.
- Further determination and prioritization of environmental factor controlling and useful in describing conditions associated with anaerobic digestion process balance or imbalance, including liquid-, solid-, and gas-phase mechanisms and parameters, as well as their individual and collective significance and utility for process development, optimization, and control.
- Translation of theoretical and empirical modeling advances into operationally diagnostic and remedial techniques, including methods to reduce uncertainty and facilitate control of routine process operations with appropriate sensors and instrumentation for evaluation of significant process variables and state conditions.
- Enhanced development of analytical techniques descriptive of biomass structure and viability, including concomitant kinetic, operational, and environmental factors establishing selection and/or dominance, temporal and spatial distribution, and associated substrate conversion patterns in processes (Fig. 10.6) or managed by physical, hydrodynamic, or biochemical techniques for phase management and control.
- Extension of the principles and practices of anaerobic digestion processes to emerging and new horizons of investigation and development, including controlled landfills, constructed wetlands, and natural soil and aqueous systems for microbial-mediated remediation, decontamination, detoxification, and emissions mitigation (Show and Lee 2008; Show et al. 2010).
- Further development and promotion of standard and consensus nomenclature and notations for clearly identifying and describing anaerobic process types and configurations; indicator parameters and analytical methods; process microbiology and biochemistry; and growth and substrate conversion patterns and kinetics, models, and control strategies.

REFERENCES

Barker H.A. (1956) Biological formation of methane. In: *Bacterial Fermentations*, Wiley, New York, p. 1.

Benjamin M. M., Ferguson J. F., Buggins M. E. (1981) Treatment of sulphite evaporator condensate with an anaerobic reactor. TAPPI Environmental Conference, New Orleans, LA, April 1–10.

Chiu Y., Chang C., Lin J., Huang S. (1997) Alkaline and ultrasonic pretreatment of sludge before anaerobic digestion. *Water Science and Technology* **36**, 155–162.

Cook E. J. (1987) Anaerobic Sludge Digestion. *Journal of the Water Pollution Control Federation*, Alexandria, VA.

Eastman J. A., Ferguson J. F. (1981) Solubilization of particulate organic carbon during the acid phase of anaerobic digestion. *Journal of the Water Pollution Control Federation* **53**, 352–366.

Heijnen J. J., Mulder A., Enger W., Hoeks F. (1989) Review on the application of anaerobic fluidized bed reactors in wastewater treatment. *Chemical Engineering Journal* **41**, 37–50.

Kugelman I. J., McCarty P. L. (1964) Cation toxicity and stimulation in anaerobic waste treatment: daily feed studies. In: Proceedings of the 19th Industrial Waste Conference, Purdue University, West Lafagette, IN.

Lawrence A. W., McCarty P. L. (1965) The role of sulphide in preventing heavy metal toxicity in anaerobic treatment. *Journal of the Water Pollution Control Federation* **37**(3), 392.

Lee D. J., Show K.Y., Su A. (2011) Dark fermentation on biohydrogen production: pure culture. *Bioresource Technology* **102**(18), 8393–8402.

Liu Y., Xu H. L., Show K. Y., Tay, J. H. (2002) Anaerobic granulation technology for wastewater treatment. *World Journal of Microbiology and Biotechnology* **18**(2), 99–113.

Mao T., Show K. Y. (2007a) Influence of ultrasonication on anaerobic bioconversion of sludge. *Water Environment Research* **79**(4), 436–441.

Mao T., Show, K. Y. (2007b) Performance of high-rate sludge digesters fed with sonicated sludge. *Water Science and Technology* **54**(9), 27–33.

Mao T., Hong S. Y., Show K. Y., Ta, J. H., Lee D. J. (2004) A comparison of ultrasound treatment on primary and secondary sludges. *Water Science and Technology* **50**(9), 91–97.

McCarty P. L. (1964) Anaerobic wastewater treatment fundamentals: 1. *Chemistry and microbiology. Public Works*, 107–112.

McCarty P. L., McKinney R. E. (1961) Volatile acid toxicity in anaerobic digestion. *Journal of the Water Pollution Control Federation* **33**, 223–232.

Metcalf & Eddy, Inc. (2003) *Wastewater Engineering: Treatment and Reuse*, 4th ed., McGraw-Hill, New York.

Mosey F. E., Hughes D. A. (1975) The toxicity of heavy metal ions to anaerobic digestion. *Journal of the Water Pollution Control Federation* **74**, 18–39.

Owen W. F. (1982) *Energy in Wastewater Treatment*, Prentice Hall, Englewood Cliffs, NJ.

Owen W. F., Stuckey D. C., Healy J. B. Jr., Young L. Y., McCarty P. L. (1979) Bioassay for monitoring biochemical methane potential and anaerobic toxicity. *Water Research* **13**, 485–492.

Show K.Y., Lee D. J. (2008) Carbon credit and emission trading: anaerobic wastewater treatment. *Journal of the Chinese Institute of Chemical Engineers* **39**(6), 557–562.

Show K. Y., Tay, J. H. (1999) Influence of support media on biomass growth and retention in anaerobic filters. *Water Research* **33**(6), 1471–1481.

Show K. Y., Tay J. H., Yang L., Wang Y., Lua C. H. (2004a) Effects of stressed loading on start-up and granulation in UASB reactors. *Journal of Environmental Engineering ASCE* **130**(7), 743–750.

Show K. Y., Wang Y., Foong S. F., Tay, J. H. (2004b) Accelerated start-up and enhanced granulation in UASB reactors. *Water Research* **38**(9), 2293–2304.

Show K. Y., Mao T., Tay J. H., Lee, D. J. (2006) Effects of ultrasound pretreatment of sludge on anaerobic digestion. *Residuals Science and Technology* **3**(1), 51–60.

Show K. Y., Mao T., Lee D. J. (2007) Optimisation of sludge disruption by sonication. *Water Research* **41**(20), 4741–4747.

Show K. Y., Ng C. A., Faiza A. R., Wong L. P., Wong, L. Y. (2010) Energy recovery and mitigation of greenhouse gas emissions from palm oil mill effluent treatment by anaerobic granular-sludge process. 3rd IWA Asia Pacific Young Water Professionals Conference: Achieving Sustainable Development in the New Era, Singapore, November 21–24.

Speece R. E., McCarty P. L. (1964) Nutrients requirements and biological solids accumulation in anaerobic digestion. Proceedings of Advances in Water Pollution Research, Oxford, UK, Vol. 2, pp. 305–322.

Tay J. H., Show K. Y. (1998) Media-induced hydraulic behaviour and performance of upflow biofilters. *Journal of Environmental Engineering ASCE* **124**(8), 720–729.

Tay J. H., Show K. Y., Jeyaseelan S. (1996a) Effects of media characteristics on the performance of upflow anaerobic packed-bed reactors. *Journal of Environmental Engineering ASCE* **122**(6), 469–476.

Tay J. H., Jeyaseelan S., Show K. Y. (1996b) Performance of anaerobic packed-bed system with different media characteristics. Water Science and Technology **34**(5–6) 453–459.

Tay J. H., Show K. Y., Jeyaseelan S. (1997) Media factors affecting the performance of upflow anaerobic packed-bed reactors. *Journal of Environmental Monitoring and Assessment* **44**, 249–261.

Van den Berg L., Lentz C. P. (1977) Food processing waste treatment by anaerobic digestion. Proceedings of the 32nd Industrial Waste Conference, Purdue University, West Lafayette, IN, May, pp. 252–258.

Wang Y., Show K. Y., Tay J. H., Sim K. H. (2004) Effects of cationic polymer on start-up and granulation in UASB reactors. *Journal of Chemical Technology and Biotechnology* **79**(3), 219–228.

Wong B. T., Show K. Y., Su A. Wong R. J., Lee D. J. (2008) Effect of volatile fatty acid composition on UASB performance. *Energy and Fuels* **22**(1), 108–112.

Zhang Z., Show K.Y., Tay J. H., Liang T., Lee D. J. (2008) Enhanced continuous biohydrogen production by immobilized anaerobic microflora. *Energy and Fuels* **22**(1), 87–92.

11

MECHANICAL PRETREATMENT-ASSISTED BIOLOGICAL PROCESSES

HÉLÈNE CARRÈRE

INRA, UR050, Laboratoire de Biotechnologie de l'Environnement, Narbonne, France

DAMIEN J. BATSTONE

Advanced Water Management Centre, The University of Queensland, Brisbane St Lucia, Queensland, Australia

ETIENNE PAUL

Université de Toulouse and Ingénierie des Systèmes Biologiques et des Procédés, Toulouse, France

11.1 INTRODUCTION

Mechanical treatment refers to methods that apply mechanical pressure or shear to a fluid, through either direct action, induction of shear, or acceleration of the luid (with or without pressure). The main mechanical methods that have been used in combination with activated sludge processes or anaerobic sludge digestion are ultrasonication, grinding, high-pressure homogenization, collision plate homogenization, and lysis centrifuge (Weemeas and Verstraete 1998; Pérez-Elvira et al. 2006; Carrère et al. 2010). Among these, ultrasonication (Khanal et al. 2007; Pilli et al. 2011) is the most investigated and has the highest current market penetration.

Biological Sludge Minimization and Biomaterials/Bioenergy Recovery Technologies, First Edition.
Edited by Etienne Paul and Yu Liu.
© 2012 John Wiley & Sons, Inc. Published 2012 by John Wiley & Sons, Inc.

11.2 MECHANISMS OF MECHANICAL PRETREATMENT

11.2.1 From Sludge Disintegration to Cell Lysis and Chemical Transformation

Mechanical pretreatment induces a number of changes in both chemistry and structure due to shearing, mechanical action, chemical reactions, and induced temperature changes. This, in turn, has an impact not only on the biodegradability, but also on handling and viscosity. The mechanisms for mechanical pretreatment are generally related to physical conditioning on a number of levels, including:

1. Change in particle size (macroscopic), resulting in more surface area. This will increase the hydrolysis rate where particle size is limiting (Jain et al. 1992; Vavilin et al. 1996). In many cases, particle size has a minimal impact on hydrolysis rate and extent (Sharma et al. 1988), and the main advantages in changes in particle size are related to materials handling and digester mixing.

2. Changes in microscopic structure (microscopic), breaking up flocs, and providing access to cells previously blocked by exocellular polymeric substances (EPS), in the case of activated sludge flocs, or degradable cellulose, in the case of lignocellulosic materials.

3. Lysis of encapsulating materials and cells (cellular). This breaks the cells up physically and releases soluble and particulate cellular material into the bulk liquid (Neis et al. 2001). This process will increase rates (Neis et al. 2001) and may increase the ultimate extent of degradation, although it is reasonable that predation and chemical attack will lyse cells under normal conditions in anaerobic digesters.

4. Induced chemical reactions (chemical). High-frequency, high-energy mechanical input, particularly sonication, can induce a range of chemical reactions, including chemical formation, cleavage, and hydrolysis reactions due to high-energy zones in cavitation bubbles, generation of peroxide and hydroxyl radicals, which have further impacts (Petrier and Casadonte 2001), and secondary chemical reactions due to localised and bulk temperature changes due to the energy input.

11.2.2 Specific Energy

The efficiency of each treatment must be compared using well-defined parameters such as the specific energy applied to the sludge [Eq. (11.1)], the treatment dose [Eq. (11.2)], the treatment density [Eq. (11.3)], or the treatment intensity [Eq. (11.4)].

$$E_S = \frac{Pt}{V \cdot \text{TS}} \tag{11.1}$$

where E_S is the specific energy (kJ kg^{-1} TS), P the applied power (kW), t the treatment duration (s), V the treated volume (m^3), and TS the total solids (kg TS m^{-3}).

$$\text{Treatment dose (kJ m}^{-3}) : \quad D = \frac{Pt}{V} \tag{11.2}$$

$$\text{Treatment density (kW m}^{-3}) : \quad De = P/V \tag{11.3}$$

$$\text{Treatment intensity (in the case of ultra sound)} : \quad I = \frac{P}{A} \tag{11.4}$$

where A is the surface area of the probe in cm^2.

As can be seen in Eq. (11.1), the consumed energy E_S is proportional to the product of applied power by the disruption time and is inversely proportional to the total solids mass of the sludge. Therefore, increasing TS improves the treatment energetic efficiency. At low E_S, primarily sludge disintegration is observed, while at higher E_S, cell rupture may occur with the release of intracellular material (Müller et al. 2000a).

11.2.3 Sonication

Sonication induces mechanical action and chemical reactions caused by applying microvibrations (sound) in the range 10 to 1000 kHz (generally less than 40 kHz) directly to the fluid via a mechanical device. Sonication has impacts at all four levels described previously. The primary mechanism is compression and expansion of the fluid, resulting in the growth and violent collapse of microbubbles (cavitation). This results in excessively localized shear rates, pressures up to 180 MPa, and localized temperatures up to 5000 K (Khanal et al. 2007). The shear rates disrupt cells and flocs, resulting in both reduction of particle sizes (see review by Pilli et al. 2011) and lysis of cells (mechanisms 1 to 3 above). This is demonstrated further in Fig. 11.1. Lower-frequency sonication ($<$ 40 kHz) results in larger cavitation bubbles, which have an increased impact for an equivalent energy input (Tiehm et al. 2001). The increased localized temperature also has an impact, due to denaturization of cell walls and cellular proteins (Wang et al. 2010). In addition, sonication induces $^{\bullet}$OH, $^{\bullet}$H, $^{\bullet}$O, and $^{\bullet}$N radicals, of which $^{\bullet}$OH is the principal form. This can have strong utility in dilute or in-situ applications for bioremediation (Petrier and Casadonte 2001). As applied to a bulk material such as waste activated or primary sludge, though, Wang et al. (2010) found, by masking $^{\bullet}$OH with NaHCO$_3$, that this mechanism only has a major impact above 100 kWh m^{-3} energy applied, which is far above the levels that would normally be applied in ultrasonic disintegration (Nickel and Neis 2007).

Numerous factors influence the cavitation phenomena (i.e., sonication density, frequency, acoustic intensity, type of ultrasound cavitation, solvent viscosity, attenuation, etc.). These factors are reviewed by Pilli et al. (2011). They are key parameters in the design of the ultrasonication device and thus influence the efficiency of sludge transformation during ultrasonication. For example, Kidak et al. (2009) studied the effect of power, contact time, and sludge concentration. They obtained the following conclusion: "High power–short retention time" is more

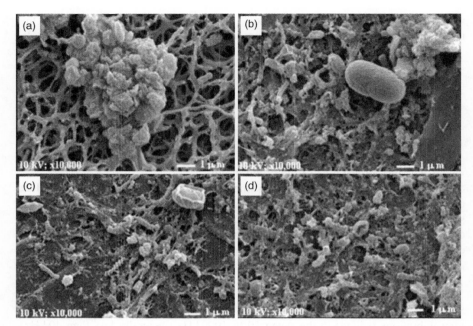

FIGURE 11.1 SEM images of undigested WAS at different sonication durations with a constant power input of 1.5 kW and a frequency of 20 kHz: (a) 0 min (control); (b) 2 min; (c) 10 min; and (d) 30 min. [From Khanal et al. (2007); used with permission.]

effective than "low power–long retention time." However, no universal value could be applied because of the variability of the sludge, and the correct combinations of power and retention must be found specifically.

A key issue is to determine whether specific energy input or ultrasonication density represents the key parameter controlling sludge disintegration efficiency. The answer to this question seems to be rather controversial. Because of attenuation, ultrasonic density may be the crucial parameter (Neis et al. 2000).

Determination of the effects of initial total solids content of sludge on floc disintegration is a key issue that will condition the economics of ultrasound sludge pretreatment. The presence of a solid phase in a solution treated by sonication has several antagonist effects (Gonze et al. 2003): By adsorbing the ultrasound wave, the particles reduce the cavitation effect, but by acting as nuclei, they decrease the threshold of cavitation and promote it. Moreover, the higher the sludge concentration, the higher the efficiency since cavitation bubbles have higher probabilities of collapsing in the vicinity of a particle. Results show that a high solids content of sludge is more efficient than a low solids content, the limiting factor probably being the contact between an imploding cavitation bubble and a sludge particle (Gonze et al. 2003). However, according to Show et al. (2007) the optimal range of solids content for sonication lies between 2.3 and 3.2% TS; if the solids concentration is too high, increased viscosity hinders cavitation bubble formation and wave propagation.

11.2.4   Grinding

The two modes of grinding that are outlined in the next section are coarse shredding (mainly for protection of mechanicals), and ball milling. The first would have only a very minor or negligible impact at level (1) (particle-size reduction) and no impact at all at levels 2 to 4. The mechanism of ball milling depends on the size of the balls and includes direct grinding due to the balls compressing sludge particles, and shear induced by high velocities. Normally, it would be expected that ball milling would mainly cause effects at levels 1 and 2: that is, reduction of coarse size and breakup of flocs. This is at odds with experimental results, however, with substantial release of soluble material (20 to 50% of total) through ball milling (Baier and Schmidheiny 1997), and solubilization levels with ball milling comparable to or higher than sonication and high-pressure homogenization (Kopp et al. 1997). These results strongly indicate that mechanisms include lysis and shearing of cells, and that energy levels in ball mills are actually quite high.

11.2.5   Shear-Based Methods: High-Pressure and Collision Plate Homogenization

Shear-based methods rely entirely on high shear rates and pressure applied directly. Mechanisms are (1) through (3), including full lysis of cells (Kopp et al. 1997), as indicated by complete deactivation of cells (Rai and Rao 2009), and release of 20% of the material to the soluble phase. The observable microscopic impacts of high-pressure homogenization are almost exactly the same as sonication (Nah et al. 2000), with substantially complete destruction of cells and flocs.

11.2.6   Lysis Centrifuge

Since lysis centrifuge is effectively centrifuge pre-thickening (to 10 to 30%), followed by shear- or grinding-based homogenization (Dohányos et al. 1997), the mechanisms are the same as those noted above for shear-based methods. Although the approximate 5000 g applied by centrifuging has a shear impact, this is minimal compared to intentional applied shear in subsequent treatment of the sludge stream. The practical outcomes are offsetting of the benefits of being able to use centrifuge kinetic energy and to operate at a higher concentration (with less energy per kilogram of dry solids), against the negative impacts of higher viscosity, higher heat impact, and non-Newtonian fluid behavior.

11.3   IMPACTS OF TREATMENT: RATE VS. EXTENT OF DEGRADABILITY

For any sludge pretreatment, two effects can be differentiated: an increase in the degradation rate and an increase in the ultimate degradability (rate vs. extent of degradation) (Batstone et al. 2009). An increase in gas production under anaerobic conditions can be related to an increase in either rate or extent, as most digesters under normal conditions will not degrade all material available. All treatment methods have a measurable, and sometimes strong impact on gas production (Thiem et al. 1997; Bougrier et al. 2005; Nickel and Neis 2007). Mechanical methods such as lysis centrifuge increase gas production not only through rate increases, but also through an effective increase in solids retention time (Dohányos et al. 1997). Based on the references cited here as well as other reviews (e.g., Carrère et al. 2010), under normal industrial conditions increases in gas production from mechanical pretreatment methods are driven by an improvement in rate rather than an improvement in ultimate degradability.

11.3.1   Grinding

Wett et al. (2010) investigated the mechanisms of a ball mill pretreatment of waste activated sludge by numerical modeling based on anaerobic digestion model 1 (ADM1) (Batstone et al. 2002). A 41% increase in the biogas production was observed compared to the control. This increase was attributed primarily to an increase in the apparent hydrolysis coefficient (k_{dis}), from $0.25\ d^{-1}$ to $1.0\ d^{-1}$, with a slight increase in the bioavailable substrate, from 39% to 49%. Baier and Schmidheiny (1997) reported that not all solubilized COD by ball milling pretreatment was converted to biogas i.e. the extent of solubilization was higher than gas production.

11.3.2   Ultrasonication

It is evident that at very high power levels, both degradability rate and extent can be increased, and this has been observed in laboratory studies (e.g., Shimizu et al. 1993), although rate increases have always been far more significant than extent increases. In general, where substantial extent increases have been found, power levels are high or not reported. The key motivation seems to be an increase in rate, and as an example, Pérez-Elvira et al. (2009) found that sonication allowed intensification by 25% while maintaining the same gas production. Other reports have generally focused on increases in gas production or decreases in retention driven by rate rather than by an increase in extent (Thiem et al. 1997; Apul and Sanin 2010). It appears that under most industrial conditions, performance increases may result from increased degradation rate rather than ultimate degradability (Carrère et al. 2010).

11.4   EQUIPMENT FOR MECHANICAL PRETREATMENT

For the purposes of enhanced rate or extent of degradation, mechanical pretreatment is almost uniformly recommended for WAS digestion, rather than primary sludge digestion (Baier and Schmidheiny 1997; Neis et al. 2001; Hogan et al. 2004). It may be applied to primary sludge for the purposes of improved dewaterability (Pilli et al. 2011), decreased viscosity, or to avoid foaming or equipment damage (Fitzpatrick 2011). Mechanical pretreatment may be applied in four configurations:

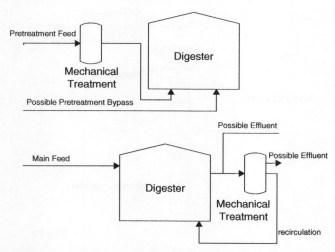

FIGURE 11.2 Possible configurations for mechanical treatment, including (top) pretreatment modes and (bottom) recirculation modes.

full input stream treatment, partial input stream treatment, recycle stream treatment, or concentrate stream return (particularly for lysis centrifuge). A layout for these configurations is shown in Fig. 11.2.

11.4.1 Sonication

Sonication may be employed in either configuration feed or recirculation mode, treating either the entire waste activated sludge (WAS) or a partial stream. The stated preference of a number of suppliers is to operate in feed mode with a partial bypass and 30 to 50% of the feed to be sonicated (Neis et al. 2001; Pérez-Evira et al. 2006; Neis et al. 2008). Sonication can be applied in mode 2 (recirculation mode), but will generally kill methanogenic biomass, particularly at higher intensities (Neis et al. 2001). Ultrasonic equipment consists of one (or more) of each of three main elements (Fig. 11.3): a transducer and power supply, a booster, transporting vibrations, the sonotrode or horn, and the reactor vessel. Units can be placed in series as shown in Fig. 11.4.

The power supply generates a high-frequency ac signal to drive the transducer, normally at 10 to 1000 kHz. Transducers can be either electromagnetic, moving in response to an induced magnetic field, or piezoelectric, moving in response to an electrical signal (Mattiat 1971). Piezoelectric transducers are the most widely used, due to high generation efficiency and simplicity.

The booster transmits vibrations to the sonotrode and allows clamping of the device at nodal points (harmonic points that do not oscillate). The wavelength (for 20 kHz in steel) is on the order of 25 cm, and for higher frequencies there will be multiple nodal points. For a given system (i.e., clamp geometry, material, booster

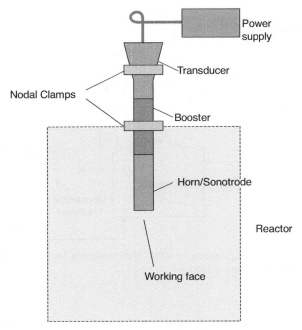

FIGURE 11.3 Sonication equipment components.

length, sonotrode, etc.), only discrete harmonic frequencies can be used that preserve positions of the nodal points; and other considerations (e.g., horn geometry) mean that in practice, frequency cannot easily be changed. The booster also provides amplification of vibrations (built-in gain) (Khanal et al. 2007). The amplification factor is dependent on the amount of mass above the nodal point as compared to the

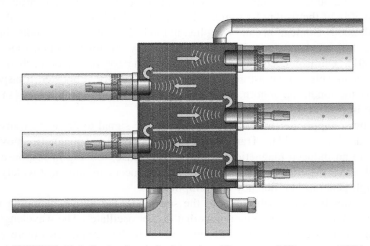

FIGURE 11.4 Sonication units in series. (Courtesy of Ultrawaves DE.)

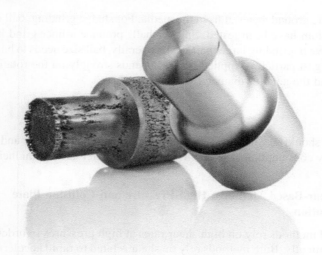

FIGURE 11.5 Worn and new transducers. (Courtesy of Ultrawaves DE.)

mass below the nodal point (i.e., sonotrode). Therefore, a booster with a large mass and a sonotrode with a small mass will provide a high level of amplification. Sonotrode design is a balance between amplification (a small tip is preferred) and transmission efficiency (a large tip area is preferred). There are a number of horn designs that emphasize the various aspects, as well as secondary design considerations (e.g., multiple actions available with doughnut horns). Sonotrodes are generally made of titanium and need regular replacement due to pitting wear from cavitation (Fig. 11.5).

11.4.2 Grinding

Sludge grinding can be used in feed or recirculation (mode 1 or 2), and in mode (1), is generally applied on the entire feed stream in order to take advantage of the improved handling properties (viscosity and general handling). Grinding equipment can be of two types:

1. *Coarse shredder grinding* (e.g., JWCE Sludge Monster–style rag removal) (Fitzpatrick 2011). This is mainly to protect downstream equipment, and grinds large particles, rags, timber, and so on, into particles or shreds of less than 2 mm. Equipment consists of interlocking rotating drums with 10 to 15 teeth (wheels) per drum. Power consumption is minimal at less than 0.02 kWh m^{-3} (17 L s^{-1} at 1.5 kW).

2. *Ball mill grinding* (Baier and Schmidheiny 1997). Ball mills are designed to grind to very small sizes (micrometer range) using ball media trapped in a rotating drum. A screen (normally on the exterior of the drum) is used to

separate ground material from the media. For sludge grinding, ball sizes of 0.2 to 1.5 mm have been tested. Smaller balls produce a finer grind but are less effective in grinding larger particles (generally, ball size needs to be larger than the largest particle). Applied power depends strongly on the rotational speed (ω) and the agitator diameter (d):

$$P = \omega^3 \, d^5 \tag{11.5}$$

which should be considered for optimizing operating conditions and scaling up. Energy consumption is $1.5 \, \text{kWh m}^{-3}$ treated (Baier and Schmidheiny 1997).

11.4.3   Shear-Based Methods: High-Pressure and Collision Plate Homogenization

Shear-based methods rely on high shear rates at high pressures in order to disrupt cells mechanically. Both methods rely on shear related to rapid acceleration of the fluid induced by pathway changes. Collision plate units operate at 10 to 50 bar, with fluid velocities of 30 to 100 m s^{-1}. As implied by the name, equipment consists of a high-pressure pump, an injection tube, and a collision plate (Fig. 11.6). The pump in particular is specialized, since it is rated high flow, high pressure (Nah et al. 2000).

High-pressure homogenization operates under a similar principle (Fig. 11.6), except that both pressure and shear rates are far higher, with shear rates on the order of 100 to 900 bar. Energy consumption ranges from $1.25 \, \text{kWh kg}^{-1}$ at 200 bar to 3 kWh at 500 bar (Rai and Rao 2009). Due to the very high energy input, active cooling is often required to maintain lower operating temperatures (Rai and Rao 2009).

(a)

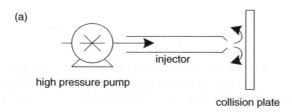

(b)

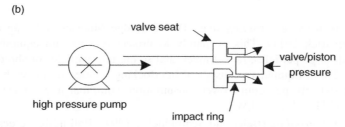

FIGURE 11.6 Shear methods: (a) collision plate homogenization; (b) high-pressure homognization.

11.4.4   Lysis Centrifuge

A lysis centrifuge is simply a high-performance centrifuge, combined with mechanical homogenization (Doháñyos et al. 1997). Homogenization is applied to the final concentrate stream from the centrifuge, and concentrate quality is therefore unaffected. Homogenization can be milling or shear-based methods, and can utilize the kinetic energy in the sludge stream to avoid the use of pumps, although pressure is limited to induced levels available from centrifugal forces. It is best applied in recirculation mode (mode 2), with the lysed concentrate returned to the digester. This therefore achieves both intensification (due to an increase in digester solids concentration) and mechanical treatment.

11.5   SIDE EFFECTS

Sludge dewaterability is affected both positively and negatively by sludge disintegration. Cake water content is affected positively due to disruption of the extracellular polymeric substances (EPS) matrix, which can contain a substantial amount of water bound to its structure. Capture of fines can be affected by floc size reduction, which can also cause clogging of the sludge cake during mechanical filtration (Laurent et al. 2009). In particular, sonication has both positive and negative effects on sludge dewaterability (Pilli et al. 2011).

Barjenbruch and Kopplow (2003) observed a decrease in sludge dewaterability after high-pressure homogenization. Kim and Kim (2003) measured sludge dewaterability after sonication at increasing times and found that dewaterability was first diminished and then improved with sonication time. In particular, Li et al. (2009) showed that sludge dewaterability was only improved when the sludge disintegration degree was 2 to 5%. In the same way, Feng et al. (2009) suggested a specific energy of $1000 \, kJ \, kg^{-1}$ TS as the optimal treatment for improving the settleability of sludge. Indeed, sludge treated with $500 \, kJ \, kg^{-1}$ TS or $1000 \, kJ \, kg^{-1}$ TS had settling velocities after 45 min of 51.62 and $57.44 \, mm \, h^{-1}$, respectively, which were faster than $8.44 \, mm \, h^{-1}$ for untreated sludge. The settling velocity of sludge treated with a specific energy higher than $1000 \, kJ \, kg^{-1}$ TS was lower than that of untreated sludge, and further increases in the specific energy led to further decreases in settling velocity. Ultrasounic treatment with high specific energies ($> 5000 \, kJ \, kg^{-1}$ TS) failed to improve sludge settleability. These results were ascribed to the fact that high specific energy treatments tend to reduce floc size and to release organic substances into the liquid phase (Feng et al. 2009). Another advantage of mechanical disintegration, such as sonication and high-pressure homogenizer, is mitigation of the sludge bulking problem and potential digester foaming, thanks to the disintegration of filamentous sludges (Wunsch et al. 2002; Müller 2000b).

Along with organic compounds, nitrogen and phosphorus compounds are solubilized during mechanical treatment of sludge. For example, Müller (2000a) observed a 10-fold increase in nitrogen concentration in the supernatant after disintegration by high-pressure homogenization (80 MPa), and a three fold increase for phosphorus. In another study (Wang et al. 2010), the sonication (intensity

$0.500\,W\ mL^{-1}$ during 1 h) of WAS originating from a biological nitrogen and phosphorus removal unit led to the release of 57% of the organic content (measured as COD), 70% of total nitrogen, and more than 60% of the phosphorus. Most released nitrogen was organic-N (84.9%), followed by NH_3-N (14.9%) and trace amounts of nitrate and nitrite. Eighty percent of the phosphorus released was in the $PO_4{}^{3-}$-P form (Wang et al. 2010).

11.6   MECHANICAL TREATMENT COMBINED WITH ACTIVATED SLUDGE

Besides the numerous applications of ultrasound on WAS to increase biogas production, another strategy consisted of using ultrasound on secondary treatment without digestion. The benefits in this case include the complete elimination of sludge bulking (or floating), improved biological nutrient removal, improved denitrification, and reduced sludge production. The mechanical disintegration unit can be associated with biological treatment in the wastewater handling unit (Fig. 11.7).

Destruction of filamentous sludge structure is caused mainly by hydromechanical effects. The remaining flocs are no longer connected by filamentous organisms and can evolve to more compact and dense structures (Müller et al. 2000b). Production of a carbon source resulting from the disintegration of the particulate COD increases the proportion of easily biodegradable organic matter useful for denitrification (Müller, 2000a,b; Kampas et al. 2007). A few studies reported experiences on coupling mechanical treatment with activated sludge process for sludge reduction (Camacho et al. 2002a,b; Strünkmann et al. 2006). At a wastewater treatment plant near Paris, France, Camacho et al. (2002a) used a pilot-plant membrane bioreactor coupled with a

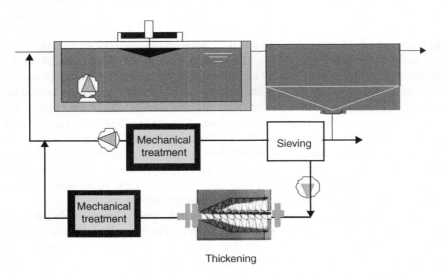

Thickening

FIGURE 11.7 Implementation of disintegration in aerobic treatment of sludge.

high-pressure homogenizer. By comparing with results obtained on a control line (the same membrane bioreactor without a homogenizer), the authors assessed the sludge reduction potential of this mechanical disintegration system at a pressure of 300, 500 and 700 bar and for a number of passages from 1 to 10. "Stress" frequency (SF, in d^{-1}), the parameter that relates the time interval during which the biomass of the sludge passes through the treatment unit, was set to 0.2 d^{-1}. The sludge reduction yield remained below 20% whatever the operating conditions used. Mineral solubilization was also observed and a significant decrease in the effluent quality was noted. Therefore, in this study, the high-pressure homogenizer mechanical treatment seemed to increase the accessibility of the particulate organic matrix without increasing its biodegradability. At a lab scale, Strünkmann et al. (2006) used three different disintegration devices—an ultrasonic homogenizer, a stirred media mill, and a high-pressure homogenizer—combined with an activated sludge process. They found better results than Camacho et al. (2002a) and have reached a reduction of excess sludge production of up to 70%. The effluent quality was affected only slightly by the mechanical treatment. Similar results (sludge reduction of 65%) were obtained previously by Kunz et al. (1996) on full-scale experiments for a period of three months in a SBR process of 1200 population equivalents (p.e.). At full scale, a demonstration of the sludge reduction potential by means of an ultrasound treatment of the return sludge was reported by Boisson et al. (2008). The test was performed at the wastewater treatment plant (WWTP) of St. Sylvain d'Anjou (France) which has a capacity of 6300 p.e. and performed nutrient removal with nitrification, predenitrification, and phosphorus removal by precipitation. Sludge production during a 264-d period where the ultrasound system was in operation was compared with conventional sludge production quantified after switching off the ultrasound unit. Switch-off of the ultrasound treatment resulted in an increase in sludge production by about 27.5%. The remaining sludge complied with the French legislation for land spreading. A cost–benefit calculation showed that ultrasound treatment was not economically feasible at the scale of the St. Sylvain plant. It was, however, deduced from this demonstration test that this technology could lead to cost savings that would generate short payback times for larger plants. An example calculation was given for a plant with a capacity of 100,000 p.e.

Drawbacks in using mechanical devices in the wastewater line include the increase in oxygen requirement and the increase in the specific energy for disintegration because of the low sludge concentration. It is the reason why only a few studies have been performed under this configuration.

11.7 MECHANICAL TREATMENT COMBINED WITH ANAEROBIC DIGESTION

11.7.1 Performances

Several papers have reviewed the performance of a combination of mechanical pretreatments and anaerobic digestion (Weemeas and Verstraete 1998; Pérez-Elvira et al. 2006; Appels et al. 2008; Carrère et al. 2010; Pilli et al. 2011).

Ultrasonication   Ultrasonication has been applied to sludge extensively as a pre-treatment prior to anaerobic digestion at both the laboratory and full scales. A linear correlation among power input, solubilization or disintegration degree, and the increase in methane production during anaerobic digestion has been shown (Wang et al. 1999; Thiem et al. 2001). Thus, the higher the power density, the higher the methane production. However, above a certain energy threshold, methane production remains more or less constant (Wang et al. 1999; Bougrier et al. 2005). Considering energy consumption and enhancement of anaerobic digestion performance, applied specific energies are usually in the range 1000 to 16,000 kJ kg^{-1} TS (0.3-4 kWh kg^{-1} dry material) (Carrère et al. 2010) or 100 to 900 kJ L^{-1}, corresponding to 30 to 250 kWh m^{-3} wet material (Pérez-Elvira et al. 2009). Increase in sludge temperature is associated to high applied energies (around a 10°C increase for energy above 50 kWh m^{-3}). In a full-scale plant, sonication-applied energy is generally lower and in the range 4 to 40 kJ L^{-1} (1 to 11) kWh m^{-3} wet material (Pérez-Elvira et al. 2009).

For a given energy, sonication is more efficient if operated with high power and low exposure time rather than high exposure time and low power (Gronroos et al. 2005). It is also generally agreed that low-frequency sonication (20 kHz) is more effective due to the formation of larger bubbles at lower frequency (Tiehm et al. 2001; Pérez-Elvira et al. 2009; Carrère et al. 2010). Total solids concentration is an important parameter for sludge sonication. Oneyche et al. (2002) showed that sonication resulted in 42 and 138% increases in biogas production for sludge concentrations of 16.3 and 48.9 g L^{-1}, respectively.

For most research studies, batch anaerobic digestion (or methane potential tests) of sonicated and unsonicated samples identifies performance improvements of 20 to 140%. In continuous or semicontinuous anaerobic digesters, sludge sonication results in 10 to 50% increases in biogas production. However, the latter may be due either to volatile solids degradability increases, an increase in rates, or higher effective loading rates (Carrère et al. 2010). An increase of anaerobic digestion rates is an important outcome of sludge sonication (Chu et al. 2002; Pilli et al. 2011). Shimizu et al. (1993) found that apparent first-order hydrolysis rates were 0.16 d^{-1} for waste activated sludge and 1.2 d^{-1} for biopolymers released during sludge sonication. Sonication therefore allows for operation of anaerobic digesters at lower retention times than would otherwise be possible (intensification). For example, Pérez-Elvira et al. (2009) applied 15 d of sludge retention time to sonicated sludge and obtained the same removal efficiency as for nonhydrolyzed sludge at a retention time of 20 d. Thiem et al. (1997) and Apul and Sanin (2010) showed that digesters operating on sonicated sludge were able to work at sludge retention times of fewer than 8 d.

Grinding   Grinding with stirred ball milling has been used as a pretreatment of anaerobic digestion of waste activated sludge (Baier and Schmidheiny 1997; Kopp et al. 1997). Operating conditions were: bead diameters ranging from 0.25 to 0.35 mm, rotation 3200 rpm or bead velocity 6 m s^{-1}, and applied specific energy 2000 kJ kg^{-1} MS. Baier and Schmidheiny (1997) showed that grinding was more beneficial on digested sludge (an increase in batch biogas production by 60%) and on WAS from an extended aeration process (24% increase) than on long-SRT activated sludge

(7% increase). The enhancement of anaerobic digestion rates by sludge grinding has been shown by short-SRT digestion runs (Kopp et al. 1997); grinding resulted in an 88% increase in volatile solids removal during 2 d of SRT digestion (fixed biomass) against 12% increase during 7 d of SRT digestion (suspended biomass).

Lysing Centrifuge   A lysing centrifuge has been used as a pretreatment of batch anaerobic digestion (Dohányos et al. 1997). It resulted in an 85% increase in biogas production from WAS and in 24% biogas production enhancement when pretreated WAS was mixed and digested with primary sludge. Biogas production in various continuous digesters increased by 15 to 26% after lysing centrifuge pretreatment (Zabranska et al. 2006).

Collision Plate and High-Pressure Homogenization   A collision plate has been employed on WAS and led to a 43% enhancement of volatile solids removal during batch anaerobic digestion (Choi et al. 1997). Moreover, when applied to continuous anaerobic digestion, collision plate homogenization allowed a decrease of sludge retention time from 14 d to 6 d without affecting anaerobic digestion performance (Nah et al. 2000).

High-pressure homogenization at 300 bar ($750 \, kJ \, kg^{-1}$ TS) of activated sludge resulted in a 60% increase in biogas production during continuous digestion at an SRT of 10 to 15 d and allowed operation of a fixed-film digester at an SRT of 2.5 d (Engelhart et al. 1999). Another study (Müller and Pelletier 1998) combined 400-bar homogenization with a fixed biomass digester at an SRT of 2.5 d. High-pressure homogenization led to a 28% increase for high load and a short sludge age (3 d of retention in an activated process) and a 87% increase for extended aeration sludge (13 d of retention in an activated process). Treating a partial stream in the recirculation mode (mode 2) at 150 bar led to a 30% increase in biogas production and a 23% reduction of sludge volume (Barjenbruch and Kopplow 2003).

11.7.2   Dewaterability

Whereas sludge dewaterability is often affected negatively by mechanical disintegration, subsequent anaerobic digestion generally alleviates this effect. Indeed, Braguglia et al. (2009) showed that dewaterability was improved substantially by the digestion of sonicated sludge, suggesting that anaerobic digestion is very effective for degrading fine dispersed particles produced by mechanical pretreatment. Nevertheless, ultrasound pretreatment did not improve the dewaterability of the digested sludge with respect to untreated digestate (Braguglia et al. 2009). Moreover, Barber (2005) found that the negative effects of sonication on dewatering could be overcome by exposing only a fraction of the secondary sludge stream to ultrasound and reblending with unsonicated material. In contrast, Pérez-Elvira et al. (2010) showed a deterioration of postdigestion dewatering for both part and full-stream sonication, and that capillary suction time values were constant (74% higher than the control digestate) compared to 30 to 100% for sonicated sludge. Kopp et al. (1997) obtained a lower-moisture cake for digestate pretreated by high-pressure homogenization or by stirred ball mill but with a higher polymer consumption than that of untreated digested sludge.

11.7.3   Full-Scale Performance and Market Penetration

Ultrasonic Treatment   Ultrasonic treatment has been carried out extensively in industry as a pretreatment for anaerobic digestion. The main suppliers of ultrasound technology for sludge applications are. Sonico Ltd. UK, Ultra WAVES GmbH, and IWE Tec GmbH (Dr Heilscher GmbH) (Pérez-Elvira et al. 2009). All these devices operate at a 20 kHz frequency. Hogan et al. (2004) provided a description of several full-scale installations using Sonix (Sonico Ltd.) around the world: Avonmouth, Wessex Water–UK (1,200,000 p.e.), Seven Trend Water–UK (150,000 p.e.), Kavlinge–Sweden, Orange County Sanitation District–U.S.A., and Beenyup–Australia (700,000 p.e.). In these installations, thickened WAS are sonicated and digested with primary sludges. Results reported were increases in volatile solids and gas production by 30 to 50%, improvement in sludge dewaterability of digested sludge and stable digester operation with a high ratio of thickened waste activated to primary sludge with the ability to treat 100% waste activated sludge (Hogan et al. 2004).

Barber (2005) reported results from 14 full-scale plants manufacturated by Dr Heilscher GmbH in Germany, Austria, Switzerland, Italy, and Japan. A 20 to 50% increase in biogas yield, a 25 to 50% increase in hydrolysis rates, the possibility of increasing organic loading rate by 20 to 30% or decreasing hydraulic retention time by 30%, a 3 to 7% improvement in dewatering, and a 10% decrease in polymer consumption were reported.

The implementation of an Ultrawaves GmbH system in 2004 in a Bamberg wastewater treatment plant (280,000 p.e., Germany) has been described by Neis et al. (2008). Two ultrasound reactors were installed to avoid the construction of another digester, due to the overload of the plant (actual load 330,000 p.e.). Sonication of 25% of total waste activated sludge led to a 23% increase of biogas production. There are clearly difficulties in assessing the true practical performance of a sludge treatment system on a real full-scale plant, and a cost–benefit study showed a very clear positive result (cost/benefit ratio: 42,106 €/120,285 €) (Wolff et al. 2007). A three-year payback time was found for the new ultrasound equipment. Ultrasound equipment (Ultrawaves GmbH) was also installed in 2005 in the Meldorf–Germany wastewater treatment plant (65,000 p.e.) to remove foaming problems in the anaerobic digester (Neis et al. 2008). A full-scale trial of ultrasonic disintegration of mixed sludge (one-third primary and two-third thickened activated) in the Ulu Pandan Water Reclamation Plant in Singapore resulted in an average 45% increase in biogas production (Xie et al. 2007).

Lysing Centrifuge   A lysing centrifuge (Lysatec GmbH) has been employed in several wastewater treatment plants as a pretreatment for anaerobic digestion: Liberec (100,000 p.e., Czech Republic), Furstenfeldbruck (70,000 p.e.), and Aachen-Soers (650,000 p.e.) in Germany (Zabranska et al. 2006). The treated sludge flow rate is 39, 12, and 200 $m^3 h^{-1}$, respectively. This resulted in a 15 to 26% increase of biogas production. Another advantage of using lysing centrifuge is the increase in pumpable solids (due to decreased viscosity) from 6% TS for untreated sludge to 9 to 11% TS.

The *Crown process* (Biogest Company) operates at 12 bar. A set proportion (25 to 100%) of the raw sludge at 3 to 6% TS concentration is fed into a relaxation tank. From there, the sludge is pumped through the Crown disintegrator using a nozzle in which hydrodynamic cavitation is produced as the medium passes through. Particles and activated sludge flocculi are broken up by the cavitation produced. The treated sludge is then fed back into the relaxation tank and mixes with the untreated sludge. The quantities transported by the eccentric worm pumps can be altered so that the sludge to be treated passes the nozzle two or three times viewed statistically. The Crown process has been installed in several full-scale facilities in Germany and Switzerland (Taunusstein, 30,000 p.e., Nierstein-Oppenheim, 22,000 p.e., Munchwilen, 30,000 p.e.). In Ingelheim (200,000 p.e.) the disintegration process is applied to the sludge originated from a pharmaceutical company. The disintegrated sludge flow rates ranged from 4 to $7\,\mathrm{m}^3\,\mathrm{h}^{-1}$, requiring 0.94 to $1.85\,\mathrm{kWh}\,\mathrm{m}^{-3}$ with an increase in biogas production ranging from 18 to 34% (Biogest 2011).

The *MicroSludge process* (Paradigm Environmental Technologies, Inc.) was applied in the Los Angeles wastewater treatment plant. In this process, sludge is first treated with caustic to pH 11 in order to weaken cell walls. A high-pressure homogenizer at 830 bar then provides cellular disruption. Treated WAS was introduced in a digester together with primary sludge, with a ratio of 68 : 32 (PS/WAS, w/w). The degradation of mixed sludge was increased from 50% to 57% (Stephenson et al. 2007). Another demonstration test was conducted at the Des Moines Metropolitan Waste-water Reclamation Facility. Codigestion of WAS and primary sludge at digestion periods ranging from 20 days down to 7 days resulted in increased methane production ranging from 16 to 22%. This indicates that the methane production from the WAS portion treated by MicroSludge was 30 to 40% higher than without MicroSludge. Also observed has been a 70% reduction in the odor of anaerobically digested sludge (Biogest 2011) and the elimination of foaming issues (Novak et al. 2007).

Cellruptor (Ecosolids) is another disintegration process with low energy require-ments. Sludge, ideally containing up to 10% solids, is compressed at pressures higher than 1 bar, and a small volume of biogas is introduced to the feed. The gas, due to its rapid rate of diffusion across the cell walls, is transported across the cell walls as a result of the high concentration gradient. The gasified sludge stream is then depressurised. Through subsequent mixing, equilibration, and depressurisation steps, the continuous process results in dissolved gases "exploding" the cellular material, releasing soluble cell components. Biogas production can be increased up to 40% and up to 25% for anaerobic digestion of WAS and mixed sludge (50:50 primary/secondary), respectively. The Cellruptor process (Ecosolids 2011) is planned to be installed at the Yorkshire Water Esholt wastewater plant in Leeds–UK as pretreatment of the anaerobic digestion.

11.7.4 Energy Balance

Investment and operation costs of lysing centrifuges are among the lowest, especially when they are implemented by adapting a lysing device to existing machinery

(Carrère et al. 2010). On the basis of sludge disintegration (solubilization) degree, Lehne et al. (2001) compared specific energy required by different mechanical disintegration methods. Whereas specific energies required by stirred ball milling and high-pressure homogenizers were of the same order of magnitude, specific energy required by ultrasound was far higher. In all cases, the lower the suspended solids concentration, the higher the specific energy. In the case of high-pressure homogenizer, Onyeche and Schafer (2003) showed that a positive energy balance can be obtained at disruption pressures below 380 bar with concentrated sludge (removal of 50% of water) and below 220 bar with nonconcentrated sludge.

According Pérez-Elvira et al. (2009), energy inputs in full-scale ultrasonication installations are far lower than on a laboratory scale: 1 to 10 kWh m^{-3} sludge against 1 to 100 kWh m^{-3} sludge, with a resulting lower performance. Considering a 40% increase in biogas production, the energy balance in lab-scale systems is positive only for sludge concentrations above 6% TS. However, the process is energetically feasible for any sludge concentration considering the typical energy consumption of 6 kWh m^{-3} for a full-scale device.

Different studies have reported the energy ratio (net energy generation divided by electricity consumption of ultrasound disintegration) of full-scale plants ranging from 2.5 to 7 (Barber 2005; Xie et al. 2007). Carrère et al. (2010) calculated theoretical energy balances in the case of conventional mesophilic and thermophilic anaerobic digestion and ultrasonication [100 W, 16 s, 30 kWh m^{-3} (Boelher and Siegrist 2006; Pérez-Elvira et al. 2009)], stirred ball milling (Boelher and Siegrist 2006), and high-pressure homogenizers [200 bar (Onyche and Schafer 2003)] pretreatments. The assumptions were that (1) the digester feed concentration was 6%; (2) the electrical requirements for the digester (mainly feed and mixing) were set to 0.12 kWh m^{-3} d^{-1}; (3) the hydraulic retention time was set to 20 and 15 d for mesophilic and thermophilic digestion, respectively; (4) VS destruction was assumed to be 40% for mesophilic digestion, and 50% for thermophilic digestion and in the case of pretreatments; (5) heating requirements for the digester were thermal capacity plus approximately 10% losses in mesophilic or 20% in thermophilic; and (6) biogas was supposed to be valorized by cogeneration, and electrical and heat energy yields were assumed to be 35 and 50% of total energy produced, respectively. The results are reported in Fig. 11.8.

According to previous assumptions, the highest net energy production (1.36 kWh kg^{-1} VS fed) is obtained with ball milling. The highest ratio of energy produced, divided by energy consumed, is also obtained by ball milling and with classical mesophilic anaerobic digestion. The highest net electricity production (0.81 kWh kg^{-1} VS fed) is obtained with conventional thermophilic digestion.

11.7.5 Nutrient Release and Recovery/Removal

As stated earlier in this chapter, substantial amounts of nitrogen and phosphorus are released due to higher VS destruction. However, due to lower sonication intensities used in full-scale plants, the release is correspondingly lower, and in field matrixes, actual effluent phosphorus concentrations may be comparable to concentrations in

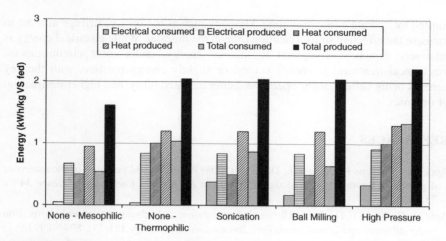

FIGURE 11.8 Impact of mechanical pretreatments on energy consumed and energy produced (electrical, heat, and total).

unsonicated digested sludge. Moreover, the decrease in soluble phosphate concentration with digestion time of disintegrated sludge has been observed and ascribed to phosphate precipitation with cations such as Mg^{2+} and Ca^{2+} (Kopp et al. 1997). Suschka et al. (2007) monitored phosphorus concentration after sludge disintegration (100 bar with recirculation through a 1.2-mm nozzle) followed by anaerobic digestion. They observed an increase in phosphate concentration from $50\,mg\,PO_4^{3-}\,L^{-1}$ to 260 to $350\,mg\,PO_4^{3-}\,L^{-1}$ after 14 days under anaerobic digestion. Sludge disintegration released polyphosphate complexes which were hydrolyzed into readily soluble orthophosphates under anaerobic conditions. Sludge disintegration (100 bar with recirculation through a 1.2-mm nozzle) followed by short (14 d) anaerobic digestion enabled removal of a substantial part of phosphorus and nitrogen in the form of precipitated struvite; at least 25% of the inflowing phosphorus load was recovered without the addition of chemicals and a higher fraction of inflowing phosphorus could be recovered with the addition of magnesium (Suschka et al. 2007). One of the advantages of enhanced pretreatment and destruction of solids streams may be much higher recovery and sustainable generation of fertilizers such as nitrogen and phosphorus.

11.8   CONCLUSION

Mechanical treatment methods, including sonication, are an effective way to increase overall performance by acting on particulate material at the macroscopic, microscopic, and chemical levels. The main mechanism at industrially reasonable levels of power input appears to be mainly via an increase in rate rather than extent. However, this increase is substantial, and readily observable, especially in systems that are limited by hydraulic retention time. Methods such as the lysis centrifuge also act to increase the effective solids retention time in the digester. While electrical energy is relatively expensive compared to thermal energy, under most circumstances, mechanical treatment is energy neutral or slightly energy positive, with the key benefits being better reactor operation, better dewaterability, and higher destruction of organics.

REFERENCES

Appels L., Baeyens J., Degreve J., Dewil R. (2008) Principles and potential of the anaerobic digestion of waste-activated sludge. *Progress in Energy and Combustion Science* **34**(6), 755–781.

Apul O. G., Sanin F. D. (2010) Ultrasonic pretreatment and subsequent anaerobic digestion under different operational conditions. *Bioresource Technology* **101**(23), 8984–8992.

Baier U., Schmidheiny P. (1997) Enhanced anaerobic degradation of mechanically disintegrated sludge. *Water Science and Technology* **36**(11), 137–143.

Barber W. P. (2005) The effects of ultrasound on sludge digestion. *Water and Environment Journal* **19**(1), 2–7.

Barjenbruch M., Kopplow O. (2003) Enzymatic, mechanical and thermal pre-treatment of surplus sludge. *Advances in Environmental Research* **7**(3), 715–720.

Batstone D. J., Keller J., Angelidaki I., Kalyuzhnyi S. V., Pavlostathis S. G., Rozzi A., Sanders W. T. M., Siegrist H., Vavilin V. A. (2002) The IWA Anaerobic Digestion Model No 1 (ADM1). *Water Science and Technology* **45**(10), 65–73.

Batstone D. J., Tait S., Starrenburg D. (2009) Estimation of hydrolysis parameters in full-scale anerobic digesters. *Biotechnology and Bioengineering* **102**(5), 1513–1520.

Biogest. (January 7, 2011) http://www.biogest.com/.

Boehler M., Siegrist H. (2006) Potential of activated sludge disintegration. *Water Science and Technology* **53**(12), 207–216.

Boisson J., Fassauer B., Friedrich H., Van der Woerd H., Jantzen J., Pottecher G. (2008) Demonstration of ultrasound technology for reducing sludge. Description and main outcome of the life environment SOUND SLUDGE project. SLUDGE, Angers, France, October 23.

Bougrier C., Carrère H., Delgenes J. P. (2005) Solubilisation of waste-activated sludge by ultrasonic treatment. *Chemical Engineering Journal* **106**(2), 163–169.

Braguglia C. M., Gianico A., Mininni G. (2009) Effect of ultrasound on particle surface charge and filterability during sludge anaerobic digestion. *Water Science and Technology* **60**(8), 2025–2033.

Camacho P., Déléris S., Geaugey V., Ginestet P., Paul E. (2002a) A comparative study between mechanical, thermal and oxidative disintegration techniques of waste activated sludge. *Water Science and Technology* **46**(10), 79–87.

Camacho P., Geaugey V., Ginestet P., Paul E. (2002b) Feasibility study of mechanically disintegrated sludge and recycle in the activated-sludge process. *Water Science and Technology* **46**(10), 97–104.

Carrère H., Dumas C., Battimelli A., Batstone D. J., Delgenès J. P., Steyer J. P., Ferrer I. (2010) Pretreatment methods to improve sludge anaerobic degradability: a review. *Journal of Hazardous Materials* **183**(1–3), 1–15.

Choi H. B., Hwang K. Y., Shin E. B. (1997) Effect on anerobic digestion of sewage sludge pretreatment. *Water Science and Technology* **35**(10), 207–211.

Chu C. P., Lee D. J., Chang B. V., You C. S., Tay J. H. (2002) "Weak" ultrasonic pre-treatment on anaerobic digestion of flocculated activated biosolids. *Water Research* **36**(11), 2681–2688.

Dohányos M., Zabranska J., Jenicek P. (1997) Enhancement of sludge anaerobic digestion by using of a special thickening centrifuge. *Water Science and Technology* **36**(11), 145–153.

Ecosolids. (January 10, 2011) http://www.ecosolids.com/.

Engelhart M., Krüger M., Kopp J., Dichtl N. (1999) Effects of disintegration on anaerobic degradation of sewage sludge in downflow stationary fixed film digester. II International Symposium on Anaerobic Digestion of Solid Waste. Barcelona, Spain, June 15–17, pp. 153–160.

Feng X., Lei H. Y., Deng J. C., Yu Q., Li H. L. (2009) Physical and chemical characteristics of waste activated sludge treated ultrasonically. *Chemical Engineering and Processing* **48**(1), 187–194.

Fitzpatrick C. (2011) New Sludge Monster offers efficient solution to end pump clogging and ragging. *Water* **21**(3).

Gonze E., Pillot S., Valette E., Gonthier Y., Bernis A. (2003) Ultrasonic treatment of an aerobic activated sludge in a batch reactor. *Chemical Engineering and Processing* **42**(12), 965–975.

Gronroos A., Kyllonen H., Korpijarvi K, Pirkonen P., Paavola T., Jokela J., Rintala J. (2005) Ultrasound assisted method to increase soluble chemical oxygen demand (SCOD) of sewage sludge for digestion. *Ultrasonics Sonochemistry* **12**(1–2), 115–120.

Hogan F., Mormede S., Clark P., Crane M. (2004) Ultrasonic sludge treatment for enhanced anaerobic digestion. *Water Science and Technology* **50**(9), 25–32.

Jain S., Lala A. K., Bhatia S. K., Kudchadker A. P. (1992) Modelling of hydrolysis controlled anaerobic digestion. *Journal of Chemical Technology and Biotechnology* **53**, 337–344.

Kampas P., Parsons S. A., Pearce P., Ledoux S., Vale P., Churchley J., Cartmell E. (2007) Mechanical sludge disintegration for the production of carbon source for biological nutrient removal. *Water Research* **41**(8), 1734–1742.

Khanal S. K., Grewell D., Sung S., van Leeuwen J. (2007) Ultrasound applications in wastewater sludge pretreatment: a review. *Critical Reviews in Environmental Science and Technology* **37**(4), 277–313.

Kidak R., Wilhelm A. M., Delmas H. (2009) Effect of process parameters on the energy requirement in ultrasonical treatment of waste sludge. *Chemical Engineering and Processing* **48**(8), 1346–1352.

Kim Y. U., Kim B. I. (2003) Effect of ultrasound on dewaterability of sewage sludge. *Japanese Journal of Applied Physics Part 1* **42**(9A), 5898–5899.

Kopp J., Müller J., Dichtl N., J. S. (1997) Anaerobic digestion and dewatering characteristics of mechanically disintegrated excess sludge. *Water Science and Technology* **36**(11), 129–136.

Kunz P., Theunert B., Wagner S. (1996) Erkenntnisse und Erfahrungen aus praktischen Anwendungen der Klärschlamm-Desintegration. *Korrespondenz Abwasser* **43**(7), 1289–1298.

Laurent J., Pierra M., Casellas M., Pons M. N., Dagot C. (2009) Activated sludge properties after ultrasonic and thermal treatments and their potential influence on dewaterability. *Journal of Residuals Science and Technology* **6**(1), 19–25.

Lehne G., Muller A., Schwedes J. (2001) Mechanical disintegration of sewage sludge. *Water Science and Technology* **43**(1), 19–26.

Li H., Jin Y. Y., Mahar R. B., Wang Z. Y., Nie Y. F. (2009) Effects of ultrasonic disintegration on sludge microbial activity and dewaterability. *Journal of Hazardous Materials* **161**(2–3), 1421–1426.

Mattiat O. E. (1971) *Ultrasonic Transducer Materials*. Springer-Verlag, London.

Müller J. (2000a) Disintegration as a key-step in sewage sludge treatment. *Water Science and Technology* **41**(8), 123–130.

Müller J. A. (2000b) Pretreatment processes for the recycling and reuse of sewage sludge. *Water Science and Technology* **42**(9), 167–174.

Müller J., Pelletier L. (1998) Désintégration mécanique des boues activées. *L'eau, l'industrie, les nuisances* **217**, 61–66.

Nah I. W., Kang Y. W., Hwang K. Y., Song W. K. (2000) Mechanical pretreatment of waste activated sludge for anaerobic digestion process. *Water Research* **34**(8), 2362–2368.

Neis U., Nickel K, Tiehm A. (2000) Enhancement of anaerobic sludge digestion by ultrasonic disintegration. *Water Science and Technology* **42**(9), 73–80.

Neis U., Nickel K., Tiehm A. (2001) Ultrasonic disintegration of sewage sludge for enhanced anaerobic biodegradation. In: Mason T. J., Tiehm A. (eds.), *Advances in Sonochemistry*, Elsevier, London; pp. 59–90.

Neis U., Nickel K., Lunden A. (2008) Improving anaerobic and aerobic degradation by ultrasonic disintegration of biomass. *Journal of Environmental Science and Health A* **43**(13), 1541–1545.

Nickel K., Neis U. (2007) Ultrasonic disintegration of biosolids for improved biodegradation. *Ultrasonics Sonochemistry* **14**(4), 450–455.

Novak J. T., Park C., Higgins M. J., Chen Y.-C., Morton R., Gary D., Forbes R. (2007) WERF odor study phase III: impacts of the MicroSludge process on odor causing compounds. In: Proceedings of the Water Environment Federation; pp. 965–978.

Onyeche T. I., Schafer S. (2003) Energy production and savings from sewage sludge treatment. *Wastewater Sludge as a Resource* 517–522.

Onyeche T. I., Schlafer O., Bormann H., Schroder C., Sievers M. (2002) Ultrasonic cell disruption of stabilised sludge with subsequant anaerobic digestion. *Ultrasonics* **40**, 31–35.

Pérez-Elvira S. I., Diez P. N., Fdz-Polanco F. (2006) Sludge minimisation technologies. *Reviews in Environmental Science and Bio/Technology* **5**(4), 375–398.

Pérez-Elvira S., Fdz-Polanco M., Plaza F.I., Garralon G., Fdz-Polanco F. (2009) Ultrasound pre-treatment for anaerobic digestion improvement. *Water Science and Technology* **60**(6), 1525–1532.

Pérez-Elvira S. I., Ferreira L. C., Donoso-Bravo A., Fdz-Polanco M., Fdz-Polanco F. (2010) Full-stream and part-stream ultrasound treatment effect on sludge anaerobic digestion. *Water Science and Technology* **61**(6), 1363–1372.

Petrier C., Casadonte D. (2001) The sonochemical degradation of aromatic and chloroaromatic contaminants. In: Mason T. J., Tiehm A. (eds.), *Advances in Sonochemistry*, Elsevier, London; pp. 91–110.

Pilli S., Bhunia P., Yan S., LeBlanc R. J., Tyagi R. D., Surampalli R. Y. (2011) Ultrasonic pretreatment of sludge: a review. *Ultrasonics Sonochemistry* **18**(1), 1–18.

Rai C., Rao P. (2009) Influence of sludge disintegration by high pressure homogenizer on microbial growth in sewage sludge: an approach for excess sludge reduction. *Clean Technologies and Environmental Policy* **11**(4), 437–446.

Sharma S. K., Mishra I. M., Sharma M. P., Saini J. S. (1988) Effect of particle size on biogas generation from biomass residues. *Biomass* **17**(4), 251–263.

Shimizu T., Kudo K., Nasu Y. (1993) Anaerobic waste-activated sludge-digestion: a bioconversion mechanism and kinetic-model. *Biotechnology and Bioengineering* **41**(11), 1082–1091.

Show K.-Y., Mao T., Lee D.-J. (2007) Optimisation of sludge disruption by sonication. *Water Research* **41**(20), 4741–4747.

Stephenson R. J., Laliberte S., Hoy P. M., Britch D. (2007) Full scale and laboratory scale results from the trial of microsludge at the joint water pollution control plant at Los Angeles County. In: Leblanc R. J., Laughton P. J., Tyagi R. (eds.), IWA specialist conferences. Moving forward wastewater biosolids sustainability, Moncton, New Brunswick, Canada, June 24–27; pp. 739–746.

Strünkmann G. W., Muller J. A., Albert F., Schwedes J. (2006) Reduction of excess sludge production using mechanical disintegration devices. *Water Science and Technology* **54**(5), 69–76.

Suschka J., Machnicka A., Grubel K. (2007) Surplus activated sludge disintegration for additional nutrients removal. *Archives of Environmental Protection* **33**(2), 55–65.

Tiehm A., Nickel K., Neis U. (1997) The use of ultrasound to accelerate the anaerobic digestion of sewage sludge. *Water Science and Technology* **36**(11), 121–128.

Tiehm A., Nickel K., Zellhorn M., Neis U. (2001) Ultrasonic waste activated sludge disintegration for improving anaerobic stabilization. *Water Research* **35**(8), 2003–2009.

Vavilin V. A., Rytov S.V., Lokshina, L.Y. (1996) A description of hydrolysis kinetics in anaerobic degradation of particulate organic matter. *Bioresource Technology* **56**:229–237.

Wang Q., Kuninobo M., Kakimoto K., Ogawa H. I., Kato Y. (1999) Upgrading of anaerobic digestion of waste activated sludge by ultrasonic pretreatment. *Bioresource Technology* **68**, 309–313.

Wang X., Qiu Z., Lu S., Ying W. (2010) Characteristics of organic, nitrogen, and phosphorus species released from ultrasonic treatment of waste activated sludge. *Journal of Hazardous Materials* **176**(1–3), 35–40.

Weemaes M., Verstraete W. (1998) Evaluation of current wet sludge disintegration techniques. *Journal of Chemistry Technology and Biotechnology* **73**(8), 83–92.

Wett B., Phothilangka P., Eladawy A. (2010) Systematic comparison of mechanical and thermal sludge disintegration technologies. *Waste Management* **30**(6), 1057–1062.

Wolff H. J., Nickel K., Houy A., Lundén A., Neis U. (2007) Two years experience on a large German STP with acoustic disintegration of waste activated sludge for improved anaerobic digestion. In: IWA (ed.), 11th World Congress on Anaerobic Digestion Bio-energy for Our Future, Brisbane, Australia, September 23–27.

Wunsch B., Heine W., Neis U. (2002) Combating bulking sludge with ultrasound. In: Neis U. (ed.), *Ultrasound in Environmental Engineering*, vol. II, TU Hamburg-Harburg Reports on Sanitary Engineering 35, pp. 201–212.

Xie R., Xing Y., Ghani Y. A., Ooi K. E., Ng S. W. (2007) Full-scale demonstration of an ultrasonic disintegration technology in enhancing anaerobic digestion of mixed primary and thickened secondary sewage sludge. *Journal of Environmental Engineering and Science* **6**(5), 533–541.

Zabranska J., Dohanyos M., Jenicek P., Kutil J. (2006) Disintegration of excess activated sludge: evaluation and experience of full-scale applications. *Water Science and Technology* **53**(12), 229–236.

12

THERMAL METHODS TO ENHANCE BIOLOGICAL TREATMENT PROCESSES

ETIENNE PAUL

Université de Toulouse; INSA, UPS, INP; LISBP, 135 Avenue de Rangueil, F-31077 Toulouse, France; INRA, UMR792, Ingénierie des Systèmes Biologiques et des Procédés, F-31400 Toulouse, France; CNRS, UMR5504, F-31400 Toulouse, France

HÉLÈNE CARRÈRE

INRA, UR050, Laboratoire de Biotechnologie de l'Environnement, Narbonne, France

DAMIEN J. BATSTONE

Advanced Water Management Centre, The University of Queensland, Brisbane St Lucia, Queensland, Australia

12.1 INTRODUCTION

Thermal treatment can be applied to either the main activated sludge treatment plant (ASTP) (sidestream treatment) or as a pretreatment to anaerobic sludge digestion (AD). The objectives are to reduce the production of waste activated sludge (WAS) or primary sludge (PS) and to enhance the conversion of sludge into biogas, respectively. In both cases, thermal treatment used to increase sludge biodegradability favors sludge degradation in the biological process. If combined with AD, thermal treatment is used to improve the sludge biodegradation extent and/or rate, allowing process intensification by decreasing sludge retention time (SRT) in the digester. If combined with ASTP, heat can also be used to develop specific microbial activities, such as hydrolytic activity and micropollutant degradation. Thermal

Biological Sludge Minimization and Biomaterials/Bioenergy Recovery Technologies, First Edition.
Edited by Etienne Paul and Yu Liu.
© 2012 John Wiley & Sons, Inc. Published 2012 by John Wiley & Sons, Inc.

treatments can be classified as low-temperature treatment ($<100°C$), which is largely biologically mediated, and high-temperature treatment ($>100°C$), which is largely physicochemical.

As compared with other types of pretreatment, the major advantage of thermal treatment is that it only needs heat. This is available at low cost where anaerobic digestion is used to generate methane, as it is produced in combined heat and power generators, and is normally available in excess. Pathogen-free biosolids can be expected from most thermal pretreatment methods, and reduced viscosity and improved dewaterability are other significant advantages of thermal treatment. Negatives include additional requirements for odor control, possible generation of colored and recalcitrant compounds, and requirements for sidestream treatment consequent on high destruction of organics.

12.2   MECHANISMS

Temperature has a fundamental impact on physicochemistry and biochemistry. At lower temperatures, it will affect biochemistry by reversible and irreversible deactivation of enzymes and cellular structural elements. This makes cellular processes less effective, and hence decreases microbial yield, as well as making cell maintenance more expensive, and directly killing cells (i.e., increasing endogenous respiration or decay). It will also increase the rate of some processes due to Arrhenius effects, and some enzymes have an elevated optimal temperature. Lower-temperature ($<80°C$) effects are largely biochemical. At higher temperatures, it has a chemical reactive impact on both mineral and organic material, as well as a physical impact due to the temperature and pressures applied. All of these factors contribute to an increase in biodegradability rate and extent, due to direct solubilization of organics, as well as an increase in accessibility to particulate material.

In this section we identify and describe mechanisms contributing to improved degradability and handling of material, including the following key issues:

- The heating effects on microbial cells through actions on cell membranes or cell constituents, including resistance mechanisms. This has further consequences on activity, deactivation, and death or lysis.
- The effect of heating on other organics. Desorption or solubilization of organic materials with or without change in chemical structure, depending on the range of temperatures applied. This results in a quantifiable change in degradability.
- At temperatures lower than $80°C$, the reactions are mainly biological.
- Changes in mineral solubilization, precipitation, and gas–liquid transfer.

12.2.1   Effects of Heating on Cells

Temperature has a fundamental impact on both processes within cells, as well as denaturation of structural elements within the cells (Farrell and Rose 1967). As temperature increases, homeostasis will be disrupted, followed by reversible dena-turation of enzymes, by irreversible denaturization, and by the breakdown of structural elements and lysis. Microbial cells have a varying capacity to maintain integrity or otherwise survive these effects. Microbes have a critical level of exposure (related to temperature and time), above which they cannot readily recover (Allwood and Russell 1970).

Action on Cell Membranes and Cell Constituents   The cell membrane, responsible for cell integrity, obviously plays a crucial role in the cell resistance to heating (Shechter 1992). The cytoplasmic membrane is composed of phospholipids which have a varying ratio of saturated to unsaturated lipids. The higher the proportion of saturated lipids, the higher the resistance to increased temperature. Proteins in the membrane will generally be more susceptible to denaturization (Rosenberg et al. 1971). Deactivation of *Escherichia coli* is observed after a few minutes at 95°C. Lang and Smith (2008) found that at 70°C, enterobacteria would be killed within a few minutes. However, Canales (1991), studying the effect of heat at 70 and 90°C on a pure culture of *Pseudomonas fluorescens*, observed two-phase response. This is demonstrated in Fig. 12.1, where N_0 is the cell concentration at t = 0 and N is the cell concentration at time t. There is a rapid 3 to 4 log reduction due to deactivation during the first 10 min, but slow response after this. A small proportion of the cells is able to withstand the temperature change in the longer term.

Cell Resistance Mechanisms   Microbial cells have evolved a number of resistance methods to short-term or extended elevated temperatures (Allwood and Russell 1970). These include formation of spores, heat-resistant proteins, and specific resistance mechanisms in the cytoplasm. Spores are characterized by low water content, a thick protein-rich membrane, and a high dipicolinic acid content. Specific defense mechanisms can remove denatured proteins and repair cells (Allwood and Russell 1970). Other factors that may increase resistance include decreased water content and low growth rates (cell division weakens cell walls) (Warth 1978). Where

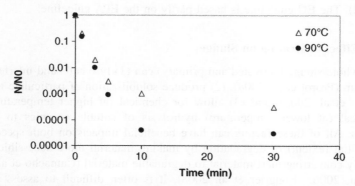

FIGURE 12.1 *Pseudomonas fluorescens* cell deactivation during heating at rather low temperature. [From Canales (1991).]

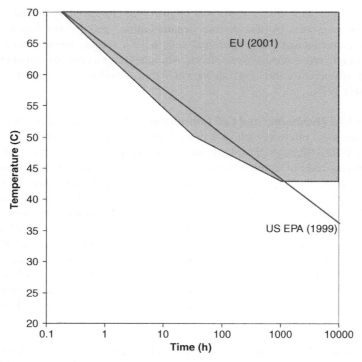

FIGURE 12.2 Temperature vs. time relationships to ensure a pathogen-free biosolids product based on EU (shaded) and U.S. EPA (line) guidelines.

cells are naturally resistant, a higher-energy input may be needed to decrease sludge production or enhance pathogen destruction. Guidelines for treatment times and temperatures have been provided by both the European Union (EU) (Carrington 2001), and the U.S. Environmental Protection Agency (EPA) (U.S. EPA 1999) (Fig. 12.2). The EU guideline is based partly on the EPA guideline.

12.2.2   Effect of Heating on Sludge

Heating whole sludge (activated and primary) can (1) lyse cells and interfere with metabolism (Prorot et al. 2008), (2) produce solubilization of particulate material (Camacho et al. 2003), and (3) allow for chemical (at higher temperature) and biochemical (at lower temperature) hydrolysis of soluble organics to smaller molecules. All of these factors can have beneficial impacts on both speed (rate) and potential (extent) of degradation by making material more accessible, or by chemically converting inert material to degradable material (Camacho et al. 2003; Paul et al. 2006a, Bougrier et al. 2008). It is often difficult to assess specific mechanisms (whether cellular or chemical), and impacts are generally assessed by the bulk method (Canales 1991; Camacho 2001; Paul et al. 2006b). Most often, to

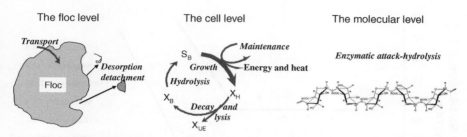

FIGURE 12.3 Different processes that may occur at different scales during heat treatment.

understand the effect of heating on sludge, solubilization of the chemical oxygen demand (COD), nitrogen, phosphorus, proteins, lipids, and carbohydrate is assessed, and specific fractions may indicate (for example) whether proteins are preferentially solubilized over carbohydrate or lipids (Camacho et al. 2003; Lu et al. 2008). The impact on soluble or colloidal materials can be distinguished using membrane and fiber filtration (Camacho 2001). Differences in release of enzymatic activities (e.g., protease activity) can also be considered together with activity measurements [biological oxygen demand (BOD) measurements and biological methane potential] to quantify both biodegradability and cell deactivation. A linkage is often assumed between degrees of solubilization and degradability. This aspect is discussed later in this chapter. Figure 12.3 summarizes different processes that may occur at the molecular, cell, or particle levels.

Organic Matter Solubilization

Effect of Treatment Temperature Although solubilization does not definitely imply degradability, it is a useful proxy for the impact of temperature. Figure 12.4 summarizes solubilization (% COD converted from particulate to soluble) from a wide range of different sludges and different conditions from literature studies. Variations include lab-scale or full-scale variation in sludge characteristics and source, and difference in heating devices. The results in Fig. 12.4 indicate that above 150°C, the major factor determining solubilization is temperature. Solubilization yields range from a few percent to around 80% of the total COD at very high temperature (>170°C). Below 150°C, the major impact is probably sludge source rather than heating temperature. Sludge heating from 25°C to 95°C induces an energy variation of 14.7 kJ for a sludge mass of 3.7 g in volatile suspended solids (VSS) and a specific heat of water (4.17 J g^{-1} K^{-1}): that is, 447 kJ mol^{-1} of VSS (weight of biomass 113 g mol^{-1}). In theory, this transferred energy by the thermal treatment is higher than the energy of a noncovalent link (20 to 30 kJ mol^{-1}). Therefore, it should be sufficient to break the noncovalent links and to destroy and modify the sludge structure. However, within the complex structure of biological flocs, synergic effect of electrostatic, ionic, and hydrogen bonds induce a significant increase in the global noncovalent energy, which may reach values near that of covalent links (Neyens and Baeyens 2003). This can explain the only partial sludge destructuration for temperatures below 100°C.

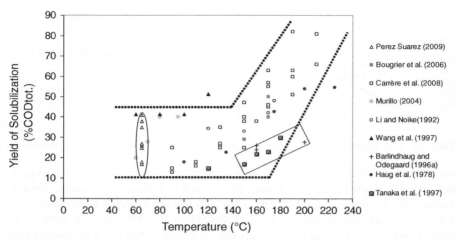

FIGURE 12.4 Effect of temperature on the yield of solubilization for different sludges. Results obtained by various authors: (Carrère et al. 2008), sludges from six different ASTPs with different organic loading rates (OLRs); (Perez Suarez 2009), sludge from an ASTP at a low OLR; (Murillo 2004), WAS and ADS from lab-scale ASTP and AD; (Bougrier et al. 2007), WAS from ASTP in the south of France; (Li and Noike 1992), WAS from an wastewater treatment plant urban; (Wang et al. 1997), WAS; (Barlindhaug and Odegaard 1996b), pilot plant fed with urban wastewater with a pre-precipitated step; (Haug et al. 1978), PS and WAS; (Tanaka et al. 1997), WAS).

A specific example is given by Carrère et al. (2008) testing five WAS samples from various urban wastewater ASTPs (Fig. 12.5). This finds that for specific samples the relationship between solubilization and temperature is linear, and that an impact can generally be seen down to 100°C. However, the slope differs strongly from sludge to sludge.

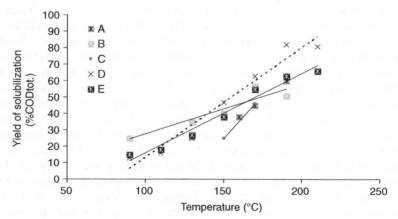

FIGURE 12.5 Effect of temperature on the solubilization yield for different WASs. [Data adapted from Carrère et al. (2008).]

This is supported by Fig. 12.4, where some sludges have very little solubilization even at 180°C [see also the Barlindhaug and Odegaard (1996a) and Tanaka et al. (1997) symbols in Fig. 12.4]. This low solubilization yield could be due to addition of inerts or hydrated mineral coagulants (Barlindhaug and Odegaard 1996b). In other examples, a large part of the COD can be solubilized even at low temperatures. At temperatures of 60 and 95°C, Murillo (2004) found that the COD released from anaerobic digested sludge (ADS) was much higher than that from activated sludge (AS) (40% vs. 15%, respectively, at 95°C for 40 min of contact time; see the gray circles in Fig. 12.4). Perez Suarez (2009) followed the COD solubilization from a WAS sampled at the same conventional ASTP during one year and found a rather wide variability of the solubilization yield (18 to 41%; see the open triangles in the oval in Fig. 12.4). Studies done during the development of the Cambi process showed after heating at 170°C strong variations of the COD solubilization yield depending on the sludge nature: around 20% for PS, from 20 to 45% for mixed sludge, from 35 to 60% for WAS, and from 50 to 75% for WAS from treatment of industrial wastewater (Kepp et al. 2000).

Effect of Treatment Duration At high temperatures, a heating duration of more than a few minutes has no further impact on COD solubilization. In general, 30 min is used in industrial applications. The situation is different at lower temperatures (<120°C). At around 70°C, Wang et al. () reported that the solubilization yield increased with treatment time. However, the impact of extended treatment times is diminished beyond 30 min (Li and Noike 1992). Around 60% of the solubilized COD is released in the first 10 min at 60°C (Wang et al. 1997). At 60 and 95°C, (Camacho 2001) confirmed rapid COD solubilization in the first 10 min but showed that the release of COD from WAS continues for up to 24 h (Fig. 12.6) with 20 to 25% release over 5 h

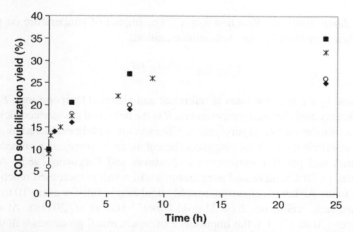

FIGURE 12.6 Time course of the COD release during batch heat treatment. (■) and (∗): WAS from an AS pilot plant treated at 95°C; (○) and (♦): full-scale ASTP with treatment at 95 and 60°C, respectively. [From Camacho (2001).]

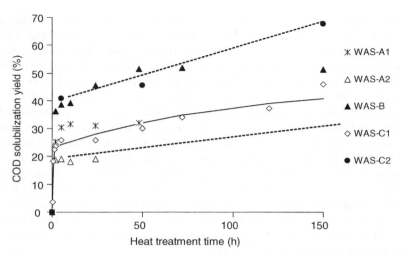

FIGURE 12.7 Long-term COD solubilization yield for various WASs along a thermal treatment at 65°C. [From Perez Suarez (2009).]

and 30 to 35% release over 24 h. At lower temperatures (65°C on five WAS samples), solubilization is prolonged, and a significant COD release continues over 150 h of treatment. Low-temperature treatment (below 100°C) induces an initial rapid COD release ($\sim$ 10%) followed by longer-term release over 24 h (20 to 30%) (Fig. 12.7). This is probably related to the different mechanisms of COD solubilization: namely, rapid techniques such as lysis occurring immediately, followed by longer-term biochemical predation and structural degradation.

Impact of Temperature on Reaction Rates   The impact of temperature on reaction rates is often described by the Arrhenius equation,

$$k_2 = k_1 e^{E_A/R(1/T_2 - 1/T_1)} \tag{12.1}$$

where k_1 and k_2 are reaction rates at reference and elevated temperatures, T_1 and T_2 are the reference and elevated temperatures, R is the universal gas law coefficient, and E_A is the activation energy. Hydrolysis coefficients are widely evaluated as apparent first-order coefficients, with the single coefficient meant to represent a complex array of sequential and parallel subprocesses (Eastman and Ferguson 1981). At lower temperatures ($<70°C$), increased temperatures will result in increased reaction rates according to the Arrhenius equation, roughly doubling in rate for every 10 to 20°C in temperature (e.g., cellulose, $E_A = 31 \pm 4$ kJ mol^{-1} (Ge et al. 2011c). At elevated temperatures (70 to 120°C), the importance of biochemical processes will diminish as hydrolytic enzymes themselves are denatured, but chemical processes will take over. At much higher temperature ($>120°C$), the reaction rate will no longer be limiting, and the only extent will depend on temperature. Apart from curve fitting to biochemical data, as done by Ge et al. (2011c), raw batch solubilization data can also be fitted on a log curve to obtain the apparent first-order coefficient:

$$\ln\left(1 - \frac{COD_{sol}}{COD_{tot}}\right) = f(t) \tag{12.2}$$

Then the logarithm of the first-order kinetic constant was plotted versus the inverse of temperature (K). The activation energy (E_A) of the COD release processes was thus calculated from the slope obtained:

$$\ln k = \frac{-E_A}{2.3R}\frac{1}{T} + \ln A \tag{12.3}$$

This work was assessed for various sludge types, and a similar order of magnitude of the activation energy was found for AS at low temperature ($<120°C$) and a much lower E_A was found for the high-temperature range (Wang et al. ; Paul et al. 2006a).

Solubilization of Specific Biochemical Compounds From the results noted earlier, variations of solubilization yield among various sludge samples apparently depend heavily on sludge origin and sludge composition. In the case of AS, the fraction of inerts depends on the SRT and on influent COD fractionation (see Chapter 2). Different compositions are also reported between AS and ADS. For example, Morgan et al. (1990) found a protein/carbohydrate ratio of 1.1 to 2.8 for digested sludge, reaching 5 for other authors, whereas this ratio is much lower (0.2 to 0.7) for PS (Lu and Arhing 2008, unpublished data). This ratio will influence response to heating. Barlindhaug and Odegaard (1996b) studied sludge thermal hydrolysis ($T = 180°C$, 30 min) in a pilot study to produce readily biodegradable substrate for denitrification. They found that carbohydrates and proteins contributed to 5 to 10% and 40 to 50%, respectively, of the solubilized COD during thermal treatment. The authors concluded that proteins were easier to solubilize than carbohydrates. Ramirez et al. (2009) observed that although COD solubilization was higher at a higher temperature (up to 220°C), protein solubilization yield was found to be similar to that obtained at 165°C (around 40%). Carbohydrate solubilization decreased strongly from 15% (at 165°C) down to 1.2% (at 220°C). They suggested that solubilization of carbohydrates would be diminished at 220°C because of the reaction of these molecules to form recalcitrant compounds such as Amadori compounds and melanoidins (a brown color was observed at $T = 220°C$ but much less at lower temperatures). This caramelization has recently been confirmed by Wilson and Novak (2009) on both WAS and PS and also on WAS by Dwyer et al. (2008), who showed that a decrease in temperature for sludge treatment from 165°C to 140°C leads to a decrease in the effluent color level but not of the sludge biodegradability. As lipids are not soluble in water, they should remain adsorbed onto organic solid fraction after thermal treatment (Bougrier et al. 2008). At 80°C, where biological reactions are negligible, Lu and Arhing (2008, unpublished data) found a high-carbohydrate release in the supernatant. Despite these efforts to analyze the link between solubilization and chemical composition, there are very few data, and given the chemical and structural complexity of the upstream components, no direct link has been found.

Thermal treatment effects on sludge cell integrity was studied at 80°C for 5, 20, 40, and 60 min and biological cell activity and viability were assessed by using correspondent staining and flow cytometry analysis before and after thermal treatment of WAS (Prorot et al. 2008). Results indicated an increase in the number of permeabilized cells and a decrease in the number of active cells, subsequent to the thermal treatment.

Heat Effect on Mineral Compounds   Temperature has a fundamental impact on most chemical processes, including precipitation and adsorption by changing chemical equilibria, according to the van't Hoff law:

$$\ln \frac{K_2}{K_1} = \frac{\Delta H^0}{R} \left(\frac{1}{T_1} - \frac{1}{T_2} \right) \tag{12.4}$$

where K_1 and T_1 are equilibrium coefficients and temperatures at reference and K_2 and T_2 those at the elevated temperature, and ΔH^0 is the heat of reaction. Exothermic reactions will become more favorable at elevated temperature. Most precipitation reactions are mildly endothermic, and hence solubility will increase with temperature. The key exception is most calcium-based compounds, where solubility will decrease slightly with temperature (Stumm and Morgan 1996) while magnesium-based compounds will be largely unaffected. Since calcium and magnesium are the major precipitating cations in wastewater, heating has no major impact on the solubilization of precipitates, especially since any dissolved precipitates resolubilize as the temperature is decreased. Murillo (2004) reported that organic material was preferentially solubilized over mineral material (Fig. 12.8), especially for temperatures above 70°C, in line with the theory discussed above.

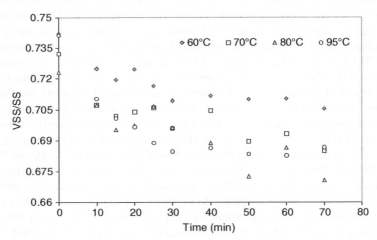

FIGURE 12.8 Variation of the VSS/suspended solids (SS) ratio against time during thermal pretreatment of a WAS at low temperatures. [From Murillo (2004).]

Due to destruction of organic and mineral compounds (e.g., polyphosphate), nitrogen and phosphorus will be released during thermal treatment (Xue and Huang 2007; Zhang and Zhang 2008). In particular, Kuroda et al. (2002) showed that nearly all the polyphosphate of WAS could be released by heating the sludge at 70°C for 1 h. For temperatures up to 70°C, orthophosphate accounted for more than 80% of total phosphorus release, and organic nitrogen was supposed to be the major component of released total nitrogen, as concentrations of NH_4^+-N, NO_3^--N, and NO_2^--N were very low (Xue and Huang 2007). Thermal pretreatment can thus be used to improve phosphorus recovery from sewage sludge (Kuroda et al. 2002; Takiguchi et al. 2004). Indeed, considering the fact that the recovery of phosphorus from urban wastewaters (Morse et al. 1998), and in particular struvite ($MgNH_4PO_4 \cdot 6H_2O$) crystallization technologies, are highly recommended (Murillo 2004; Marti et al. 2008; Zhang et al. 2009), the increased concentrations of soluble nitrogen and phosphorus become very interesting and make this process feasible, in contrast to waterline struvite recovery. However, the stoichiometry of struvite precipitation means that only small amounts of nitrogen are removed.

Changes in Biodegradability Extent and Rate   A beneficial outcome in terms of material biodegradability is the main objective when implementing a pre- or co-treatment. As discussed in Chapter 3, there are two levels behind the term *bio-degradability:* an enhancement of the total COD that can be biodegraded and/or an increase in the biodegradation rate. The first essentially increases the amount of food that is available, while the second changes the speed at which it is consumed. Taking this differentiation into account, methods to evaluate the aerobic or anaerobic biodegradability enhancement after a treatment are discussed in Chapter 3.

Several papers have reviewed the performances of a combination of thermal pretreatment methods and AD Weemaes and Verstraete 1998; Camacho et al. 2005; Pérez-Elvira et al. 2006; Appels et al. 2008). In this section we consider successively results obtained at low temperatures (<100°C) and those obtained at higher temperatures (>100°C). This separation is supported by the differences in COD solubilization yield observed for the two temperature ranges and because, at low temperature, there is an additional biochemical impact.

Low Temperature   By using short-term respirometric tests (considering maximal growth yield equal to 0.63 g COD g^{-1} COD), Paul et al. (2006b) found a percentage of biodegradable COD after thermal treatment of WAS at 95°C around 50 to 60% of the COD released, depending on the type of sludge. In addition, when running a continuous AS process with an online thermal co-treatment at 95°C, they obtained up to 60% of excess sludge production (ESP) compared to a control when presettled wastewater was used. However, only 12% of ESP was reached when raw wastewater was fed to the pilot (Perez Suarez 2009). The authors concluded that this thermal co-treatment gave a reduction yield of ESP similar to that of a conventional anaerobic sludge digestion of WAS. Seemingly, heating does not act identically on WAS, whether or not primary settlement is carried out. The removal of PS led to an increase in the performance of the thermal treatment. Perez Suarez (2009) studied, for three

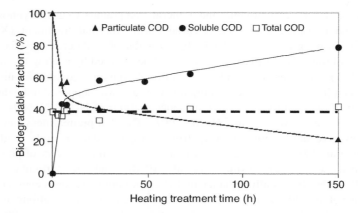

FIGURE 12.9 Variations of the biodegradable COD fractions along a 65°C heat treatment for a WAS. The soluble and particulate biodegradable fractions are expressed as a percentage of the total biodegradable fraction. [From Perez Suarez (2009).]

WASs, the variations in biodegradability [long-term biological methane potential (BMP)] of the total, the particulate, and the soluble COD fractions during a 65°C heat treatment. Figure 12.9 gives the results for one of the WASs considered. No change in the total biodegradability was observed. The increase in the soluble fraction biodegradability corresponded to the decrease in the particulate fraction biodegradability. Thus, the biodegradable molecules are simply solubilized but the nonbiodegradable material remained refractory. Moreover, the COD biodegradation yield was found proportional to the COD solubilization yield, as shown in Fig. 12.10.

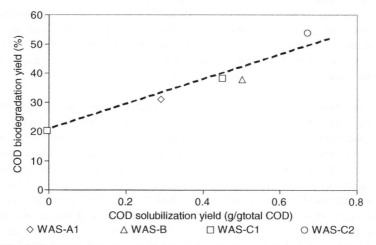

FIGURE 12.10 Relationship between the COD anaerobic biodegradation yield and the solubilized COD yield obtained after a thermal treatment of different WASs at 65°C, 150 h. [From Perez Suarez (2009).]

Using batch experiments, Gavala et al. (2003) compared the anaerobic biodegradability of PS or WAS at 60, 70, and 80°C with and without addition of sodium azide, an inhibitor for microorganisms. Using this stratagem they were able to quantify the specific contributions of biology and heating on degradation. They were able to conclude that solubilization is primarily (more than 65% at 60 or 70°C) or exclusively (80°C) due to chemical effects. However, biological reactions still contributed to increased degradability below 80°C. Gavala et al. (2003) investigated with batch experiments the 70°C thermal pretreatment effect on mesophilic digestion of PS or WAS and thermophilic digestion of PS or WAS. The methane potential was increased only slightly (20% of that of a control) when WAS were pretreated and sent to a mesophilic reactor. Similar results were obtained by Ferrer et al. (2008), who reported a 30% methane production increase during thermophilic continuous AD of mixed sludge pretreated at 70°C. According to Ge et al. (2011c), assessing continuous digestion of pretreated PS, improved performance (25% enhancement in methane production after 2 days of treatment at 50 to 70°C) was due to an increased hydrolysis coefficient rather than an increased inherent degradability. A similar study treating WAS continuously arrived at a similar result, with the hydrolysis coefficient changing from 0.2 to $1.0\,d^{-1}$ but no significant change in degradability (Ge et al. 2011b). The hydrolysis coefficient was increased progressively from 55°C (no impact as compared to 35°C control) to 70°C (a five fold increase over control).

Batch experiments can simulate thermal pretreatment performed before AD. However, bacteria acclimatization to the pretreatment conditions is a long-term process, and only a few studies report long-term experiments on continuous or semicontinuous treatment systems. Ge et al. (2011b) operated a continuous thermophilic parent reactor for the purposes of batch testing (Ge et al. 2011c) and found results from two-stage batch testing in line with continuous WAS testing. That is, thermophilic conditions up to 70°C result largely in an increase in rate rather than extent. The impact of pH, retention time, and temperature were also evaluated, and it was found that depressed pH values and extended retention time had no impact, whereas performance improved continuously at higher temperatures (Ge et al. 2011a–c). A thermophilic (65°C) microaerobic process coupled with a mesophilic (35°C) digester was evaluated for WAS degradation and compared to a conventional mesophilic digester by Dumas et al. (2010). The combined process led to a maximum 30% increase in the maximal biodegradability potential, making it possible to reach a biodegradation yield of $61 \pm 1\%$, which is unconventionally high for WAS produced at a high SRT. As the extra degraded COD was oxidized in the thermophilic aerobic reactor, it was proposed that complementary hydrolytic capacities between hyperthermophilic aerobic and mesophilic anaerobic microorganisms had developed in this combined process. These complementarities were the consequence of the co-treatment, the anaerobically biodegradable COD first being degraded completely in the anaerobic digester, with an SRT of 40 d.

Based on the review above, below 100°C, the hydrolysis rate increases, probably due to the release of material due to desorption or floc destructuration. However, this does not result in an increase in the biodegradability extent (or potential), as the energy provided is not enough for a sufficient change in the chemical structure of the organic matter. As a consequence, when only a thermal effect is expected (80 to 100°C), coupling a thermal (pre- or co-) treatment at low temperature with a post-biodegradation reactor should not increase the biodegradability potential. This was confirmed previously by Camacho et al. (2003) using thermal/AS co-treatment on a pilot scale. Moreover, this analysis is also in good agreement with the fact that the heating effect differs for PS and WAS, the former being less affected than the latter.

While pure energetic contributions cannot result in an increase in fundamental degradability, thermophilic biological activities could result in an increase in degradability extent. Dumas et al. (2010) effectively found an increase in extent, while Ge et al. (2011a,b) found that only rate was increased. In the first case, it is likely that aerobic thermophiles were contributing additional hydrolytic capabilities compared to the anaerobic microbes employed in the second case. In any case, it is likely that the impact of thermal treatment is being leveraged additionally by the presence of microbes to provide additional benefits.

High Temperature   All studies report a positive impact on biodegradability resulting from treatment at higher temperatures (>100°C). However, the optimum conditions and magnitude of improvement vary considerably, depending on a wide range of factors, including temperature, feed type, and upstream sludge age (see below).

Figure 12.11 reports on a compilation of literature values about the enhancement degree in methane production depending on temperature. Generally, authors observed both an increase in the biodegradability potential and an increase in

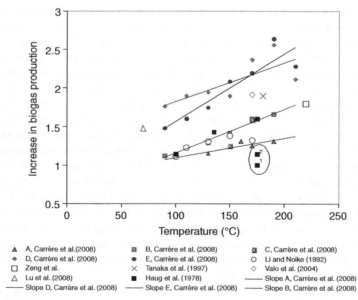

FIGURE 12.11 Increase in biogas production compared to a control for sludge submitted to thermal pretreatment, depending on the temperature used. Results from various authors. Within the circle: index[1] corresponds to PS and index[2] to a 1: 1 mixture of WAS and PS.

biodegradation rate. This result demonstrates that thermal treatment at high temperature induces substantial modifications in molecule chemical or physical structures that help biodegradation.

Testing thermal pretreatment (in the range 90 to 220°C) to increase methane production from various WASs, Carrère et al. (2008) found a linear relationship between treatment temperature and biodegradation (CH$_4$ production) (Fig. 12.11). However, it can be seen that the slope and improvement in performance are strongly dependent on the sludge origin. Results from other authors are included in the range defined by the results from Carrère et al. (2008) (see Fig. 12.11). The impact of thermal hydrolysis is generally higher for WAS than for mixed sludge, and is low or negligible for primary sludge. For example, Haug et al. (1978) compared different sludges with pretreatment of 170 to 175°C and subsequent continuous AD (SRT of 15 d). Primary sludge was not improved by pretreatment, while mixed sludge had a 14% improvement, and WAS was improved by 62%. Among different WAS samples, Carrère et al. (2008) showed that the lower the initial sludge biodegradability, the higher the efficiency of thermal treatment. Moreover, the lower the SRT in the digester, the higher the impact of thermal pretreatment (consistent with an improvement in rate). Graja et al. (2005) reduced the SRT in the digester to 2.9 d by using a fixed-film reactor which was fed with the liquid fraction of pretreated (175C) sludge. Batstone et al. (2009) found that both degradability and rate were greatly improved (145 to 165C) for WAS, but that degradability was dependent on upstream sludge age, and degradability decreased at a sludge age of more than 20 d. Below 20 d there was no relationship between sludge age and degradability.

The link between biodegradability enhancement and COD solubilization has been well established, but the two terms are not intimately linked, as shown in Fig. 12.12 (Carrère et al. 2008). The increase in biodegradability appears proportional to the

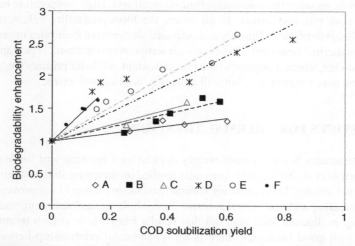

FIGURE 12.12 Relationship between biodegradability enhancement and COD solubilization yield for six WASs [Adapted from Carrère et al. (2008).]

solubilized COD, but again the proportionality is strongly sludge dependent and decouples at higher temperature, due to the production of recalcitrant soluble organic material (Dwyer et al. 2008).

Modelling is a valuable tool to evaluate data consistency and to help understand fundamental changes, as illustrated by Ramirez et al. (2009). This work altered parameters in the IWA anaerobic digestion model 1 (Batstone et al. 2002) to determine modifications of the COD fractions after pretreatment of sludge at 110, 165, and 220°C compared to untreated sludge. The fraction of the composite biodegradable particulate substrate (X_c) changed from 3.19 kg COD m^{-3} for untreated sludge to 3.44, 3.01, and 2.01 kg COD m^{-3} for thermally pretreated sludge at 110, 165, and 220°C, respectively. However, the highest methane production was observed for pretreatment at 165°C. Therefore, it can be concluded that the content of the composites in terms of carbohydrates, proteins, and lipids—together with the availability of these substrates to the microorganisms—is at least as important as the concentration of composites in itself. This result can also explain the variability of the biodegradability increase depending on the sludge origin. Another example is the work of Batstone et al. (2009), in which a full-scale process was modeled to evaluate whether improvements in performance could be related to increases in rate or extent. It was found that both were improved substantially compared to low-temperature treatment (Ge et al. 2011a,b).

12.2.3 Mechanisms of Thermal Pretreatment

We have reviewed two principal methods of thermal pretreatment: low-temperature treatment (<80°C), where the mechanism is both biochemical and chemical, and high-temperature treatment (>140°C), where the mechanism is purely chemical. Low-temperature pretreatment will generally increase rate but not biodegradability extent. Extent may be enhanced by microaerophilic co-treatment. High-temperature treatment enhances both rate and extent. In all cases, the biodegradability enhancement is strongly sludge dependent. Primary and activated sludge have their rates improved by low-impact thermal treatment. However, high-temperature treatment is best applied to activated sludge, where it improves both rate and extent, while for primary sludge, high temperature may improve rate but will generally not improve extent.

12.3   DEVICES FOR THERMAL TREATMENT

Thermal treatment has been most widely applied as a pretreatment for WAS (see above; Carrère et al. 2010), and is generally applied on the entire sludge stream rather than a partial stream. This is true for several reasons, including (1) improvements in material handling and viscosity that result from whole stream treatment, and (2) the consistency in digester feed material that results from whole stream treatment. In addition, with good insulation there is no fundamental relationship between pre-treatment retention time and energy consumption, and energy consumption is related to feed stream heating rather than heat losses from the digester (Carrère et al. 2010) (see later). The major negative impacts of increased reactor size are higher capital costs, increased mixing in the reactor, and potential production of recalcitrant or undesirable products (e.g., melanoidins) (Dwyer et al. 2008). However, equipment used for low- and high-temperature pretreatment vary dramatically, with these two systems being completely different.

12.3.1 Low-Temperature Pretreatment

Since low-temperature pretreatment occurs below <80°C, it is at atmospheric pressure, below the temperature level at which there are significant occupational health and safety considerations, and at a temperature where material considerations are minor to moderate. This means that vessel design generally involves standard stirred tanks, although plug-flow reactors can be used to provide a defined retention time where proof of pathogen kill is important (v.s. EPA 2002). Methods of heating can be divided into either heat exchange (with issues similar to those of normal digester sludge heating; (Metcalf & Eddy, Inc. 2003) or direct chemical or thermal heating. Heat exchange–based methods include:

- *Heating of the feed stream.* This is commonly used where mixing is by gas lift or by mechanical impeller. Advantages include the ability to recover effluent heat, and to work at a greater ΔT between the hot and cold sides; disadvantages include low heat-transfer coefficients due to high fluid viscosities and fluid velocity, as well as the potential for sludge to coat the surface of the heat exchanger, especially where feed is intermittent (which it normally is).

- *Recirculation heating.* This is commonly used where hydraulic mixing is used. It will have a better heat transfer coefficient due to better fluid properties, but normally works at a lower ΔT. Efficiency is highly and inherently dependent on the temperature differential between the inlet and the outlet of the heat exchanger.

Methods for direct heating may include:

- *Direct hot water injection.* This is generally not used, due to dilution of the sludge and hence a decrease in volumetric loading.

- *Direct steam injection.* This is normally not used, due to the considerable additional operational and safety requirements when generating steam.

- *Biochemical production of heat by autothermal aerobic digestion.* The exothermic nature of aerobic digestion is utilized by first operating under aerobic conditions to raise temperature, then removing the air supply to operate under anaerobic digestion. This requires a higher-solids feed and readily degradable primary substrate (Layden et al. 2007).

The other major issue for low-temperature pretreatment is the pretreatment reactor configuration. Fixed-volume continuous or semibatch thermal is preferred from a process point of view, as storage is not required, and an increase in sludge production rate can be addressed by increasing the feed flow. However, since the particle distribution follows a continuously stirred tank reactor (CSTR) profile, a fixed retention time cannot be guaranteed for the entire feed quantity. Where a specific retention time must be guaranteed, batch or plug flow must be used. The first requires feed buffering and volume management, while the second has increased capital costs and an increased possibility of total failure due to profile breakthrough (Richardson et al. 2002). Generally, where it can be shown that a fixed-volume reactor will achieve adequate performance, one will be used.

12.3.2 High-Temperature Pretreatment

All commercially available high-temperature treatment systems currently available are batch systems, which is acceptable in this context due to the relatively short retention times (normally, <1 h). They are normally also multivessel, with both the Veolia and Cambi systems utilizing a 130 to 160°C multiple-effect heating system (steam is generated in the second reactor to heat the first reactor). Most also utilize a flash vessel, which allows rapid depressurization to less then 130°C to cause further disruption and cavitation due to boiling. Different systems vary in implementation details, with the Cambi system using physically separated vessels (preheat, react, flash; Panter and Kleiven 2005), whereas the Veolia system places all three processes in the same vessel, with multiple vessels being staged to share the steam regenerated (Chauzy et al. 2007). Veolia has also been piloting a continuous thermal hydrolysis process that promises to avoid staging and many of the mechanical operations. All commercial systems so far have used direct steam injection in the main (high-temperature) stage as primary source of heat, and most rely on preconcentration of sludge to approximately 12% to achieve an optimal energy balance. That means that these systems are inherently dependent on generation of at least 6-bar steam, with its consequent increased operational and training requirements. While the most common application has been whole feed stream treatment, thermal hydrolysis has also been applied on the digestate side, with treated sludge recirculated into the digester (Zabranska et al. 2006).

12.4 APPLICATIONS OF THERMAL TREATMENT

12.4.1 Thermal Treatment Combined with Activated Sludge

Very few references have been found that evaluate the integration of thermal pretreatment with the main activated sludge line. This is because concentrations in return activated sludge loops are relatively low. Canales et al. (1994) evaluated a sludge thermal treatment loop in a membrane bioreactor. Sludge was heated at 90°C for 3 h, leading to nearly 100% cell death. Experiments were performed at two values of SRT and hydraulic retention time, and results were compared to that obtained on a control membrane bioreactor. A 2.5-fold decrease in the growth yield observed (from 0.42 to 0.17 g g^{-1} COD at a net specific growth rate of 0.1 h^{-1}) was obtained as explained by an increase in the maintenance coefficient by a factor of 3.

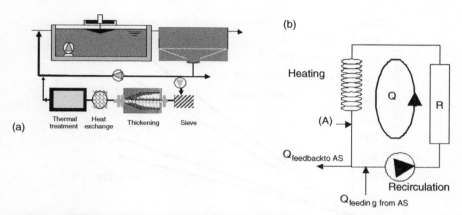

FIGURE 12.13 Thermal treatment system combined with an AS reactor as used by Camacho (2001). (a) Overall system and (b) the heating reactor with the heating device and the recirculation.

This thermal treatment (95°C)–membrane bioreactor concept was applied at a pilot scale fed with real urban wastewater by Camacho et al. (2003) (Fig. 12.13).

The treatment frequency, f_{treat} [Eq. (12.5)], was used to characterize the process:

$$f_{treat} = \frac{\text{daily mass of treated sludge}(gd^{-1})}{\text{mass of sludge in the system}(g)} \quad (12.5)$$

$$N = f_{treat} \cdot SRT \quad (12.6)$$

$$D_S = \frac{f_{treat} \cdot CT}{\text{treated VSS}} \quad (12.7)$$

N in Eq. (12.6) represents the number of times the sludge undergoes thermal treatment before leaving the system, and D_S in Eq. (12.7) represents the specific thermal "dose" applied. The contact time (CT) is the time during which the sludge is heated. Multiplying Eq. (12.6) by Eq. (12.7) gives the total thermal dose applied for one mass of sludge during the SRT. It is important to notice that if a reduction of ESP is achieved, the SRT will increase automatically. Results obtained by Camacho (2001) are presented in Fig. 12.14, where the SS or VSS produced is plotted versus the COD removed for combined AS–thermal treatment at 95°C. In the work of Camacho et al. (2003), the variable volume and the possibility to change the feeding rate of the thermal treatment allowed working with a treatment frequency between 0.3 and 3 d^{-1} and a contact time up to 1 h for a 24 h/24 h operation. Normalized reduction yields were calculated using data from the control and the treatment line. For the conditions $T = 59°C$, $f_{treat} = 0.2\,d^{-1}$, and a CT of 36 min, the sludge production yield observed (Y_{obs}) was 28 and 35% for SS and VSS, respectively. In the case $T = 95°C$, $0.03 < f_{treat}\,(d^{-1}) < 0.4$, and $5 < CT\,(min) < 435$ (7 h 30 min), the reduction yield was 21 to 59% and 20 to 63% for SS and VSS, respectively (Fig. 12.15).

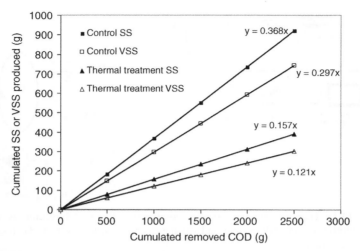

FIGURE 12.14 SS or VSS produced versus COD removed for combined AS–thermal treatment at 95°C. [From Camacho (2001).]

The following preliminary conclusions can be drawn from Fig. 12.15: a low treatment frequency is ineffective for VSS reduction even if the CT is increased drastically (CT 450 min). The optimal treatment frequency is between 0.2 and $0.4\,d^{-1}$, with a contact time between 20 and 30 min.

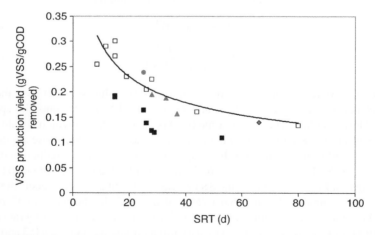

FIGURE 12.15 Change in the VSS production yield depending on sludge age for the combined AS–95°C thermal treatment for various heating conditions and compared to a control line. Open square control line with no thermal treatment; black square, $60°C < T < 95°C$, $0.2\ d^{-1} < f_{treat} < 0.4\,d^{-1}$, 20 min < CT < 36 min; gray triangle, $T = 95°C$, $0.1\,d^{-1} < f_{treat} < 0.2\,d^{-1}$, CT = 5 min; gray diamond $T\,(°C) = 95°C$, $f_{treat} = 0.06\ d^{-1}$, CT = 36 min; gray circle $T = 95°C$, $f_{treat} = 0.03\ d^{-1}$, CT = 450 min; black line, power law to simulate control behaviour. [From Paul et al. (2006b).]

Up to a 60% reduction in sludge production compared to a control was reached with presettled wastewater but only 12% with raw wastewater. The comparison of these results with those of Canales et al. (1994) obtained on a pure culture of *Pseudomonas fluorescens* and synthetic substrate and those from Camacho (2001) obtained on both real settled and raw sludge underlines the strong influence on the heating effect of the material from the wastewater. It confirms that the efficiency of heating on sludge reduction is really sludge-quality dependent.

Treatment Efficiency The system resulted in additional release in soluble microbial products, with up to double that in a normal treatment plant (38 ± 6 mg L^{-1}). This was not related to thermal treatment dosage (stress frequency). While nitrification was maintained, respirometric analyses of the ammonia uptake rate (mg $N\text{-}NH_4^+$ g^{-1} VSS h^{-1}) demonstrated that thermal treatment induced a decrease of nitrification kinetics in correlation to the sludge reduction rate [more information is available in Paul et al. (2006b)]. Because of high energy consumption and equal or lower performance compared to that of a conventional ASTP, it has not been applied in full scale.

Sakai et al. (2000) combined the conventional AS process with that of a thermophilic aerobic sludge digester, in which excess sludge is solubilized by thermophilic enzymes and called a digester S-TE reactor (Fig. 12.16). At the origin, solubilizing thermophilic aerobic bacteria were isolated from composted sludge and seeded to the biological pretreatment reactor. The co-digestion conditions selected were a temperature of 65°C and an SRT of 1 d. Total elimination of excess sludge was achieved when three times the excess sludge generated from influent BOD was recirculated into the S-TE reactor and solubilized. Accumulation of inorganic matter contents in the system was not observed. The authors claimed a reduction in operating costs of 40 to 50% compared to that of a conventional sludge-handling unit.

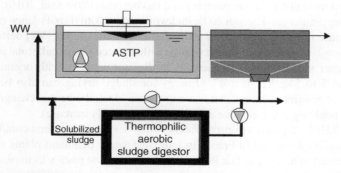

FIGURE 12.16 Configuration of the thermophilic aerobic digestor proposed by Sakai et al. (2000).

12.4.2 Thermal Pretreatment to Anaerobic Digestion

Operating Conditions and Performances Both high- and low-energy thermal treatment have been applied widely to anaerobic digestion at full scale, with performance information given in detail in the foregoing sections. Lower-temperature anaerobic digestion has been employed with retention times from 2 d (Lu et al. 2008; Ge et al. 2010) to 7 d (Gavala et al. 2003), and down to 9 h (70°C) (Ferrer et al. 2008). High-temperature treatment is also a mature technology, with optimal treatment temperatures from 160 to 180°C and pressure varying from 600 to 2500 kPa. Treatments at excessively high temperatures (higher than 170 to 190°C) or long treatment times lead to decreased sludge biodegradability despite achieving high solubilization efficiencies.

Industrial Application Low-temperature pretreatment has been applied widely, but since the technology is relatively uncomplicated and low risk, it is not normally implemented as a specialized commercial product. This may change in the future as the process is better understood and optimized.

High-temperature thermal hydrolysis has a higher process risk and has been commercialized in proprietary industrial processes such as Cambi (Kepp et al. 2000), Veolia *Bio*THELYS (Chauzy et al. 2002, 2004, 2007), and more recently, Veolia Exelys DLD. The three processes consist of treatment at 150 to 180°C for 30 to 60 min, with steam injection as a primary heat source. The first Cambi process was implemented in 1995 at the HIAS wastewater treatment plant (90,000 population equivalents (p.e.) of Hamar (Norway), and more than 20 plants are currently in operation worldwide (http://www.cambi.no). Cambi plant capacities ranging from 1600 metric tons of dry matter per year (Næstved, Danemark) to 91,000 tons dry matter per year (Davyhulme, UK). Pre-dewatered solids, up to 15% solids concentration, are added to the feed tank. This high solids content allows reduction of tank volumes and energy consumption and hence of capital and operating costs. The temperature is also reduced by flashing, to 100°C, and subsequent cooling (normally with feed sludge) to a digester feed temperature of 37°C. By the addition of the water in the steam and due to solublilization, the resulting solids concentration to digestion is 10 to 12%. The thermal hydrolysis process decreases viscosity dramatically, reducing pumping and mixing costs (Ross et al. 2010). The main outcomes are (Panter and Kleiven 2005; Pickworth et al. 2006) (Fdz-Polanco et al. 2008) (1) an increase in biogas production and volatile (organic) solids (VS) destruction of around 60%; (2) a reduction in sludge volume with digested sludge cake total solids (TS) content higher than 30%; (3) an increase in digester capacity with organic loading greater than 3 to 5 kg VS m^{-3} d^{-1}. Energy for sludge drying can also be reduced. Formation of gelatinous lumps that can sometimes block the heat exchangers can be limited by applying a hot alkaline solution (leading to pH increase).

The *Bio*THELYS process (Veolia Waters: http://www.veoliawaterst.com/biothelys/en/) has been implemented in France in four wastewater treatment plants sized from 30000 (Ternier) to 80000 p.e. (Le Pertuiset SIVO). The first plant was implemented in 2006 at the urban wastewater treatment plant of Saumur-France (62000 p.e., 1400 t TS yr^{-1} of sludge from an extended aeration tank). The *Bio*THELYS thermal hydrolysis works with dewatered sludge to 12 to 16% TS. The system is composed of lines of two or three thermal hydrolysis reactors working in parallel. Each reactor is working in batch mode, and a complete cycle lasts for 120 to 165 min:

1. The reactor is filled.
2. The sludge is preheated with recycled steam coming from another reactor.
3. Live steam is injected in order to reach hydrolysis temperature.
4. The sludge is exposed to the required temperature (160°C) under pressure (approximately saturated vapor pressure) during the retention time (30 min).
5. The steam is released (the flash) from the reactor to another reactor (flash allows energy recovery via steam recycling and a decrease in the treated sludge temperature).
6. The reactor is emptied using the residual pressure. The results were an increase in TS removal from 25 to 45% and an increase in sludge cake TS content from 22% to 30%, corresponding to a 46% reduction in sludge volume compared to conventional digestion (Chauzy et al. 2007). More recently, Veolia Water has initiated commercialization of the Exelys process (165°C, 9 to 12 bar of pressure) with two reference sites in France (Versailles and Lille) and one in Denmark near Copenhagen. An original configuration DLD (digestion, lysis, and further digestion) in the continuous mode leads to the best efficiency in terms of methane recovery and sludge reduction. Other configurations are also available.

Energy Balance   Several studies have shown positive energy balance with either 70° or 165 to 190°C pretreatments. Carrère et al. (2010) calculated the theoretical energy balances in the case of conventional mesophilic and thermophilic AD and 70 and 170°C pretreatments. The results are reported in Fig. 12.17. The following assumptions were made:

1. The digester feed concentration was 6%, except after 170°C treatment when it can be increased to 9%.
2. Electrical requirements (mainly feed and mixing) were set to 0.12 kWh m^{-3} d^{-1}.
3. Hydraulic retention time was set to 20 and 15 d for mesophilic and thermophilic digestion, respectively.
4. VS destruction was assumed to be 40% for mesophilic digestion and 50% for thermophilic digestion in the case of 70°C pretreatment, and 60% for 170°C pretreatment.
5. Heating requirements were thermal capacity plus approximately 10% losses in mesophilic or 20% in thermophilic digestion.
6. Biogas was supposed to be valorized by cogeneration, and electrical and heat energy yields were assumed to be 35 and 50% of total energy produced, respectively.

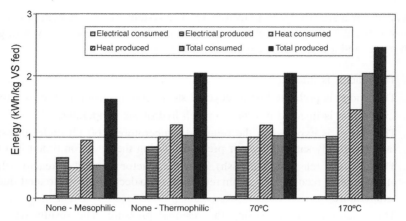

FIGURE 12.17 Impact of thermal pretreatments on energy consumed and energy produced (electrical, heat, and total).

According to the previous assumptions, the highest net energy production (1.075 kWh kg^{-1} VS fed) and the highest ratio of energy produced divided by energy consumed (2.99) are obtained with conventional mesophilic AD. However, the highest energy recovery (2.47 kWh kg^{-1} VS fed) and electricity production (1.02 kWh kg^{-1} VS fed) are achieved with 170°C pretreatment. Figure 12.17 also shows that both 70 and 170°C pretreatments need more heat energy than that produced. An option can be direct use of a fraction of biogas produced for thermal treatment, the fraction remaining being used for cogeneration (Kepp et al. 2000). However, heat consumption can easily be optimized by thickening sludge before thermal hydrolysis (Chauzy et al. 2007; Fdz-Polanco et al. 2008) and the recovery of heat from hot streams (Bougrier et al. 2007; Fdz-Polanco et al. 2008). In this way, Fdz-Polanco et al. (2008) proposed a 170°C pretreatment system that is energetically self-sufficient; the entire increase in biogas production can be utilized for electricity generation. This can be achieved by (1) a high concentration of sludge to limit the amount of energy wasted heating water, and (2) the exploitation of the high temperature and enthalpy of streams such as vapor produced in the flash, hydrolyzed sludge, exhaust gases, and hot water from the gas engine (Fdz-Polanco et al. 2008).

Ferrer et al. (2009) showed that the theoretical net energy production from mixed sludge is almost doubled by implementing a 70°C pretreatment step to thermophilic digesters operating at a short SRT of 10 d. Lu et al. (2008) implemented a 70°C pretreatment before thermophilic AD (SRT of 13 d, 15 d without pretreatment); net electricity and heat productions were 0.67 and 1.5 kJ d^{-1}, respectively.

In the case of high-temperature (165°C) pretreatments, an energy balance performed on the full-scale HIAS plant showed that thermal hydrolysis of dewatered sludge (10 g TS L^{-1}) led to a 27% increase in net electricity production, from 175 kW to 233 kW (Kepp et al. 2000). 85% of biogas was used for the combined heat and power (CHP) engine. Steam is produced from the CHP flue gas and the remaining

15% of biogas. Heat from steam and treated sludge is then used to heat the digester and to produce hot water (Kepp et al. 2000). Energy balance details from sludge treatment using the Cambi process are provided by Kepp et al. (2000) and Pickworth et al. (2006).

Nutrient Release and Management As seen above, the use of sludge thermal pretreatment leads to the solubilization of organic matter, nitrogen, and phosphorus. The improvement in digester performance also results in an increase in nitrogen and phosphorus concentrations, and generation of inert solubles and small particles increases organics in the supernatants or dewatering reject streams of digested sludge. For example, Yang et al. (2010) measured an increase in concentration of total nitrogen in the liquid phase after AD upflow anerobic sludge blanket (UASB) of thermally treated (200°C) WAS (769 mg L^{-1}) as compared to conventional AD of WAS (424 mg L^{-1}), the nitrogen being in ammonium form at more than 90%. In contrast, a thermal treatment–UASB process resulted in a decrease in the digested sludge liquid phosphorus concentration (0.2 mg L^{-1} against 17 mg L^{-1} for conventional AD) and in higher total phosphorus concentrations in the residue. This was ascribed to the combined effects of redissolution, refixation, and utilization on anaerobic sludge growth.

Supernatants of digested sludge are generally returned to the main activated sludge treatment stream to treat solubilized carbon, nitrogen, and phosphorus compounds. Higher amounts of pollution, mainly carbon and nitrogen, have thus to be treated in the ASTP or BNPR process if thermal hydrolysis is used. The digested sludge solids are generally used in land application as a fertilizer and as a soil improvement agent. A study with 160 to 180°C pretreated sludge from the full-scale HIAS plant showed that nitrogen and phosphorus in sludge had an equivalent agronomic impact on chemical fertilizer (Fjærgaard and Sander 2001). Moreover, the comparison over two different time periods of hydrolyzed and digested sludge analysis with digested sludge analysis showed a decrease in volatile solids (60% against 73%), no variation in nitrogen level (38 to 40 g N kg^{-1} TS), an increase in the phosphorus level (25 g P kg^{-1} TS) against 15 g P kg^{-1} TS, and an increase in some heavy metals whose concentration remained under accepted levels.

Side Effects Sludge sanitation is a key advantage of thermal treatment. A report from the European Commission (Carrington 2001) indicates that thermophilic temperatures are lethal to pathogens if they are exposed for a sufficient time, such as 7 min at 70°C, 30 min at 65°C, or 4 h at 55°C in digesting conditions. However, plant design constraints indicate that the minimum time for exposure should be 30 min. In the United States, class A biosolids can be land-applied without any pathogen-related restrictions at the site. To satisfy class A requirements, the fecal coliform density must be less than 1000 most probable number (MPN) per gram of total solids, the *Salmonella* density must be less than 3 MPN per 4 g of TS, enteric viruses must be less than 1 CFU (colony-forming unit) per 4 g of TS, and helminths must be less than one viable organism per 4 g of TS (U.S. EPA 2002). These requirements may be achieved by a temperature and time process, with a temperature higher than 50°C (e.g., thermophilic AD). The minimum process time is given by

$$D = \frac{131,700,000}{10^{0.14t}} \tag{12.8}$$

where D is the time in days and t is the temperature in Celsius degrees. If TS $< 7\%$ and time > 30 min, Eq. (12.8) is replaced by

$$D = \frac{50,070,000}{10^{0.14t}} \tag{12.9}$$

Several processes to further reduce pathogens are listed (U.S. EPA 2002). Among them, the pasteurization process consists of maintaining the temperature of the sewage sludge at 70°C or higher for 30 min or longer, and the heat treatment process consists of heating liquid sewage sludge to a temperature of 180°C or higher for 30 min.

Another advantage of thermal hydrolysis is the improvement in sludge dewater-ability, as thermal treatment allows degradation of the sludge gel structure and release of linked water. Sludge has to be heated at temperatures higher than 150°C (Anderson et al. 2002; Neyens and Baeyens, 2003) and the higher the temperature (up to 225°C), the better the dewaterability (Haug et al. 1978). However, thermal treatments at low temperatures in the range 90 to 130°C have been reported to alter WAS dewaterability (Bougrier et al. 2008). Heat treatment industrial plants (Porteous and Zimpro processes) developed from the 1940s to the 1970s to optimize sludge dewatering before incineration. Temperatures were typically 200 to 250°C. However, even if thermally pretreated digested sludge presents better dewatering properties than digested sludge (Haug et al. 1978), subsequent digestion of thermally treated sludge alters their dewaterability (Haug et al. 1983) and reduces the impact of thermal treatment.

Thermal hydrolysis is also effective in improving sludge settling properties and in decreasing their apparent viscosity. Bougrier et al. (2008) showed that sludge apparent viscosity and sludge volume indexes were reduced first with temperature and then remained almost constant for temperatures higher than 150°C.

12.5   CONCLUSIONS

Sludge heating can lead to an increase in the maximal biodegradation potential as defined by a long-term biological methane potential (>40 d). This increase in biodegradation can be obtained at high temperature (around 140 to 170°C), pre-sumably due to chemical hydrolysis of the organic matter. This results in an increase in both the potential (extent) and speed (rate) of degradation. Higher temperatures result in production of inhibitory and refractory compounds. Improvement in biodegradation can also be reached at low temperatures (65 to 80°C), but the increase in biodegradation is related primarily to an increase in degradation rate rather than an increase in attainable potential. Potential is further enhanced with additional treatment, such as aerobic co-treatment.

Both low- and high-intensity treatment therefore have the potential to increase gas production significantly by treating sludge and coupling with AD. However, the effectiveness of thermal treatment to increase the maximal biodegradation potential is strongly sludge dependent, with, in particular, primary sludge being minimally improved by thermal hydrolysis. Hence, more research is needed to understand the behavior during heat treatment of the organic matter, depending on its nature and its interaction with minerals.

Heat can be generated in a wastewater treatment plant and therefore sludge heating can easily be achieved by using heat exchangers or by injection of steam. Implementation of both low-temperature (65 to 80°C) and high-temperature (140 to 170°C) treatments before anaerobic digestion has shown positive energy balance; however, sludge concentration should be high enough and heat should be recovered from different streams. The degree of maturity of thermal treatment is thus rather good. This process is integrated preferentially in the sludge-handling units and a high solids content should be privileged to reduce the specific energy consumption for heating. Various objectives, such as improving methane production, decreasing sludge production, handling costs, and increasing sludge quality, to reach class A standards led recently to the development and commercialization of new thermal hydrolysis processes. Thermal treatment is an established and mature technology, but needs further research and optimization, particularly at lower temperatures.

REFERENCES

Allwood M. C., Russell A. D. (1970) Mechanisms of thermal injury in nonsporulating bacteria. *Advances in Applied Microbiology* **12**, 89–119.

Anderson N. J., Dixon D. R., Harbour P. J., Scales P. J. (2002) Complete characterisation of thermally treated sludges. *Water Science and Technology* **46**(10), 51–54.

Appels L., Baeyens J., Degreve J., Dewil R. (2008) Principles and potential of the anaerobic digestion of waste-activated sludge. *Progress in Energy and Combustion Science* **34**(6), 755–781.

Barlindhaug J., Odegaard H. (1996a) Thermal hydrolysate as a carbon source for denitrification. *Water Science and Technology* **33**(12), 99–108.

Barlindhaug J., Odegaard H. (1996b) Thermal hydrolysis for the production of carbon source for denitrification. *Water Science and Technology* **34**(1–2), 371–378.

Batstone D. J., Keller J., Angelidaki I., Kalyuzhnyi S. V., Pavlostathis S. G., Rozzi A., Sanders W. T. M., Siegrist H., Vavilin V. A. (2002) Anaerobic digestion model no. 1 (ADM1). In: ITGfMMoAD (ed.), *Processes*, IWA Publishing, London.

Batstone D. J., Tait S., Starrenburg D. (2009) Estimation of hydrolysis parameters in full-scale anerobic digesters. *Biotechnology and Bioengineering* **102**(5), 1513–1520.

Bougrier C., Delgenes J. P., Carrère H. (2006) Combination of thermal treatments and anaerobic digestion to reduce sewage sludge quantity and improve biogas yield. *Process Safety Environment Protection* **84**(B4), 280–284.

Bougrier C., Delgenes J. P., Carrère H. (2007) Impacts of thermal pre-treatments on the semi-continuous anaerobic digestion of waste activated sludge. *Biochemical Engineering Journal* **34**(1), 20–27.

Bougrier C., Delgenes J. P., Carrère H. (2008) Effects of thermal treatments on five different waste activated sludge samples solubilisation, physical properties and anaerobic digestion. *Chemical Engineering Journal* **139**(2), 236–244.

Camacho P. (2001) Etude de procédés de réduction de la production de boues par couplage de traitements physique ou chimique et biologique. INSA, Toulouse, France.

Camacho P., Ginestet P., Audic J. M. (2003) Pilot plant demonstration of reduction technology during activated sludge treatment of wastewater. In: WEFTEC'03, Los Angeles, October 11–15.

Camacho P., Ginestet P., Audic J. M. (2005) Understanding the mechanisms of thermal disintegrating treatment in the reduction of sludge production. *Water Science and Technology* **52**(10–11), 235–245.

Canales A. (1991) Croissance cryptique en bioréacteur à membrane: application au traitement des eaux résiduaires urbaines. University of Toulouse, INSA, Toulouse, France.

Canales A., Pareilleux A., Rols J. L., Goma G., Huyard A. (1994) Decreased sludge production strategy for domestic waste-water treatment. *Water Science and Technology* **30**(8), 97–106.

Carrère H., Bougrier C., Castets D., Delgenes J. P. (2008) Impact of initial biodegradability on sludge anaerobic digestion enhancement by thermal pretreatment. *Journal of Environmental Science and Health A* **43**(13), 1551–1555.

Carrère H., Dumas C., Battimelli A., Batstone D. J., Delgenes J. P., Steyer J. P., Ferrer I. (2010) Pretreatment methods to improve sludge anaerobic degradability: a review. *Journal of Hazardous Materials* **183**(1–3), 1–15.

Carrington E. G. (2001) *Evaluation of Sludge Treatments for Pathogen Reduction.* Office for Official Publications of the European Communities, Luxembourg. http://ec.europa.eu/environment/waste/sludge/....

Chauzy J., Crétenot D., Fernandes P., Patria L. (2002) Bio THELYS, a new process for sludge minimization and sanitization. In: 7th European Biosolids and Organic Residuals Conference, Wakefield, UK. November, 18–20.

Chauzy J., Graja S., Gerardin F., Crétenot D., Patria L., Fernandes P. (2004) Minimisation of excess sludge production in a WWTP by coupling thermal hydrolysis and rapid anaerobic digestion. *Water Science and Technology* **52**(10–11), 255–263.

Chauzy J., Cretenot D., Bausseon A., Deleris S. (2007) Anaerobic digestion enhanced by thermal hydrolysis: First reference Biothelys® at Saumur, France. In: Facing Sludge Diversities: Challenges, Risks and Opportunities, Antalya, Turkey.

Dohányos M., Zábranská J., Kutil J., Jenícek P. (2004) Improvement of anaerobic digestion of sludge. *Water Science and Technology* **49**(10), 89–96.

Dumas C., Perez S., Paul E., Lefebvre X. (2010) Combined thermophilic aerobic process and conventional anaerobic digestion: effect on sludge biodegradation and methane production. *Bioresource Technology* **101**, 2629–2636.

Dwyer J., Starrenburg D., Tait S., Barr K., Batstone D. J., Lant P. (2008) Decreasing activated sludge thermal hydrolysis temperature reduces product colour, without decreasing degradability. *Water Research* **42**, 4699–4709.

Eastman J. A., Ferguson J. F. (1981) Solubilization of particulate organic carbon during the acid phase of anaerobic digestion. *Journal of the Water Pollution Control Federation* **53**, 352–366.

Farrell J., Rose A. (1967) Temperature effects on microorganisms. *Annual Review of Microbiology* **21**, 101–120.

Fdz-Polanco F., Velazquez R., Pérez-Elvira S. I., Casas C., del Barrio D., Cantero F. J., Fdz-Polanco M., Rodriguez P., Panizo L., Serrat J. (2008) Continuous thermal hydrolysis and energy integration in sludge anaerobic digestion plants. *Water Science and Technology* **57**(8), 1221–1226.

Ferrer I., Ponsa S., Vazquez F., Font X. (2008) Increasing biogas production by thermal (70 degrees C) sludge pre-treatment prior to thermophilic anaerobic digestion. *Biochemical Engineering Journal* **42**(2), 186–192.

Ferrer I., Serrano E., Ponsa S., Vazquez F., Font X. (2009) Enhancement of thermophilic anaerobic sludge digestion by 70 degrees C pre-treatment: energy considerations. *Journal of Residuals Science and Technology* **6**(1), 11–18.

Fjærgaard T., Sander O. (2001) Five years' experience with the Cambi process at HIAS: In: Nordic Conference, Copenhagen, Denmark, January 17–19.

Gavala H. N., Yenal U., Skiadas I. V., Westermann P., Ahring B. K. (2003) Mesophilic and thermophilic anaerobic digestion of primary and secondary sludge: effect of pre-treatment at elevated temperature. *Water Research* **37**(19), 4561–4572.

Ge H. Q., Jensen P. D., Batstone D. J. (2010) Pre-treatment mechanisms during thermophilic-mesophilic temperature phased anaerobic digestion of primary sludge. *Water Research* **44**(1), 123–130.

Ge H., Jensen P., Batstone D. J. (2011a) Relative kinetics of anaerobic digestion under thermophilic and mesophilic conditions Water Science and Technology **64**(4), 848–853.

Ge H., Jensen P. D., Batstone D. J. (2011b) Increased temperature in the thermophilic stage in temperature phased anaerobic digestion (TPAD) improves degradability of waste activated sludge. *Journal of Hazardous Materials* **187**(1–3), 355–361.

Ge H., Jensen P. D., Batstone D. J. (2011c) Temperature phased anaerobic digestion increases apparent hydrolysis rate for waste activated sludge. *Water Research* 45(**4**), 1597–1606.

Graja S., Chauzy J., Fernandes P., Patria L., Cretenot D. (2005) Reduction of sludge production from WWTP using thermal pretreatment and enhanced anaerobic methanisation. *Water Science and Technology* **52**(1–2), 267–273.

Haug R., Stuckey D. C., Gossett J. M., McCarty P. L. (1978). Effect of thermal pre-treatment on digestibility and dewaterability of organic sludge. *Journal of the Water Pollution Control Federation* **50**(1), 73–85.

Haug R. T., Lebrun T. J., Tortorici L. D. (1983) Thermal pretreatment of sludges: a field demonstration. *Journal of the Water Pollution Control Federation* **55**(1), 23–34.

Kepp U., Machenbach I., Weisz N., Solheim OE. (2000) Enhanced stabilisation of sewage sludge through thermal hydrolysis: three years of experience with full scale plant. *Water Science and Technology* **42**(9), 89–96.

Kuroda A., Takiguchi N., Gotanda T., Nomura K., Kato J., Ikeda T., Ohtake H. (2002) A simple method to release polyphosphate from activated sludge for phosphorus reuse and recycling. *Biotechnology and Bioengineering* **78**(3), 333–338.

Lang N. L., Smith S. R. (2008) Time and temperature inactivation kinetics of enteric bacteria relevant to sewage sludge treatment processes for agricultural use. *Water Research* **42**(8–9), 2229–2241.

Layden N. M., Kelly H. G., Mavinic D. S., Moles R., Bartlett J. (2007) Autothermal thermophilic aerobic digestion (ATAD): II. Review of research and full-scale operating experiences. *Journal of Environmental Engineering and Science* **6**(6), 679–690.

Li Y. Y., Noike T. (1992) Upgrading of anaerobic-digestion of waste activated-sludge by thermal pretreatment. *Water Science and Technology* **26**(3–4), 857–866.

Lu J., Arhing B. K. (2008) Biological and thermal effects of thermophilic anaerobic pre-treatment on the hydrolysis of organic solids in sewage sludge. Unpublished results.

Lu J. Q., Gavala H. N., Skiadas I. V., Mladenovska Z., Ahring B. K. (2008) Improving anaerobic sewage sludge digestion by implementation of a hyper-thermophilic prehydro-lysis step. *Journal of Environmental Management* **88**(4), 881–889.

Marti N., Ferrer J., Seco A., Bouzas A. (2008) Optimisation of sludge line management to enhance phosphorus recovery in WWTP. *Water Research* **42**(18), 4609–4618.

Metcalf & Eddy, Inc. (2003) *Wastewater Engineering, Treatment and Reuse*, McGraw-Hill, New York.

Morgan J. W., Forster C. F., Evison L. (1990) A comparative-study of the nature of biopolymers extracted from anaerobic and activated sludges. *Water Research* **24**(6), 743–750.

Morse G. K., Brett S. W., Guy J. A., Lester J. N. (1998) Review: Phosphorus removal and recovery technologies. *Science of the Total Environment* **212**(1), 69–81.

Murillo M. (2004) Couplage d'un procédé d'oxydation et d'une boue activée pour la réduction de la production de boues. Toulouse University, INSA, Toulouse, France.

Neyens E., Baeyens J. (2003) A review of thermal sludge pre-treatment processes to improve dewaterability. *Journal of Hazardous Materials* **98**(1–3), 51–67.

Panter K., Kleiven H. (2005) Ten years experience of full scale thermal hydrolysis projects. In: 10th European Biosolids & Biowastes Conference, 13–16th November 2005, Wakefield, UK.

Paul E., Camacho P., Lefebvre D., Ginestet P. (2006a) Organic matter release in low temperature thermal treatment of biological sludge for reduction of excess sludge produc-tion. *Water Science and Technology* **54**(5), 59–68.

Paul E., Camacho P., Spérandio M., Ginestet P. (2006b) Technical and economical evaluation of a thermal, and two oxidative techniques for the reduction of excess sludge production. *Process Safety and Environmental Protection* **84**(B4), 247–252.

Perez Suarez S. (2009) Réduction de la production de boues par couplage d'une digestion aérobie thermophile et anaérobie. Toulouse University, INSA., Toulouse, France.

Pérez-Elvira S. I., Nieto Diez P. N., Fernandez-Polanco F. (2006) Sludge minimisation technologies. *Reviews in Environmental Science and Bio/Technology* **5**(4), 375–398.

Pickworth B., Adams J., Panter K., Solheim O. E. (2006) Maximising biogas in anaerobic digestion by using engine waste heat for thermal hydrolysis pre-treatment of sludge. *Water Science and Technology* **54**(5), 101–108.

Prorot A., Eskicioglu C., Droste R., Dagot C., Leprat P. (2008) Assessment of physiological state of microorganisms in activated sludge with flow cytometry: application for monitoring sludge production minimization. *Journal of Industrial Microbiology and Biotechnology* **35**(11), 1261–1268.

Ramirez I., Mottet A., Carrère H., Déléris S., Vedrenne F., Steyer J-P. (2009) Modified ADM1 disintegration/hydrolysis structures for modeling batch thermophilic anaerobic digestion of thermally pretreated waste activated sludge. *Water Research* **43**(14), 3479.

Richardson J. F., Coulson J. M., Harker J. H., Backhurst J. R. (2002) *Coulson and Richardson's Chemical Engineering: Particle Technology and Separation Processes*. Butterworth-Heinemann, Oxford. http://books.google.com.au/books?id=ottGCe1CDUoC.

Rosenberg B., Kemeny G., Switzer R. C., Hamilton T. C. (1971) Quantitative evidence for protein denaturation as the cause of thermal death. *Nature* **232**, 471–473.

Ross D., Shrive C., Chauvin D., Harnum D., Constantine T. (2010) The power of sludge maximizing energy recovery at the Woodward Avenue WWTP in Hamilton, Residuals and Biosolids 2010, Savannah International Trade and Convention Center Savannah, Georgia Conference: May 23–26, 2010 Ontario, Savannah, GA, May 23–26, pp. 1144–1152.

Sakai Y., Aoyagi T., Shiota N., Akashi A., Hasegawa S. (2000) Complete decomposition of biological waste sludge by thermophilic aerobic bacteria. *Water Science and Technology* **42**(9), 81–88.

Shechter E. (1992) *Biochimie et biophysique des membranes: aspects structuraux et fonctionnels*, Masson, Paris.

Stumm W., Morgan J. J. (1996) *Aquatic Chemistry: Chemical Equilibria and Rates in Natural Waters*. 3rd ed. Wiley-Interscience, New York.

Takiguchi N., Kishino M., Kuroda A., Kato J., Ohtake H. (2004) A laboratory-scale test of anaerobic digestion and methane production after phosphorus recovery from waste activated sludge. *Journal of Bioscience and Bioengineering* **97**(6), 365–368.

Tanaka S., Kobayashi T., Kamiyama K., Bildan M. (1997) Effects of thermochemical pretreatment on the anaerobic digestion of waste activated sludge. *Water Science and Technology* **35**(8), 209–215.

U.S. EPA (Environmental Protection Agency) (1999) *Environmental Regulations and Technology: Control of Pathogens and Vector Attraction in Sewage Sludge*, EPA/625/R-92/013, EPA, Washington, DC.

U.S. EPA (Environmental Protection Agency) (2002) *Biosolds Applied to Land: Advancing Standards and Practices*, EPA, Washington, DC.

Valo A., Carrère H., Delgenes J. P. (2004) Thermal, chemical and thermo-chemical pretreatment of waste activated sludge for anaerobic digestion. *Journal of Chemical Technology and Biotechnology* **79**(11), 1197–1203.

Wang Q., Noguchi C., Hara Y., Sharon C., Kakimoto K., Kato Y. (1997) Studies on anaerobic digestion mechanism: influence of pretreatment temperature on biodegradation of waste activated sludge. *Environmental Technology* **18**(10), 999–1008.

Wang W. H. M., Takeda N., Sakai S., Goto N., Okajima S. (1988) Solubilization of sludge solids in thermal pretreatment for anaerobic digestion. *Proc. Environ. Sanit. Eng. Res.*, **24**, 41–51.

Warth A. D. (1978). Relationship between the heat resistance of spores and the optimum and maximum growth temperatures of *Bacillus* species. *Journal of Bacteriology* **134**, 699–705.

Weemaes M. P. J., Verstraete W. H. (1998) Evaluation of current wet sludge disintegration techniques. *Journal of Chemical Technology and Biotechnology* **73**(2), 83–92.

Wilson C. A., Novak J. T. (2009) Hydrolysis of macromolecular components of primary and secondary wastewater sludge by thermal hydrolytic pretreatment. *Water Research* **43**(18), 4489–4498.

Xue T., Huang X. (2007) Releasing characteristics of phosphorus and other substances during thermal treatment of excess sludge. *Chinese Journal of Environmental Science* **19**, 1153–1158.

Yang X. Y., Wang X., Wang L. (2010) Transferring of components and energy output in industrial sewage sludge disposal by thermal pretreatment and two-phase anaerobic process. *Bioresource Technology* **101**(8), 2580–2584.

Zabranska J., Doháyos M., Jenicek P., Kutil J. (2006) Disintegration of excess activated sludge: evaluation and experience of full-scale applications. *Water Science and Technology* **53**(12), 229–236.

Zhang G. M., Zhang P. Y. (2008) Comparison of different methods for sludge lysis. *Research Journal of Chemistry and Environment* **12**(3), 12–17.

Zhang Z. C., Huang X., Yang H. J., Xiao K., Luo X., Sha H., Chen Y. M. (2009) Study on P forms in extracellular polymeric substances in enhanced biological phosphorus removal sludge by P-31-NMR spectroscopy. *Spectroscopy and Spectral Analysis* **29**(2), 536–539.

Zheng J., Kennedy K. J., Eskicioglu C. (2009) Effect of low temperature microwave pretreatment on characteristics and mesophilic digestion of primary sludge. *Environmental Technology* **30**(4), 319–327.

13

COMBUSTION, PYROLYSIS, AND GASIFICATION OF SEWAGE SLUDGE FOR ENERGY RECOVERY

YONG-QIANG LIU

Institute of Environmental Science and Engineering, Nanyang Technology University, Singapore

JOO-HWA TAY

Department of Environmental Science and Engineering, Fudan University, Shanghai, China

YU LIU

Division of Environmental and Water Resources Engineering, School of Civil and Environmental Engineering, Nanyang Technological University, Singapore

13.1 INTRODUCTION

With the increase in world population, urbanization, and more stringent wastewater discharge standards in wider areas, more and more wastewater treatment facilities will be needed. In present wastewater treatment plants, most soluble pollutants in wastewater are converted into biomass through complex biochemical reactions. Thus, excessive sludge accumulated in a wastewater treatment process must be handled, treated, and disposed of in a safe and effective manner. Generally, the costs of sewage sludge treatment often represent more than 50% of the total wastewater treatment costs.

The sewage sludge produced annually in the world is enormous: around 6.5 million metric tons of dry sludge was produced in the United States in 2003 (www.werf.org), 9.0 in Europe (Tarantini et al. 2007), and 2.0 in Japan (www.pwri.go.jp) in 2005,

Biological Sludge Minimization and Biomaterials/Bioenergy Recovery Technologies, First Edition.
Edited by Etienne Paul and Yu Liu.
© 2012 John Wiley & Sons, Inc. Published 2012 by John Wiley & Sons, Inc.

respectively. In many developing countries, however, the bulk of domestic and industrial wastewater is discharged without any treatment or after primary treatment only, and the sewage volume treated per capita is much lower than that of developed countries. The sewage sludge produced is thus lower. For example, the annual dry sludge production in China is 1.9 in 2003 and 2.9 million metric tons in 2007, although the population of town and city reached 0.6 billion (Yu et al. 2007; Wang et al. 2010). However, with the rapid urbanization and stricter discharge standards of wastewater, wastewater treatment coverage will definitely be extended, and the amount of annual dry sludge production in China will increase substantially in the near future. A similar situation can be expected in other developing and developed countries.

Several methods for sludge treatment and disposal have been developed, such as sludge dumping into sea, use of sludge as fertilizer, sludge disposal to landfills, anaerobic digestion, and thermal treatment of sludge. With the increased ecological awareness, sludge dumping into the sea has been forbidden in almost all countries, whereas utilization of sludge as fertilizer has been debated for years due to concern regarding contaminants, especially heavy metals in sludge. It is likely that utilization of sludge for agriculture will be phased out completely in the future. Disposal of sewage sludge to landfills has been practiced worldwide (Werthera and Ogadab 1999). However, it may cause serious environmental problems, such as emissions of odor, methane and leachate, and underground water contamination.

Alternative methods have been sought for sludge management, among which thermal treatment of sludge for reduction of sludge volume and heat recovery is the most promising and attractive method for future sludge disposal. According to the European Waste Management Policy of Sustainable Development, the waste management priorities should be in the order minimization, recycling, incineration with energy recovery, and landfilling (Davis 1996). In addition to incineration of sludge, other thermal treatment technologies (e.g., pyrolysis and gasification for both heat and fuel recovery) have also been developed (Fytili and Zabaniotou 2008). Therefore, in this chapter we provide general insights into current thermal treatment technologies for sludge with a focus on energy recovery.

13.2 CHARACTERISTICS AND DEWATERING OF SEWAGE SLUDGE

According to the U.S. Environmental Protection Agency (EPA), sewage sludge includes solids, semisolids, or liquid residue generated by the processes of domestic treatment works. Sewage sludge is a heterogeneous medium consisting largely of water (>90%) and solids (<10%) (Amuda et al., 2008). To treat sludge effectively and efficiently, sludge composition needs to be determined, as it is related to potential gas emission and the quality of products. According to Rulkens and Bien (2004), sludge composition is characterized by five groups of components:

- Nontoxic organic carbon compounds, Kjeldahl-N, phosphorus-containing components

TABLE 13.1 Elemental Dry Composition of Biologically Stabilized Sewage Sludge[a]

	Sludge 1	Sludge 2	Sludge 3	Sludge 4
Component (wt %)				
C	40.57	29.75	39.48	39.48
H	5.36	4.12	6.19	5.91
O	23.50	18.35	25.46	16.54
N	4.50	3.55	3.93	4.51
S	1.20	1.32	1.45	2.56
Ash	24.83	42.83	23.51	31.00
Heating value (MJ kg^{-1})	15.10	7.56	12.00	17.43

[a] Sludge 1, world (average) (Werle and Wilk 2010); sludge 2, Bialystok (POL) (Werle and Wilk 2010); sludge 3, Turkey (Dogru et al. 2002) sludge 4, Singapore.

- Toxic pollutants, such as heavy metals, polychlorinated biphenyls, polycyclic aromatic hydrocarbons, dioxins, pesticides, endocrine disrupters, linear alkyl-sulfonates, and nonylphenoles
- Pathogens and other microbiological pollutants
- Inorganic compounds, such as silicates, aluminates, calcium, and magnesium
- Water content

Table 13.1 shows the ultimate analysis of stabilized sewage sludge from different countries. It appears that all sludge has a high ash content, which needs to be disposed of after thermal treatment and energy recovery. In addition, nitrogen and sulfur in sludge affect negatively the quality of gases emitted after thermal treatment.

The metals in ash are harmful to the environment and human health if they are not managed or disposed of properly, especially toxic heavy metals such as arsenic, mercury, and lead. Sewage sludge contains a large quantity of water, generally higher than 95%. As such, dewatering of sludge is essential for further handling. For composting, landfilling, or thermal treatment, the moisture content of sludge should be reduced to at least 50 to 60%. A big challenge is how to reduce the water content cost effectively. According to Vesilind (1994) and Carberry et al. (1983), water in sludge can be classified into the following five categories:

- Free water: water not associated with solid particles
- Interstitial water: water trapped inside crevices and interstitial spaces of flocs and organisms
- Surface (or vicinal) water: water held onto the surface of solid particles by adsorption and adhesion
- Hydration water
- Water trapped in the polymeric matrix

Carberry et al. (1983) reported a quantitative water distribution for concentrated sludge, indicating that 70% of the total water was interstitial water, 22% was surface and capillary water, and 8% was cellular water. However, it is still difficult to identify the most suitable dewatering technology for sludge. Direct thermal drying (evaporative processes) can result in a nearly entirely dry sludge, while the energy input is high. Compared with thermal dewatering of sludge, a mechanical method is often selected first, due to its low energy requirement (Vaxelaire et al. 1999). Generally, mechanical dewatering can remove about 15 to 30% of water from sludge with a water content of 95%, because only free water is removed (Wang et al. 2010). For other types of water (e.g., bound water) removal, energy consumption was high, which is one of the main limiting factors in practical dewatering of sludge.

One way to improve the dewaterability of sludge is to change the sludge structure and release more bound water. Several methods for improving sludge dewaterability have been developed so far.

1. Chemical pretreatment using polymer or inorganic coagulant (Wu et al. 1997; Chu and Lee 1999; Arvand et al. 2010). The free water amount can be increased by the addition of some chemical conditioners, although the reason behind is still unclear. The overdose of chemical conditioners, however, could increase the bound water content. The selection of chemicals is dependent on the device used for dewatering and on the nature of the sludge (Marinetti et al. 2009).

2. Mechanical disintegration using ultrasound, mills, homogenizers, magnetic fields (Eichholz et al. 2008), electric fields (Hwang and Min 2003; Mahmoud et al. 2010), and others, where the necessary energy is provided as pressure, translational, or rotational energy (Neyens and Baeyens 2003; Yin et al. 2004).

3. Freezing and thawing. By alternately freezing and thawing activated sludge, the floc structure will be changed irreversibly into a more compact form, the bound water content will be reduced, and therefore the sludge dewaterability can be improved significantly (Hellstrom and Kvarnstrom 1997; Kawasaki et al. 2004).

4. Biological hydrolysis with or without enzyme addition (Thomas et al. 1993; Guellil et al. 2001). The enzymatic lysis cracks the compounds of the cell wall by an enzyme-catalyzed reaction. Autolytic processes with or without addition of external enzymes can be employed at ambient temperature (Neyens and Baeyens 2003).

5. Thermal or hydrothermal pretreatment in the temperature range from 40 to 180°C (Barjenbruch et al. 1999; Kepp et al. 2000; Wang et al. 2010). It can effectively break down the sludge gel network and decrease the water affinity of the sludge solid for easier dewatering. The cell wall could also be destroyed by thermal treatment, and protein would be degraded as easy as carbohydrate and lipid.

13.3 ENERGY RECOVERY FROM SLUDGE

13.3.1 Incineration

Incineration of sludge is aimed at a complete oxidation of organic sludge compounds at high temperature (Braguglia et al. 2003), which has been commonly used as an energy recovery and waste minimization method in highly populated municipalities (e.g., about 70% of sewage sludge is incinerated in Japan) (Murakami et al. 2009). The incineration process is a natural extension of the drying process, converting the sludge through combustion into an inert ash (Paul 1994). Combustion is a rapid chemical reaction with oxygen and fuel producing light and liberating large quantities of heat. The combustion occurs only above the ignition temperature, while oxidation takes place at any temperature. The sludge incineration system usually contains a dewatering device, such as a vacuum filter, centrifuge, or belt press; an incinerator (e.g., a multiple-hearth furnace or fluidized bed); a sludge feeding system; an ash-handling system, and air pollution and other control devices (U.S. EPA 1978).

Effects of Sludge Moisture Sludge dewatering has a significant impact on subsequent sludge incineration. Sludge with a high water content requires more energy to dry off the moisture, leading to a low combustion efficiency. Often-used mechanical dewatering devices, such as vacuum filters, centrifuges, and belt presses normally help to reduce the water content of sewage sludge to about 80%. At this moisture content, sludge cannot be autocombusted. The supplementary fuel must be supplied to further reduce the sludge water content. The quantity of the supplementary fuel required depends on the moisture content, type of sludge, and temperature of the combustion air. It has been reported that for wet sludge with 20 to 25 wt% dry content, around 100 to 200 kg oil per ton of dry sludge is required if the combustion air is preheated to about 450°C. In contrast, 200 to 400 kg oil per ton of dry sludge is needed if the combustion air is not preheated (Werthera and Ogadab 1999). Moreover, the evaporated water results in an increased quantity of flue gas, which in turn affects the sizes of the flue gas treatment and handling equipment. The moisture content of sludge is also an important design parameter, especially for dimensioning the combustion chamber, whereby for a good operation, an evaporation capacity falls into the range 300 to 800 kg steam per hour per square meter of the cross section of the combustor's grate (Muhlhaus 1991). These seem to suggest that the moisture content of sewage sludge needs to be reduced in order to mitigate the aforementioned disadvantages.

During the drying process, the sewage sludge experiences an important physical change in terms of fluidity. When the dry solids content in sewage sludge is low, the sludge is free-flowing and can easily be spread onto a heated tube. However, sludge becomes pasty when dry solids in sludge increase to around 60 to 65% by further drying. Beyond 60 to 65% dry solids, sludge becomes crumbly in nature and mixes freely (Werthera and Ogadab 1999). Therefore, it is impossible to dry sewage sludge completely in a single unit because of the sticky zone it has to pass through. Generally, the predried sludge is mixed with the dewatered cake in a certain ratio so as to achieve a solids content beyond the sticky phase.

Incinerator Type The most used sludge incinerators so far are the multiple-hearth (MH) furnace or fluidized-bed (FB) furnace, while other types of incinerators are also available, including rotary kilns, electric furnaces, cyclones, or smelting furnaces. Compared to multiple-hearth units, fluidized-bed furnaces are known to have fewer

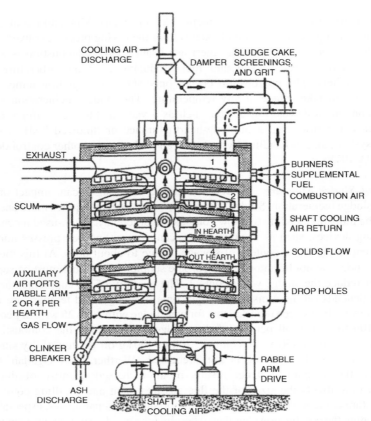

FIGURE 13.1 Cross section of multiple-hearth sludge incinerator. (U.S. EPA 1979.)

problems with emissions because of more uniform combustion of biosolids. The first multiple-hearth furnace for sludge incineration was built in 1935 in Dearborn, Michigan. From then until the late 1960s, the multiple-hearth furnace had been the main technique choice for sludge thermal disposal. In 1962, the first sludge multiple-hearth furnace type of incinerator was built in Europe (Werthera and Ogadab 1999), adapted primarily from U.S. furnaces. Nowadays, hundreds of aging or upgraded multiple-hearth furnaces are still in operation.

A cross-sectional diagram of a typical multiple-hearth incinerator is shown in Fig. 13.1. Four to 12 horizontal hearths are enclosed in a vertical cylindrical refractory-lined steel shell furnace. A rotating shaft with rabble arms cantilevered out over each hearth for sweeping sludge in each hearth is mounted in the center of the furnace. Cooling air is introduced into the shaft from the bottom. Sludge enters the top hearth and flows downward through the annular space between the hearth and the center shaft. The retention time of the sludge in the multiple–hearth incinerator ranges from 0.5 to 3 h.

Basically, a multiple-hearth furnace could be divided into three zones (Dangtran et al. 2000). The upper hearths comprise the drying zone, in which sludge moisture and some organic volatiles are evaporated. The heat for sludge drying is mainly from the sludge combustion in the second zone in combination with energy from burners mounted on most hearths. The temperature in this zone is typically in the range 430 to 540°C. The second zone is composed of middle hearths, which is the combustion zone (or pyrolysis). The temperature in this zone is typically from 820 to 1000°C. The lower hearths form the cooling zone, in which the formed ash is cooled by the combustion air introduced with a countercurrent flow for energy recovery and easy ash handling. Temperature in this zone ranges from 180 to 200°C.

A multiple-hearth furnace has the advantage of good internal energy usage because the hot flue gas comes directly into contact with the sludge (Dangtran et al. 2000). However, the multiple-hearth furnace is sensitive to the change in feed sludge and satisfactory performance can only be obtained with the stable feed rate and moisture content. A multiple-hearth furnace is used primarily to treat wet sludge with a dry solids content of around 20% after mechanical dewatering. Sludge drying is conducted in the upper zone of the incinerator, and the auxiliary fuel is thus necessary in most cases for a multiple-hearth furnace because the heating value of wet sludge is too low to be self-combusted. The cost of auxiliary fuel is an important factor affecting the use of multiple-hearth furnaces. Another important factor influencing the choice of multiple-hearth furnace is the gaseous emission from the incinerator. It appears from Table 13.2 that the pollutant emission limits for an existing multiple-hearth furnace is much higher than that of existing fluidized-bed incinerators, due to the technical constraints of the multiple-hearth furnace itself. However, for new multiple-hearth and fluidized-bed furnaces, the same pollutant emission limits were proposed by the EPA.

TABLE 13.2 Proposed Emission Limits for Both Existing and New Sewage Sludge Incinerators by the EPA in 2010

Pollutant (units)	Existing MH Incinerators	Existing FB Incinerators	New MH and FB Incinerators
Cadmium (mg/dscm)	0.095	0.0019	0.00051
Mercury (mg/dscm)	0.02	0.0033	0.0010
Lead (mg/dscm)	0.3	0.0098	0.00053
Carbon monoxide (ppmvd)	3900	56	7.4
Hydrogen chloride (ppmvd)	1.0	0.49	0.12
Nitrogen oxides (ppmvd)	210	63	26
Sulfur dioxide (ppmvd)	26	22	2.0
Particular matter (mg/dscm)	80	12	4.1
Dioxins and furans			
Toxic equivalency (ng/dscm)	0.32	0.056	0.024
Total mass (ng/dscm)	5.0	0.61	0.0022
Opacity (%)	10	0	0

Source: www.epa.gov/ttn/oarpg/t3/fr_notices/ssi_atec_093010.pdf.

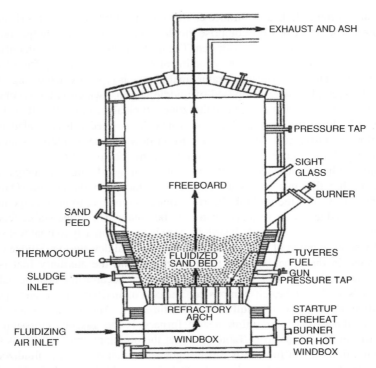

FIGURE 13.2 Cross section of a fludized-bed sludge incinerator. [From U.S. EPA (1979).]

In the 1970s, the fluidized-bed furnace became the preferred technique choice for sludge incineration, primarily because of tighter emission regulations and the increasing cost of auxiliary fuel. The Lynwood, Washington, wastewater treatment plant installed the first fluidized bed for sludge incineration in 1962. Since then, the application of fluidized-bed furnaces has been increasing rapidly.

There are two types of fluidized-bed incinerators: bubbling fluidized bed (BFB) and circulating fluidized bed (CFB). Figure 13.2 shows the cross section of a typical bubbling fluidized-bed sludge incinerator, which is composed of four parts (Dangtran et al. 2000). The lower part, called a *windbox*, is used to receive combustion air, and air can go in the fluidized sand bed through the refractory arch distributor. The air is distributed homogeneously across the bed by alloy tuyeres or nozzles on the refractory arch distributor. The arch separates the bed from the windbox. The third part above the refractory arch distributor is the main body of the incinerator (i.e., the bed area), in which combustion occurs. Sand is a fluidizing medium, which also enhances heat transfer to create the uniform temperature distribution in the bed. The part above the bed is called the *freeboard* or *disengagement zone*. It is typically 4.5 m high and usually is expanded laterally along its height to maximize residence time and to reduce sand use while the height of the fluidized sand bed is typically 1 m. The freeboard can provide a gas residence time of 6 to 7 s, in which the combustion of any volatile hydrocarbons escaping from the bed can be completed; thus, it indeed acts as an afterburner.

In a fluidized-bed incinerator, one of the most important operational parameters is the superficial air velocity. If the superficial air velocity is too high, the sludge fed will float to the top of the freeboard. Otherwise, sand cannot be fluidized enough for uniform mixing and heat transfer. Normally, the superficial air velocity at the bottom of the bed of a BFB is controlled at 0.5 to 1 m s^{-1} (U.S. EPA 1979).

CFB is the latest fluidized-bed type for sludge incineration due to more uniform temperature in the furnace and a lower temperature for combustion. Compared with a BFB, a CFB has a much smaller diameter and higher height-to-diameter ratio, which can create higher superficial air velocity in the bed. Typically, superficial air velocity in CFB can reach 4 to 6m s^{-1}. The sand medium, air, and sludge are thus in an intensified turbulent state, which allows the height of combustion zone to be raised, resulting in improved combustion efficiency and reduced excess air ratio for combustion. In CFB combustion, sand or other bed materials and unburned char are carried out from the furnace by high superficial air velocity to the cyclone, which is connected to the furnace. The solid part would be circulated into the furnace for the second combustion or supply of bed materials. The circulation of materials from cyclone to furnace is a feature of a CFB and makes it different from a BFB. CFBs are becoming popular, and more and more CFBs have been built.

The basic design concept for multiple-hearth and fluidized-bed incinerators is different. For a multiple-hearth incinerator, the design is based on the sludge drying, combustion, and cooling, while the design of a fluidized-bed combustor is based on intense mixing, excellent heat transfer, short sludge detention time, long detention of gases, moderate combustion temperature, and low excess air (Dangtran et al. 2000). Due to such differences in design, a fluidized-bed combustor has the following advantages over multiple-hearth incinerators (Dangtran et al. 2000):

- Lower NO$_x$ formation due to a typical combustion temperature of 850°C for fixed-bed and 950°C for multiple-hearth combustors
- Lower CO formation
- Lower total hydrocarbon formation
- Suitable for intermittent operation
- Feed variability and avoidance of thermal shock
- Easy control and automation
- Lower auxiliary fuel use
- Reduced maintenance cost
- A smaller gas treatment system

However, a fluidized-bed incinerator also has some drawbacks compared with multiple hearth incinerators: high power requirements, harder ash removal from the flue gas, sand requirements, and higher ash disposal costs (Dangtran et al. 2000).

Pollutants from Incineration System

Formation of NO_x and N_2O   Sewage sludge contains large quantities of nitrogen and phosphorus. Normally, the nitrogen content in sewage sludge is around 6 to 8% by weight. During combustion, nitrogen is converted to NO_x (NO and NO_2) and N_2O. NO_x is a type of ozone-depleting chemical (Crutzen 1970), while N_2O is known as a greenhouse gas. Apart from ozone destruction and global warming, NO_x and N_2O are also harmful to human health.

Sewage sludge also contains ash, which can be as high as 30 to 40% in some cases. The metal oxide, such as iron oxide, calcium oxide, and magnesium oxide, in sludge ash could influence NO_x and N_2O production positively or negatively. It has been speculated that a lower NO_x and N_2O ratio from sewage sludge combustion than from coal combustion may be attributed to the high contents of CaO and Fe_2O_3 in sewage sludge, which are effective in the reduction of NO_x and N_2O (Werthera and Ogadab, 1999). However, several studies showed that the accumulation of sludge ash would significantly increase NO_x emission in both a bubbling fluidized-bed combustor and a circulating fluidized-bed combustor in a manner similar to coal combustion (Shimizu and Toyono, 2007, Shimizu et al. 2007). The pretreatment of sewage sludge, the excess air ratio of combustor, and the combustion temperature may also influence NO_x and N_2O emissions. Increasing excess air ratio and combustion temperature may lead to high NO_x and N_2O emissions. That is the reason that a fluidized-bed combustor can reduce NO_x and N_2O emission compared with a multiple-hearth combustor due to the higher combustion temperature and excess air ratio in multiple-hearth combustor. The reduced air-to-sewage sludge ratio in a large-scale sewage sludge fluidized-bed combustor also produces less nitrous oxide (Korving et al. 2010).

Ash and Heavy Metal   The ash produced from incinerator includes bottom ash and fly ash, which are mainly noncombustible residues of sludge. Bottom ash accumulates in the incinerator and might form clinkers. They could be discharged from the bottom of the incinerator. Fly ash typically consists of fine particles and can escape with exhaust gas. The particulate matters in exhaust gas from an incinerator needs to be lower than a certain value (Table 13.2) to meet the environmental requirements. The capture of fly ash from exhaust gas is thus necessary. Venturi scrubbers, ionizing wet scrubbers, and electrostatic precipitators are conventional ash removal devices (Lee and Chun 1993). It was reported that a combined venturi scrubber and electrostatic precipitator resulted in almost one order of magnitude of increase in particulate removal compared to a venturi scrubber alone (Myer et al. 2007).

Compositions of incinerated ash from sewage sludge include mainly inorganic metal compounds (Sizawa 1999; Japan Sewage Works Association 2001), which are similar to those found in clay. Therefore, incinerated sludge ash has a potential use in such construction products as concrete, ceramic materials, cement, fine aggregate for concrete products, and the manufacture of synthetic coarse aggregate. In addition, the existence of nutrients such as phosphorus, calcium, potassium, and magnesium in sludge ash implies that sludge ash can be used as fertilizer for farmland. However, incinerated sludge ash also contains hazardous heavy metals that could be released. This limits the application of incinerated sludge ash if no pretreatment is conducted to stabilize or reduce heavy metals in ash. The poisoning effect of heavy metals has been well documented (Amer 2002; Reijinders 2005). Heavy metals in sewage sludge often exist in the form of hydroxides, carbonates, phosphate, silicates, and sulfates (Ødegaard et al. 2002). At the high combustion temperature in the incinerator, most of the heavy metal compounds are vaporized, but they can be condensed on the surface of the ash particles in the cooler part of the steam evaporator and subsequently removed with the ash (Hirth et al. 1990). The heavy metals in ash may be aqueous leaching to give rise to environmental pollution again. Several possible solutions to immobilize heavy metals have been proposed (Hirth et al. 1990). In addition, forced extraction of heavy metals in ash has been advocated as a contribution to the supply of metals and to leaching (Nugteren et al. 2001; Amer 2002; Pedersen et al. 2003; Shen and Forssberg, 2003).

Dioxins and Furans　The term *dioxins* and *furans* refer to a class of compounds of 75 chlorinated dibenzo-*p*-dioxins (PCDDs) and 135 chlorinated digenzofurans (PCDFs) substituted with one to eight chlorine atoms (Liem and van Zorge 1995). They are also called PCDD/Fs. PCDD/Fs are the most toxic and stable by-products from incineration and can cause human diseases related with immune, nervous, endocrine, reproductive, carcinogenic, and mutagenic potential (Yazawa et al. 1999; Tan et al. 2001). Many countries have thus set the emission standards of PCDD/Fs in the last decades (U.S. EPA 1996; Mohr et al. 1998; Tuppurainen et al. 2003). Intensive investigation has been conducted on the formation mechanisms of PCDD/Fs and the reduction of PCDD/Fs. Although the specific formation mechanism of PCDD/Fs is not very clear, it is generally speculated that PCDD/Fs are formed through the following possible routes (Werthera and Ogadab 1999; Lin and Chang 2008):

- Formation due to incomplete destruction in the combustion chamber of compounds containing PCDD/Fs
- Formation from the chlorine compounds (e.g., chlorophenols, chlorobenzenes, or polychlorinated diphenyl ethers)
- Decomposition/cleavage reaction of polycyclic aromatic compounds
- Reformation of PCDD/Fs from inorganic chlorine compounds and organic compounds: de novo synthesis

For waste incineration it is believed that compositions and properties of waste, incinerator design, and operational parameters influence the formation and emission of PCDD/Fs. Temperature is one of the most important parameters that influence the formation of PCDD/Fs. Based on the postulated formation mechanisms, PCDD/Fs could be formed in two temperature ranges: 500 to 800°C by a "homogeneous" route and 200 to 400°C by a "heterogeneous" route (Stanmore 2004). Dioxins and furans could be destroyed completely at temperatures above 800°C; thus, the combustion temperature is recommended to be higher than this critical value. However, the temperature range in off-gas treatment systems, including fabric filters, electrostatic precipitators, and waste heat recovery boilers, is generally low, which may lead to the formation of PCDD/Fs. Metallic compounds in ash, such as copper chloride, oxide and sulfate, and oxides of iron, zinc, nickel, and aluminum, have been reported as catalysts for PCDD/Fs formation (Kilgroc 1996). It appears that the removal of ash at higher temperature favors the reduction of PCDD/Fs formed. Chlorine also affects significantly the formation of PCDD/Fs through the route of de novo synthesis as a reactant (Kuzuhara et al. 2003; Wikström et al. 2003; Ryu et al. 2004). The higher chlorine content may result in the higher emission of PCDD/Fs (Chang 1996; Huotari and Vesterinen 1996). The presence of sulfur or nitrogen compounds, such as sulfur dioxide and urea, could poison the catalysts for PCDD/Fs formation and thus reduce the emission of PCDD/Fs (Stanmore 2004; Shao et al. 2010). It has been reported that increasing the S/Cl ratio could reduce the concentration of PCDD/Fs (Geiger et al. 1992). To control the PCDD/F concentration in flue gas, several strategies have been proposed (Buekens and Huang 1998). The best way is to prevent or reduce the formation of PCDD/F during the combustion or in an off-gas treatment system. To reduce the PCDD/F formed in flue gas, adsorption by activated carbon has been applied and considered as the most effective technique (Lin and Chang 2008). Another promising technique is the catalytic oxidation of PCDD/Fs using oxidation or reduction catalysts (Buekens and Huang 1998; Bonte et al. 2002; Goemans et al. 2004). For PCDD/Fs in fly ash, thermal treatment of ash at 600°C or chemical treatment by catalyzed decomposition of PCDD/F had been reported (Buekens and Huang 1998).

13.3.2   Pyrolysis and Gasification

Since incineration produces a large amount of flue gas and ash containing PCDD/F, heavy metal, NO_x, SO_2, and so on, there is a great environmental concern about the incinerator, and more stringent emission standards have been implemented. This unavoidably increases the cost of an off-gas cleaning system of incineration, further to the entire incineration system. Furthermore, public acceptance is of another concern about pollutant emission from the incineration process. Therefore, alternative technologies are needed to improve the thermal conversion process. Pyrolysis and gasification, called advanced thermal technologies, have been developed and widely applied for reducing the quantity of ash and flue gas volume as well as recovering energy.

Pyrolysis is a thermal process to break down organic waste at high temperature and converts organics to solid, liquid, and gas in the absence of oxygen. To differentiate pyrolysis from incineration, no visible flame is essential for pyrolysis. Gasification is another thermal process in which organic waste is exposed to some oxygen, but not enough for combustion to occur. Gasification produces hydrogen, carbon monoxide, carbon dioxide, and water by partial combustion. Gasification also produces hydrocarbons, particularly in the lower–temperature ranges in fluidized-bed reactors. The amounts of solid, liquid, and gaseous fractions formed from the thermal processes are markedly dependent on the process variables, as are the distribution of products within each solid, liquid, and gas phase produced. Compared with incineration, pyrolysis and gasification can produce more useful products (e.g., gas, oil, and solid char) as fuels and feedstock for petrochemicals and other applications. Energy generation by syngas from pyrolysis and gasification is more efficient than that by steam turbine used in incineration. In addition, the low temperature of pyrolysis can help to eliminate the formation of SO_2 and NO_x (Kaminsky and Ying 1993; Caballero et al. 1997), and the second emission is less than incineration, especially when melting technology is used. It should be noted that there are limited large-scale facilities on sludge pyrolysis and gasification so far. Capital and operating costs are the main concerns for its application. Most works still focuse on process understanding or demonstration of a specific pyrolysis or gasification technology. Further investigation on sludge pyrolysis and gasification is strongly needed for successful large-scale commercial implementation.

Pyrolysis Pyrolysis technology can be classified into slow pyrolysis and fast pyrolysis (flash pyrolysis). Slow pyrolysis occurs in a vapor residence time of 5 to 30 min (Bridgwater 1994, 1990; Bridgwater et al. 2001); which has been used in the production of charcoal for centuries (Mohan et al. 2006). The heating rate in slow pyrolysis is typically much slower than that in fast pyrolysis. Fast pyrolysis takes place within a vapor residence time of 2 s and thus requires good heat transfer in the reactor and continuous or frequent char removal. Due to the long residence time of vapor in the slow pyrolysis process, the components in the vapor phase continue to react with each other as the solid char and liquid are being formed. However, for fast pyrolysis, the rapid heating rate, rapid vapor removal and rapid condensation of vapor are unfavorable to the breakdown of higher-molecular-weight species into the gaseous products and thus produce the maximum liquid fraction. According to Bridgwater (2003), fast pyrolysis has four important features: (1) very high heating and heat transfer rates are used, which usually require a finely ground biomass feed; (2) pyrolysis reaction is controlled at around 500°C and vapor-phase temperature at 425 to 500°C; (3) vapor residence time is typically less than 2 s; and (4) pyrolysis vapors are cooled rapidly to produce bio-oil. Pyrolysis is the first step in the combustion and gasification processes, followed by total or partial oxidation of the primary products (Bridgwater 2003). A lower process temperature and longer vapor residence time favor charcoal production. A higher temperature and longer residence time enhance biomass conversion to gas, whereas moderate temperature and short vapor residence time may lead to the production of liquids. All pyrolysis products indeed have commercial values. For example, the pyrolysis char and gases can be used as a potential fuel, while oil can serve as a fuel and a useful chemical material. For the design of a fast pyrolysis system, such parameters as feed, drying, particle size, pretreatment, reactor configuration, heat supply, heat transfer, heating rates, reaction temperature, vapor residence time, secondary cracking, char separation, ash separation, and liquid collection all need to be considered (Bridgwater 1999). It should be noted that the liquid product from pyrolysis can be easily stored and transported, while heat recovered from incineration or syngas from gasification need to be used on site for further energy production.

Since the 1980s, extensive research has been carried out to investigate the conversion of sewage sludge to bio-oil through pyrolysis, which is considered a promising technology for sludge disposal (Piskorz et al. 1986; Stammbach et al. 1989; Caballero et al. 1997; Conesa et al. 1998; Silveira et al. 2002; Shen and Zhang 2003). The yield, quality, and stability of bio-oil produced from sludge pyrolysis are closely related to characteristics of sludge, sludge size, pretreatment of sludge, ash content, reactor type and configuration, feed rate, heating rate, pyrolysis temperature, and vapor residence time. For both slow and fast pyrolysis, char and oil yields are much higher than gas yield, which is normally lower than 20% (Inguanzo et al. 2002; sáncheza et al. 2009; Park et al. 2010). The ash content of sludge has an obvious effect on sludge pyrolysis (i.e., the high ash content of sludge may result in a high gas yield but low oil and char yields) (Fonts et al. 2009a). The pyrolysis product distribution and oil properties are also related to sludge source (e.g., the higher volatile content of sludge may lead to a higher liquid yield) (Fonts et al. 2009a,b). With the increase of final pyrolysis temperature, the char yield decreases and the gas yield increases), while the liquid yield remains nearly unchanged (Inguanzo et al. 2002; Sáncheza et al. 2009). In addition, improved oil yield was observed when the reported temperature was increased from 300°C to 500°C (Kim and Parker 2008). However, some studies showed that the heating rate is important only at low final pyrolysis temperature and had no significant effect on the oil yield at temperatures higher than 650°C (Inguanzo et al. 2002). The smaller or larger feed size affects oil production adversely (Sancheza et al. 2009). It was also found that metal oxide catalysts (e.g., CaO, La_2O_3) would cause increased water content and chlorine removal from bio-oil (Sancheza et al. 2009).

Gasification   Gasification is a partial oxidation process conducted with different gasifying agents, such as air, oxygen, and steam, which may produce gases with different heating values (Bridgwater 2003). If air is used for gasification, the product is a mixture of CO, CO_2, H_2, CH_4, N_2 and tar which has a low heating value of about 5 MJ m^{-3}, leading to difficulty in combustion, particularly in a gas turbine. If oxygen is used as a gasifying agent, N_2 is absent from the gas product, and the heating value of mixed gases can reach a heating value of about 10 to 12 MJ m^{-3}. Although the use of oxygen as a gasifying agent is costly compared to air, a better-quality fuel gas can compensate for such extra cost. Use of steam as a gasifying agent probably makes changes to the ratio of components in the gas phase, and in turn maximizes the methane and hydrocarbon contents in the mixed gas. As the result, the heating value of a mixed gas can be as high as 15 to 20 MJ m^{-3}. During gasification, evaporation of moisture in feedstock is the first step, followed by pyrolysis for the production of gas, vaporized tars or oils, and solid char residue (Bridgwater 2003). Subsequently, the solid char, pyrolysis tars, and pyrolysis gases are gasified or partially oxidized. In general, pyrolysis proceeds faster than gasification (i.e., the latter is the rate-controlling step of the entire process). Since the liquid products from pyrolysis cannot be fully utilized, the residual tar exists in the final gas product. This leads to some serious problems and much research work has focused on the tar cracking or removal in gas cleanup. As temperature for gasification is often higher than that for pyrolysis, the tar produced in gasification tends to be refractory and difficult to remove by thermal, catalytic, or physical treatment. It should be noted that tar is a considerable technical barrier for gasification. Different types of gasifier reactors or processes have an impact on the quality of the gas product. Fixed and fluidized-bed reactors have been widely adopted for gasification. A circulating fluidized-bed gasifier is preferable for large-scale application, while a bubbling fluidized-bed gasifier is competitive at medium scale, and a downdraft fixed-bed gasifier is most suitable for small-scale applications (Bridgwater 2003).

Like pyrolysis, operational conditions can affect the gasification and gas product quality. The syngas with the higher hydrogen and lower carbon dioxide contents has the higher heating value. Optimization of operational conditions is thus essential for minimizing the yield of carbon dioxide and maximizing the syngas yield. Temperature is one of the most important operational parameters for syngas production. Higher temperature contributed to higher hydrogen production and syngas yield (Li et al. 2009) (e.g., the hydrogen yield at 1000°C was found to be 0.076 g gas g^{-1} sample; Nipattummakul et al. 2010). Moreover, it was shown that increased syngas production and H_2 content with increasing temperature was accompanied by lowered tar and char yield and reduced amounts of CO and CH_4 in the syngas (Wei et al. 2007). Steam as a gasifying agent can improve syngas quality and yield, and the optimal ratio of steam to base material was found to be 1.33 (Li et al. 2009). Compared with air as a gasifying agent, the use of steam can increase the hydrogen yield threefold under similar operational conditions (Nipattummakul et al. 2010). Syngas production is also related to feedstock size (e.g., increased dry syngas yield, hydrogen yield, and carbon conversion efficiency were achieved with small feedstock particles; Luo et al. 2009). One of the main issues in sludge gasification is the formation of tar (Manyà et al. 2005). Tar is a complex mixture of condensable hydrocarbons, including single- and multiple-ring aromatic compounds, along with other oxygen-containing hydrocarbons and complex polycyclic aromatic hydrocarbons (Simell and Bredenberg 1990; Devi et al. 2005). These organic impurities can cause clogging of pipelines, filters, and engines. For elimination of tar, catalysts have been used in gasification. de Andrés et al. (2011) reported that dolomite has the highest efficiency in tar elimination, followed by alumina and olivine. In addition to tar control, the use of catalysts can also increase the H_2 content in the gases by nearly 60%. K_2CO_3, CaO, NiO, and Fe_2O_3 had also reported to be capable of enhancing the steam gasification rate and carbon conversion (Zhu et al. 2008).

13.3.3 Wet Oxidation

Wet oxidation in the aqueous phase at a high temperature and high pressure is useful for the treatment of sewage sludge (Mishra et al. 1995). The high pressure is essential for preventing boiling at the high temperatures required for wet oxidation. Dissolved oxygen in water oxidized organics in sludge (e.g., carbohydrates, proteins, lipids, and fibers) to simple and soluble organic compounds, such as sugars, amino acids, and fatty acids, finally, to easily biodegradable oxygenated products, carbon dioxide, inorganic salts, and water after complete oxidation (Bernardi et al. 2010). Depending on the temperature and pressure used, wet oxidation is classified into two types: subcritical and supercritical wet oxidation. Subcritical wet oxidation takes place at subcritical conditions of below 374°C and a pressure of 10 MPa, while supercritical wet oxidation occurs at a temperature and pressure above the supercritical point of water (374°C and 22.1 MPa) (Werthera and Ogadab 1999; Rulkens 2008). Subcritical conditions can be achieved easily and the reaction under such conditions is controllable (Werthera and Ogadab 1999), while supercritical water has superior ability to dissolve oxygen and organic compounds. Under supercritical conditions, the oxidation rate is much higher, and all organic compounds can be destroyed completely. Energy recovery from a wet oxidation process can be realized by direct heat exchange. One of the most obvious advantages of wet oxidation is that dewatering of sewage sludge before oxidation is not necessary. Although a large-scale subcritical wet oxidation system for sewage sludge is available (Boon and Thomas 1996), supercritical wet oxidation has not yet been fully commercialized after over 20 years of technology development (Svanstrom et al. 2005). Several small supercritical wet sludge oxidation plants have been reported in the United States (Griffith and Raymond 2002), Sweden (Gidner and Stenmark 2001; Patterson et al. 2001), and Japan (Gidner et al. 2001).

13.3.4   Thermal Plasma Pyrolysis and Gasification

Plasma is considered the fourth state of matter, after solids, liquids and gases. In fact, plasma is an ionized gas resulting from an electrical discharge (Huang and Tang 2007). Thermal plasma technology has been widely used in metallurgical processing, materials synthesis, and so on (Pfender 1988; Matsuda 1998; Pfender 1999), while it is still under active development for sludge treatment (Bogaerts et al. 2002). At extremely high plasma temperature, waste materials are completely decomposed to very simple molecules (Imris et al. 2005). In addition, the pollutant emission from off-gas and slag from thermal plasma process is much less than from incineration. The principal advantages of the thermal plasma process include (Heberlein 1992; Heberlein 1993; Heberlein and Murphy 2008) (1) rapid heating and reactor startup, high heat and reactant transfer rates, smaller installation for a given waste throughput, melting of high-temperature materials and high quench rates to obtain nonequilibrium compositions or metastable materials, and (2) use of electricity as the energy source, resulting in decoupling of the heat generation from the oxygen potential and the mass flow rate of the oxidant or air; control of the processing environment; more options for the process chemistry; a lower off-gas flow rate and, consequently, lower gas cleaning costs, and the possibility of producing salable co-products.

Pilot- and full-scale plasma gasification facilities had been developed for conversion of waste to energy in Japan, the United States, Canada, and Europe (Ludwig et al. 2003; Mountouris et al. 2008). The full-scale facility of plasma gasification in Utashinai city, Japan is able to produce 7.9 MW gross electrical energy (4.1 MW net electrical energy) from 183 tons of municipal solid waste per day (Cyranoski 2006). The case study on plasma gasification conducted in the Athens' Central Wastewater

Treatment Plant on Psittalia Island showed that plasma treatment of 250 td^{-1} sewage sludge with 68% moisture could produce 2.85 MW of electrical energy. However, the thermal plasma-associated cost is unfavorable compared with traditional incineration at the current stage.

REFERENCES

Amer A. M. (2002) Processing of Egyptian boiler ash for extraction of vanadium and nickel. *Waste Management* **22**, 515–520.

Amuda O. S., Deng A., Alade A. O., Hung, Y. T. (2008) Conversion of sewage sludge to biosolids, biosolids engineering and management. *Handbook of Environmental Engineering* **7**, 65–119.

Arvand M., Shemshadi R., Zeynalov N. A., Efondiov A.A. (2010) Application of chemical coagulants and biopolymers for sewage sludge dewatering. *Asian Journal of Chemistry* **22**, 6147–6154.

Barjenbruch M., Hoffmann H., Tränker J. (1999) Minimizing of foaming in digesters by pretreatment of the surplus sludge. *Water Science and Technology* **42**, 235–242.

Bernardi M., Cretenot D., Deleris S., Descorme C., Chauzy J., Besson M. (2010) Performances of soluble metallic salts in the catalytic wet air oxidation of sewage sludge. *Catalysis Today* **157** (1–4) 420–424.

Bogaerts A., Neyts E., Gijbels R., Van der Mullen J. (2002) Gas discharge plasmas and their applications. *Spectrochimia Acta B* **57**(4), 609–658.

Braguglia C. M., Mininni G., Marani D., Lotito V. (2003) Sludge incineration: good practice and environmental aspects. *Wastewater Sludge as a Resource*, 523–530.

Bridgwater A. V. (1990) A survey of thermochemical biomass processing activities. *Biomass* **22** (1–4) 279–290.

Bridgwater A. V. (1994) Catalysis in thermal biomass conversion. *Applied Catalysis A* **116** (1–2) 5–47.

Bridgwater A. V. (1999) Principles and practice of biomass fast pyrolysis processes for liquids. *Journal of Analytical and Applied Pyrolysis* **51**, 3–22.

Bridgwater A. V. (2003) Renewable fuels and chemicals by thermal processing of biomass. *Chemical Engineering Journal* **91**, 87–102.

Bridgwater A. V., Czernik S., Piskorz J. (2001) An overview of fast pyrolysis. In: Bridgwater A. V., (Ed). *Progress in Thermochemical Biomass Conversion*, Vol. 2, Blackwell Science, London, pp. 977–997.

Bonte J. L., Fritsky K. J., Plinke M. A., Wilken, M. (2002) Catalytic destruction of PCDD/F in a fabric filter: experience at a municipal waste incinerator in Belgium. *Waste Management* **22**, 421–426.

Boon A., Thomas V. (1996) Resource or rubbish? *Chemical Engineering London* **612**, 25–30.

Buekens A., Huang H. (1998) Comparative evaluation of techniques for controlling the formation and emission of chlorinated dioxinsrfurans in municipal waste. *Journal of Hazardous Materials* **62**, 1–33.

Caballero J. A., Front R., Marcilla A., Conesa, J. A. (1997) Characterization of sewage sludges by primary and secondary pyrolysis. *Journal of Analytical and Applied Pyrolysis* **40–41**, 433– 50.

Carberry J. B., Englande A. J. (1983) *Sludge Characteristics and Behavior*, Martinus Nijhoff, Boston.

Chang D. P. Y. (1996) Chlorine in waste combustion. *Hazardous Waste and Hazardous Materials* **13**(1), U3–U5.

Chu C. P., Lee D. J. (1999) Moisture distribution in sludge: effects of polymer conditioning. *Journal of Environmental Engineering* **125**(4), 340–345.

Conesa J. A., Marcilla A., Moral R., Moreno-Caselles J., Perez-Espinosa A. (1998) Evolution of the gases in the primary pyrolysis of different sewage sludges. *Thermochimica Acta* **313** 63–73.

Crutzen P. J. (1970) The influence of nitrogen oxides on the atmospheric ozone content. *Quarterly Journal of the Royal Meteorological Society* **96**(408), 320–325.

Cyranoski D. (2006) Waste management: One man's trash. . . . *Nature* **444**, 262–263.

Dangtran K., Mullen J. F., Mayrose D. T. (2000) A comparison of fluid bed and multiple hearth biosolids incineration. In: *14th Annual Residuals and Sludge Management Conference*, Boston.

Davis R. D. (1996) The impact of EU and UK environmental pressures on the future of sludge treatment and disposal. *Journal of the Chartered Institution of Water and Environmental Management* **10**(1), 65–69.

de Andrés J. M., Narros A., Rodriguez M. E. (2011) Behaviour of dolomite, olivine and alumina as primary catalysts in air-steam gasification of sewage sludge. *Fuel* **90**, 521–527.

Devi L., Ptasinski K. J., Janssen F. J. J. G., van Paasen S. V. B., Bergman P. C. A., Kiel J. H. A. (2005) Catalytic decomposition of biomass tars: use of dolomite and untreated olivine. *Renewable Energy* **30**, 565–587.

Dogru M., Midilli A., Howarth C. R. (2002) Gasification of sewage sludge using a throated downdraft gasifier and uncertainty analysis. *Fuel Processing Technology* **75**, 55–82.

Eichholz C., Stolarski M., Gortz V., Nirschl H. (2008) Magnetic field enhanced cake filtration of superparamagnetic PVAc particle. *Chemical Engineering Science* **63**(12), 3193–3200.

Fonts I., Azuara M., Gea G., Murillo M. B. (2009a) Study of the pyrolysis liquids obtained from different sewage sludge. *Journal of Analytical and Applied Pyrolysis* **85**, 184–191.

Fonts I., Juan A., Gea G., Murillo M. B., Arauzo J. (2009b) Pyrolysis in a fluidized bed: 2. Influence of operating conditions on some physicochemical properties of the liquid product. *Industrial and Engineering Chemistry Research* **48**(4), 2179–2187.

Fytili D., Zabaniotou A. (2008) Utilization of sewage sludge in EU application of old and new methods: a review. *Renewable and Sustainable Energy Reviews* **12**(1), 116–140.

Geiger T., Hagenmaier H., Hartmann E., Römer R., Seifert H. (1992) Einfluß des Schwefels auf die Dioxin-und Furanbildung bei der Klärschlammverbrennung [Influence of sulfur on the formation of dioxins and furans during sewage sludge combustion]. *VGB Kraftwerktechnik* **72**(2), 159–165.

Gidner A., Stenmark L. (2001) Supercritical water oxidation of sewage sludge: state of the art. In: *Proceedings of the IBC's Conference on Sewage Sludge and Disposal Options*, Birmingham, UK, March 26–28.

Gidner A., Stenmark L., Carlsson K. (2001) Treatment of different wastes by supercritical water oxidation. In: *Proceedings of the Twentieth IT3 Conference*, Philadelphia, May, 14–18.

Goemans M., Clarysse P., Joannès J., De Clercq P., Lenaerts S., Matthys K., Boels K. (2004) Catalytic NO$_x$ reduction with simultaneous dioxin and furan oxidation. *Chemosphere* **54**, 1357–1365.

Griffith J. W., Raymond D. H. (2002) The first commercial supercritical water oxidation sludge processing plant. *Waste Management* **22**, 453–459.

Guellil A., Boualam M., Quiquampoix H., Ginestet P., Audic P., Block J. C. (2001) Hydrolysis of wastewater colloidal enzymes extracted from activated sludge flocs. *Water Science and Technology* **43**, 33–40.

Heberlein J. (1992) Thermal plasmas for the destruction of hazardous wastes. *Proceedings of Plasma Technologies for Hazardous Waste Destruction*, Como, Italy. In: Bonizzoni, G. (ed.), Editrice Compositori, Bologna, Italy, pp. 59–76.

Heberlein J. (1993) Thermal plasmas for the destruction of hazardous wastes. *Industrial Applications of Plasma Physics*, In: Bonizzoni, G. (ed.), Italian Physical Society, Bologna, Italy, pp. 219–235.

Heberlein J., Murphy, A. B. (2008) Thermal plasma waste treatment. *Journal of Physics D* **41**, 053001, pp. 1–20.

Hellstrom D., Kvarnstrom E. (1997) Natural sludge dewatering: 1. Combination of freezing, thawing, and drying as dewatering methods. *Journal of Cold Regions Engineering* **11**, 1–14.

Hirth H., Jochum J., Jodeit H., Wieckert C. (1990) Ein thermisches Entgiftungsverfahren fur Filterstaub aus Müllverbrennungsanlagen [A thermal process for decontaminating fly ash from waste incinerators]. *Chemical Engineering Technology* **62**(12), 1054–1055.

http://www.werf.org/am/template.cfm?section=Search_Research_and_Knowledge_Areas&template=/cm/ContentDisplay.cfm&ContentID=7008. http://www.pwri.go.jp/eng/activity/pdf/reports/ozaki.070603.pdf.

http://www.epa.gov/ttn/oarpg/t3/fr_notices/ssi_atec_093010.pdf.

Huang H., Tang L. (2007) Treatment of organic waste using thermal plasma pyrolysis technology. *Energy Conversion and Management* **48**, 1331–1337.

Huotari J., Vesterinen R. (1996) PCDD and PCDF emissions from co-combustion of RDF with peat wood waste and coal in FBC boilers. *Journal of Hazardous Waste and Hazardous Materials* **13**(1), 1–10.

Hwang S. C., Min K. S. (2003) Improved sludge dewatering by addition of electro-osmosis to belt filter press. *Journal of Environmental Engineering and Science* **2**(2), 149–153.

Imris I., Klenovcanova A., Molcan P. (2005), Energy recovery from waste by plasma gasification. *Archives of Thermodynamics* **26**, 3–16.

Inguanzo M., Domínguez A., Menéndez J. A., Blanco C. G., Pis J. J. (2002) On the pyrolysis of sewage sludge: the influence of pyrolysis conditions on solid, liquid and gas fractions. *Journal of Analytical and Applied Pyrolysis* **63**, 209–222.

Japan Sewage Works, Association., (2001) *Manuals for Using Sewage Sludge as Construction Material, JSWA*, Tokyo.

Kaminsky W., Ying Y. (1993) Chemicals from biomass pyrolysis in a fluidized bed. In: A.V. Brigdwater (ed.), *Advances in Thermochemical Biomass Conversion*, Vol. 2, Blackie, London.

Kawasaki K., Matsuda A., Yamashita H. (2004) The effect of freezing and thawing treatment on the solid liquid separation characteristics of bulking activated sludge, *Kagaku Kogaku Ronbunshu* **30**(5), 587–591.

Kepp U., Machenbach I., Weisz N., Solheim O. E. (2000) Enhanced stabilization of sewage sludge through thermal hydrolysis: 3 years of experience with full-scale plant. *Water Science Technology* **42**, 89–96.

Kilgroc J. D. (1996) Control of dioxin, furan and mercury emissions from municipal waste combustors. *Journal of Hazardous Materials* **47**, 163–194.

Kim Y., Parker W. (2008) A technical and economic evaluation of the pyrolysis of sewage sludge for the production of bio-oil. *Bioresource Technology*, **99**, 1409–1416.

Korving L.D., Schilt C., De Jong W. (2010) Reduction of nitrous oxide emission by a smaller air to fuel ratio in a large-scale sewage sludge fluidized bed combustor. In : *5th International Conference on Waste Management and the Environment*, Tallinn, Estonia.

Kuzuhara S., Sato H., Kasai E., Nakamura T. (2003) Influence of metallic chlorides on the formation of PCDD/Fs during low-temperature oxidation of carbon. *Environmental Science and Technology* **37**, 2431–2435.

Lee K. J., Chun S. A. (1993) Two-stage swirl flow fluidized bed incineration of sewage sludge. In: Rubow L.N. (ed.), *Proceedings of the 12th International Conference on Fluidised Bed Combustion*, San Diego, CA, pp. 1181–1188.

Li J., Yin Y., Zhang X., Liu J., Yan, R. (2009) Hydrogen-rich gas production by steam gasification of palm oil waste over support tri-metallic catalyst. *International Journal of Hydrogen Energy* **34**, 9108–9115.

Liem D. A., van Zorge J. A. (1995) Dioxins and related compounds, status and regulatory aspects. *Environmental Science and Pollution Research* **21**, 46–55.

Lin K. S., Chang N. B. (2008) Control strategy of PCDD/Fs in an industrial fluidized bed incinerator via activated. *Petroleum Science and Technology* **26**, 764–789.

Ludwig C., Hellweg S., Stucki S. (eds.) (2003) *Municipal Solid Waste Management Strategies and Technologies for Sustainable Solutions*, Springer-Verlag, Berlin.

Luo S., Xiao B., Hu Z., Liu S., Guo X., He M. (2009) Hydrogen-rich gas from catalytic steam gasification of biomass in a fixed bed reactor: influence of temperature and steam on gasification performance. *International Journal of Hydrogen Energy* **34**, 2191–2194.

Mahmoud A., Olivier J., Andrew V. J., Hoadley F. A. (2010) Electrical field: a historical review of its application and contributions in wastewater sludge dewatering. *Water Research* **44**, 2381–2407.

Manyà J.J., Sánchez J.L., Gonzalo A., Arauzo J. (2005) Air gasification of dried sewage sludge in a fluidized bed: effect of the operating conditions and in-bed use of alumina. *Energy Fuels* **19**, 629–636.

Marinetti M., Malpei F., Bonomo, L. (2009) Relevance of expression phase in dewatering of sludge with chamber filter presses. *Journal of Environmental Engineering ASCE* **135**, 1380–1387.

Matsuda A. (1998) Plasma and surface reactions for obtaining low defect density amorphous silicon at high growth rates. *Journal of Vacuum Science and Technology A* **16**(1), 365–368.

Mishra V. S., Mahajani V. V., Joshi J. B. (1995) Wet oxidation. *Industrial and Engineering Chemistry Research* **34**(1), 2–48.

Mohan D., Charles U., Pittman Jr., P. H. (2006) Pyrolysis of wood/biomass for bio-oil: a critical review. *Energy and Fuels* **20**, 848–889.

Mohr K., Nonn C., Kolenda J., Gass H., Menke D., Jager, J. (1998) Innovations in continuous measuring methods for the determination of PCDD/PCDF in stack gas of incinerators and thermal processes. *Chemosphere*, **37** 2409–2424.

Mountouris A., Voutsas E., Tassios D. (2008), Plasma gasification of sewage sludge: process development and energy optimization. *Energy Conversion and Management* **49**, 2264–2271.

Muhlhaus L., Verbrennung von Klarschlamm im Wirbelschichtofen (1991) [Combustion of sewage sludge in a fluidized bed]. In: *VDI-Seminar, Klärschlammentsorgung II*. Düsseldorf, germany.

Murakami T., Suzuki Y., Nagasawa H., Yamamoto T., Koseki T., Hirose, H., Okamoto, S. (2009) Combustion characteristics of sewage sludge in an incineration plant for energy recovery. *Fuel Processing Technology* **90**, 778–783.

Myer J. W., Mullen J. F., Dangtran K. (2007) *Thirty years of satisfactory fluid bed sludge incineration: the Northwest Bergen County Utilities Authority experience*, http://www.infilcodegremont.com/images/pdf/Session_15A.pdf.

Neyens E., Baeyens J. (2003) A review of thermal sludge pre-treatment processes to improve dewaterability. *Journal of Hazardous Materials*, **B98**, 51–67.

Nipattummakul N., Ahmed I. I., Kerdsuwan S., Gupta A. K. (2010) Hydrogen and syngas production from sewage sludge via steam gasification. *International Journal of Hydrogen Energy* **35**, 11738–11745.

Nugteren H. W., Janssen-Jurkovicova M., Scarlett B. (2001) Improvement of environmental quality of coal fly ash by applying forced leaching. *Fuel* **80**, 873–877.

Ødegaard H., Paulsrud B., Karlsson I. (2002) Wastewater sludge as a resource: sludge disposal strategies and corresponding treatment technologies aimed at sustainable handling of wastewater sludge. *Water Science and Technology* **46**, 295–303.

Park H. J., Heo H. S., Park Y. K., Yim J.-H., Jeon J.-K., Park J., Ryu C., Kim S.-S. (2010) Clean bio-oil production from fast pyrolysis of sewage sludge: effects of reaction conditions and metal oxide catalysts. *Bioresource Technology* **101**, S83–S85.

Patterson D. A., Stenmark L., Hogan, F. (2001) In: *Proceedings of the Sixth European Biosolids and Organic Residuals Conference*, Wakefield, UK, November 11–14.

Paul N. C. (1994) *Sludge Management and Disposal*, Prentice Hall, Upper Saddle River, NJ.

Pedersen A. J., Ottosen L. M., Villumsen A. (2003) Electrodialytic removal of heavy metals from different fly ashes. *Journal of Hazardous Materials* **100**, 65–78.

Pfender E. (1988) Thermal plasma processing in the nineties. *Pure and Applied Chemistry* **60**(5), 591–606.

Pfender E. (1999) Thermal plasma technology: Where do we stand and where are we going? *Plasma Chemistry and Plasma Processing* **19**(1), 1–31.

Piskorz J., Scott D. S., Westerberg I. B. (1986) Flash pyrolysis of sewage sludge. *Industrial Engineering Chemical Process Design and Development*, **25**, 265–270.

Reijnders L. (2005) Disposal, uses and treatments of combustion ashes: a review. *Resources Conservation and Recycling* **43**, 313–336.

Rulkens W. (2008) Sewage sludge as a biomass resource for the production of energy: overview and assessment of the various options. *Energy and Fuels*, **22**, 9–15.

Rulkens W. H., Bien, J. D. (2004) Recovery of energy from sludge: comparison of the various options. *Water Science and Technology* **50**, 213–221.

Ryu J. Y., Mulholland J. A., Dunn J. E., Iino F., Gullett B. K. (2004) Potential role of chlorination pathways in PCDD/F formation in a municipal waste incinerator. *Environmental Science and Technology* **38**, 5112–5119.

Sáncheza M. E., Menéndezb J. A., Domínguezb A., Pisb J. J., Martíneza O., Calvoa L. F., Bernadc P. L. (2009) Effect of pyrolysis temperature on the composition of the oils obtained from sewage sludge. *Biomass and Bioenergy* **33**, 33–940.

Shao K., Yan J. H., Li X. D., Lu S. Y., Wei Y. L., Fu M. X., (2010) Inhibition of de novo synthesis of PCDD/Fs by SO_2 in a model system. *Chemosphere* **78**(10), 1230–1235.

Shen H.T., Forssberg E. (2003) An overview of recovery of metals from slags. *Waste Management* **23**, 933–949.

Shen L., Zhang D.-K. (2003) An experimental study of oil recovery from sewage sludge by low temperature pyrolysis in a fluidized bed. *Fuel* **82**, 465–472.

Shimizu T., Toyono M. (2007) Emissions of NO_x and N_2O during co-combustion of dried sewage sludge with coal in a circulating fluidized bed combustor. *Fuel* **86**, 2308–2315.

Shimizu T., Toyono M., Ohsawa H. (2007) Emissions of NO_x and N_2O during co-combustion of dried sewage sludge with coal in a bubbling fluidized bed combustor. *Fuel* **86**, 957–964.

Silveira I. C. T., Rosa D., Monteggia L. O., Romeiro G. A., Bayer E., Kutubuddin M. (2002) Low temperature conversion of sludge and shavings from leather industry. *Water Science and Technology* **46**(10), 277–283.

Simell P., Bredenberg J. B. (1990) Catalytic purification of tarry fuel gas. *Fuel* **69**, 1219–1225.

Sizawa H. (1999) Use of dehydrated biosolids in cement manufacturing. In: *Sewage Works in Japan*, Japan Sewage Works Association, Tokyo.

Stammbach M. R., Kraaz B., Hagenbucher R. Richarz W. (1989) Pyrolysis of sewage sludge in a fluidized bed. *Energy and Fuels* **3**, 255–259.

Stanmore B. R. (2004) The formation of dioxins in combustion systems. *Combustion and Flame* **136**, 398–427.

Svanstrom M., Froling M., Olofsson M., Lundin M. (2005) Environmental assessment of supercritical water oxidation and other sewage sludge handling options. *Waste Management and Research* **23**(4), 356–366.

Tan P., Hurtado I., Neuschütz, D. (2001) Thermodynamic modeling of PCDD/Fs formation in thermal processes. *Environmental Science and Technology* **35**, 1867–1874.

Tarantini M., Buttol P., Maiorino L. (2007) An environmental LCA of alternative scenarios of urban sewage sludge treatment and disposal. *Thermal Science* **11**(3), 153–164.

Thomas L., Jungschaffer G., Sprössler B. (1993) Improved sludge dewatering by enzymatic treatment. *Water Science and Technology* **28**, 189–192.

Tuppurainen K., Asikainen A., Ruokojärvi P., Ruuskanen J. (2003) Perspectives on the formation of polychlorinated dibenzo-*p*-dioxins and dibenzofurans during municipal solid waste (MSW) incineration and other combustion processes. *Accounts of Chemical Research* **36**, 652–658.

U.S. EPA Environmental Protection Agency (1978) *Field Manual for Performance Evaluation and Troubleshooting at Municipal Wastewater Treatment Facilities*, EPA/430/9-789-001, EPA, Washington, DC.

U.S. EPA Environmental Protection Agency (1979) *Process Design Manual for Sludge Treatment and Disposal*, EPA, Cincinnati, OH.

U.S., EPA Environmental Protection Agency (1996) Proposed rule: Revised standards for hazardous waste combustors maximum achievable emissions control proposal. EPA Office of Solid Waste, GI Federal Register 17358-536, U.S. Government Printing Office, Washington, DC.

Vaxelaire J., Bongiovanni J. M., Puiggali J. R. (1999) Mechanical dewatering and thermal drying of residual sludge. *Environmental Technology* **20**(1), 29–36.

Vesilind P.A. (1994) The role of water in sludge dewatering. *Water Environment Research* **66**(1), 4–11.

Wang W., Luo Y. X., Qiao W. (2010) Possible solutions for sludge dewatering in China, *Frontiers of Environmental Science and Engineering China* **4**, 102–107.

Wei L., Xu S., Zhang L., Liu C., Zhu H., Liu S. (2007) Steam gasification of biomass for hydrogen-rich gas in a free-fall reactor. *International Journal of Hydrogen Energy* **32**, 24–31.

Werle S., Wilk R. K. (2010) A review of methods for the thermal utilization of sewage sludge: the Polish perspective. *Renewable Energy* **35**(9), 1914–1919.

Werthera J., Ogadab T. (1999) Sewage sludge combustion, *Progress in Energy and Combustion Science* **25**(1), 55–116.

Wikström E., Ryan S., Touati A., Telfer M., Tabor D., Gullett B. (2003) Importance of chlorine speciation on de novo formation of polychlorinated dibenzo-*p*-dioxins and polychlorinated dibenzofurans. *Environmental Science and Technology* **37**, 1108–1113.

Wu C. C., Huang C., Lee D. J. (1997) Effects of polymer dosage on alum sludge dewatering characteristics and physical properties, *Colloids and Surfaces A* **122** (1–3) 89–96.

Yazawa A., Nakazawa S., Menad N. (1999) Thermodynamic evaluations on the formation of dioxins and furans in combustion gas. *Chemosphere* **38**, 2419–2432.

Yin X., Han P. F., Lu X. P., Wang Y. R. (2004) A review on the dewaterability of bio-sludge and ultrasound pretreatment. *Ultrasonics Sonochemistry* **11**, 337–348.

Yu J., Tian N., Wang K., Ren Y. (2007) Analysis and discussion of sludge disposal and treatment of sewage treatment plants in China. *Chinese Journal of Environmental Engineering* **1**, 82–86.

Zhu, X. Y., Song, B. H., Kim, D., Kang, S. K., Lee, S., Jeon, S., Choi, Y., Byoun, Y., Moon, W., Lee J., Kim H., Lee H., Shim J. (2008) Kinetic study on catalytic gasification of a modified sludge fuel. *Particuology* **6**(4), 258–264.

14

AEROBIC GRANULAR SLUDGE TECHNOLOGY FOR WASTEWATER TREATMENT

BING-JIE NI AND HAN-QING YU

Department of Chemistry, University of Science and Technology of China, Hefei, China

14.1 INTRODUCTION

In the last decade, intensive research has demonstrated that aerobic granular sludge technology is a novel and promising development in the field of biological wastewater treatment (Morgenroth et al. 1997; Beun et al. 1999; 2002; Jiang et al. 2002; 2006; Jang et al. 2003; de Bruin et al. 2004; de Kreuk et al. 2005a,b; Adav et al. 2007, 2008a; Yilmaz et al. 2008; Liu et al. 2009). The Aerobic granulation process is usually completed in sequencing batch reactors (SBRs), with a cycle configuration chosen such that a strict selection for fast-settling sludge and frequent repetition of distinct feast and famine conditions occur. In an SBR, wastewater is mixed with the aerated activated sludge in a pulse-feed mode. Then the sludge and input substrate "react" in a form of batch treatment. This highly dynamic feed regime leads to the growth of stable and dense granules (Liu and Tay 2002; 2004; Su and Yu 2005; Zheng et al. 2005; 2006; Liu et al. 2009) (Fig. 14.1). Compared to the conventional activated sludge flocs, aerobic granules have several advantages. An outstanding feature is their excellent settling ability (Fig. 14.2), which is a prerequisite for good solids–liquid separation. Moreover, aerobic granular sludge provides a high and stable rate of metabolism, resilience to shocks and toxins due to protection by a matrix of extracellular polymeric substances (EPSs), long biomass residence times, biomass immobilization inside granules, and therefore, the possibility for bioaugmentation (Su and Yu 2005; Lemaire et al. 2008a,b; Yilmaz et al. 2008).

Biological Sludge Minimization and Biomaterials/Bioenergy Recovery Technologies, First Edition.
Edited by Etienne Paul and Yu Liu.
© 2012 John Wiley & Sons, Inc. Published 2012 by John Wiley & Sons, Inc.

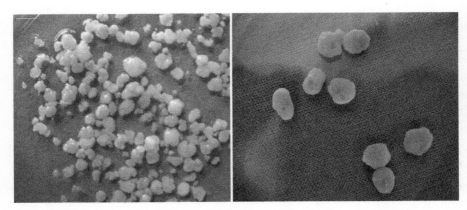

FIGURE 14.1 Image of aerobic granular sludge. [From Yang et al. (2008) and Ni and Yu (2010b).]

To facilitate and promote its practical application for wastewater treatment, researchers worldwide have extensively investigated the fundamentals of aerobic granulation. Analysis of the great body of literature published in the last decade shows that the properties of aerobic granules formed in SBRs are influenced by many factors, including substrate composition, organic loading, hydrodynamic shear force, feast–famine regime, feeding strategy, dissolved oxygen (DO), reactor configuration, solids retention time, cycle time, settling time, and volume exchange ratio. Several

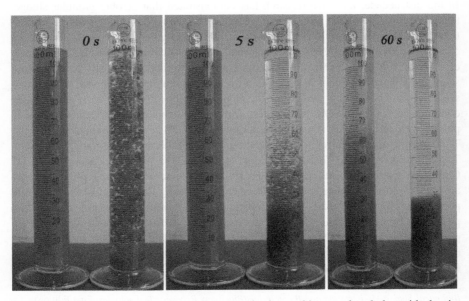

FIGURE 14.2 Comparison of the settling capacity in aerobic granular sludge with that in conventional activated sludge flocs.

review papers have been published in the past five years, and most aspects of microbial granulation have been covered by them. Liu and Tay (2004) and Maximova and Dahl (2006) gave the most encompassing reviews of the bioaggregation processes. Hulshoff Pol et al. (2004), de Kreuk et al. (2007a), Adav et al. (2008b), Liu et al. (2009), and Ni and Yu (2010a) have provided reviews on the state of art for the anaerobic and aerobic granules.

From extensive laboratory-scale investigations into this system and its scaling up (Schwarzenbeck et al. 2005; de Kreuk and van Loosdrecht 2006; Zheng et al. 2006; Ni et al. 2009), it has been concluded that the system holds considerable promise for full-scale implementation. Therefore, in this chapter, the technological starting points of the aerobic granules (cultivation), the mechanisms of aerobic granulation process, the microbial and physicochemical characteristics of aerobic granules, and the modeling of granule-based reactor are delineated. An overview of the bioremediation of wastewaters with aerobic granular sludge technology is also presented. The aim is to provide knowledge of aerobic granular sludge to facilitate the engineering and use of this novel technology.

14.2 TECHNOLOGICAL STARTING POINTS: CULTIVATING AEROBIC GRANULES

14.2.1 Substrate Composition

Aerobic granules have been cultivated with a wide variety of wastewaters, as shown in Table 14.1. Generally, aerobic granulation is independent of substrate type. However, the morphology and microstructure of aerobic granules are highly dependent on the composition of the wastewater on which they are grown. As an example, the structural instabilities of aerobic granules occurred due to filamentous outgrowth in the treatment of dairy wastewater (Schwarzenbeck et al. 2005). The outgrowth of filamentous organisms was related to the fact that in the dairy wastewater, easily biodegradable substances were slowly released at a low concentration attributed to slow hydrolysis of the initial polymeric substrates.

It is recognized that carbohydrates in wastewater and a low DO level lead to flocculation, due to the favored growth of filamentous microorganisms (Gaval and Pernell 2003; Martins et al. 2003). The glucose-grown aerobic granules exhibit a filamentous structure, while acetate-grown aerobic granules have a nonfilamentous and very compact bacterial structure in which a rodlike species predominates (Tay et al. 2001a). At a high potential growth rate on certain substrates, it is more difficult to cultivate aerobic granules. It is easier to obtain compact granule structure on methanol than on acetate, because the growth rates of the microorganisms is lower on methanol than on acetate. The only exception observed was the growth of granular sludge on glucose. Usually, microorganisms have a high growth rate on glucose, but in biofilm and granule systems, populations are found to have a low growth rate on glucose, and therefore dense and smooth structures are formed (de Kreuk et al. 2005a). Aerobic nitrifying granules can be cultivated with an inorganic carbon

TABLE 14.1 Types of Substrate Used for Cultivation of Aerobic Granules

Substrate	Organic Loading Rate (kg COD m^{-3} d^{-1})	Cultivation Time (d)	Filamentous Outgrowth?	Size (mm)	Reference
Molasses	0.42–1.20	70	Yes	2.35	Morgenroth et al. (1997)
Ethanol	2.5–7.5	63	Yes	3.2 ± 0.9	Beun et al. (1999)
Glucose	6.0	21	Yes	2.4	Tay et al. (2001a)
Acetate	2.5	37	No	2.5	Beun et al. (2002)
Soybean-processing wastewater	6.0	60	No	1.22 ± 0.85	Su and Yu (2005)
Sucrose	3.75	60	No	1.0	Zheng et al. (2005)
Phenol	3.6	33	No	0.5–0.6	Jiang et al. (2002)
p-Nitrophenol/glucose	2.5	79	No	0.386 ± 0.016	Yi et al. (2006)
2,4-Dichlorophenol/glucose	2.8	39	No	1.0–2.0	Wang et al. (2007)
Chloroanilines/glucose/acetate	1.0–3.6	100	No	0.45–2.0	Zhu et al. (2005)
Dairy wastewater	2.4	105	Yes	2.0–3.0	Schwarzenbeck et al. (2005)
Brewery wastewater	3.0	63	No	2.0–7.0	Wang et al. (2007)
Domestic wastewater	1.0–1.6	36	Yes	0.5–2.0	de Kreuk and van Loosdrecht (2006)
Abattoir wastewater	2.6	76	No	1.7	Cassidy and Belia (2005)

432

source (Tsuneda et al. 2003, 2006). The nitrifying granules show excellent nitrification ability.

14.2.2   Organic Loading Rate

The accumulated evidence suggests that aerobic granules can form across a very wide range of organic loading rates (OLRs), from 0.4 to 15 kg COD $m^{-3} d^{-1}$ (Morgenroth et al. 1997; Moy et al. 2002; Liu and Tay 2004). This indicates that the formation of aerobic granules in an SBR is substrate-concentration independent. However, it has been reported that kinetic behavior and the morphology of aerobic granules are also related to the applied substrate loading (Moy et al. 2002; Zheng et al. 2006). The mean size of aerobic granules increases from 1.6 to 1.9 mm, with an increasing OLR from 3 to 9 kg COD $m^{-3} d^{-1}$ (Liu and Tay 2004). Furthermore, OLR could affect the stability of aerobic granules. Zheng et al. (2006) reported that bacteria-dominated aerobic granules with a mean diameter of 1 mm could be cultivated in an SBR at a high OLR of 6 kg COD $m^{-3} d^{-1}$ in 30 d. However, under such high-loading conditions, the bacteria-dominated granules were not stable and readily transited into large-sized filamentous granules. The instability of aerobic granules may be attributed to the mass-transfer limitation and possible presence of anaerobes in the large aerobic granules.

14.2.3   Seed Sludge

In most studies regarding aerobic granular sludge, SBRs were seeded with conventional activated sludge flocs. The important factors governing the quality of seed sludge for aerobic granulation appear to include the macroscopic characteristics, settleability, surface properties, and microbial activity (Liu and Tay 2004). Little information on the role of seed sludge in aerobic granulation is available. Hu et al. (2005) cultivated aerobic granules in SBRs by seeding anaerobic granular sludge using acetate-based synthetic wastewater. In their experiments, the inoculated anaerobic granules experienced a process of disintegration–recombination – growing up. The disintegrated anaerobic sludge might play the role of a nucleus for the aerobic granulation. The bacterial community residing in activated seed sludge was important for the aerobic granulation process, as the hydrophilic bacteria would be less likely to attach to sludge flocs compared with the hydrophobic counterpart, which constitutes the majority of free bacteria in the effluent from full-scale treatment plants. The greater the number of hydrophobic bacteria in the seed sludge, the faster the aerobic granulation, with excellent settleability.

14.2.4   Reactor Configuration

The Reactor configuration influences the flow pattern of liquid and microbial aggregates in reactors (Beun et al. 1999; Liu and Tay 2002). Until now, all aerobic granules are cultivated in pneumatically agitated reactors, including the bubble column and airlift reactor with a sequencing batch operational. An important operational factor in aerobic granulation and reactor operation is superficial air velocity. It exerts an influence on aerobic granules through the oxygen supply and hydrodynamic shear stress. In a column-type upflow reactor a higher ratio of reactor height to diameter (H/D) can ensure a longer circular flow trajectory, which in turn provides a more effective hydraulic attrition to aerobic granules. However, at a higher H/D, the aerobic granules at the top face low shear stress and will grow out more readily with filametous and/or fingertype structure. In this case, no granules would be formed (de Kreuk et al. 2005a).

Shear stress provided by aeration rate depends on reactor configuration as well as reactor scale. Beun et al. (2000) reported that much more dense granules with a smaller diameter were obtained in an airlift reactor than in a bubble column at the same substrate loading rate. To reduce the aeration rate to a reasonable value, Liu and Tay (2007) designed a novel airlift loop reactor with divided draft tubes for aerobic granulation.

14.2.5   Operational Parameters

The positive role of a high hydrodynamic shear force in providing a great aeration rate in the stable operation of biofilm and aerobic granule systems has been widely recognized (Liu and Tay 2002). Chen et al. (2007) found that at shear forces of 2.4 and $3.2 \, \text{cm s}^{-1}$, granules could maintain a robust and stable structure. Granules developed in low shear forces of 0.8 and $1.6 \, \text{cm s}^{-1}$ deteriorated to large filamentous ones with an irregular shape and loose structure, and resulted in poor performance and operational instability. Granules cultivated under high shear forces of 2.4 and $3.2 \, \text{cm s}^{-1}$ stabilized with clear morphology, dense and compact structure, and good performance in 120-d operation. In most studies on aerobic granulation, the upflow air superficial velocity in reactors is much higher than $1.2 \, \text{cm s}^{-1}$. However, high aeration rate means high energy consumption.

Adav et al. (2007) reported that the production of extracellular polysaccharides was closely associated with the shear force and the stability of aerobic granules. The extracellular polysaccharides content increased with the increasing shear force estimated in terms of superficial upflow air velocity. Thus, a high shear force stimulates bacteria to secrete more extracellular polysaccharides (Ramasmy and Zhang 2005).

The cyclic operation of an SBR consists of influent filling, aeration, settling, and effluent removal. The settling time and exchange ratio of liquid volumes at the end of each cycle present the main screening step to remove nongranular biomass from the reactor. A shorter cycle time results in a shorter hydraulic retention time (HRT), which provides stronger selective pressure. Sludge loss is observed through hydraulic washout at a short cycle time because bacterial growth is unable to compensate (Pan et al. 2004). Liu and Tay (2007) reported the influence of cycle time on the kinetic behavior of aerobic granules. The specific biomass growth rate of aerobic granules observed decreased from $0.266 \, \text{d}^{-1}$ to $0.031 \, \text{d}^{-1}$, while the biomass growth yield of granular sludge observed decreased from $0.316 \, \text{g VSS g}^{-1} \, \text{COD}$ to $0.063 \, \text{g VSS g}^{-1} \, \text{COD}$ when the cycle time was increased from 1.5 h to 8 h.

The settling time acts as a major hydraulic selection pressure on a microbial community in SBRs. A short settling time preferentially selects for the growth of rapid-settling bacteria, and the sludge with a poor settleability is washed out. It is recognized that the selection pressure imposed by a short settling time should be more important in fully aerobic granule systems, but in anaerobic–aerobic alternative systems with phosphate-accumulating organisms (PAOs), the settling time seemed to be less important because of the inherent tendency of PAOs to aggregate (de Kreuk et al. 2005a), meanwhile, Meyer et al. (2003) cultivated aerobic granules-containing glycogen accumulating organisms at a settling time of 25 min.

The unique feature of an SBR over a continuous-flow activated sludge reactor is its cycle operation, which in turn results in a periodical starvation phase during the operation. It is proposed that such a periodical starvation would be somehow important to the aerobic granulation (Tay et al. 2001b). Although starvation is proposed not to be a prerequisite for aerobic granulation (Liu et al. 2007), the increase in hydrophobicity on carbon starvation has been reported (Sanin et al. 2003).

McSwain et al. (2004) enhanced aerobic granulation by intermittent feeding. In fact, pulse feeding to the SBR contributes to compact aerobic granules. Li et al. (2006) observed that the aerobic granulation process was initiated by starvation and cooperated by shear force and anaerobic metabolism. A shorter starvation time resulted in faster granulation (Yang et al. 2005).

Aerobic granules are cultivated successfully at a DO concentration above $2 \, mg \, L^{-1}$ (Yang et al. 2005; Adav et al. 2007). However, Peng et al. (1999) observed that small granules (diameter of 0.3 to 0.5 mm) were agglomerated into big flocs during settling in an SBR at a DO of $1 \, mg \, L^{-1}$. Mosquera-Corral et al. (2005) reported that reducing the oxygen saturation to 40% caused deterioration, a decreased density, and finally, breaking of the granules. Based on the literature available, DO concentration is not a dominating factor for aerobic granulation.

The biological process rates depend on temperature. Most studies on aerobic granular sludge were carried out at room temperatures (20 to 25°C). In an investigation into the effect of temperature changes on the conversion processes and the stability of aerobic granular sludge, de Kreuk et al. (2005a) found that temperature change could affect the performance of an aerobic granular sludge reactor to a large extent. The startup of a reactor at low temperatures led to the presence of organic COD in the aeration phase, deterioration of granule stability, and even biomass washout. Once a reactor was started up at a higher temperature, it was possible to operate a stable aerobic granular sludge system at a lower temperature. Thus, they concluded that startup should take place preferentially during warm summer periods, and that decreased temperatures during winter periods should not be a problem for granule stability and pollutant removal in a granular sludge system (de Kreuk et al. 2005a).

In microbial growth, pH is an important environmental factor. However, information regarding the effect of pH on species selection and aerobic granulation is still limited. Yang et al. (2008) evaluated the effect of feeding alkalinity and pH on the formation of aerobic sludge granules. In an SBR with a low alkalinity of 28.7 mg $CaCO_3 \, L^{-1}$ in the influent and a reactor pH of 3.0, rapid formation of fungi-dominating granules was achieved in 1 week. In another SBR with a high alkalinity of 301 mg $CaCO_3\,L^{-1}$ and a reactor pH of 8.1, formation of bacteria-dominating granules was achieved after 4 weeks of operation. These results suggest that microbial communities and structural features of aerobic granules could be formed through controlling the feeding alkalinity and reactor pH.

It appears from the above that aerobic granulation is a very complex phenomenon with numerous internal interactions among process variables. All of them have significant effects on the overall reactor performance. Thus, cultivating aerobic granules with wastewaters with a complex composition (e.g., soybean-processing and fatty acids–rich wastewaters) needs to be explored further. More work should be performed to answer how the dynamic aerobic granulation process can be characterized quantitatively regarding these complex internal interactions. In addition, the review results indicate that many factors are involved in the granulation of activated sludge, but most studies concerning aerobic granule have been focused on well-controlled lab-scale reactors with high- or middle-strength synthetic wastewaters. Is it feasible to cultivate aerobic granules for the treatment of low-strength municipal wastewater in a pilot-scale SBR? What should be the key factors in the granulation of activated sludge grown on such a low-concentration wastewater in an SBR? These questions need to be answered.

14.3 MECHANISMS OF THE AEROBIC GRANULATION PROCESS

14.3.1 Granulation Steps

The most definitive list of aerobic granulation steps is provided by Liu and Tay (2002) and Adav et al. (2008b). Microbial aggregation was a hypothesis in biology that occurred by intra-, inter-, and multigeneric cell-to-cell attachment through cell surface receptors such as protein saccharide or protein–protein interaction (Kolenbrander et al. 1999; Palmer et al. 2001). Tay et al. (2001a) recognized that aerobic granulation was a process of microbial self-immobilization without carrier support. Liu and Tay (2002) and Adav et al. (2008b) proposed that the following four steps corresponded to the aerobic granulation process: (1) Microbe-to-microbe contact to form aggregates by hydrodynamic, diffusion, gravity, and/or thermodynamic forces; (2) initial attraction to form aggregates by physical (van der Waals, opposite charge, thermodynamic forces), chemical (ionic pairing, triplet ionic pairing, interparticulate bridging), or biochemical (cell membrane fusion, cell receptor attraction, cell surface dehydration) forces; (3) microbial forces to form aggregates by biological glue such as cellular clustering and secretion of EPS; and (4) a hydrodynamic shear force to stabilize the three-dimensional structure of the granule.

Using Confocal Scanning Laser Microscopy (CSLM) coupled with different specific florochromes, fluorescent microspheres, and oligonucleotide probes, the interior of bioaggregates collected during aerobic granulation process was examined (McSwain et al. 2005; Adav et al. 2007, 2008b). The CLSM images for seed flocs and mature granules using the multicolor fluorescent technique recently developed by Chen et al. (2006, 2007) and Yang et al. (2008) are shown in Fig. 14.3. The results demonstrated that microbial aggregation served as an initial step in granule formation

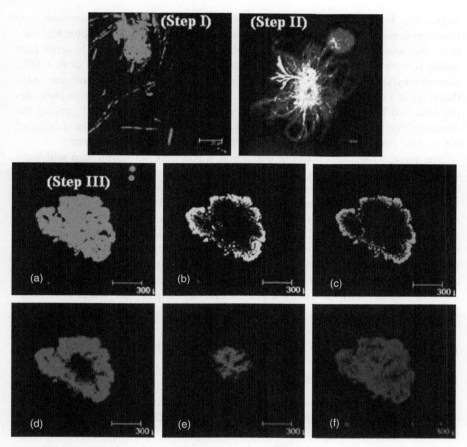

FIGURE 14.3 CLSM images of bioaggregates in different stages. The bioaggregates were cultivated in a sequential batch reactor with synthetic wastewater containing $500\,\mathrm{mgL}^{-1}$ phenol and stained for EPS [(a) proteins (green): FITC; (b) lipids (yellow): Nile red; (c) α-polysaccharide (light blue): Con A rhodamine; (d) total cells (red): SYTO 63; (e) dead cells (violet): Sytox blue; (f) β-polysaccharide (blue): calcofluor white]. step I: nowflocculated cells; step II: flocculated sludge floc of puffy structure, and step III: young granule with dead cells at the granule core. [From Adav et al. (2008b).]

(step II). The aggregated bacteria secreted EPS at the attachment site, multiplied, and grew as large sludge flocs (step III). The sludge flocs then grew due to proliferation of the attached bacteria and reunion, forming granules. This granulation model took into account the noted changes in morphology and interior structure.

14.3.2 Selective Pressure

In SBR operation, only particles that settle within a given time frame could be retained in the reactor, while those with poor settleability were washed out of the system.

Apparently, borrowed from biological evolution theory, this physical screening step was considered to provide "selection pressure" to the biomass in the reactor, and only those that adapted to this challenge (to become big and dense enough to settle fast) would survive and be retained in the reactor (Liu and Tay 2002). Tay et al. (2002) studied nitrifying bacterial granulation at different selection pressures and concluded that there is a need of strong selection forces for granulation. The selection pressures required had been created by keeping a constant column height and varying the discharge port height (Wang et al. 2004). Wang et al. (2007) noted that the stability of the granule could be enhanced with stepwise increased selection pressure.

The physical settling–washing out action was a pure screening step without a demand for the microbes to respond to, or to make changes in, the fluid carryout, hence having a different intended meaning through biological evolution theory. Microorganisms in high-shear environments adhered by secreting EPS to resist damage to suspended cells by environmental forces (Trinet et al. 1991). Experimental proof was needed to justify how cells communicated with each other and tried to respond to the high liquid upflow in order to become large enough to remain in the reactor. Moreover, those tiny flocs that were washed out initially had no chance to evolve with the environmental changes; hence, the selection is not fair. Nonetheless, the screening step cultivated aerobic granules successfully in SBRs (Beun et al. 2002; Liu et al. 2005a).

14.4   CHARACTERIZATION OF AEROBIC GRANULAR SLUDGE

14.4.1   Biomass Yield and Sludge Reduction

Yield is a stoichiometric parameter to describe the amount of a product that is obtained from specified amounts of reactants, including biomass growth yield coefficients, extracellular polymer yield coefficients, and cell-internal storage yield coefficients. The yield coefficients reported for aerobic storage and biomass growth in aerobic granules by Ni and Yu (2008) are 0.79, 0.61, and $0.67\,g\,COD\,g^{-1}$ COD, respectively. In the approach of Ni and Yu (2008), substrate electrons are diverted to both microbial storage products and active biomass simultaneously, and the heterotrophs grow on storage products rather than directly on the soluble substrates. In a follow-up study to Ni and Yu (2008), Ni et al. (2008) further reported a set of stoichiometric parameters for the anoxic storage and growth of the denitrifiers in aerobic granules. They are estimated to be 0.55, 0.40, and $0.67\,g\,COD\,g^{-1}$ COD, respectively, which are much lower than their aerobic counterparts.

Ni and Yu (2010b) also reported that the storage formation coefficient is estimated to be $0.26\,g\,COD_{STO}\,g^{-1}\,COD_S$, while the EPS formation coefficient is determined to be $0.23\,g\,COD_{EPS}\,g^{-1}\,COD_S$. Therefore, electrons from the external substrate are distributed in this order when a storage polymer is produced: new biomass synthesis 39%, storage polymer 26%, and EPSs 23%. More substrate electrons are diverted to the storage polymers, but less is distributed to produce EPSs when sufficient substrate is available.

Fang et al. (2009) reported the yield coefficient for ammonia-oxidizing bacteria (AOB) in aerobic granules is $0.21\,g\,COD\,g^{-1}\,N$, whereas the corresponding value for nitrite-oxidizing bacteria (NOB) is 0.05 g COD g^{-1} N. The yield coefficients obtained for AOB and NOB in aerobic granules were similar to the values reported by de Kreuk et al. (2007b) and in the range of 0.03 to 0.13 g VSS g^{-1} N for the AOB and 0.02 to 0.07 g VSS g^{-1} N for the NOB (Sin et al. 2008). It has been observed that a portion of the energy obtained from catabolism is spent on cell maintenance rather than cell growth, resulting in lower apparent biomass growth yield values than the true values.

As we know, one of the most serious problems encountered in the application of activated sludge process is the production of a huge amount of excess sludge. The daily production of excess sludge from a conventional activated sludge process plant is around 15 to 100 kg^{-1} BOD_5 d^{-1} (BOD: biological oxygen demand), in which over 95% is water (Liu and Tay 2001). The expenses of sludge disposal account for 25 to 65% of the total plant operation costs (Low and Chase 1999; Liu and Tay 2001). Furthermore, employment of landfill and incineration for sludge disposal may cause severe secondary pollution. Thus, reducing the production of sludge in a wastewater treatment process is a better option than disposing of sludge after its generation.

Various methods are available for controlling the accumulation of excess sludge, such as utilization of an extended aeration process, changing operating conditions (Chen et al. 2001, 2003), promoting microorganism predation on bacteria, and introducing bacterial parasites or phages (Rensink and Rulkens 1997; Mayhew and Stephenson 1998). However, these methods require either a large energy input or strict operational control. As mentioned above, under normal conditions, the catabolism of microorganisms is coupling with anabolism through energy transfer, and the chemicals released from catabolism are used for anabolic processes such as cell growth and maintenance (Green and Reiblet 1975). However, in light of a newly developed theory of metabolism uncoupling (Russell and Cook 1995), catabolism could be uncoupled with anabolism so as to decrease the production of excess cells under particular conditions (Low and Chase 1999; Liu and Tay 2001; Wei et al. 2003). In this case, microorganisms cannot adjust their energy level of catabolism to acclimate to that of anabolism. Accordingly, the link between energy-yielding reactions and the energy-consuming reactions of biosynthesis will change to a certain extent, and then energy spilling occurs (Russell and Cook 1995). Since energy is partially lost to nongrowth reactions, the energy generated from catabolism for cell growth is decreased. As a result, the cell yield is decreased and the amount of excess sludge from aerobic granules process could be reduced accordingly. Consequently, the methods developed from the metabolism uncoupling, such as the utilization of a chemical uncoupler, provide an alternative way of reducing the amount of excess sludge from aerobic granule–based reactors. Various chemicals, including 2,4-dinitrophenol (dNP), p-nitrophenol (pNP), 2,4-dichlorophenol (dCP), 3,3′,4′,5- tetrachlorosalicylanilide (TCS), and rotenone, can be used as an uncoupler. TCS and 4-chloro-2-nitrophenol (CNP) were identified as the most effective uncouplers among 12 uncouplers (Strand et al. 1999). Mayhew and Stephenson (1998) tested eight different chemicals to uncouple the metabolism. The addition of rotenone, dNP, or quinacrine reduced the sludge yield significantly. TCS was found to be effective for limiting sludge growth rate, and the sludge yield could be reduced by around 40% at TCS concentrations of 0.8 to 1.0 mg L^{-1} (Chen et al. 2002). When dNP was selected as an uncoupler to reduce sludge production, the sludge yield decreased with an increasing ratio of initial uncoupler concentration to initial biomass concentration (Liu et al. 1998).

14.4.2 Formation and Consumption of Microbial Products

EPSs are a major component of the matrix material in granules (McSwain et al. 2005; Sheng et al. 2006). EPSs are sticky solid materials secreted by cells, and they are involved in adhesion phenomena, formation of the matrix structure, controlling the microbial physiology, and the long-term stability of the granules (Tay et al. 2001a, Sheng et al. 2006). In addition to EPSs, all bacteria convert a fraction of the organic substrate into soluble microbial products (SMPs), which account for the bulk of the soluble organic carbon in reactor effluents (de Silva and Rittmann 2000a,b; Benjamin et al. 2006). On the other hand, aerobic granules are usually subjected to alternative feast and famine conditions in an SBR (Arrojo et al. 2004; Su and Yu 2005) and are able to take up carbon substrate in wastewater rapidly and to store it as intracellular storage products when the substrate is in excess (Beun et al. 2001; Su and Yu 2006a). The storage of the carbon sources as internal storage products (X_{STO}), such as poly(hydroxyalkanoates), lipids, and polysaccharides, is likely to play a significant role in the carbon turnover (van Loosdrecht et al. 1997; Majone et al. 1999; Pratt et al. 2004). The EPS, SMP, and X_{STO} are important sinks for electrons and carbon derived from the original substrate. The microorganisms in aerobic granules may promote the accumulation of X_{STO}, EPS, or both.

Ni and Yu (2010b) demonstrated that the external substrate in aerobic granules is used primarily by active biomass for the generation of new biomass. An excess amount of substrate available is converted to X_{STO}. After the consumption of the primary external substrate, the secondary growth process occurs on the stored X_{STO} in the famine phase. Figure 14.4 illustrates a consistent approach to the fate of the substrate electrons, which enter a cell directly. There are four possible ways. Part of the external substrate is used for biomass synthesis. Other substrate electrons are diverted to the formation of utilization-associated products (UAPs) and EPSs. UAPs are released to the aqueous solution, where as EPSs are released as a solid to form the aggregate matrix. The hydrolysis of EPSs produces biomass-associated products (BAPs), which are soluble. Substrate oxidation and respiration of the electrons to reduce O_2 and generate the energy needed to fuel the formation of active biomass, EPSs, and UAPs. In a feasting period, some of the external substrate is converted to X_{STO}. Because the formation of X_{STO} competes with the usual biomass synthesis, the formation of X_{STO} occurs only when the substrate concentration is high. The active biomass decays in two ways. First, the active biomass is oxidized through endogenous respiration to yield energy for maintenance. Second, the decay also produces residual inert biomass, which is not biodegradable. Since both UAP and BAP are biodegradable, some of their electrons can also be used by the microorganisms as "recycled" substrate, while the remaining electrons also go to the electron acceptor for energy generation. X_{STO} is also biodegradable and can be utilized by the active biomass under famine conditions. Some of the electrons in X_{STO} are used for the biomass synthesis, while the other electrons are respired for energy generation.

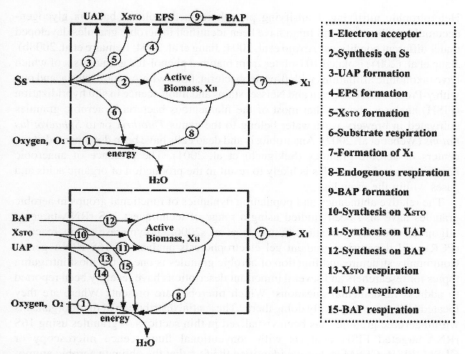

FIGURE 14.4 Schematic of electron flows from the external substrate (upper panel on the left), and formation of active and inert biomass, EPSs, SMPs and X_{STO} (underside panel on the left) in aerobic granules.

Ni and Yu (2010b) also underlined the importance of the initial substrate and biomass concentrations for the overall formation and consumption of EPS, SMP and X_{STO} in aerobic granules. A higher substrate concentration results in a greater concentration of EPSs, SMPs, and X_{STO}. An accumulation of biomass in an aerobic granular sludge system leads to an increased production rate of EPSs, SMPs and X_{STO}. However, there is no direct correlation between the biomass concentration and the total content of the EPSs, SMPs, and X_{STO}.

14.4.3 Microbial Structure and Diversity

The recent development of modern molecular biology techniques is providing new insight into the structure and function of microbial communities in natural and engineered systems, including biological wastewater treatment reactors. Microbial community structure analysis of aerobic granules, based primarily on 16S rRNA gene sequencing (Arrojo et al. 2004; Tsuneda et al. 2006), is becoming the most powerful tool for investigating the microbial populations present in aerobic granular reactors. The microbial diversity of aerobic granules is closely related to the composition of culture media in which they are developed and the structure of aerobic granules.

Heterotrophic, nitrifying, denitrifying, phosphorus-accumulating bacteria, glycogen-accumulating bacteria, and fungi have been identified in aerobic granules developed under different conditions (Arrojo et al. 2004; Jiang et al. 2004; Lemaire et al. 2008b). Jiang et al. (2004) isolated 10 isolates from matured phenol-fed granules six of which have taxonomic affiliations with β-proteobacteria, three with Actinobacteria, and one with γ-Proteobacteria. Gram and Neisser stains and fluorescence in situ hybridization (FISH) analyses showed that most of the filamentous bacteria in aerobic granules cultivated in brewery wastewater belong to the genus *Thiothrix* or to *Sphaerotilus natans* (Weber et al. 2007). Anaerobiosis and dead cells have been documented at the centers of aerobic granules (Sekiguchi et al. 2001). The presence of anaerobic bacteria in aerobic granules is likely to result in the production of organic acids and gases within the granules.

The relative abundancy and population dynamics of functional groups in aerobic granules have also been studied using a range of techniques: 16S rRNA-targeted oligonucleotide hybridization (Tsuneda et al. 2006), polymerase chain reaction (PCR), and denaturing gradient gel electrophoresis analysis of 16S rRNA genes. Community structure and function of aerobic granules is one of the most intriguing topics for researchers and several important descriptions have recently been reported to address fundamental questions: Which microbes are present? Where are they located? What are they really doing there? The spatial distribution of microorganisms within aerobic granules has been visualized in thin sections of granules using 16S rRNA-targeted FISH analysis with conventional fluorescence microscopy or CLSM. FISH–CLSM technique identified the fact that the obligate aerobic ammonium-oxidizing bacterium *Nitrosomonas* spp. was mainly at a depth of 70 to 100 μm from the granule surface, while the anaerobic bacterium *Bacteroides* spp. was detected at a depth of 800 to 900 μm from the granule surface (Yuan and Blackall 2002). Lemaire et al. (2008b) reported that in granules above 500 mm in diameter, *Accumulibacter* spp. were dominant in the outermost 200-mm region of the granule while *Competibacter* spp. dominated in the granule central zone, as shown in Fig. 14.5. The stratification of these two populations between the outer aerobic and inner anoxic part of the granule was highly significant ($p < 0.003$). They concluded that the glycogen-accumulating organisms (GAOs) *Competibacter* spp., not the phosphorus-accumulating organisms (PAOs) *Accumulibacter* spp., were responsible for denitrification in this SBR. This is undesirable for simultaneous nitnification, denitrification, and phosphorus removal, as savings in carbon demand cannot be fulfilled, with phosphorus removal and denitrification being achieved by different groups of bacteria. Thus, these techniques are bridging the gap between engineers (reactor operation) and microbiologists (culture-based study) and lead to interactive communication between them for optimizing microbial population and improving reactor performance (de Kreuk et al. 2007b).

14.4.4 Physicochemical Characteristics

Morphology   The morphology of aerobic granules varies substantially, depending on substrate types and cultivation conditions (de Kreuk et al. 2005a). However, many

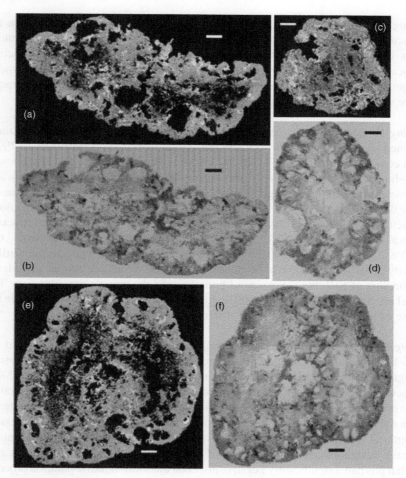

FIGURE 14.5 Reconstructed CLSM images of FISH micrographs (A, C, and E) and Nile blue stain micrographs (B, D, and F) of entire granule sections. In (A), (C), and (E) *Accumulibacter* spp. cells are cyan (overlay of blue PAOmix and green EUBmix), *Competibacter* spp. Cells are yellow (overlay of red GAOmix and green EUBmix) and other bacteria are green (green EUBmix). In (B), (D), and (F), overlays were of transmitted light images (black and white) and Nile blue–stained PHAs in red. Subsequent granule sections (7 mm apart) of two different granules are presented in (A)–(B) and (E)–(F). (C) and (D) are not images of the same granules. The granules were sampled at the end of the anaerobic (A–B and C) and at the end of the aerobic (D and E–F) periods. Scale bar = 100 mm. [From Lemaire et al. (2008b).]

studies confirm that the morphology of aerobic granules is completely different from that of sludge flocs (Morgenroth et al. 1997; Beun et al. 1999, 2002; Jiang et al. 2002, 2006; Jang et al. 2003; de Bruin et al. 2004; de Kreuk et al. 2005a,b; Adav et al. 2007, 2008a; Yilmaz et al. 2008; Liu et al. 2009). Aerobic granules have a well-defined appearance and are visible as separate entities larger than 0.1 mm in diameter after settling, as shown in Fig. 14.1. The granule size is an important parameter in the characterization of aerobic granulation. The average diameter of aerobic granules varies in the range 0.2 to 5 mm. For quantitative differentiation of the structure characteristic and morphology of aerobic granules, Su and Yu (2005) used fractal geometry to describe their characteristics. The matured aerobic granules had a fractal nature with a fractal dimension of 1.87 ± 0.34.

Settling Properties   An evident advantage of aerobic granules over conventional activated sludge flocs is their excellent settling properties (Morgenroth et al. 1997; Beun et al. 1999, 2002; Jiang et al. 2002, 2006), which determine the efficiency of solid–liquid separation and are essential to the stable operation of wastewater treatment systems. The sludge volume index (SVI) of aerobic granules can be lower than $50 \, \text{mL} \, \text{g}^{-1}$, which is much lower than that of conventional sludge flocs. The settling velocity of aerobic granules is associated with granule size and structure and is as high as 30 to $100 \, \text{m} \, \text{h}^{-1}$, while that of flocs is usually lower than $9 \, \text{m} \, \text{h}^{-1}$ (Su and Yu 2005). Liu et al. (2005b) developed a new model to describe the settling velocity of aerobic granules. In this model the settling velocity of aerobic granules is the function of SVI, the mean size of granules, and the granule concentration. The model established could satisfactorily match the experimental results obtained in the course of aerobic granulation under different conditions.

Strength   The strength of aerobic granules is essential for their stability and for solid–liquid separation of effluent from reactors. Granules with excellent physical strength could withstand compression and high shear (abrasion). Zheng (2006) characterized the compressive strength of aerobic granules in the diameter range 1 to 4 mm using a novel device. They found that aerobic granules with a diameter of 2 mm exhibited the best compressive properties and could withstand a compressive strength of $24 \, \text{N} \, \text{cm}^{-2}$. The abrasion experimental results demonstrated that an increase in size enhanced the erosion of primary particles at a certain shear rate and that this had a significantly negative effect on the solid–liquid separation process.

Cell Surface Hydrophobicity   Cell surface hydrophobicity plays a key role in the self-immobilization and attachment of cells to a surface (Liu et al. 2004). In a thermodynamic sense, an increase in cell hydrophobicity causes a simultaneous decrease in the excess Gibbs energy of the surface, which promotes the self-aggregation of bacteria from the liquid phase to form a new solid phase (Liu et al. 2004) (i.e., microbial granules). The hydrophobic binding force is of prime importance in the cell-to-cell approach and interaction, and the cell hydrophobicity can act is a driving force for the initiation of cell-to-cell aggregation, which is the first STEP toward aerobic granulation and also keeps the aggregated bacteria tightly together (Mu and Yu 2006).

Rheology   Rheology is a powerful tool for characterizing the non-Newtonian properties of sludge suspensions, as it can quantify flow behaviors in real processes on a scientific basis (Su and Yu 2005). Rheological parameters are very important in sludge management, not only as design parameters for transporting, storing, land-filling, and spreading operations, but also as monitoring parameters in many biological treatment processes (Su and Yu 2005). Su and Yu (2005) characterized the non-Newtonian rheological behavior of aerobic granules and demonstrated that the granules containing liquor were shear thinning, and their rheological character-istics could be described using the Herschel–Buckley equation. The suspended solids concentration, pH, temperature, diameter, settling velocity, specific gravity, and sludge volume index all had an effect on the apparent viscosity of the mixed liquor of aerobic granules.

Permeability   Unlike microbial flocs and suspended cells, the dense aerobic granules may encounter problems associated with the limited diffusion of substrates into and metabolites out of the granules. The pore-size distribution and permeability of aerobic granules are closely related to substrate and metabolite transport (Zheng and Yu 2007). Therefore, their permeability feature has a significant influence on substrate and product transportation in granules. The pore-size distribution and available porous volume to which substrate can penetrate are the main factors governing granule activity. To evaluate the porosity and permeability of aerobic granules quantitatively, Zheng and Yu (2007) used size-exclusion chromatography, in which poly(ethylene glycols) and distilled water were used as solute and mobile phase, respectively. The porosity of the aerobic granules varied from 68 to 93%. The EPSs of the granules might clog the pores and might be responsible for the reduced porosity.

The porosity and permeability also influence the settling velocity of aerobic granules and the settling velocity of a particle depends greatly on its drag coefficient. Thus, Mu et al. (2008) provided a reliable approach to evaluate the drag coefficient of porous and permeable microbial granules. It was realized by taking the porosity and permeability of the granules into consideration. The drag coefficient of the microbial granules was found to be less than that of smooth rigid spheres and biofilm-covered particles. In addition, this study demonstrates that the drag coefficient of microbial granules depended heavily on their permeability and porosity. A fractal-cluster model was found to be able to predict the distribution of the primary particles in the microbial granules.

Mass Transfer   Aerobic granules have a dense surface layer and compact interior core that can generate significant mass-transfer resistance to oxygen and nutrient intake. In a biodegradation process, substrates and DO are initially transferred from the bulk liquid to the external surface of aerobic granules, before diffusing or being carried by an advective flow into the interior for biodegradation. Oxygen diffusivity is commonly used as an input parameter for modeling the transport processes in granules. Morgenroth et al. (1997) assumed that the granule center is anaerobic, although the surrounding liquid has a relatively high DO content. Liu et al. (2005a) noted a decline in the specific substrate removal rate from large granules, revealing the inhibition induced by mass-transfer resistance. Oxygen limitation, if it occurred, produced an anaerobic core in aerobic granules. Anaerobic bacteria were found to exist in the anaerobic core for large aerobic granules.

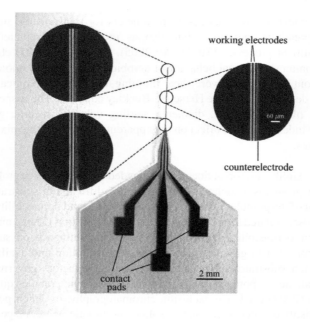

FIGURE 14.6 Innovative microelectrode and three magnified microscopic images of different sections of the needle. [From Liu et al. (2007).]

Recently, the microelectrode method has been adopted to evaluate the microtransport processes in aerobic granules. Chiu et al. (2006) estimated the oxygen diffusivity in acetate- and phenol-grown aerobic granules by probing the DO level at the granule center using microelectrodes, with a sudden change in the DO of the bulk liquid. The flow velocity across the granule was set such that the external mass-transfer resistance was negligible. They also measured the steady-state and transient DO with step changes in surrounding DO levels at various depths in granules using microelectrodes. A marked decrease in DO was also observed over this surface layer. No aerobic oxidation could occur beneath the active layer, indicating the oxygen transfer limitation. Liu et al. (2007) successfully fabricated a novel microelectrode using photolithography to determine the DO distribution in aerobic nitrifying granules (Fig. 14.6). It was found that the main active part of the nitrifying granule was the upper 150-μm layer. Consequently, Liu et al. (2008) manufactured a solid-state microelectrode through electrochemical co-deposition of Pt–Fe nanoparticles on a gold microelectrode fabricated using photolithography for in situ nitrite determination in aerobic nitrifying granules. At the outside of the granular surface, the nitrite concentration dropped rapidly because of its diffusion from the granular surface to the bulk solution. Jang et al. (2003) explored ion gradients in aerobic granules by microelectrode. DO and NH_4^+-N concentrations tended to decrease from the surface. The nitrification rates decreased dramatically when the concentration of DO was reduced to zero. Thus, DO had a strong influence on the nitrification rate, as mentioned above. The oxygen concentration due to diffusion limitations is likely to have occurred at 300 mm into the granule thickness. Most of the nitrification is likely to be restricted to the upper and middle layers of the granule. To obtain a high nitrification rate, therefore, it seems vital to maintain a higher degree of oxygen after forming granules.

14.5 MODELING GRANULE-BASED SBR FOR WASTEWATER TREATMENT

14.5.1 Nutrient Removal in Granule-Based SBRs

Beun et al. (2001) have developed a simulation model to evaluate the effects of several operating factors on nitrogen removal in a granule-based SBR. The SBR performance was described using a model made in Aquasim (Reichert 1998). This model is based on balance equations connecting conversion processes and transport processes, and thus it is able to predict the N-conversion processes in the reactor under different conditions. This model used one linear equation to describe acetate uptake, biomass growth, poly(β-hydroxybutyrate) (PHB) production, and mainte-nance for the feast period:

$$-r_S = \frac{1}{Y_{SX}}r_X + \frac{1}{Y_{SP}}r_P + m_S X \qquad (14.1)$$

and one linear equation to describe PHB consumption, biomass growth, and maintenance for the famine period:

$$-r_P = \frac{1}{Y_{PX}}r_X + m_P X \qquad (14.2)$$

where r_S is the acetate uptake rate, r_X the biomass growth rate, r_P the PHB production rate, Y_{SX} and Y_{SP} yields of biomass and PHB on acetate, respectively, Y_{PX} the yield of biomass on PHB, and m_S and m_P maintenance coefficients for growth on acetate and PHB, respectively. In addition, X represents active biomass concentration.

The Aquasim program does not allow formation of hollow structures in the biofilm. Therefore, it was assumed that decay of biomass resulted in formation of inert particulate compounds. It has been shown that nitrification, denitrification, and removal of COD can occur simultaneously in such a granule-based SBR and that the exact location of the autotrophic biomass influences the net nitrogen removal. The distribution of the autotrophs in granules is influenced by the DO in the reactor. It is also found that storage and subsequent degradation of PHB benefit denitrification. In particular, PHB is stored in bacteria situated in deeper layers of granules, below where the autotrophic growth occurs, and serves as a carbon source for denitrification.

A granule-based SBR is a complex bioreactor with numerous internal interactions among process variables and sludge characteristics. In addition to the biological reactions, mass transfer, the hydrodynamic of reactors, and the characteristics of granules have been proven in be influential in the overall performance of a granule-based SBR. Su and Yu (2006a,b) have established a generalized model to simulate a granule-based SBR with considerations of biological processes, reactor hydrodynamics, mass transfer, and diffusion. A discretization of time, size, and segment of sludge has been employed for the discontinuous expressions of different processes. Granules in the SBR are first classified into various size fractions, and each granule is then sliced up along the radius. The concentrations of model components and biological reactions are calculated based on each slice of granules in each size fraction.

Input values of the model include the influent composition, reactor configuration, operating conditions, and characteristics of granules. With these given values, the mass transfer and diffusion, as well as the biological reaction kinetics, could be determined. Thus, the concentrations of components (substrate, ammonia, and nitrate) in the bulk liquid at any operating time could be calculated. The SBR is considered to be a series of continuously stirred tank reactors (CSTRs) in time sequence. For CSTR(t), the influent substrate concentration is $S^i(t - \Delta t)$, and that of effluent is $S^i(t)$, which can be calculated using

$$
\begin{aligned}
S^i(t) &= S^i(t - \Delta t) + k^i(t) \quad \Delta t \\
S^i(0) &= S_0^i \qquad \text{for } t = 0
\end{aligned}
\tag{14.3}
$$

In the calculation of the reaction rate $k^i(t)$, the unknown $S^i(t)$ is considered to be equal to $S^i(t - \Delta t)$, because the value of $S^i(t)$ is close to that of $S^i(t - \Delta t)$, as Δt is sufficiently short.

The reaction rate of component i in the bulk liquid is the sum of reaction rates of all slices in all granules:

$$
k^i(t) = \sum_{m=1}^{M} \left[\left(\sum_{n=1}^{N} k_{m,n}^i f_{V,m,n} \right) f_{V,m} \right]
\tag{14.4}
$$

where N is the number of slices for a granule, M the number of granule size fractions, and $f_{V,m}$ and $f_{V,m,n}$ the volume fractions of the granules belonging to the mth size fraction and those of the nth slice.

In a granule-based SBR, the rates of gas–liquid oxygen transfer are assumed to be proportional to the difference in the oxygen concentration between the gas–liquid interfaces. The proportionality factor is the volumetric oxygen transfer coefficient $k_L a$. On the granule surface, oxygen transferred from the gas phase is equal to that diffused into granules. There is a mass balance equation,

$$
D_e a \frac{\partial S}{\partial R}\bigg|_{R=R_m} = J_{\text{sur}} a = k_L a (S_{\text{gas}} - S_b)
\tag{14.5}
$$

where S_{gas} is the oxygen concentration in the gas phase, S_b the oxygen concentration in the bulk liquid; J_{sur} the oxygen flux on the granule surface, and a the gas–liquid interfacial area per unit liquid volume. Here, the liquid–solid oxygen transfer resistance (external mass transfer) is ignored.

Activated sludge model 1 is modified and used to describe the biological reactions. On the basis of the difference between the results calculated and those measured, the model structure is improved further through the introduction of simultaneous consumption of soluble substrates by storage and heterotroph growth with a changeable reaction rate. The established model is verified with the experimental results for four granule-based SBRs with various granule sizes fed with different wastewaters (Su and Yu, 2006b). The verification results show that the established model is appropriate to simulate and predict nitrogen and chemical oxygen demond (COD) removal in the granule-based SBRs.

A mathematical model has also been developed by de Kreuk et al. (2007b) to simulate the performance of a granule-based SBR for the simultaneous removal of COD, nitrogen, and phosphate. A combination of completely mixed reactor and biofilm reactor compartments is used to simulate the mass transport and conversion processes occurring in the bulk liquid and in the SBR. The biological conversion processes are described using stoichiometric and kinetic parameters from Hao et al. (2001, 2002) and Meijer (2004). The Aquasim software does not allow the volume of the bulk liquid in the biofilm compartment to vary in time. To sort out this problem and simulate the fill and discharge process, two linked compartments have to be defined. A completely mixed liquid compartment with variable volume is connected to the biofilm compartment. A high fluid circulation rate ($Q_{exchange}$) between the two compartments ensures the same bulk liquid concentrations in both compartments (Fig. 14.7).

The model describes the experimental data well. The effect of process parameters on the nutrient removal rates of aerobic granules could be evaluated reliably using this model. The oxygen penetration depth in combination with the position of the autotrophic biomass plays a crucial role in the conversion rates of the various components and thus on the overall nutrient removal efficiency. The ratio between the aerobic and anoxic volumes in the granule strongly determines the N-removal efficiency, as is shown by model simulations with varying oxygen concentration,

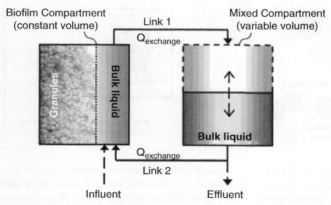

FIGURE 14.7 Schematic of the model setup in Aquasim. Each compartment contains the soluble components and particulate components involved in the metabolic processes. All soluble and particle components are found in effluent and recirculation links. [From de Kreuk et al. (2007b).]

temperature, and granule size. The optimum granule diameter for maximum N and P removal at a DO value of $2\,mg\,L^{-1}$ and 20°C is found between 1.2 and 1.4 mm, and the optimum COD loading rate is $1.9\,kg\,COD\,m^{-3}\,d^{-1}$. When all ammonia is oxidized, oxygen diffused to the granule core inhibits the denitrification process. To optimize the process, anoxic phases can be implemented in the SBR-cycle configuration, leading to more efficient overall N removal. Phosphate removal efficiency depends primarily on the sludge age. At an SRT longer than 30 days, insufficient sludge is removed from the system to keep effluent phosphate concentrations low.

14.5.2   Multiscale Modeling of Granule-Based SBR

Xavier et al. (2007) have developed a multiscale model to describe the complex dynamics of populations and nutrient removal in granule-based SBRs. In this model, the bulk concentrations and effluent composition in six solutes (oxygen, acetate, ammonium, nitrite, nitrate, and phosphate) are described at a macro scale. At a finer scale of one granule (1.1 mm in diameter), the two-dimensional spatial arrangement of four bacterial groups [heterotrophs, ammonium oxidizers, nitrite oxidizers, and polyphosphate-accumulating organisms (PAOs)] is described using individual-based modeling (IbM) with species-specific kinetic models. Initially, Kreft et al. (1998) introduced IbM to microbial populations. This framework has been extended by Xavier et al. (2007) to describe granule-based SBRs.

The multiscale model considers three spatial scales (Fig. 14.8), and the individual scale describes the metabolism of individual biomass elements. The granule scale

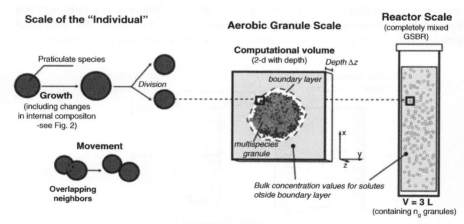

FIGURE 14.8 Spatial and temporal scales of the multiscale model. Spatial scales range from individual biomass elements, at a scale of a few micrometers, to dynamics of multiple bacterial groups in the "aerobic granule scale," in the millimeter scale, to the full system (a 3-L lab-scale granule-based SBR). The two-dimensional computational domain represents a small sub-volume inside the reactor containing a single granule. The number of granules in the reactor (n_g) is a multiplier used to scale-up the granule-scale mass balances to the bulk concentrations dynamics. [From Xavier et al. (2007).]

describes the spatial structure of the aerobic granule, whereas the reactor scale describes dynamics of the entire reactor (i.e., bulk concentration of all solutes and total amount of biomass). The kinetic model for the bioconversions is based on the ASM1 with the inclusion of a metabolic description of PAOs and a separate description of ammonium- and nitrite-oxidizing bacteria (de Kreuk et al. 2007b). The model for PAOs includes three internal storage compounds: polyhydroxyalkanoates, polyphosphate, and glycogen. The computational domain represents a two-dimensional median cross section of a single granule. Simulations start with 10 equally sized particles of each of the four microbial groups, constituting a granule of 120 μm. Spatial solute distributions can be calculated from a steady-state diffusion-reaction equation for each of the solutes, since diffusion is much faster than microbial growth.

For a granule-sludge-based SBR, both the emptying and refilling operations are assumed to be instantaneous; that is, the substrate concentration becomes the volume-weighted average of the substrate concentrations in influent and that remaining in the reactor. The dynamics of the bulk concentrations of each solute in each cycle are described generally as

$$\frac{dS_{i,\text{bulk}}}{dt} = n_g r_i(t) \tag{14.6}$$

where n_g is the number of granules in the reactor and r_i is the global conversion rate of solute i in a single granule. Conversions by nongranular biomass suspended in bulk liquid are neglected.

Simulations of long-term reactor operation show how the microbial population and activity depend on the operating conditions. The short-term dynamics of solute bulk concentrations could be generated with results comparable to the experimental data from laboratory-scale reactors. The multiscale modeling results suggest that N removal in granule-based SBRs occurs mostly via alternating nitrification and denitrification rather than simultaneous nitrification and denitrification, supporting an alternative strategy to improve N removal in this promising wastewater treatment process. This multiscale modeling work demonstrates the application of IbM to granule-based SBRs. The simulations provide insight into the many bioconversion processes occurring while describing both short-term dynamics and long-term reactor operation. For the first time this novel model integrates the dynamics of microbial metabolisms, granule-scale diffusion reaction with two-dimensional spatial organization and larger-scale SBR operation. By being computationally demanding, these models are still far from having a disseminated application in process control. Nevertheless, they already constitute a valuable research tool in academic and industrial research settings to study spatial temporal dynamics in the long-term development of multispecies microbial communities. The use of two- and three-dimensional models can often produce unexpected theoretical results that could not be predicted from one-dimensional models (Batstone et al. 2006). Nevertheless, simpler one-dimensional biofilm models, such as that in the popular Aquasim software (Reichert 1998), which presently runs effortlessly in off-the-shelf desktop computers, have demonstrated the power of simulation for bioprocess design in aerobic granular sludge technologies (Beun et al. 2001; de Kreuk et al. 2007b; Ni and Yu 2008). With the foreseeable increase in affordable computing power and efficient numerical methods, multiscale individual-based models might be a common tool for the future application of aerobic granular sludge processes.

14.6   BIOREMEDIATION OF WASTEWATERS WITH AEROBIC GRANULAR SLUDGE TECHNOLOGY

14.6.1   Organic Wastewater Treatment

Granulation of activated sludge can lead to high biomass retention in reactors because of its compact and dense structure. Biomass concentrations as high as 6.0 to $12.0 \, g \, L^{-1}$ have been obtained in SBRs operated with a volumetric exchange ratio of 50% (Tay et al. 2004). Thus, aerobic granular sludge is advantageous for wastewater treatment over conventional activated sludge. A considerable amount of work has been conducted to the treatment of synthetic wastewater using aerobic granules, as shown in Table 14.1. The feasibility of applying aerobic granulation technology to the treatment of an industrial wastewater was demonstrated by Schwarzenbeck et al. (2005), who examined the ability of aerobic granules to treat dairy wastewater. Aerobic granular sludge can be cultivated successfully in an SBR treating dairy wastewater. After complete granulation and the separation of biomass from the effluent, removal efficiencies of 90% total COD, 80% total nitrogen, and 67% total phosphorus were achieved at a volumetric exchange ratio of 50% and a cycle duration of 8 h. Wang et al. (2004) cultivated aerobic granules with brewery wastewater. After granulation, high and stable removal efficiencies of 88.7% COD and 88.9% NH_4^+-N were achieved at a volumetric exchange ratio of 50% and a cycle duration of 6 h. However, Schwarzenbeck et al. (2005) and Arrojo et al. (2004) found that a significant fraction of suspended solids was present in the reactor effluents. Thus, a post-treatment step is required.

14.6.2   Biological Nutrient Removal

In a biological nutrient removal process, inorganic nitrogen in the form of ammonium is removed through aerobic, autotrophic nitrification followed by anoxic, heterotrophic denitrification. The process is normally split into two stages, as the environmental conditions required for each process are very different. In a granular sludge system, the substrate is supplied in a short period of time. A high substrate concentration in the bulk liquid causes penetration of substrate deeper into granules than oxygen penetration. During the period in which the external substrate is available (feast period), oxygen is quickly consumed in the outer layers by growth, substrate storage, and nitrification. Oxygen has only a limited penetration depth in this period. Acetate storage [as poly(β-hydroxybutyrate) or (PHB)] and growth occur aerobically in the outermost layer or anoxically inside the granule (Beun et al. 2001). During the period without an external substrate (famine period), growth takes place on the internally stored PHB at a much lower growth rate (Beun et al. 2001). The oxygen penetration depth during the famine period will be higher because of this decreased respiration rate of the heterotrophs, but will still be limited, due to the increased nitrification relative to the feast phase (Beun et al. 2001). The nitrate produced can simultaneously be denitrified inside the granules using the stored PHB as an electron donor. Tsuneda et al. (2003) investigated the granulation of nitrifying bacteria in an aerobic upflow fluidized-bed reactor for the treatment of an inorganic wastewater containing $500 \, mg \, L^{-1}$ of NH_4^+-N. The ammonia removal rate reached $1.5 \, kg \, N \, m^{-3} \, d^{-1}$, suggesting that the nitrifying granules were able to achieve stable and efficient nitrification.

Phosphorus can be removed biologically through biological phosphorus removal processes, exploiting the ability of PAOs to take up P in excess of metabolic requirements and to accumulate it intracellularly as polyphosphate. Lin et al. (2003) cultivated phosphorus-accumulating granules at different substrate P/COD ratios in the range $1:100$ to $10:100$ by weight in SBRs. The soluble COD and PO_4^--P profiles showed that the granules had typical P-accumulating characteristics, with a concomitant uptake of soluble organic carbon and the release of phosphate in the anaerobic stage, followed by rapid phosphate uptake in the aerobic stage.

Recent research work on aerobic granules suggests that granules could be beneficial for simultaneous nitrification, denitrification, and phosphorus removal (SNDPR). In granules there is an oxygen mass-transfer limitation that is important in facilitating the aerobic and anoxic zones required for SNDPR. Lemaire et al. (2008b) cultivated aerobic granules for SNDPR and observed that simultaneous phosphorus removal and nitrification occurred throughout the SBR operation. Good phosphorus removal and nitrification occurred throughout the SBR with a dominancy of *Accumulibacter* spp. (PAOs) and *Competibacter* spp. (GAOs). *Accumulibacter* spp. were dominant in the outermost 200-μm region of the granule, while *Competibacter* spp. dominated in the granule central zone. Yilmaz et al. (2008) investigated the biological removal of nitrogen and phosphorus from nutrient-rich abattoir wastewater using granular sludge. It is demonstrated that the granules could be sustained and indeed developed further using of abattoir wastewater. The organic, nitrogen, and phosphorus loading rates used were $2.7 \, kg \, COD \, m^{-3} \, d^{-1}$, $0.43 \, kg \, N \, m^{-3} \, d^{-1}$ and $0.06 \, kg \, P \, m^{-3} \, d^{-1}$, respectively. The removal efficiency of soluble COD, nitrogen, and phosphorus was 85%, 93%, and 89%, respectively. However, the amount of high suspended solids in the effluent limited the overall removal efficiency to 68%, 86%, and 74% for total COD, total N, and total P, respectively. *Accumulibacter* spp. were found to be responsible for most of the denitrification, further reducing the COD requirement for nitrogen and phosphorus removal. Mineral precipitation was evaluated and was not found to contribute significantly to the overall nutrient removal. An anaerobic feeding phase combined with low DO (10 to 20% saturation) in the aerated period in aerobic granular reactor favor N, P, and COD removal by the aerobic granules. The aforementioned feeding pattern proved to generate more stable granules than with a pulse feed of 3 min. This was due to the selection of relatively slow growing PAOs. These organisms store acetate as PHB during the anaerobic feeding period, while releasing phosphate, while during the aerated period, PAOs use the stored PHB as a carbon source and again take up the released phosphate. During aeration, ammonia is converted to nitrate, which can serve as an electron acceptor for PAOs in the core of the granules, where oxygen is depleted. To enlarge the anoxic zone volume within granules, a low DO was used (20%). At these conditions, high COD-, N-, and P-removal efficiencies were reached and amounted to 100%, 98%, and 99%, respectively.

14.6.3   Domestic Wastewater Treatment

For aerobic granules, Tay et al. (2004) reported that it was difficult to form granules with an OLR lower than $2\,kg\ COD\,m^{-3}\,d^{-1}$. It is expected that a low-strength wastewater will result in the difficulties of granulation or a long startup of the aerobic granular system from activated sludge. Thus, the possibility of forming aerobic granules on domestic sewage in an SBR should be explored. De Kreuk and van Loosdrecht (2006) studied aerobic granulation with presettled sewage as influent. After 20 days of operation at a high COD loading rate (about $2\,g\,COD\,L^{-1}\,d^{-1}$ with a 2-h cycling time), heterogeneous aerobic granules were formed, with an SVI after 10 min of settling of $38\,mL\,g^{-1}$ and an average diameter of 1.1 mm. Utilization of a high COD load was found to be critical to the formation of aerobic granules on low-strength domestic wastewater. Therefore, a short cycle time is preferred to form granules in an SBR when domestic wastewater is used as the influent.

14.6.4   Xenobiotic Contaminant Bioremediation

The aggregation of microorganisms into compact aerobic granules has additional benefits, such as protection against predation and resistance to chemical toxicity (Jiang et al. 2004). Because cell self-immobilization creates a diffusional resistance and establishes a concentration gradient that shelters the microbial cells beneath the protective barrier by diluting the toxic chemical below some threshold value to allow continued microbial activity and substrate utilization. Tay et al. (2004) and Jiang et al. (2004) investigated the feasibility of treating phenol-containing wastewater with aerobic granular sludge. The granules displayed an excellent ability to degrade phenol. Adav et al. (2008a) reported that aerobic granules could degrade phenol at $1.18\,g\,phenol\,g^{-1}\,VSS\,d^{-1}$. Jiang et al. (2004) isolated 10 bacterial strains from aerobic phenol-degrading granules and identified their potential to degrade phenol. The PG-01 strain, a member of the α-proteobacteria, is common in granules and is the predominant strain in phenol degradation. Another strain affiliated with β-proteobacteria, PG-08, has minimal phenol degradation capability and a high propensity for self-aggregation. Adav et al. (2007) isolated the yeast strain *Candida tropicalis* from their phenol-degrading granules and reported it to be a functionally dominant strain in the granules. Hence, different strains on aerobic granules may have specific roles in granule structural integrity and phenol degradation.

Cultivated phenol-fed aerobic granules were also able to degrade pyridine. The granules completely degraded 250 to $1500\,mg\,L^{-1}$ pyridine at a constant rate with no time lag, and with 12- and 15-h time lags at 2000 and $2500\,mg\,L^{-1}$ pyridine concentration, respectively (Adav et al. 2007). Yi et al. (2006) developed aerobic granules for co-metabolic transformation of p-nitrophenol and 2,4-dichlorophenol, respectively, with glucose as a co-substrate. It was found that glucose could promote aerobic granulation and facilitate the biodegradation of recalcitrant xenobiotics. Nancharaiah et al. (2006) cultivated aerobic granules successfully for the biodegradation of nitrilotriacetic acid. Development of aerobic granules for the biological degradation of 2,4-dichlorophenol (2,4-DCP) in a sequencing batch reactor was reported by Wang et al. (2004). After operation for 39 d, stable granules with a diameter range of 1 to 2 mm and a clearly defined shape and appearance were obtained. After granulation, the effluent 2,4-DCP and COD concentrations were 4.8 and 41 mg L^{-1}, with high removal efficiencies of 94% and 95%, respectively. Specific 2,4-DCP biodegradation rates in the granules followed the Haldane model for substrate inhibition, and peaked at 39.6 mg 2,4-DCP g^{-1} VSS h^{-1} at a 2,4-DCP concentration of 105 mg L^{-1}. Efficient degradation of 2,4-DCP, nitrilotriacetic acid, and phenol by the aerobic granules suggests their potential application in the treatment of industrial wastewater containing chlorophenols and other xenobiotic contaminants.

14.6.5   Removal of Heavy Metals or Dyes

Liu et al. (2002) developed aerobic granules using synthetic wastewater for the bioaccumulation of zinc. The biosorption of zinc as Zn(II) was governed by the concentration of Zn(II). This phenomenon had also been seen with other biosorbents such as marine algae (Liu et al. 2002; Taniguchi et al.). The maximum biosorption capacity of Zn(II) by aerobic granules was 270 mg g^{-1} (Liu et al. 2002). In another study, Liu investigated the biosorption of Ni by aerobic granules, and in this study, the Ni^{2+} biosorption was investigated with release of Ca^{2+}, Mg^{2+}, and K$^+$. The study found that the Ca^{2+} released (0.52 meq g^{-1}) was much higher than Mg^{2+} (0.045 meq g^{-1}) and K$^+$ (0.061 meq g^{-1}) for a Ni^{2+} uptake of 0.76 meq g^{-1} dry weight. They concluded that Nickel biosorption onto aerobic granules involved an ion-exchange mechanism, not chemical precipitation of Ni^{2+}. The study also found that Ni^{2+} was distributed uniformly from the surface to the inner core of aerobic granules (Liu and Xu 2007). Zhang et al. (2005) also investigated cerium (Ce) adsorbed by aerobic granules. Ce ions adsorbed onto the granules increased gradually with respect to time, and this was observed at various initial Ce ion concentrations (Zhang et al. 2005). Ce biosorption was attributed to functional groups or biopolymers, and can be described as a physicochemical process that obeyed first-order reversible kinetics as seen with cadmium (Cd) biosorption (Liu et al. 2003; Zhang et al. 2005). Yao et al. (2009) found that Cr^{3+} biosorption capacity increased with increasing pH at a pH range of 2 to 6. At an initial Cr^{3+} concentration of 50 mg L^{-1} and pH 5, the maximum biosorption capacity of aerobic granules is 37.8 mg g^{-1}. They argued that the predominance of negatively charged functional groups such as carboxyl, amine, and phosphate groups had drawn Cr^{3+} ions. At a pH greater than 5, precipitation of Cr(OH)$_3$ occurred and competed with functional groups on biosorption (Yao et al. 2009). Later, Liu et al. (2003, 2004) extended the heavy metal study to multielements and introduced cadmium and copper in addition to zinc. They found that maximum biosorption capacities of Cd^{2+}, Zn^{2+}, and Cu^{2+} by aerobic granules were 625, 204, and 52.9 mg g^{-1}, respectively, and these values were much higher than those of other biosorbents. In addition, aerobic granules have a settling velocity 5 to 10 times higher than that of microbial flocs, which made aerobic granules an excellent heavy metal biosorbent (Liu et al. 2003, 2004).

Recently, Sun and co-workers studied the feasibility of treating malachite green wastewater with aerobic granules (Sun et al. 2008). They revealed that malachite green removal was rapid in the initial stage, but decreased with time. They argued that in the initial phase, the aerobic granules surface was available and that this explained the fast rate of biosorption. After the initial phase, fewer sorption sites remained available on the aerobic granule surface. They found the biosorption equilibrium to be comparable to the adsorption of dyes by activated sludge, sawdust, and activated powdered carbon. The malachite green biosorption is a single curve, and this may be because of monolayer coverage of malachite green on the aerobic granule surface. The study also found that the initial concentration was the driving force that overcame the mass-transfer resistance of the dye with respect to the aqueous and solid phases. A higher initial concentration of malachite green enhanced the biosorption process in aerobic granules (Sun et al. 2008). In the same study it was found that malachite green biosorption increased with increasing pH. They postulated that low biosorption of malachite green by aerobic granules under acidic conditions could be attributed to the development of cations on the biosorbent, which prevented biosorption of malachite green onto the surface of aerobic granules. The presence of excessive H ions would also compete with the positively charged malachite green for negatively charged biosorption sites (Sun et al. 2008). The formation of dimers when the pH increased also enhanced malachite green biosorption onto an aerobic granule surface by electrostatic interactions between malachite green and the granule surface (Sun et al. 2008). The maximum biosorption capacity of malachite green onto aerobic granules was 56.8 mg g^{-1} (Sun et al. 2008).

14.7   REMARKS

Aerobic granulation is a very promising technology from both an engineering and an economic point of view and offers an attractive alternative for the treatment of different types of wastewater. In many cases, this granular system makes possible a more stable operation, and the treatment of larger loads, the removal of multiple toxic pollutants, lower volumes for the settling systems, and the production of better-quality effluents than do conventional systems. Aspects related to aerobic granules, including cultivation, formation mechanisms, microbial and physicochemical characteristics, modeling of granule-based systems, and practical applications of this technology have been presented.

Over the years, our knowledge of aerobic granulation has improved significantly, due largely to the high number of valuable studies from various disciplines. However, unanswered questions about this technology remain in relation to some issues. Work in the following areas is necessary to gain a greater understanding of aerobic granulation technology. Although aerobic granulation technology is a compact reactor technology, it still has limitations, such as a relatively high suspended solids concentration in the effluent. Thus, further research is needed to investigate the feasibility of being coupled to a post-treatment unit. For further improvements in aerobic granulation biotechnology, we need to expand our knowledge of microbial communities and population dynamics related to their function in aerobic granules. Linking the microbial population with the operational factors that influence aerobic granules is likely to be the major problem to be resolved. To acquire this knowledge, detailed molecular surveys of microbial communities in aerobic granules are required.

REFERENCES

Adav S. S., Lee D. J., Ren N. Q. (2007) Biodegradation of pyridine using aerobic granules in the presence of phenol. *Water Research* **41**, 2903–2910.

Adav S. S., Chang C. H., Lee D. J. (2008a) Hydraulic characteristics of aerobic granules using size exclusion chromatography. *Biotechnology and Bioengineering* **99**, 791–799.

Adav S. S., Lee D. J., Show K. Y., Tay J. H. (2008b) Aerobic granular sludge: recent advances. *Biotechnology Advances* **26**, 411–423.

Arrojo B., Mosquera-Corral A., Garrido J. M., Mendez R. R. (2004) Aerobic granulation with industrial wastewater in sequencing batch reactors. *Water Research* **38**, 3389–3399.

Batstone D. J., Picioreanu C., van Loosdrecht M. C. M. (2006) Multi-dimensional modelling to investigate interspecies hydrogen transfer in anaerobic biofilms. *Water Research* **40**, 3099–3108.

Benjamin S., Magbanua J. R., Bowers A. R. (2006) Characterization of soluble microbial products (SMP) derived from glucose and phenol in dual substrate activated sludge bioreactors. *Biotechnology and Bioengineering* **93**, 862–870.

Beun J. J, Hendriks A., van Loosdrecht M. C. M, Morgenroth E., Wilderer P. A., Heijnen J. J. (1999) Aerobic granulation in a sequencing batch reactor. *Water Research* **33**, 2283–2290.

Beun J. J., van Loosdrecht M. C. M., Heijnen J. J. (2000) Aerobic granulation. *Water Science and Technology* **41**, 41–48.

Beun J. J, Heijnen J. J, van Loosdrecht M. C. M. (2001) N-removal in a granular sludge sequencing batch airlift reactor. *Biotechnology and Bioengineering* **75**, 82–92.

Beun J. J., van Loosdrecht M. C. M., Heijnen J. J. (2002) Aerobic granulation in a sequencing batch airlift reactor. *Water Research* **36**, 702–712.

Cassidy D. P., Belia E. (2005) Nitrogen and phosphorus removal from an abattoir wastewater in a SBR with aerobic granular sludge. *Water Res* **39**, 4817–4823.

Chen G. H., Yip W. K., Mo H. K., Liu Y. (2001) Effect of sludge fasting/feasting on growth of activated sludge cultures. *Water Research* **35**(4), 1029–1037.

Chen G. H., Mo H. K., Liu Y. (2002) Utilization of a metabolic uncoupler, 3,3′,4′,5-tetrachilrosalicylanilide (TCS) to reduce sludge growth in activated sludge culture. *Water Research* **36**(8), 2077–2083.

Chen G. H., An K. J., Saby S., Brois E., Djafer M. (2003) Possible cause of excess sludge reduction in an oxic-settling-anaerobic activated sludge process (OSA process). *Water Research* **37**(16), 3855–3866.

Chen M. Y., Lee D. J., Yang Z., Peng X. F. (2006) Fluorescent staining for study of extracellular polymeric substances in membrane biofouling layers. *Environmental Science and Technology* **40**, 6642–6646.

Chen Y., Jiang W., Liang D. T., Tay J. H. (2007) Structure and stability of aerobic granules cultivated under different shear force in sequencing batch reactors. *Applied Microbiology and Biotechnology* **76**, 1199–1208.

Chiu Z. C., Chen M. Y., Lee D. J., Tay S. T. L., Tay J. H., Show K. Y. (2006) Diffusivity of oxygen in aerobic granules. *Biotechnology and Bioengineering* **94**, 505–513.

de Bruin L. M. M., de Kreuk M. K., de Roest H. F. R., van der Uijterlinde C., van Loosdrecht M. C. M. (2004) Aerobic granular sludge technology: alternative for activated sludge? *Water Science and Technology* **49**, 1–7.

de Kreuk M. K., van Loosdrecht M. C. M. (2006) Formation of aerobic granules with domestic sewage. *Journal of Environmental Engineering* **132**, 694–697.

de Kreuk M. K., Heijnen J. J., van Loosdrecht M. C. M. (2005a) Simultaneous COD, nitrogen, and phosphate removal by aerobic granular sludge. *Biotechnology and Bioengineering* **90**, 761–769.

de Kreuk M. K., Pronk M., van Loosdrecht M. C. M. (2005b) Formation of aerobic granules and conversion processes in an aerobic granular sludge reactor at moderate and low temperatures. *Water Research* **39**, 4476–4484.

de Kreuk M. K., Kishida N., van Loosdrecht M. C. M. (2007a) Aerobic granular sludge: state of the art. *Water Science and Technology* **55**, 75–81.

de Kreuk M. K., Picioreanu C., Hosseini M., Xavier J. B., van Loosdrecht M. C. M. (2007b) Kinetic model of a granular sludge SBR: influences on nutrient removal. *Biotechnology and Bioengineering* **97**, 801–815.

de Silva D. G. V., Rittmann B. E. (2000a) Interpreting the response to loading changes in a mixed-culture completely stirred tank reactor. *Water Environment Research* **72**, 566–573.

de Silva D. G. V., Rittmann B. E. (2000b) Nonsteady-state modeling of multispecies activated-sludge processes. *Water Environment Research* **72**, 554–565.

Fang F., Ni B. J., Li X. Y., Sheng G. P., Yu H. Q. (2009) Kinetic analysis on the two-step processes of AOB and NOB in aerobic nitrifying granules. *Applied Microbiology and Biotechnology* **83**, 1159–1169.

Gaval G., Pernell J. J. (2003) Impact of the repetition of oxygen deficiencies on the filamentous bacteria proliferation in activated sludge. *Water Research* **37**, 1991–2000.

Green D. E., Reiblet S. (1975) Paired moving charges in mitochondrial energy coupling: II. universality of the principles for energy coupling in biological systems. *Proceedings of the National Academy of Sciences USA* **72**(1), 253–257.

Hao X., van Loosdrecht M. C. M., Meijer S. C. F., Heijnen J. J., Qian Y. (2001) Model based evaluation of denitrifying P removal in a two-sludge system. *Journal of Environmental Engineering* **127**, 112–118.

Hao X., Heijnen J. J., van Loosdrecht M. C. M. (2002) Model-based evaluation of temperature and inflow variations on a partial nitrification ANAMMOX biofilm process. *Water Research* **36**, 4839–4849.

Hu L., Wang J., Wen X., Qian Y. (2005) The formation and characteristics of aerobic granules in sequencing batch reactor (SBR) by seeding anaerobic granules. *Process Biochemistry* **40**, 5–11.

Hulshoff Pol L. W., de Castro Lopes S. I., Lettinga G., Lens P. N. L. (2004) Anaerobic sludge granulation. *Water Research* **38**, 1376–1389.

Jang A., Yoon Y. H., Kim I. S., Kim K. S., Bishop P. L. (2003) Characterization and evaluation of aerobic granules in sequencing batch reactor. *Journal of Biotechnology* **105**, 71–82.

Jiang H. L., Tay J. H., Tay S. T. L. (2002) Aggregation of immobilized activated sludge cells into aerobically grown microbial granules for the aerobic biodegradation of phenol. *Letters in Applied Microbiology* **35**, 439–445.

Jiang H. L., Tay J. H., Maszenana M., Tay S. T. L. (2004) Bacterial diversity and function of aerobic granules engineered in a sequencing batch reactor for phenol degradation. *Applied Environmental Microbiology* **70**, 6767–6775.

Jiang H. L., Tay J. H., Maszenan A. M., Tay S. T. L. (2006) Enhanced phenol biodegradation and aerobic granulation by two coaggregating bacterial strains. *Environmental Science and Technology* **40**, 6137–6142.

Kolenbrander P. E., Andersen R. N., Clemans D. L., Whittaker C. J., Klier C. M. (1999) Potential role of functionally similar coaggregation mediators in bacterial succession. In: Newman H. N., Wilson M. (eds.), *Dental Plaque Revisited: Oral Biofilms in Health and Disease*. Bioline, Cardiff, UK pp. 171–186.

Kreft J. U., Booth G., Wimpenny J. W. T. (1998) BacSim, a simulator for individual-based modeling of bacterial colony growth. *Microbiology SGM* **144**, 3275–3287.

Lemaire R., Webb R. I., Yuan Z. (2008a) Micro-scale observations of the structure of aerobic microbial granules used for the treatment of nutrient-rich industrial wastewater. *ISME Journal* **2**, 528–541.

Lemaire R., Yuan Z., Blackall L., Crocetti G. (2008b) Microbial distribution of *Accumulibacter* spp. and *Competibacter* spp. in aerobic granules from a lab-scale biological nutrient removal system. *Environmental Microbiology* **10**, 354–363.

Li Z. H., Kuba T., Kusuda T. (2006) The influence of starvation phase on the properties and the development of aerobic granules. *Enzyme Microbial Technology* **38**, 670–674.

Lin Y. M., Liu Y., Tay J. H. (2003) Development and characteristics of phosphorus-accumulating microbial granules in sequencing batch reactors. *Applied Microbiology and Biotechnology* **62**, 430–435.

Liu S. Y., Liu G., Tian Y. C., Chen Y. P., Yu H. Q, Fang F. (2007) An innovative microelectrode fabricated using photolithography for measuring dissolved oxygen distributions in aerobic granules. *Environmental Science and Technology* **41**, 5447–5452.

Liu S. Y., Chen Y. P., Fang F., Liu S. H., Ni B. J., Liu G., Tian Y. C., Xiong Y., Yu H. Q. (2008) An innovative solid-state microelectrode for nitrite determination in a nitrifying granule. *Environmental Science and Technology* **42**, 4467–4471.

Liu X. W., Sheng G. P., Yu H. Q. (2009) Physicochemical characteristics of microbial granules. *Biotechnology Advances* **27**, 1061–1070.

Liu Y., Tay J. H. (2001) Strategy for minimization of excess sludge production from the activated sludge process. *Biotechnology Advances* **19**(2), 97–107.

Liu Y., Tay J. H. (2002) The essential role of hydrodynamic shear force in the formation of biofilm and granular sludge. *Water Research* **36**, 1653–1665.

Liu Y., Tay J. H. (2004) State of the art of biogranulation technology for wastewater treatment. *Biotechnology Advances* **22**, 533–563.

Liu Y. Q., Tay J. H. (2007) Cultivation of aerobic granules in a bubble column and an airlift reactor with divided draft tubes at low aeration rate. *Biochemical Engineering Journal* **34**, 1–7.

Liu Y., Xu H. (2007) Equilibrium thermodynamics and mechanisms of Ni^{2+} biosorption by aerobic granules. *Biochemical Engineering Journal* **35**(2), 174–182.

Liu Y., Yang S. F., Tay J. H., Liu Q. S., Qin L., Li Y. (2004) Cell hydrophobicity is a triggering force of biogranulation. *Enzyme and Microbial Technology* **34**, 371–379.

Liu Y., Chen G. H., Paul E. (1998) Effect of the S0/X0 ratio on energy uncoupling in substrate-sufficient batch culture of activated sludge. *Water Research* **32**(10), 2883–2888.

Liu Y., Wang Z. W., Qin L., Liu Y. Q, Tay J. H. (2005a) Selection pressure-driven aerobic granulation in a sequencing batch reactor. *Applied Microbiology and Biotechnology* **67**, 26–32.

Liu Y., Wang Z. W., Liu Y. Q., Qin L., Tay J. H. (2005b) A generalized model for settling velocity of aerobic granular sludge. *Biotechnology Progress* **21**, 621–626.

Liu Y. Q., Wu W. W., Tay J. H., Wang J. L. (2007) Starvation is not a prerequisite for the formation of aerobic granules. *Applied Microbiology and Biotechnology* **76**, 211–216.

Low E. W., Chase H. A. (1999) Reducing production of excess biomass during wastewater treatment. *Water Research* **33**(5), 1119–1132.

Majone M., Dircks K., Beun J. J. (1999) Aerobic storage under dynamic conditions in activated sludge processes: the state of the art. *Water Science and Technology* **39**, 61–73.

Martins A. M. P., Heijnen J. J., van Loosdrecht M. C. M. (2003) Effect of dissolved oxygen concentration on sludge settleability. *Applied Microbiology and Biotechnology* **62**, 586–593.

Maximova N., Dahl O. (2006) Environmental implications of aggregation phenomena: current understanding. *Current Opinions in Colloid and Interface Science* **11**, 246–266.

Mayhew M., Stephenson T. (1998) Biomass yield reduction: Is biochemical manipulation possible without affecting activated sludge process efficiency? *Water Science and Technology* **38**(8–9) 137–144.

McSwain B. S., Irvine R. L., Wilderer P. A. (2004) The influence of settling time on the formation of aerobic granules. *Water Science and Technology* **50**, 195–202.

McSwain B. S., Irvine R. L., Hausner M., Wilderer P. A. (2005) Composition and distribution of extracellular polymeric substances in aerobic flocs and granular sludge. *Applied Environmental Microbiology* **71**, 1051–1057.

Meijer S. C. F. (2004) Theoretical and practical aspects of modelling activated sludge processes. Ph. D. dissertation, Technical University, Delft, The Netherlands.

Meyer R. L., Saunders A. M., Zeng R. J., Keller J., Blackall L. L. (2003) Microscale structure and function of anaerobic–aerobic granules containing glycogen accumulating organisms. *FEMS Microbiology Ecology* **45**, 253–261.

Morgenroth E., Sherden T., van Loosdrecht M. C. M., Heijnen J. J., Wilderer P. A. (1997) Aerobic granular sludge in a sequencing batch reactor. *Water Research* **31**, 3191–3194.

Mosquera-Corral A., de Kreuk M. K., Heijnen J. J., van Loosdrecht M. C. M. (2005) Effects of oxygen concentration on N-removal in an aerobic granular sludge reactor. *Water Research* **39**, 2676–2686.

Moy B. Y. P., Tay J. H., Toh S. K., Liu Y., Tay S. T. L. (2002) High organic loading influences the physical characteristics of aerobic sludge granules. *Letters in Applied Microbiology* **34**, 407–412.

Mu Y., Yu H. Q. (2006) Rheological and fractal characteristics of granular sludge in an upflow anaerobic reactor. *Water Research* **40**, 3596–3602.

Mu Y., Ren T. T., Yu H. Q. (2008) Drag coefficient of porous and permeable microbial granules. *Environmental Science and Technology* **42**, 1718–1723.

Nancharaiah Y. V., Schwarzenbeck N., Mohan T. V. K., Narasimhan S. V., Wilderer P. A. (2006) Biodegradation of nitrilotriacetic acid (NTA) and ferric–NTA complex by aerobic microbial granules. *Water Research* **40**, 1539–1546.

Ni B. J., Yu H. Q. (2008) Growth and storage processes in aerobic granules grown on soybean wastewater. *Biotechnology and Bioengineering* **100**, 664–672.

Ni B. J., Yu H. Q. (2010a) Mathematical modeling of aerobic granular sludge: a review. *Biotechnology Advance* **28**, 895–909.

Ni B. J., Yu H. Q. (2010b) Modeling and simulation of the formation and utilization of microbial products in aerobic granular sludge. *AIChE Journal* **56**, 546–559.

Ni B. J., Yu H. Q., Xie W. M. (2008) Storage and growth of denitrifiers in aerobic granules: Part II. *Model calibration and verification. Biotechnology and Bioengineering* **99**, 324–332.

Ni B. J., Xie W. M., Yu H. Q., Wang Y. Z., Wang G., Dai X. L. (2009) Granulation of activated sludge in a pilot-scale sequencing batch reactor for the treatment of low-strength municipal wastewater. *Water Research* **43**, 751–761.

Palmer R. J., Kazmerzak K., Hansen M. C., Kolenbrander P. E. (2001) Mutualism versus independence: strategies of mixed-species oral biofilms in vitro using saliva as the sole nutrient source. *Infection and Immunology* **69**, 5794–5704.

Pan S., Tay J. H., He Y. X., Tay S. T. L. (2004) The effect of hydraulic retention time on the stability of aerobically grown microbial granules. *Letters in Applied Microbiology* **38**, 158–163.

Peng D. C., Bernet N., Delgenes J. P., Moletta R. (1999) Aerobic granular sludge: a case report. *Water Research* **33**, 890–893.

Pratt S., Yuan Z., Keller J. (2004) Modelling aerobic carbon oxidation and storage by integrating respirometric, titrimetric, and off-gas CO_2 measurements. *Biotechnology and Bioengineering* **88**, 135–147.

Ramasmy P., Zhang X. (2005) Effects of shear stress on the secretion of extracellular polymeric substances in biofilms. *Water Science and Technology* **52**(7), 217–223.

Reichert P. (1998) *Aquasim 2.0-User Manual: Computer Program for the Identification and Simulation of Aquatic Systems*, EAWAG, Dübendorf, Switzerland.

Rensink J. H., Rulkens W. H. (1997) Using metazoa to reduce sludge production. *Water Science and Technology* **36**(11), 171–179.

Russell J., Cook G. M. (1995) Energetic of bacterial growth: balance of anabolic and catabolic reaction. *Microbiology Reviews* **59**(1), 48–63.

Sanin S. L., Sanin F. D., Bryers J. D. (2003) Effect of starvation on the adhesive properties of xenobiotic degrading bacteria. *Process Biochemistry* **38**, 909–914.

Schwarzenbeck N., Borges J. M., Wilderer P. A. (2005) Treatment of dairy effluents in an aerobic granular sludge sequencing batch reactor. *Applied Microbiology and Biotechnology* **66**, 711–718.

Sekiguchi Y., Kamagata Y., Harada H. (2001) Recent advances in methane fermentation technology. *Current Opinions Biotechnology* **12**, 277–282.

Sheng G. P., Yu H. Q., Li X. Y. (2006) Stability of sludge flocs under shear conditions: roles of extracellular polymeric substances (EPS). *Biotechnology and Bioengineering* **93**, 1095–1102.

Sin G., Kaelin D., Kampschreur M. J., Takacs I., Wett B., Gernaey K. V., Rieger L., Siegrist H., van Loosdrecht M. C. M. (2008) Modeling nitrite in wastewater treatment systems: a discussion of different modeling concepts. *Water Science and Technology* **56**, 1155–1171.

Strand S. E., Harem G. N., Stensel D. (1999) Activated-sludge yield reduction using chemical uncouplers. *Water Environment Research* **71**(4), 454–458.

Su K. Z., Yu H. Q. (2005) Formation and characterization of aerobic granules in a sequencing batch reactor treating soybean-processing wastewater. *Environmental Science and Technology* **39**, 2818–2828.

Su K. Z., Yu H. Q. (2006a) A generalized model of aerobic granule-based sequencing batch reactor: I. Model development. *Environmental Science and Technology* **40**, 4703–4708.

Su K. Z., Yu H. Q. (2006b) A generalized model for aerobic granule-based sequencing batch reactor: II. Parametric sensitivity and model verification. *Environmental Science and Technology* **40**, 4709–4713.

Sun X. F., Wang S. G., Liu X. W., Gong W. X., Bao N., Gao B. Y., Zhang H. Y. (2008) Biosorption of Malachite Green from aqueous solutions onto aerobic granules: kinetic and equilibrium studies. *Bioresource Technology* **99**(9), 3475–3483.

Tay J. H., Liu Q. S., Liu Y. (2001a) The role of cellular polysaccharides in the formation and stability of aerobic granules. *Letters in Applied Microbiology* **33**, 222–226.

Tay J. H., Liu Q. S., Liu Y. (2001b) The effects of shear force on the formation, structure and metabolism of aerobic granules. *Applied Microbiology and Biotechnology* **57**, 227–233.

Tay J. H., Yang S. F., Liu Y. (2002) Hydraulic selection pressure-induced nitrifying granulation in sequencing batch reactors. *Applied Microbiology and Biotechnology* **59**, 332–337.

Tay J. H., Pan S., He Y. X., Tay S. T. L. (2004) Effect of organic loading rate on aerobic granulation: I. Reactor performance. *Journal of Environmental Engineering* **130**, 1094–1101.

Trinet F., Heim R., Amar D., Chang H. T., Rittmann B. E. (1991) Study of biofilm and fluidization of bioparticles in a three-phase fluidized-bed reactor. *Water Science and Technology* **23**, 1347–1354.

Tsuneda S., Nagano T., Hoshino T., Ejiri Y., Noda N., Hirata A. (2003) Characterization of nitrifying granules produced in an aerobic upflow fluidized bed reactor. *Water Research* **37**, 4965–4973.

Tsuneda S., Ogiwara M., Ejiri Y., Hirata A. (2006) High-rate nitrification using aerobic granular sludge. *Water Science and Technology* **53**(3), 147–154.

van Loosdrecht M. C. M., Pot M., Heijnen J. J. (1997) Importance of bacterial storage polymers in bioprocesses. *Water Research* **35**, 41–47.

Wang Q., Du G., Chen J. (2004) Aerobic granular sludge cultivated under the selective pressure as a driving force. *Process Biochemistry* **39**, 557–563.

Wang X. H., Zhang H. M., Yang F. L., Xia L. P., Gao M. M. (2007) Improved stability and performance of aerobic granules under stepwise increased selection pressure. *Enzyme Microbiology and Technology* **41**, 205–211.

Weber S. D., Ludwig W., Schleifer K. H., Fried J. (2007) Microbial composition and structure of aerobic granular sewage biofilms. *Applied Environmental Microbiology* **73**, 6233–6240.

Wei Y. S., van Houten R. T., Borger A. R., Eikelboom D. H., Fan Y. B. (2003) Minimization of excess sludge production for biological wastewater treatment. *Water Research* **37**(18), 4453–4467.

Xavier J. B., de Kreuk M. K., Picioreanu C., van Loosdrecht M. C. M. (2007) Multi-scale individual-based model of microbial and bioconversion dynamics in aerobic granular sludge. *Environmental Science and Technology* **41**, 6410–6417.

Yang S. F., Tay J. H., Liu Y. (2005) Effect of substrate N/COD ratio on the formation of aerobic granules. *Journal of Environmental Engineering* **131**, 86–92.

Yang S. F., Li X. Y., Yu H. Q. (2008) Formation and characterisation of fungal and bacterial granules under different feeding alkalinity and pH conditions. *Process Biochemistry* **43**, 8–14.

Yao L., Ye Z. F., Tong M. P., Lai P., Ni J. R. (2009) Removal of Cr^{3+} from aqueous solution by biosorption with aerobic granules. *Journal of Hazardous Materials* **165**(1–3) 250–255.

Yi S., Zhuang W. Q., Wu B., Tay S. T. L, Tay J. H. (2006) Biodegradation of *p*-nitrophenol by aerobic granules in a sequencing batch reactor. *Environmental Science Technology* **40**, 2396–2401.

Yilmaz G., Lemaire R., Keller J., Yuan Z. (2008) Simultaneous nitrification, denitrification, and phosphorous removal from nutrient-rich industrial wastewater using granular sludge. *Biotechnology and Bioengineering* **100**, 529–541.

Yuan Z., Blackall L. L. (2002) Sludge population optimisation: a new dimension for the control of biological wastewater treatment systems. *Water Research* **36**, 482–490.

Zhang L. L., Feng X. X., Xu F., Xu S., Cai W. M. (2005) Biosorption of rare earth metal ion on aerobic granules. *Journal of Environmental Science and Health A* **40**(4), 857–867.

Zheng Y. M. (2006) The cultivation and characterization of aerobic granular sludge. Ph. D. dissertation, University of Science and Technology of China, Hefei, China.

Zheng Y. M., Yu H. Q. (2007) Determination of the pore size distribution and porosity of aerobic granules using size-exclusion chromatography. *Water Research* **41**, 39–46.

Zheng Y. M., Yu H. Q., Sheng G. P. (2005) Physical and chemical characteristics of granular activated sludge from a sequencing batch airlift reactor. *Process Biochemistry* **40**, 645–650.

Zheng Y. M., Yu H. Q., Liu S. J., Liu X. Z. (2006) Formation and instability of aerobic granules under high organic loading conditions. *Chemosphere* **63**, 1791–1800.

Zhu L., Xu X. Y., Zheng Y. (2005) Acta Scientiae Circumstantiae **25**, 1148 (in Chinese).

15

BIODEGRADABLE BIOPLASTICS FROM FERMENTED SLUDGE, WASTES, AND EFFLUENTS

ETIENNE PAUL

Université de Toulouse; INSA, UPS, INP; LISBP, 135 Avenue de Rangueil, F-31077 Toulouse, France; INRA, UMR792, Ingénierie des Systèmes Biologiques et des Procédés, F-31400 Toulouse, France; CNRS, UMR5504, F-31400, Toulouse, France

ELISABETH NEUHAUSER

Université Paul Sabatier, Laboratoire de Biologie Appliquée à l'Agroalimentaire et à l'Environnement, Auch, France

YU LIU

Division of Environmental and Water Resources Engineering, School of Civil and Environmental Engineering, Nanyang Technological University, Singapore

15.1 INTRODUCTION

15.1.1 Context of Poly(hydroxyalkanoate) Production from Sludge and Effluents

Large volumes of effluents and organic wastes are produced from industrial and urban systems. The removal of such pollution is costly and consumes great quantities of energy. Effluents and sludge can thus be considered to be troublesome wastes. In a context of petroleum depletion and climate change, the possibility of recovering material from wastewater and sludge is an appealing solution that may reduce the

Biological Sludge Minimization and Biomaterials/Bioenergy Recovery Technologies, First Edition.
Edited by Etienne Paul and Yu Liu.

impact of waste treatment. Energy and materials contained in the wastes could be turned into resources with substantial added value. Currently, valorization strategies include production of a variety of carbon-based materials, such as nutrients, bricks, coagulant, pumice, slag, and activated carbon. However, this attractive objective faces some strong constraints, such as the relatively low carbon substrate concentration, the variability of the resource and its low availability, which make it difficult to degrade, and the use of nonoptimal culture conditions, since the broth cannot be controlled. Nevertheless, works are currently in progress to assess the feasibility of some waste valorization routes (Gurieff and Lant 2007).

Interest is currently focused on the use of mixed microbial cultures coming from wastewater and waste treatment plants, with the aim of turning waste materials into resources. The merits of mixed culture (MC) fermentation are the utilization of organic wastes as the substrate and the absence of a requirement for septic processing. Moreover, an MC may be more robust than a pure culture in the context of an open culture because it can grow on various organic compounds and adapts easily to the variable substrate composition of the wastes and to the variable environments.

Biological transformations by MC fermentation offer a wide-ranging potential for chemical or energy production from effluents, wastes, and residues. Kleerebezem and van Loosdrecht (2007) have considered the opportunity of using MC fermentation for bioenergy production. The solutions proposed include the well-known example of anaerobic digestion with methane or hydrogen as end products, and also the production of acetone, butanol, and ethanol mixtures. In cases where no methane reinjection or direct exploitation can be implemented, production of poly(hydroxyalkanoate) (PHA) as an energy carrier could be an attractive alternative. For instance, in the case of wastewater treatment, transformation of the chemical oxygen demand (COD) into PHA by a microbial population could lead to a sludge containing more than 70 wt% of volatile suspended solids (VSS) as PHA (Gurieff and Lant 2007; Serafim et al. 2008). This enriched sludge could be then dehydrated or dried for subsequent use and polyhydroxybutyrate (PHB)-enriched cells could be used for direct combustion or transformation into methane.

Chemical production from wastewater and waste by MC fermentation can also be considered. The question then arises as to what chemical should be chosen and how "green" the process will be. Moreover, the amount and availability of the waste must be checked, as must the existence of a market for the final product. Among the most promising biomaterials to be produced from wastes are again polyesters of hydroxyalkanoates (PHAs). PHAs are attractive because they are biodegradable and also because their properties are very close to those of polyethylene or polypropylene. Moreover, a large number of copolymer blends are possible, allowing for the production of a wide variety of polymers (natural PHA plastics are highly versatile). Their broad range of physical properties means that PHAs can be rigid to highly elastic, have very good gas and liquid barrier properties, and are resistant to hot water and grease. PHAs can thus replace petrochemical-derived plastics in a large variety of applications: fibers, textiles, films, adhesives, starting material for the synthesis of chiral compounds, packaging materials, prostheses, disposable items, surgical sutures, and wound dressings (Lee 1996a). Bioplastics from PHAs are less porous to oxygen than are conventional plastics. Therefore, when they are used to cover food products, antioxidant consumption can be reduced. In addition, biocompatibility and biodegradability are important features, for example, in the biomedical field.

The objective is therefore to convert organic matter from concentrated effluents and sludge into PHA. Thus, both COD valorization and sludge reduction can be targeted. A recent life-cycle assessment and a financial analysis of PHA production from sludge or concentrated effluents by mixed cultures have shown the very promising potential of PHA production (Gurieff and Lant 2007).

PHAs are mono- or heteropolyesters that can be synthesized and stored in the form of intracellular granules by numerous microbial species. They are carbon and energy storage molecules that can be produced by many bacteria under external/or internal growth-limiting conditions (Anderson and Dawes 1990; Anderson et al. 1990). More than 300 different microorganisms have been found to be able to store PHAs, whose composition in 3-hydroxyfatty acids varies depending on the carbon substrate provided (Anderson et al. 1990; Dias et al. 2006). The role of PHAs as metabolic intermediates in microbial processes for wastewater treatment was recognized early (Cech and Chudoba 1983; van Loosdrecht et al. 1997) and has been thoroughly investigated in such anaerobic–aerobic systems as enhanced biological phosphorus removal (Cech and Hartman 1990; Cech and Hartman 1993; Satoh et al. 1999). For the last decade, there has been growing interest in an evaluation of the potential use of MC fermentation for PHA production from waste streams. Complex substrates with high organic carbon concentrations, previously fermented and converted to volatile fatty acids (VFAs), appear to be good candidates: food wastes (Rhu et al. 2003), olive and palm oils (Din et al. 2006; Dionisi et al. 2006a; Becarri et al. 2009), mill and paper mill effluents (Bengtsson et al. 2008a), sugarcane molasses (Albuquerque et al. 2007), fruit and tomato cannery effluents (Gurieff 2007; Liu et al. 2008), and municipal sludges (Coats et al. 2007b; Mengmeng et al. 2009). With regard to overall environmental impact, Gurieff and Lant (2007) studied how PHA production could outperform that of synthetic plastics by using a theoretical effluent with different organic loads. Considering PHA production from organic sludge by MC fermentation, Gurieff and Lant (2007) suggested that this strategy would not only help solve an expensive solids disposal problem, but could also produce a valuable "green" product.

15.1.2 Industrial Context for PHA Production

Up to now, industrial production of PHAs has used pure culture fermentation. Table 15.1 lists various companies involved in PHA production and the names of the corresponding products they market. A major problem is the high production cost of these PHAs compared to the final cost of petroleum-derived plastics, for which prices around $4.90\,kg^{-1}$, $5.58\,kg^{-1}$, and as low as $4.75\,kg^{-1}$ can be found in the literature, the lowest price being obtained for production on a scale of 1 million metric tons per year (Choi and Lee 1997). These prices are much lower than those of PHA polymers, sold at $16\,kg^{-1}$ in 1996 (Lee 1996b). Fortunately, the PHA polymer cost can be minimized by the high performance of the process in terms of productivity

TABLE 15.1   Some Companies Involved in PHA Production

Company	Products
Berlin Packaging Corp. (U.S.)	Zeneca/ICI Biopol
Bioscience Ltd. (Finland)	Medical applications of PHAs
Bioventures Alberta, Inc. (Canada)	PHA produced by recombinant *Escherichia coli*
Metabolix, Inc. (U.S.)	PHB, P(HB : HV) (Mirel)
Metabolix/ADM	Transgenic plant PHAs
Monsanto (U.S.)	Transgenic plant PHAs
Polyferm, Inc. (Canada)	PHAs from hemicellulose; use of *Burkholderia cepacia* on xylose
Monsanto-Metabolix (U.S.)	Biopol from *Cupriavidus necator*
Nodax Procter and Gamble (U.S.)	PHBHx, PHBO, PHBOd (Nodax)
Tianan Biologic Material Co (China)	PHB and P(HB : HV) (Enmat)
Tianjin GreenBio Materials Co., Ltd. (GreenBio) (China)	Sogreen
Biocycle Copersucar (Brasil)	PHB and P(HB : HV) (Biocycle)
Biomer (Germany)	PHB and P(HB : HV) (Biomer L)
BIO-ON (Italy)	Minerv-PHA (from sugar beets)
NatureWorks LLC (U.S.)	Ingeo biopolymer
Micromidas	Constructed microbial population able to adapt to a variety of materials, including waste

and yield. Choi and Lee (1999b) reported a P(HB:HV) (copolymer of hydroxybutyrate and hydroxyvalerate) concentration of 158.8 g L^{-1}, corresponding to a P(HB:HV) content of 78.2 wt% with an HV fraction of 10.6 mol% obtained in 55.1 h; this results in a productivity of $2.88 \text{ g P(HB:HV) L}^{-1} \text{ h}^{-1}$. In the same way, a very high productivity of $4.94 \text{ g PHB L}^{-1} \text{ h}^{-1}$ was achieved from a laboratory fed-batch system using *Alcaligenes latus*. This would lead to a production cost as low as $2.6 kg^{-1} PHB (Lee and Choi 1998), which could open up a significant market for fermentation-based PHAs. Nevertheless, because the PHB production yield is low (around 0.4 g PHB g S^{-1}), the origin and availability of the substrate strongly influence the final production cost. Considering the cheapest organic substrate, a value of $0.22 kg^{-1} of PHA can be compared to the value of $0.185 kg^{-1} obtained for polypropylene (Kothuis and Schelleman, 1998, cited by Salehizadeh and van Loosdrecht 2004). Therefore, it would be possible to decrease the final cost significantly by using agricultural wastes such as whey and molasses. The use of MCs may also bring some cost decrease because of their low investment cost and the absence of a requirement for axenic conditions. In their life-cycle assessment and financial analysis of PHA production, Gurieff and Lant (2007) reported a promising internal rate of return (25%) in the case of PHA production in a MC with concentrated effluents. Their results showed clear benefits when highly concentrated feed and improved PHA production technology were used. In the case of MC and organic matter from wastes, the authors also pointed out that energy rather than substrate represented the main operating cost. They also stressed the impact of the production technology chosen,

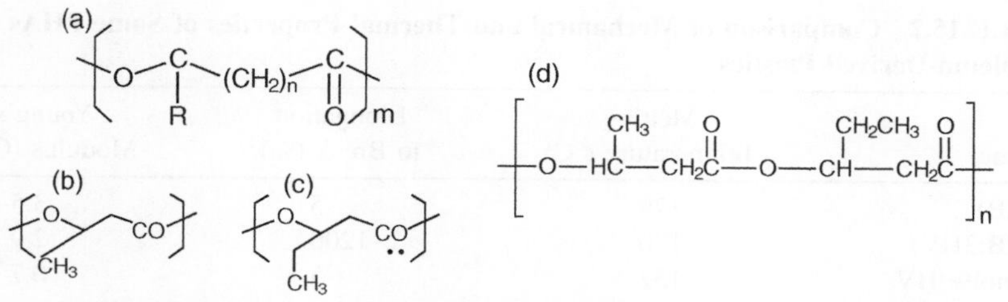

(a)

(b)

(c)

(d)

CH_3 O CH_2CH_3 O
—O—HC—CH_2C—O—CH—CH_2C—

FIGURE 15.1 PHA structure: (a) general structure; (b) poly(3-hydroxybutyrate) ($CH_{1.5}O_{0.5}$, $m = 21.5$ g $Cmol^{-1}$); (c) poly(3-hydroxyvalerate) (PHV; $CH_{1.6}O_{0.4}$, $m = 20$ g $Cmol^{-1}$); and (d) poly(3-hydroxybutyrate-*co*-3-hydroxyvalerate) [P(3HB:3HV); $CH_{1.56}O_{0.44}$, $m = 20.67$ g $Cmol^{-1}$].

which must be as simple as possible to reduce the capital cost of the plant and for a sustainable, efficient recovery process.

15.2 PHA STRUCTURE

More than 300 different microorganisms have been identified as PHA producers and around 100 different monomer units was found to be constituents of PHA (Lee 1996b). Two categories of PHAs are generally considered: short-chain-length PHAs (SCL-PHAs), composed of short carbon chains ($C_4 \rightarrow C_5$) as in Fig. 15.1, and medium-chain-length PHAs (MCL-PHAs), with longer carbon chains ($C_6 \rightarrow C_{14}$) that may contain aromatic rings when produced under specific growth conditions (Witholt and Kessler 1999; Kim et al. 2007).

PHAs have optical properties (Lee and Choi 1999; Reddy et al. 2003) since the monomers are all in the R chiral configuration, due to the stereospecificity of the enzyme involved in the biosynthesis. Physical properties of PHA plastics depend strongly on the chemical nature of the monomers included in the polymer (Table 15.2). PHB in its pure form is rigid, breaks easily, and has a high processing temperature which is very close to the degradation temperature, whereas the copolymer P(3HB:3HV) gives a softer and tougher product with properties similar to those of polypropylene. This is due to a decrease in the crystallinity and the melting temperature. Flexibility and processability are thus improved when the copolymer P(3HB:3HV) is formed. As a consequence of their low degree of crystallinity and low melting temperature, MCL-PHAs are elastic or tacky materials showing more flexibility and elastomeric properties than are shown by SCL-PHAs (Kim et al. 2007).

15.3 MICROBIOLOGY FOR PHA PRODUCTION

Both pure cultures and recombinant microorganisms are used for PHA industrial production. For example, genera of prokaryotic microorganisms capable of

TABLE 15.2   Comparison of Mechanical and Thermal Properties of Some PHAs and Petroleum-Derived Plastics

Polymer	Melting Temperature (°C)	Elongation to Break (%)	Young's Modulus (GPa)
P(3HB)	179	5	3.5
P(3HB:3HV)	170	>1200	2.9
3 mol% HV	137	5	0.7
25 mol% HV	77		
55 mol% HV	83		
71 mol% HV			
P(4HB)	53	1000	149
Polypropylene	170	400	1.7
Polyethylene-terephtalate	262	7300	2.2
Polystyrene	110	3.1	

accumulating PHA has been thoroughtly studied (Koller et al. 2010). First, *Azotobacter* spp. were chosen because of their capacity to use saccharose and glucose as carbon sources. However, the PHA production was found to be unstable since polysaccharides were produced instead of PHA, reducing the conversion yield (Anderson and Dawes 1990). Wild species' capacity to use molasses from beet or malt was improved so as to increase the production yield (Page and Knosp 1989). *Alcaligenes latus* is able to use various substrates and is characterized by high specific rates of growth and production (Hrabak 1992; Lee and Choi 1998). The *Pseudomonas* genus can develop and produce PHB on substrates with long carbon chains which are not soluble in water. *Cupriavidus necator* is one of the best PHA-storing bacteria for use in PHA industrial production, due to its high yield, rapid production rate, and ability to grow from renewable sources (Byrom 1987). Cells were first grown under nonlimiting nutrient conditions with the aim of biomass generation and polymer accumulation was then achieved by applying a nutrient (nitrogen, phosphate, oxygen, etc.) limitation.

Recombinant strains have been built by cloning the PHA biosynthesis genes from various wild organisms into *Escherichia coli* strains. These strains were selected for their high PHA productivity, their high PHA content (up to 90 wt%), their ability to use several inexpensive substrates, and a notable ease of PHA extraction, thanks to the fragility of their cell walls and the absence of PHA degradation during the culture, due to their lack of intracellular depolymerase (Lee 1997). Li et al. (2007) have recently reviewed the use of recombinant organisms for PHA production and give a comparison of the capacity of several production processes using recombinant *E. coli* strains. In particular, Table 1 of that review synthesizes the productivity and PHA content obtained with the *E. coli* strains.

An open MC is also widely used for treating wastes and effluents. The actual microbial composition of such MCs is generally unknown, but by applying the right selection pressure (operational and environmental parameters), it is possible to impose microbial transformations. Storage of organic compounds in activated sludge has been described by various authors (Cech and Chudoba 1983). It has been studied widely in the case of phosphate-accumulating organisms (PAOs) and glycogen-accumulating organisms (GAOs). However, the proportion of PHA-storing organisms in activated sludge may be low, and the enrichment of activated sludge in PHA-storing organisms would therefore be a key issue to provide an economically feasible process based on open cultures. Three systems are used for enrichment of the microbial population in PHA-storing organisms: the anaerobic–aerobic system, which involves PAOs and/or GAOs; the micro-aerophilic system; and aerobic dynamic feeding. These systems and approaches are presented and discussed in Sections 15.4 and 15.7. However, up to now, very few studies have focused on characterizing the microbial community of MCs for PHA production. Generally, authors follow the PHA production capacity by culturing and sampling sludge during a batch experiment. However, the real increase in PHA production capacity due to enrichment is not quantified, certainly because the methods for quantifying PHA-storing organisms in a mixed population are not yet available. Studies and characterization of microbial consortia were begun recently. Dionisi et al. (2005a) used denaturing gradient gel electrophoresis applied to sludge to follow the dynamics of the microbial community against time. This strategy allowed Dionisi et al. (2006b) to provide a clone library from the total DNA of a mixed culture. Clones were also screened, and the relevant ones were sequenced for organism identification. A review of these results is available in Dias et al. (2006). Unpublished data (Paul 2010) from the ISBP laboratory at the University of Toulouse deal with fed-batch cultures with P-limiting growth conditions using activated sludge from wastewater treatment plants as inocula. Figure 15.2 shows the polymorphisms observed by these researchers in a PHB-accumulating MC after 60 h of culture.

Thus, the question of whether it is better to use a pure culture or an MC for PHA production from wastes and concentrated wastewater is still open. The answer will depend partly on our capacity to implement either the strain selected or the consortium selected for PHA production, and make it reliable.

15.4 METABOLISM OF PHA PRODUCTION

Understanding the metabolic pathways involved in PHA synthesis is of great interest since it allows the ways that polymer accumulates in the cell to be predicted and helps in the control of PHA composition. In MCs, various micro-organisms are involved, each of which may have metabolic specificities. In the case of PHA synthesis, different storing behaviors have been reported, depending on the type of microorganisms and the substrate used (Anderson and Dawes 1990). In cases where the same carbon source and growth conditions are used, it has often been hypothesized that PHA metabolism in MCs is similar to that reported for pure cultures. Nevertheless, this hypothesis has not yet been fully confirmed.

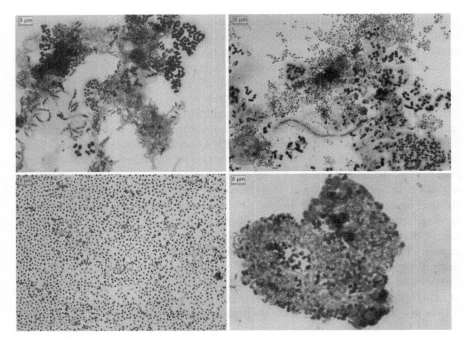

FIGURE 15.2 Cell polymorphisms in a fed-batch or continuous cultures seeded with activated sludge and conducted with a phosphorus growth limitation. Specific black coloration of PHB granules (Sudan black staining).

15.4.1 PHB Metabolism

Most of the organisms that accumulate PHB can synthesize the polymer from acetyl coenzyme A (acetyl-CoA) by a sequence of three reactions, as described in Fig. 15.3. The enzymes involved are: 3-ketothiolase, which catalyzes the condensation of two molecules of acetyl-CoA; acetoacetyl-CoA reductase, which catalyzes the reduction of acetoacetyl-CoA into 3-hydroxybutyryl-CoA; and poly(3-hydroxybutyrate) synthase, which includes the activated monomer in the PHB polymer.

CoA is the key effector metabolite controlling PHB biosynthesis. Acetyl-CoA can be oxidized via the tricarboxylic acid (TCA) cycle or can serve as a precursor for PHB synthesis, depending on the cell environmental conditions. When the NAD(P)H/NAD(P) ratio increases, some enzymes of the TCA cycle are inhibited and acetyl-CoA is partially diverted to PHB synthesis. Moreover, a high concentration of CoA–SH leads to competitive inhibition of the 3-ketothiolase, thereby preventing PHB synthesis. Thus, PHB may be seen as a carbon reserve but also as a sink of reducing power and can therefore be considered as a redox regulator for cells (Senior and Dawes 1971). Various factors may explain an increase in the NAD(P)H/NAD(P) ratio or a decrease in the CoA/acetyl-CoA ratio in the cell. Growth limitation by controlled availability of oxygen or other nutrients, such as nitrogen, phosphate, sulphur, or magnesium, and also excess of a carbon compound for

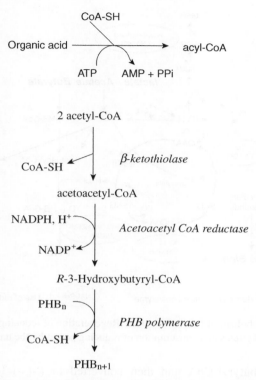

FIGURE 15.3 Steps involved in the production of PHB. Activation of an organic acid, VFAs like to give the acyl-CoA is also described in the upper part of the figure.

growth, are the most common factors leading to PHB accumulation (Braunegg et al. 2004). Operating conditions with dynamic feeding can also lead to PHB accumulation, as a consequence of what is often called "unbalanced growth" (Anderson and Dawes 1990).

Different substrates can be used to produce PHB. When refined single-carbon sources are used, glucose and organic acids are the most conventional substrates. Glucose as the carbon source in a culture is broken down following the glycolysis pathway, which leads to acetyl-CoA and energy production. When Volatile fatty acids are used, the organic acid must cross the cell membrane to be activated into its corresponding acyl-CoA form (Fig. 15.3). PHB synthesis from butyric or valeric acids does not involve acetyl-CoA and can proceed directly via acetoacetyl-CoA involving a nondegradative pathway (Anderson and Dawes 1990). This nondegradative pathway can be seen in Fig. 15.4.

In addition, PHB-storing organisms express some differences in their metabolism of PHB synthesis. In *Rhodospirillium rubrum*, five steps are described. The pathway is similar to that determined for *cupriavidus necator,* but in that case, acetoacetyl-CoA is reduced by a NADPH-dependent reductase into

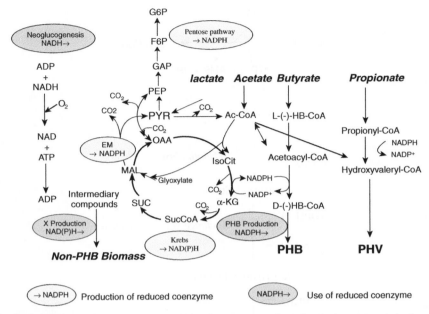

FIGURE 15.4 Metabolism of PHA production. Regeneration of reducing power is indicated by the lightly shaded circles and consumption of reducing power by the darkly shaded circles.

S-(+)-3-hydroxybutyryl-CoA and then converted to R-(−)-3-hydroxybutyryl-CoA by two enoyl-CoA hydratases.

In another metabolic pathway, encountered in the major *Pseudomonas* species, intermediary compounds from the β-oxidation pathway lead to medium-chain-length-hydroxyalkanoates (MCL-PHAs). For example, *P. oleovorans* accumulates mainly 3-hydroxyoctanoate (3HO) and 3-hydroxyhexanoate (3HHx) when grown on octane, octanol, or octanoate.

Alternatively, *Pseudomonas* species can also synthesize copolymers of MCL-PHAs (3-hydroxydecanoate), and in that case the precursors are derived from the fatty acid de novo synthesis pathway.

The reducing power (NADPH, H$^+$) required for PHB synthesis is provided through the Entner–Doudoroff pathway (also called the pentose phosphate pathway) [Eq. (15.1)] and through the activities of two NADP-dependent enzymes: isocitrate dehydrogenase activity [Eq. (15.2)] or malic enzyme activity (see Fig. 15.4) (Anderson and Dawes 1990):

$$\text{glucose} + \text{ATP} + 2\text{NADP}^+ \rightarrow \text{ribulose-5-P} + \text{CO}_2 + \text{ADP} + 2\text{NADPH}, \text{H}^+$$

$$(15.1)$$

$$\text{glucose} + \text{NADP}^+ \rightarrow \text{NADPH}, \text{H}^+ + \text{pyruvate} + \text{3-P-glyceraldehyde} \quad (15.2)$$

Equation (15.3) describes the elongation of PHB polymer in the case of *C. necator* employing the Entner–Doudoroff pathway. Energy is generated (ATP) but decarboxylation occurs. Consequently, less than 2.1 g of glucose is required per gram of PHB produced, notably due to the need for substrate to generate new cells.

$$PHB_n + glucose + ADP + P_i + 3NAD^+ \rightarrow PHB_{n+1} + ATP + 3NADH, H^+ + 2CO_2$$

$$(15.3)$$

15.4.2 Metabolism for Other PHA Production

Numerous polymers can be synthesized by microorganisms, depending on the culture conditions and on the substrate type. It is generally accepted that the various polymers are formed to allow the cells to balance the redox equivalents produced and needed for the conversion of substrate to PHA.

When propionic acid is used as the carbon source, one propionyl-CoA molecule is condensed with one acetyl-CoA molecule to form 3-ketovaleryl-CoA. This molecule is reduced to 3-hydroxyvalerate, which can be included in the polymer by PHA synthase. If acetyl-CoA is present or formed from the breakdown of propionyl-CoA (which always occurs to some extent), 3HB is also formed. In consequence, both 3HB and 3HV units are always produced from propionic acid but the 3HV/3HB ratio increases when the level of propionic acid compared to acetyl-CoA-generating substrate increases. A polymer P(3HB:3HV) (60 : 40) can be obtained when propionic acid is the only carbon source. When two molecules of propionyl-CoA condense, 3-hydroxy-2-methylvaleryl-CoA is produced, leading to poly(3-hydroxy-2-methylvalerate).

In comparison to experiments performed under either oxygen excess or a restricted oxygen supply (1 to 4% of air saturation), a co-supplementation of glucose and propionic acid leads to an increase in the rate and the yield of 3HV production from propionic acid. This is due to the fact that the unwanted oxidative loss of CO_2 from propionyl-CoA can be avoided by restricting the oxygen supply.

Butyric and valeric acids proceed via the nondegradative pathway. Butyrate leads to PHB production, while valerate is transformed into both 3HV and 3HB. An increased percentage of 3HV in the polymer is observed when valerate is used as precursor instead of propionic acid. When valeric acid is the sole carbon source, *R. eutropha* is able to synthesize a copolyester with 90 mol% of 3HV monomers (Braunegg et al. 2004). VFAs containing an even number of carbon atoms lead primarily to the formation of HB monomers, whereas VFAs containing an odd number of carbon atoms lead to the formation of a copolymer with HV monomers.

MCL–hydroxyalkanoate production relies on three metabolic routes: (1) the de novo fatty acid biosynthesis pathway, giving (R)-3-hydroxyacyl-CoA precursors from carbon sources such as glucose, (2) fatty acid degradation by β-oxidation, and, (3) chain elongation (acyl-CoA extended by incorporation of acetyl-CoA) (Witholt and Kessler 1999).

TABLE 15.3 PHB Production Yield and Volumetric Productivity Obtained Depending on the Nutrient Limitation Type and Degree

	PHB Yield, Y_{PHB} (g PHB g^{-1} glucose)	Volumetric Productivity (g PHB L^{-1} h^{-1})
P starvation	0.31	2.21
N starvation	0.27	0.45
N limitation	0.32	1.16

Source: Aragao et al. (1996).

15.4.3 Nutrient Limitations

Under oxygen limitation, the NADH/NAD$^+$ ratio increases due to the lack of final electron acceptor. Consequently, acetyl-CoA cannot totally enter the TCA cycle, which leads to a decrease in CoA–SH concentration. Inhibition of the β-ketothiolase is thus removed and PHB can be synthesized. One useful parameter to describe the oxygen limitation level is the *relative respiration rate* (RRR), defined as the ratio between the respiration rate under oxygen limitation and the respiration rate measured at the end of the exponential growth phase (Vollbrecht and Schlegel 1979). Values of 0.25 (Gaudin 1998) or 0.45 (Vollbrecht and Schlegel 1979) have been proposed for this parameter.

Under nutrient limitation such as nitrogen and phosphate limitation, ATP excess is observed because of reduced activity of the anabolic pathways; therefore, acetyl-CoA accumulates with consequences similar to those observed under oxygen limitation. However, drastic starvation in one nutrient should be avoided because growth is necessary to maintain PHA storage capacity. Table 15.3 presents the PHB production yields, which depend on the type and level of nutrient limitation (Aragao et al. 1996). Figure 15.5 further illustrates the evolution of the specific PHB production rate with the specific growth rate (μ). Clearly, an optimum value of μ can be defined.

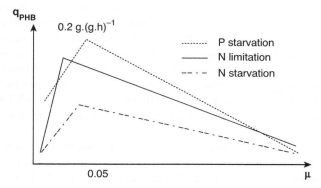

FIGURE 15.5 Relationship between q_{PHB} and μ, depending on the nutrient limitation applied. [From Aragao et al. (1996)].

As shown in Fig. 15.5, PHB accumulation under nutrient limitation is correlated with the decrease in the specific growth rate, and the maximum specific PHB production rate (q_{PHB}^{max}) is higher for P limitation than for N limitation. This may be correlated with the fact that phosphorus does not enter the protein composition and thus has less consequence on cell anabolism. Phosphorus forms part of membrane, RNA, and nucleotide components. It is thus frequently included in phosphorylated metabolic intermediaries and thus appears more easily transferable than nitrogen from one component to another due to cell reorganization.

15.4.4 PHA Metabolism in Mixed Cultures

PHA storing capacity was observed in alternating anaerobic–aerobic bioreactors when a selector was placed prior to the activated sludge process or when dynamic aerobic feeding was imposed on the bioreactor. These conditions are in good agreement with the limitation described earlier that led to PHA storage in pure culture.

PHB Production in PAOs and GAOs The first study reporting PHA production by MCs in the wastewater field was by Wallen and Rohwedder (1974). During phosphorus removal, they observed the storage of a copolymer containing HV and HB units and HHx. Two groups of microorganisms were then identified for their capacity to store PHA under dynamic conditions, notably in alternating anaerobic–aerobic processes. These two groups have been named PAOs and GAOs. PAOs have the capacity to utilize the energy stored as poly-P, for PHB accumulation when there is no external electron acceptor (oxygen or nitrate) in the medium. In another way, GAOs are not able to store poly-P, but they can accumulate glycogen and use this internal reserve to produce PHB. According to Mino et al. (1998), PAOs and GAOs can use similar metabolisms to produce energy and reducing power from the degradation of internal glycogen. However, in the case of PAOs, reducing power is provided mainly by glycogen degradation via the Entner–Doudoroff pathway, whereas for GAOs, ATP is produced mainly via the Embden–Meyerhoff–Parnas pathway. Moreover, when microaerophilic conditions are imposed, the microorganism may be able to get enough energy for assimilative activities (synthesis of proteins, glycogen, etc.) and for taking up organic substrates. The schematic description of the metabolism of PHA production by PAOs and GAOs can be found in Salehizadeh and van Loosdrecht (2004).

Various metabolic models were developed in the case of MCs operating under alternating anaerobic–aerobic conditions. These models were reviewed recently by Oehmen et al. (2007). Alternating anaerobic and aerobic conditions with electron donor excess favors the selection of PAOs and GAOs. These conditions have been used for the selection of PHA-storing organisms but also to produce PHAs (Satoh et al. 1996; Satoh et al. 1998a; Takabatake et al. 2000; Chua et al. 2003). Specific selection of GAOs has also been done and a high fraction of 3HV monomers and even of 3-hydroxy-2-methylvalerate, in the copolymer could be obtained (Bengtsson 2009). Glycogen formation and its conversion to PHA could explain this metabolic behavior (Bengtsson et al. 2008a; Dai et al. 2008).

PHB Production Under Aerobic Dynamic Feeding   Beun et al. (2000a) proposed that the PHB storage capacity observed during feast and famine regimes may be related to the notion of unbalanced growth, described previously by some authors for pure cultures (Anderson et al. 1992). Under aerobic dynamic feeding (ADF) conditions, cells have a given conversion capacity for anabolic reactions, closely linked to the intracellular level of the anabolic enzymes. When the substrate uptake rate is larger than this conversion rate, PHB storage occurs. In contrast, when no substrate is available, PHB degradation takes place, leading to new cell growth and consequently to dilution of the anabolic enzymes. Metabolic models for PHA storage under ADF have been reviewed by Dias et al. (2006). ADF is currently the most widely used technique for the selection of PHA-storing organisms and it can also be adapted for industrial PHA production.

15.4.5   Effect of Substrate in Mixed Cultures

As already mentioned, the chemical nature of the substrate conditions the composition of the (co-) polymer produced. Some studies describe PHA production by mixed cultures using propionate, butyrate, lactate, succinate, pyruvate, malate, or ethanol (Satoh et al. 1992; Majone et al. 2001; Beccari et al. 2002), while others report the use of glutamate, aspartate (Satoh et al. 1998b), or glucose (Yu 2001; Hollender et al. 2002) as the carbon substrate (Tables 15.4 and 15.5).

The formation of copolymers containing C_4 and C_5 3-hydroxyacids has been described when using glucose and propionic acid. In MCs, some PHV can also be produced even if acetate is used as the sole substrate because glycogen is converted to PHA through propionyl-CoA in order to satisfy the redox balance (Satoh et al. 1994). The general fatty acid metabolism can also generate 3-hydroxyacyl-CoAs. Unlike pure cultures, MCs tend to transform carbohydrate substrates mostly into glycogen rather than PHA (van Loosdrecht et al., 1997; Carta et al. 2001; Dircks et al. 2001). Beun et al. (2000a) explained this behavior by the difference in the energy required

TABLE 15.4   Composition of PHA Polymers Produced by MCs Under Alternating Anaerobic–Aerobic Systems Depending on the Substrate Used[a]

Substrate	Polymer Composition (PHA%) (HB/HV/HMB/HMV)	PHB Content (%)	Reference
Acetate	93:7:0:0	41	Dai et al. (2008)
Fermented food waste	77:23:0:0	60	Rhu et al. (2003)
Fermented diluted paper mill wastewater	62:29:0:9	25	Bengtsson et al. (2008b)
Sugar cane molasses	Short- and medium-chain-length monomers	17	Pisco et al. (2009)
Fermented wastewater	50:50:0:0	40	Coats et al. (2007a)

[a] PHA content in g PHA (g biomass^{-1}) $\times$ 100; PHA composition in mol%.

TABLE 15.5 Composition of PHA Polymers Produced by MCs in ADF Systems, Depending on the Substrate Used[a]

Substrate	Polymer Composition (PHA%) (HB/HV/HMB/HMV)	PHB Content (%)	Reference
Acetate	100:0:0:0	65	Serafim et al. (2004a)
Acetate and N limitation	—	89	Johnson et al. (2010a)
Propionate	12:61:0:27	13.6	
Propionate and acetate	54:33:0:13	25.4	Lemos et al. (2006)
Valerate	32:52:0:16	14.3	
Fermented molasses	83:17:0:0	33	Albuquerque et al. (2008)
Fermented diluted paper mill wastewater	39:61:0:0	48	Bengtsson et al. (2008a)
Fermented POME	—	44.5	Din et al. (2006)
Fermented OME	89:11:0:0	54	Dionisi et al. (2005b)
Fermented primary sludge	35:65:0:0	32	Gurieff (2007)
Tomato cannery wastewater	100:0:0:0	20	Liu et al. (2008)
Fermented brewery wastewater	—	38	Mato et al. (2008)

[a] PHA content in g PHA (g biomass^{-1}) × 100; PHA composition in mol%.

for substrate storage: 0.17 mol ATP (C mol G6P)$^{-1}$ against 0.25 mol ATP (C mol acetyl-CoA)$^{-1}$. For glucose or starch feeding, glycogen is produced instead of PHA when a mixed culture is used (Goel et al. 1999). Storage capacities reach 45% when acetate was used (PHB storage), while these capacities reached 68% and 36% when glucose and starch (glycogen storage) were used, respectively. Although acetate is consumed more slowly than glucose, no diauxie was observed when biomass developed on a mixture of acetate and glucose. Yields observed were similar to those obtained on pure substrates, with values around 0.6 C mol C mol^{-1} for Y_{PHB} and around 0.7 mol C mol^{-1} C for Y_{Gly} (Carta et al. 2001). The authors concluded that the conversion efficiency under mixed substrate conditions was the sum of the conversion efficiencies obtained with the individual substrates.

15.5 PHA KINETICS

Performance levels obtained with pure cultures are useful to assess the capacity of MC to compete with current industrial production. Results of PHB production by *C. necator* and *A. latus* are summarized in Table 15.6. Productivities as high as 2.42 g L^{-1} h^{-1} and PHB contents up to 88% are reported.

TABLE 15.6 Characteristics of Cultures for PHB Production by Industrial Strains of *C. necator* and *A. latus*

Organism	Substrate	Culture Mode	Performance[a]	Reference
Cupriavidus necator	Glucose	Fed-batch	$X_f = 164$ g L^{-1}; $PHB_f = 121$ g L^{-1} (PHB = 76%); $r_{PHB} = 2.42$ g L^{-1} h^{-1}	Kim et al. (1994)
	Glucose	Two-stage continuous	% PHB = 72.1%	Du et al. (2001)
	Oleic acid	Fed-batch	PHB final = 32.5 g L^{-1} (60 h)	Eggink et al. (1992)
	Acetic acid + lactic acid	Fed-batch	$X_f = 75$ g L^{-1}; $PHB_f = 54.8$ g L^{-1} (PHB = 73.1%); $r_{PHB} = 1.33$ g L^{-1} h^{-1}	Tsuge et al. (2001)
Alcaligenes latus	Saccharose (N limited)	Batch	$X_f = \sim 80$ g L^{-1}; PHB = 83% $q_{PHB} = 0.87$ g g^{-1} h^{-1}	Wang and Lee (1997)
	Saccharose (N-limited)	Fed-batch	$X_f = 111.7$ g L^{-1}; PHB = 88 % $q_{PHB} = 0.44$ g g^{-1} h^{-1}; $Y_{PHB} = 0.42$ g g^{-1}	Wang and Lee (1997)
	Saccharose	Fed-batch	$X_f = 24.7$ g L^{-1}; PHB = 63% $\mu = 0.265$ h^{-1}; $Y_{PHB} = 0.32$	Grothe and Chisti (2000)

[a] X_f, total cell concentration; PHB_f, PHB final concentration; r_{PHB}, PHB productivity; q_{PHB}, PHB specific production rate.

In MCs, specific productivity calculated as the amount of PHA produced per amount of active biomass and per hour (g COD PHA g^{-1} COD h^{-1}) is presented in the review by Serafim et al. (2008). Values are extremely dispersed, from around 0.008 to around 0.7 g COD PHA g^{-1} COD h^{-1}. Although enrichment strategies were used in these studies, this dispersion certainly reflects differences both in the proportion of PHA-storing organisms in the MCs and in the performance of the accumulation strategy adopted.

PHB storage yield on acetate substrate mostly varied between 0.53 and 0.84 g COD-PHA g^{-1} COD-acetate, the latter value representing the theoretical value calculated by Dias et al. (2005). Expressed in C mol per C mol, PHB storage yield under aerobic conditions is around 0.6 C mol PHB (C mol acetate)$^{-1}$. The lowest PHA yield values were obtained when real wastewater was used as the substrate. Serafim et al. (2008) mention a slightly higher PHA yield for the anaerobic–aerobic process than for the ADF process.

15.6 PHA STORAGE TO MINIMIZE EXCESS SLUDGE PRODUCTION IN WASTEWATER TREATMENT PLANTS

Depending on the operating conditions, cells can adopt two ways of substrate utilization, as schematized in Fig. 15.6. One way is direct growth on the substrate; the other supposes prior conversion of the substrate into a storage compound and then growth on this stored polymer. A question thus arises: Does the intermediate production of PHB induce a decrease in the net growth yield and thus a minimization of excess sludge production? To answer this question, the metabolic model developed by vanAalastvanLeeuwen et al. (1997) can be used. Using this model, Beun et al. (2000a) compared the biomass growth yield for the two routes: when direct cell growth was adopted (Y_{SX}^{max}) or when PHB was first stored and then used for cell growth (Y_{SX}^{max})$_{PHB}$. If acetate was used as the substrate, a reduction of between 10 and 4% in the net biomass yield was observed for Y_{SX}^{max}PHB compared to Y_{SX}^{max}, depending on the efficiency of the oxidative phosphorylation (δ with $1 < \delta < 3$).

It can be concluded that the PHB storage mechanism is energetically efficient, and consequently, the minimization of excess sludge production will be marginal. It must also be considered that not all the COD from wastewater could be stored as PHB.

Considering the PHB storage capacity of activated sludge, PHA accumulation in the cells should lead to an increase rather than a decrease in the amount of

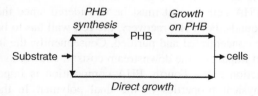

FIGURE 15.6 Two ways to use a substrate for growth.

activated sludge produced. Nevertheless, the overall carbon conversion in the wastewater treatment plant should be considered. If anaerobic digestion is present this excess sludge amount will be transformed into methane. Using the storage strategy, less oxygen will be consumed in the activated sludge process and more methane will be produced. Storing PHA on the wastewater line could therefore be an appealing solution for transferring a part of the COD to the sludge treatment line in order to form methane and to improve the overall energy balance of the treatment system (van Loosdrecht et al. 1997). However, the global requirement of treatment must be regarded, notably, when denitrification has to be performed. As stored PHA can be degraded in the aerobic tank instead of in the denitrification tank, COD will be lost for denitrification. This degradation will be exacerbated when the aerobic sludge retention time is long. Beun et al. (2000b) indicate that for a feast and famine process, the required influent COD/N ratio for denitrification can be increased by 70% because of storage. The aerobic sludge retention time should therefore be reduced. To keep the high nitrification efficiency, the use of fixed biofilm for nitrification, or a moving bed, is recommended (Odegaard et al. 2000; Paul et al. 2007).

In the case of concentrated industrial wastewater with a high COD/N ratio, PHB production will lead to a biomass with a high PHA content that can yield added value. Biotechnological polymer production occurs in aerobic processes, however, so only about 50% of the main carbon sources, and an even lower percentage of the precursors used for production of copolyesters, find their way into the desired products.

15.7   CHOICE OF PROCESS AND REACTOR DESIGN FOR PHA PRODUCTION

15.7.1   Criteria

If the PHA production processes are to be described and analyzed further, some key parameters for process characterization and optimization need to be known. First, the PHA production yield (Y_{PHA}) must be maximized to make the best use of the substrate. Y_{PHA} depends on the nature of the substrate used, on maintenance requirements, and on various environmental parameters. Second, the volumetric PHA productivity, calculated as the concentration of PHA produced per hour, determines the efficiency of the reactor volume. Aspects concerning the resistance of the cells and the inhibition by organic acids must be optimized. Third, PHA concentration or PHA cell content must be considered since these products are intracellular compounds. For PHA recovery, the cell wall has to be broken and the PHA must then be concentrated and purified. Consequently, the intracellular PHA content has a direct impact on the downstream costs: the lower its value, the higher the polymer extraction costs. Fourth, PHA composition is important because it determines the physical properties of the final polymer. In the case of MCs, competition between PHA-storing organisms and the other organisms must lead to enrichment of the MCs in the PHA-storing organisms. Given these objectives, the best process must achieve a high cell concentration with a high proportion of PHA-accumulating organisms and a high substrate conversion yield. As substrates come from complex feedstocks, the microbial population must be able to use the highest proportion of substrates and convert them to polymers with the desired composition. Optimally, the process should be robust and stable even when variations of the feedstock composition and microbial contamination occur. Generally, previous fermentation of the organic fraction of the waste is necessary in order to feed the PHA production system with the highest possible concentration of VFAs. Tohyama and Shimizu (1999), for example, proposed an innovative two-stage process based on glucose fermentation by *Lactobacillus delbrueckii* to produce lactic acid that was then used by *C. necator* for PHA accumulation. Thus, the choice between pure culture and MCs to produce PHA is still under debate. The option chosen will certainly depend on the context: the type and concentration of substrates, the sterilization requirements, and the type of products to be recovered. The substrate may often be fermented prior to PHA production, and in the following, only PHA production using MC is considered.

An analysis of the specialized literature reveals that three main processes are used to enrich a MC or to produce PHA from an MC: the anaerobic–aerobic (AN/AE) process, the feast and famine process (i.e., ADF system), and the fed-batch culture with growth limitation by a nutrient component. In this list, production processes are based mostly on enriched cultures obtained from AN/AE or ADF systems. The distinction between reactors for production and for culture selection is not always clear in the various studies. Figure 15.7 presents the possible systems for PHA production by open mixed cultures from wastewater or from lixiviates produced from solid wastes.

15.7.2 Anaerobic–Aerobic Process

The complete AN/AE system for PHA production in an activated sludge treatment plant (ASTP) is shown in Fig. 15.7. It includes a culture enrichment step performed in the ASTP (the AN/AE system) followed by an accumulation step for PHA production that is performed in a reactor fed with fermented substrate containing VFAs. PHA extraction and recovery is the last step in the process. In the AN/AE process, during the anaerobic phase there is an external growth limitation due to the absence of a mineral electron donor (oxygen or nitrate). Under these conditions the carbon source supplied is stored by PHA-accumulating bacteria (PAOs and GAOs). This system has been studied widely in the case of enhanced biological phosphorus removal involving PHA, glycogen, and poly-P storage. The PHA amount accumulated in these systems was generally low, not exceeding 20% (Satoh et al. 1996), so efforts were made to improve accumulation. Satoh et al. (1998b) proposed supplying a limited amount of oxygen to the anaerobic zone of an AN/AE system, allowing the cells to obtain energy from substrate oxidation. Maximum PHA content thus increased to 62%. After comparing the AN/AE activated sludge, a microaerophilic–aerobic activated sludge, and a fully aerobic activated sludge, Takabatake et al. (2000) found a

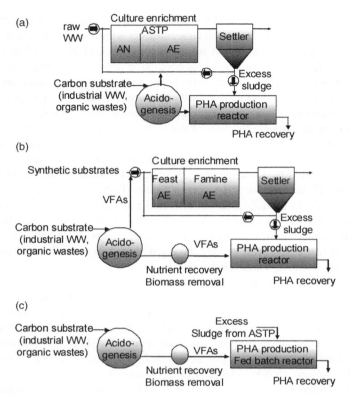

FIGURE 15.7 Different strategies for PHA production. (a) AN/AE activated sludge system with PHA production; (b) three-step system with waste acidogenesis, ADF system, and batch reactor for PHA production; and (c) direct PHA production by fed-batch reactor with nutrient limitation using excess sludge from ASTP. [Part (a) from Chua et al. (2003); part (c) from Paul (2010).]

maximum PHA content of 57% for the AN/AE system. However, under these conditions, PHA production proved to be unstable throughout the reactor operation, while a higher stable PHA content (33 to 50%) was obtained using the microaerophilic–aerobic activated sludge system. Chua et al. (2003) used the AN/AE process with SBR operating conditions consisting of a cycle of 4 h, including a supernatant decanting step (15 min), an influent feeding step (5 min), an anaerobic step (1 h), an aerobic step (2 h), and a settling period (40 min). They studied the influence of the acetate concentration in the feed, the SRT, and the pH value on the storage capacity of the selected biomass. When they used acetate-supplemented municipal wastewater, PHA contents of up to 31% of sludge dry weight were reached, while only 21% of PHA content was achieved when municipal wastewater was used without the supplement. In addition, an SRT of 3 days gave 10% more PHA content than an SRT of 10 days. Two main reviews have presented results selected from the literature and have summarized the performances of this AN/AE process (Dias et al. 2006;

Serafim et al. 2008). However, comparison remains somewhat difficult since the results may have been influenced by the different operating conditions applied in the works compiled. There is a need to find a way to dissociate an increase in PHA due to the MC enrichment in PHA-storing organisms from an increase in PHA due to metabolic forcing.

15.7.3 Aerobic Dynamic Feeding Process

ADF is a fully aerobic process where sludge is subjected to consecutive periods of external substrate excess (feast) and starvation (famine). The effect of dynamic feeding was discovered by Majone et al. (1996), who operated in an aerobic system with a previous selector for bulking control. The residence time in selectors is calculated in order to achieve complete removal of easily biodegradable COD from the liquid phase. In these conditions, the COD taken up in the selector is stored as PHA, which is then consumed in the following reactor. ADF is now widely used for culture selection and PHA production (Beun et al. 2000a; Serafim et al. 2004a; Dias et al. 2006; Dionisi et al. 2006a; Lemos et al. 2006; Serafim et al. 2008).

The most probable explanation for PHA accumulation in the ADF process is based on the "unbalanced growth" concept. Under conditions of excess of both external carbon source and electron acceptor, unbalanced growth appears to be due to internal growth limitation. Internal limitation can be the result of insufficient availability of enzymes or RNA for the growth metabolism compared to the complete substrate consumption that would be necessary for optimal growth. Consequently, PHA accumulation is achieved rather than new cell growth (Anderson and Dawes 1990; Beun et al. 2000a).

The kinetics and the effects of operating parameters on ADF performance for PHA accumulation were studied mainly using synthetic substrates [see the review by Dias et al. (2006)]. Beun et al. (2002) studied the ADF process at 20°C with addition of acetate at various concentrations. One major finding in this work was the dependence of the PHB production yield ($Y_{PHB/S}$) on SRT. $Y_{PHB/S}$ reached a high value and remained constant for SRT > 2.5 days but decreased rapidly for SRT < 2.5 days. This SRT threshold value gives a μ_{obs} of $0.017\,h^{-1}$, which is in good agreement with theoretical considerations on PHB metabolism indicating that growth must be limited to allow PHB accumulation. Another interesting point is that the specific rate, μ_{obs}, obtained in the famine period depends on the cell PHB fraction. It was concluded that in the ADF system, cells would adjust their mean fraction of PHB so that the cell growth could balance cell wastage.

ADF is operated primarily using a sequential batch reactor (SBR) process because of the high modularity of this system (Beun et al. 2002; Serafim et al. 2004a; Dionisi et al. 2005a; Albuquerque et al. 2007). The length of feast and famine periods can be fixed as desired, as the entire cycle, including sludge settling and liquid withdrawal periods, takes place in a single reactor. The substrate feeding mode also means that a high-carbon-source gradient occurs during a cycle. Moreover, in an SBR reactor, the SRT can be varied independent of the HRT, which is an important consideration when the PHA volumetric productivity is to be maximized while maintaining high PHA production yield.

In many cases, the ADF–SBR process is used primarily for culture selection to reach a high proportion of PHA-storing organisms. New cells of PHA-storing organisms can develop during the famine period by consuming the internal carbon reserve. This process should lead to culture enrichment. Then excess sludge from the ADF process is used for PHA accumulation in a batch or fed-batch reactor (Johnson et al. 2010a). The global PHA production process based on an ADF-SBR is illustrated in Fig. 15.7.

When a continuous process is required, two reactors can be set up in series, followed by a separation system for cell concentration and recycling toward the first reactor. This system has been described by Salehizadeh and van Loosdrecht (2004) and has been used in practice by Bengtsson et al. (2008a). The first reactor, of the plug-flow type, is designed to provide the feast conditions. The hydraulic residence time (HRT) is thus designed for complete depletion of the easily biodegradable carbon substrate. The second reactor, a continuously stirred tank reactor (CSTR), is designed for cell starvation and a significant PAH degradation for cell growth and maintenance. A part of the cell is withdrawn, providing the cells for PHA production, and the other part is recycled for further PHA accumulation. Performances of ADF–SBRs and continuous systems are considered similar but the continuous process should be more suitable for upgrading existing industrial wastewater treatment plants (Serafim et al. 2008).

ADF is the most studied system for PHA production by MCs. The duration of the total feast and famine cycle varies greatly from one author to another, notably because of different substrate concentrations in the feed. Nevertheless, a feast length must be chosen for complete substrate consumption, and a famine length must be long enough to allow significant depletion of the previously accumulated PHA. Examples of ADF cycles in SBRs can be found in Dias et al. (2006) or in Serafim et al. (2008), and the performances obtained with ADF systems are synthesized in various well-documented tables.

ADF in SBR is considered as the most promising strategy for industrial production of PHAs because of the high and stable PHA accumulation obtained (Salehizadeh and van Loosdrecht 2004). Optimization of the process has led to a selected culture able to reach PHA content in the cells of up to 65% when no nutrient limitation is imposed (Serafim et al. 2004b) or up to 89% when nitrogen starvation is applied (Johnson et al. 2010a). As for any transient process, the feeding rate must be controlled properly. By performing online calculation of the oxygen uptake rate or following the online pH dynamic profile, it is possible to detect the time when the carbon substrate becomes exhausted, and thus adapt the length of the feast phase. Then the famine phase can be started so as to reach a significant cell starvation time.

15.7.4 Fed-Batch Process Under Nutrient Growth Limitation

Various studies have reported that an excess of nutrients has detrimental effects on cell PHA content (Serafim et al. 2004b; Dionisi et al. 2005a; Bengtsson et al. 2008a;

Johnson et al. 2009). In fed-batch accumulation experiments, Johnson et al. (2010a) made a detailed study of the effect of the nitrogen limitation degree (i.e., starvation, ammonium limitation or ammonium excess) on PHA production. They obtained a PHB content of 89 wt% under N starvation but only 77 wt% under N limitation and concluded that nitrogen depletion in the feed is the best strategy for reaching the highest PHB percentage. This is probably true when the goal of the fed-batch process is only PHA accumulation in previously formed cells. On the other hand, if any increase in cell concentration is desired, nitrogen is required (see section 15.4) and the right N limitation must thus be found.

Fed-batch cultures are very efficient when concentrated substrates can be used. Using concentrated acetate as carbon source and controlling a phosphorus growth limitation, Paul (2010) found a PHB content of 60 wt% in 60 h, starting from an activated sludge inoculum. This experience was repeated with inocula from different activated sludges. In the case of wastewater, as low COD concentration is present, mixed liquor dilution occurs, reducing final biomass and PHB concentrations.

15.8　CULTURE SELECTION AND ENRICHMENT STRATEGIES

Substrate consumption and storage rates by activated sludge are usually considered as very low. This is because the fraction of active cells in the sludge is particularly low when the SRT values are high and also because the percentage of PHA-storing organisms may be small (Dircks et al. 2001; Beccari et al. 2002). In fact, the fraction of PHA-storing organisms in sludge can vary greatly depending on the operating conditions of the activated sludge treatment plant. Obviously, for a cost-effective industrial application of the process using mixed culture, it is worth obtaining a microbial community with a high content of PHA-storing cells. Consequently, in open cultures, the choice of the inoculum and the enrichment procedure must be addressed.

The selection procedure must lead to a microbial population where the highest proportion of cells possesses a high storage capacity but not necessarily a high PHA content. An increase in the proportion of PHA-storing organisms in an MC can be achieved by applying an adequate environmental selective pressure. Substrate must be consumed preferentially by PHA-storing organisms, which must grow faster than the other organisms. This may be possible if the substrate consumption rate for PHA production is faster than the consumption rate for growth (Reis et al. 2003; Johnson et al. 2009). Although enrichment is a key factor in improving PHA productivity and PHA production yield, very few studies have quantified the real increase in PHA production capacity (Dionisi et al. 2004b; Serafim et al. 2004a). The existing studies focus on either the AN/AE or ADF–SBR process.

AN/AE　Enrichment of PAOs and GAOs has been achieved in enhanced biological phosphorus removal systems or equivalent systems. Nevertheless, GAOs are believed to be more robust, reaching higher PHA contents and easily producing copolymers of P(3HB:3HV) from simple carbon substrates (Dai et al. 2007; Oehmen et al. 2007). Dai et al. (2007) obtained a microbial population composed of 75% of GAOs containing the copolymer 70 : 30 P(3HB:3HV), but the PHA content of the biomass reached only 14% of the dry biomass. Bengtsson et al. (2008b) selected a biomass with GAOs producing the complex polymer 33 : 60 : 5 P(3HB:3HV:3H2MV) with a PHA content of up to 30% of the cell dry weight in anaerobic conditions and up to 25% of the cell dry weight in aerobic conditions. Pisco et al. (2008) worked with fermented molasses and obtained P(3HB:3HV:3HHx) and a PHA content of 37%. More recently, Bengtsson (2009) has used an SBR reactor with anaerobic–aerobic sequences to enrich the mixed microbial culture in GAOs. Elevated temperature (30°C) and phosphorus limitation (COD/P = 107) led to unfavorable conditions for PAOs, which were thus found in very low concentrations in the MC. This confirms previous findings by Lopez-Vazquez et al. (2007). Then a value of 49% PHA in total suspended solids (TSS), with a copolymer containing 3HB and 27 mol% 3HV, was obtained under anaerobic conditions and using acetate as a carbon source in a batch reactor developed by Bengtsson (2009). In this case, high anaerobic production of PHA was possible because of the high glycogen content (36% of TSS) in the cells sampled from the SBR. Operating conditions of the SBR could thus be optimized to increase the intracellular glycogen content, and so the potential for anaerobic PHA accumulation. When similar batch productions were conducted under aerobic conditions, PHA contents of up to 60% of TSS with a maximum specific production rate of $0.44 \, C \, mol \, C \, mol^{-1} \, h^{-1}$ were obtained.

In conclusion, compared to the ADF process, selection of GAOs for mixed-culture PHA production leads to specificities in terms of PHA content, process stability, microbial mixed-culture enrichment, and downstream recovery.

ADF   The clear distinction between the use of ADF for cell selection or for PHA production is relatively recent (Serafim et al. 2008). Selection under ADF conditions is based, first, on the preferential consumption of the substrate by PHA-storing organisms, and second on their capacity for growth on polymers accumulated previously. Both storage and growth must be supported. Under dynamic feeding, the storage metabolism is dominant ($\geq 70\%$ on a C mol basis) compared to growth (Majone et al. 1999; Serafim et al. 2004b). This is because during the conversion of acetate to PHA, the energy required for storage is lower than the energy required for biomass growth (Beun et al. 2000a). Consequently, a higher specific substrate uptake rate can be achieved by PHA-storing microorganisms in the feast condition, allowing selection of these organisms by SRT during the process (Reis et al. 2003). The real improvement in the PHA production potential is not clearly quantified in the literature. For example, depending on the inoculum and the operating parameters of the ADF process, the optimal experiment duration required to maximize the concentration of PHA-storing organisms is neither given nor studied. Moreover, very few studies have provided insights into the microbiology associated with PHA production in the ADF process (Dionisi et al. 2005a; Serafim et al. 2006). However, a PHA content of up to 89% dry weight has been obtained in fed-batch production under nitrogen starvation (Johnson et al. 2010a). As this value is close to the maximum PHA cell content reported for pure cultures, a very high proportion of storing organisms can obviously be selected by the ADF process.

Most often, the selection procedure has used single synthetic substrates, but some studies relate the use of mixed substrates (Dionisi et al. 2004a) or real complex substrates Dionisi et al. 2005b; Bengtsson et al. 2008a). These works have been reviewed by Dias et al. (2006).

Supplementation in nutrients should be given during the enrichment period in order to make new cell growth efficient. This is particularly true when low SRT is maintained to produce cells for the accumulation step. A decrease in nutrients will affect cell productivity and enrichment. Temperature must also be controlled. As it greatly influences biological kinetics, a change in this parameter will change the ratio between the feast time and the famine time. This may affect the enrichment capacity of the ADF process. Examples of the effect of temperature on culture enrichment can be found in Johnson et al. (2010b).

15.9 PHA QUALITY AND RECOVERY

As seen previously, the type of VFAs used to feed an MC greatly influences the PHA composition and thus determines the mechanical and thermal properties of the polymer extracted. Consequently, the VFA spectra obtained after fermentation of wastes and wastewater must be controlled. Tables 15.3 and 15.4 show the potential offered for the production of copolymers containing at least HB and HV from a mixture of acetate, propionate, butyrate, and valerate obtained from fermented wastes.

It is known that recovery and purification of the polymer account for a huge part of the PHA total production cost. Consequently, PHA recovery is a key issue to make the global process economically and environmentally acceptable. Recovery methods for PHAs of various purities from microorganisms have received attention (Moo-Young et al. 1998; Tamer et al. 1998a,b). The method to be chosen must lead to high extraction yield and high polymer purity, and PHA degradation must be minimized or nullified during extraction. Moreover, it must be a simple, fairly cheap process that does not lead to environmental or health hazards.

Two goals are targeted for efficient recovery of the internal stored polymers: cell membrane disruption and solubilization of the polymer for its separation, concentration, and purification. Cell disruption may be achieved through the use of solvents, acids, alkalis, surfactants, enzymes, heat shock, or mechanical processes (Lee 1996b; Choi and Lee 1999a). A high cellular PHA content may favor the PHA recovery process because a smaller quantity of chemicals would be required and also because cells accumulating large amounts of PHA become very fragile (Lee et al. 1994; Lee 1996a; Lee and Lee 1996). Extraction and cell disruption can also be combined.

The most popular recovery methods are certainly the solvent extraction method, employing chloroform and methanol, or the sodium hypochlorite method, which solubilizes the cell material. In contrast to the solvent-based method, the use of sodium hypochlorite, with its strong oxidant property, leads to polymer degradation. The release of chlorine also represents a significant drawback. Sodium hydroxide appears as a method of choice for PHA recovery because of its low cost and its good recovery yield of highly purified PHA. Low endotoxin levels have also been reported, which are more important for medical and food uses (Choi and Lee 1999a; Lee et al. 1999). With these conventional methods, recovery efficiencies of 95 to 97% are generally reported for pure cultures. Although there is no evidence for it yet, some differences in sensitivity to the recovery treatment processes may exist between pure cells and mixed cells from MCs.

More gentle methods are under development, such as the use of enzymatic treatments that may be combined with heat shock or the use of dispersion solutions (such as the anionic detergent sodium dodecyl sulfate). Proteases such as the commercial alcalase prepared with subtilisin (a bacterial enzyme with broad protein digestion specificity) or peptidoglycan hydrolases such as lysosyme are often used (Kapritchkoff et al. 2006). Induction of lysis by phage infection has also been used for cell wall destruction.

15.10   INDUSTRIAL DEVELOPMENTS

To our knowledge up to now there has been no full-scale application of PHB production from wastes or concentrated wastewater using MCs. However, promising research on real effluents and wastes has recently been reported for various feedstocks: food waste (Rhu et al. 2003), olive and palm oils (Dionisi et al. 2005b; Din et al. 2006; Beccari et al. 2009), mill and paper mill effluents (Bengtsson et al. 2008a,b), sugarcane molasses (Albuquerque et al. 2007, 2008, 2010a,b), fruit and tomato cannery effluents (Gurieff 2007; Liu et al. 2008), or municipal sludges (Coats et al. 2007b; Mengmeng et al. 2009; Paul 2010). Practical demonstrations of the three-step concept described in Fig. 15.7 and development of technologies are in progress. Very recently, PHA production from fermented primary and waste activated sludges has received attention from both research laboratories and wastewater treatment companies (Coats et al. 2007b; Gurieff 2007; Paul 2010). The use of fermented sludge for PHA production is very attractive because it is a relatively abundant source of waste organics that induces high treatment and disposal costs for elimination when methane production is not desired. Interestingly, the financial feasibility of converting primary sludge to PHA has been demonstrated by Gurieff and Lant (2007).

At the industrial scale, either MC or enriched culture with a specific PHA producer can be used. For example, Carole et al. (2004), in their study, mentioned the interest shown by I-PHA BioPolymers, a Hong Kong–based company, for a two-step process developed at the Hawaii Natural Energy Institute, University of Hawaii. The aim of this two-step process is to transform wastes into PHA, which must be produced from around 60% of the initial organic material, the remaining 40% leading to fertilizers. The PHA production step used an enriched culture of *C. necator* and led to a PHA content of 72.6 wt%. It was fed with dialyzed VFAs produced by fermentation of the waste. The estimated PHA production cost was between \$2.20 and \$4.40 kg^{-1}. The use of pure culture of *C. necator* and MC is also being compared in studies at INSA–University of Toulouse, France (Paul 2010).

The high energy consumption required for aeration, mixing, and other operations necessary for each process of the PHA production chain will entail high costs and high environmental impacts. In contrast to PHA production with pure culture and refined substrate, this high cost is caused by low cellular and PHA concentrations, due to low substrate concentrations. Continuous processes should thus be preferred to fed-batch culture when the feed used is too diluted.

From the few reported studies dealing with the use of complex wastes and from our knowledge of PHA metabolism, it is reasonable to think that product quality (i.e., the polymer composition and properties) could be controlled by using the right organic substrate mixture. This mixture must therefore be produced by a previous digestion process (biological, chemical, or physical). Special attention must be paid to digestion processes in order to deliver the right VFA spectra. For example, pH and redox potential must be controlled during the acidogenic step of the fermentation process. Supplementation of specific VFA could also be carried out and no polymer degradation should occur during PHA recovery.

In conclusion, complex waste fermentation followed by PHA production may be an attractive way of adding value to organic matter while treating the corresponding pollution, even if no reduction of the amount of sludge is achieved. Under similar conditions, the PHA production route is certainly complementary to anaerobic digestion with methane production. More research and development work is needed, however, to better understand the effect of complex organics and nutrients on PHA production potential. The control of MCs for PHA production should also be improved together with the sustainability of the PHA recovery process. In the case of primary sludge exploitation and considering life-cycle assessment and financial analysis, Gurieff and Lant (2007) believe that the next improvement should target the PHA production process to make it more competitive. Although this study was directed toward primary sludge, the following recommendations can obviously be applied to other feedstocks:

- Increase the biodegradability of wastes to be fermented to obtain higher organic matter concentrations; adequate pretreatment can be used to improve the organics availability.
- Increase the organic load for PHA production. This can be achieved by centralizing biosolids management infrastructure.
- Decrease the energy cost, which accounts for the majority of process costs and environmental impact: cheap renewable energy should be used.
- Manage the quality control and recovery of PHA.

REFERENCES

Albuquerque M. G. E., Eiroa M., Torres C., Nunes B. R., Reis M. A. M. (2007) Strategies for the development of a side stream process for polyhydroxyalkanoate (PHA) production from sugar cane molasses. *Journal of Biotechnology* **130**(4), 411–421.

Albuquerque M. G. E., Torres C., Bengtsson S., Werker A., Reis M. A. M. (2008) Strategies for culture selection in a three-stage PHA production process from sugar cane molasses. In: Proceedings II of the 4th IWA Specialised Conference on Sequencing Batch Reactor Technology (SBR4) Rome, April 7–10, pp.; 2–4.

Albuquerque M. G. E., Bengtsson S., Martino V., Pollet E., Reis M. A. M. (2010a) Eco-engineering of mixed microbial cultures to develop a cost-effective bioplastic (PHA) production process from a surplus feedstock—sugar molasses. *Journal of Biotechnology* **150**, S70–S70.

Albuquerque M. G. E., Concas S., Bengtsson S., Reis M. A. M. (2010b). Mixed culture polyhydroxyalkanoates production from sugar molasses: the use of a 2-stage CSTR system for culture selection. *Bioresource Technology* **101**(18), 7123–7133.

Anderson A. J., Dawes E. A. (1990) Occurrence, metabolism, metabolic role, and industrial uses of bacterial polyhydroxyalkanoates. *Microbiological Reviews* **54**(4), 450–472.

Anderson A. J., Haywood G. W., Dawes E. A. (1990) Biosynthesis and composition of bacterial poly(hydroxyalkanoates). *International Journal of Biological Macromolecules* **12**(2), 102–105.

Anderson A. J., Williams D. R., Taidi B., Dawes E. A., Ewing D. F. (1992) Studies on copolyester synthesis by *Rhodococcus-ruber* and factors influencing the molecular mass of polyhydroxybutyrate accumulated by *Methylobacterium-extorquens* and *Alcaligenes-eutrophus*. *FEMS Microbiology Reviews* **103**(2–4), 93–101.

Aragao G. M. F., Lindley N. D., Uribelarrea J. L., Pareilleux A. (1996). Maintaining a controlled residual growth capacity increases the production of polyhydroxyalkanoate copolymers by *Alcaligenes eutrophus*. *Biotechnology Letters* **18**(8), 937–942.

Beccari M., Dionisi D., Giuliani A., Majone M., Ramadori R. (2002) Effect of different carbon sources on aerobic storage by activated sludge. *Water Science and Technology* **45**(6), 157–168.

Beccari M., Bertin L., Dionisi D., Fava F., Lampis S., Majone M., Valentino F., Vallini G., Villano M. (2009) Exploiting olive oil mill effluents as a renewable resource for production of biodegradable polymers through a combined anaerobic–aerobic process. *Journal of Chemical Technology and Biotechnology* **84**(6), 901–908.

Bengtsson S. (2009) The utilization of glycogen accumulating organisms for mixed culture production of polyhydroxyalkanoates. *Biotechnology and Bioengineering* **104**(4), 698–708.

Bengtsson S., Werker A., Christensson M., Welander T. (2008a) Production of polyhydrox-yalkanoates by activated sludge treating a paper mill wastewater. *Bioresource Technology* **99**(3), 509–516.

Bengtsson S., Werker A., Welander T. (2008b) Production of polyhydroxyalkanoates by glycogen accumulating organisms treating a paper mill wastewater. *Water Science and Technology* **58**(2), 323–330.

Beun J. J., Paletta F., van Loosdrecht M. C. M., Heijnen J. J. (2000a) Stoichiometry and kinetics of poly-beta-hydroxybutyrate metabolism in aerobic, slow growing, activated sludge cultures. *Biotechnology and Bioengineering* **67**(4), 379–389.

Beun J. J., Verhoef E. V., van Loosdrecht M. C. M., Heijnen J. J. (2000b) Stoichiometry and kinetics of poly-beta-hydroxybutyrate metabolism under denitrifying conditions in activated sludge cultures. *Biotechnology and Bioengineering* **68**(5), 496–507.

Beun J. J., Dircks K., Van Loosdrecht M. C. M., Heijnen J. J. (2002) Poly-beta-hydroxybutyrate metabolism in dynamically fed mixed microbial cultures. *Water Research* **36**(5), 1167–1180.

Braunegg G., Bona R., Koller M. (2004) Sustainable polymer production. *Polymer Plastics Technology and Engineering* **43**(6), 1779–1793.

Byrom D. (1987) Polymer synthesis by microorganisms: technology and economics. *Trends in Biotechnology* **5**(9), 246–250.

Carole T. M., Pellegrino J., Paster M. D. (2004) Opportunities in the industrial biobased products industry. *Applied Biochemistry and Biotechnology* **113**, 871–885.

Carta F., Beun J. J., van Loosdrecht M. C. M., Heijnen J. J. (2001) Simultaneous storage and degradation of PHB and glycogen in activated sludge cultures. *Water Research* **35**(11), 2693–2701.

Cech J. S., Chudoba J. (1983) Influence of accumulation capacity of activated-sludge microorganisms on kinetics of glucose removal. *Water Research* **17**(6), 659–666.

Cech J. S., Hartman P. (1990) Glucose-induced break down of enhanced biological phosphate removal. *Environmental Technology* **11**(7), 651–656.

Cech J. S., Hartman P. (1993) Competition between polyphosphate and polysaccharide accumulating bacteria in enhanced biological phosphate removal systems. *Water Research* **27**(7), 1219–1225.

Choi J. I., Lee S. Y. (1997) Process analysis and economic evaluation for poly(3-hydroxybutyrate) production by fermentation. *Bioprocess Engineering* **17**(6), 335–342.

Choi J. I., Lee S. Y. (1999a) Efficient and economical recovery of poly(3-hydroxybutyrate) from recombinant *Escherichia coli* by simple digestion with chemicals. *Biotechnology and Bioengineering* **62**(5), 546–553.

Choi J. I., Lee S. Y. (1999b) High-level production of poly(3-hydroxybutyrate-*co*-3-hydroxyvalerate) by fed-batch culture of recombinant *Escherichia coli*. *Applied and Environmental Microbiology* **65**(10), 4363–4368.

Chua A. S. M., Takabatake H., Satoh H., Mino T. (2003) Production of polyhydroxyalkanoates (PHA) by activated sludge treating municipal wastewater: effect of pH, sludge retention time (SRT), and acetate concentration in influent. *Water Research* **37**(15), 3602–3611.

Coats E. R., Loge F. J., Smith W. A., Thompson D. N., Wolcott M. P. (2007a) Functional stability of a mixed microbial consortium producing PHA from waste carbon sources. *Applied Biochemistry and Biotechnology* **137**, 909–925.

Coats E. R., Loge F. J., Wolcott M. P., Englund K., McDonald A. G. (2007b) Synthesis of polyhydroxyalkanoates in municipal wastewater treatment. *Water Environment Research* **79**(12), 2396–2403.

Dai Y., Yuan Z. G., Wang X. L., Oehmen A., Keller J. (2007) Anaerobic metabolism of *Defluviicoccus vanus* related glycogen accumulating organisms (GAOs) with acetate and propionate as carbon sources. *Water Research* **41**(9), 1885–1896.

Dai Y., Lambert L., Yuan Z., Keller J. (2008) Characterisation of polyhydroxyalkanoate copolymers with controllable four-monomer composition. *Journal of Biotechnology* **134**(1–2), 137–145.

Dias J. M. L., Lemos P. C., Serafim L. S., Oliveira C., Eiroa M., Albuquerque M. G. E., Ramos A. M., Oliveira R., Reis M. A. M. (2006) Recent advances in polyhydroxyalkanoate production by mixed aerobic cultures: from the substrate to the final product. *Macromolecular Bioscience* **6**(11), 885–906.

Din M. F. M., Ujang Z., van Loosdrecht M. C. M., Ahmad A., Sairan M. F. (2006) Optimization of nitrogen and phosphorus limitation for better biodegradable plastic production and organic removal using single fed-batch mixed cultures and renewable resources. *Water Science and Technology* **53**(6), 15–20.

Dionisi D., Majone M., Papa V., Beccari M. (2004a) Biodegradable polymers from organic acids by using activated sludge enriched by aerobic periodic feeding. *Biotechnology and Bioengineering* **85**(6), 569–579.

Dionisi D., Renzi V., Majone M., Beccari M., Ramadori R. (2004b) Storage of substrate mixtures by activated sludges under dynamic conditions in anoxic or aerobic environments. *Water Research* **38**(8), 2196–2206.

Dionisi D., Beccari M., Di Gregorio S., Majone M., Papini M. P., Vallini G. (2005a) Storage of biodegradable polymers by an enriched microbial community in a sequencing batch reactor operated at high organic load rate. *Journal of Chemical Technology and Biotechnology* **80**(11), 1306–1318.

Dionisi D., Carucci G., Papini M. P., Riccardi C., Majone M., Carrasco F. (2005b) Olive oil mill effluents as a feedstock for production of biodegradable polymers. *Water Research* **39**(10), 2076–2084.

Dionisi D., Majone M., Levantesi C., Bellani A., Fuoco A. (2006a) Effect of feed length on settleability, substrate uptake and storage in a sequencing batch reactor treating an industrial wastewater. *Environmental Technology* **27**(8), 901–908.

Dionisi D., Majone M., Vallini G., Di Gregorio S., Beccari M. (2006b) Effect of the applied organic load rate on biodegradable polymer production by mixed microbial cultures in a sequencing batch reactor. *Biotechnology and Bioengineering* **93**(1), 76–88.

Dircks K., Henze M., van Loosdrecht M. C. M., Mosbaek H., Aspegren H. (2001) Storage and degradation of poly-beta-hydroxybutyrate in activated sludge under aerobic conditions. *Water Research* **35**(9), 2277–2285.

Du G. C., Chen J., Yu J., Lun S. Y. (2001) Kinetic studies on poly-3-hydroxybutyrate formation by *Ralstonia eutropha* in a two-stage continuous culture system. *Process Biochemistry* **37**(3), 219–227.

Eggink G., Preusting H., Huijberts G., Huisman G., Witholt B. 1992. Synthesis of poly-3-hydroxy-alkanoates (phas) by pseudomonase–substrates polymerases, bioreactor configurations, and products. Abstracts of Papers of the American Chemical Society 204, 73-PMSE.

Gaudin P. (1998) Contribution de la synthèse de poly-β-hydroxybutyrate (PHB) à la croissance de *Ralstonia eutropha*. Doctorat, INSA, Toulouse, France.

Goel R., Mino T., Satoh H., Matsuo T. (1999) Modeling hydrolysis processes considering intracellular storage. *Water Science and Technology* **39**(1), 97–105.

Grothe E., Chisti Y. (2000) Poly(β-hydroxybutyric acid) thermoplastic production by *Alcaligenes latus*: behavior of fed-batch cultures. *Bioprocess and Biosystems Engineering* **22**(5), 441.

Gurieff N. B. (2007) Production of biodegradable polyhydroxyalkanoate polymers using advanced biological wastewater treatment process technology. University of Queensland, Australia.

Gurieff N., Lant P. (2007) Comparative life cycle assessment and financial analysis of mixed culture polyhydroxyalkanoate production. *Bioresource Technology* **98**, 3393–3403.

Hollender J., van der Krol D., Kornberger L., Gierden E., Dott W. (2002) Effect of different carbon sources on the enhanced biological phosphorus removal in a sequencing batch reactor. *World Journal of Microbiology and Biotechnology* **18**(4), 355–360.

Hrabak O. (1992) Industrial-production of poly-beta-hydroxybutyrate. *FEMS Microbiology Reviews* **103**(2–4), 251–255.

Johnson K., Jiang Y., Kleerebezem R., Muyzer G., van Loosdrecht M. C. M. (2009) Enrichment of a mixed bacterial culture with a high polyhydroxyalkanoate storage capacity. *Biomacromolecules* **10**(4), 670–676.

Johnson K., Kleerebezem R., van Loosdrecht M. C. M. (2010a) Influence of the C/N ratio on the performance of polyhydroxybutyrate (PHB) producing sequencing batch reactors at short SRTs. *Water Research* **44**(7), 2141–2152.

Johnson K., van Geest J., Kleerebezem R., van Loosdrecht M. C. M. (2010b) Short- and long-term temperature effects on aerobic polyhydroxybutyrate producing mixed cultures. *Water Research* **44**(6), 1689–1700.

Kapritchkoff F. M., Viotti A. P., Alli R. C. P., Zuccolo M., Pradella J. G. C., Maiorano A. E., Miranda E. A., Bonomi A. (2006) Enzymatic recovery and purification of polyhydroxybutyrate produced by *Ralstonia eutropha*. *Journal of Biotechnology* **122**(4), 453–462.

Kim B. S., Lee S. C., Lee S. Y., Chang H. N., Chang Y. K., Woo S. I. (1994) Production of poly(3-hydroxybutyric-*co*-3-hydroxyvaleric acid) by fed-batch culture of *Alcaligenes-eutrophus* with substrate control using online glucose analyzer. *Enzyme and Microbial Technology* **16**(7), 556–561.

Kim D. Y., Kim H. W., Chung M. G., Rhee Y. H. (2007) Biosynthesis, modification, and biodegradation of bacterial medium-chain-length polyhydroxyalkanoates. *Journal of Microbiology* **45**(2), 87–97.

Kleerebezem R., van Loosdrecht M. C. M. (2007) Mixed culture biotechnology for bioenergy production. *Current Opinion in Biotechnology* **18**(3), 207–212.

Koller M., Salerno A., Dias M., Reiterer A., Braunegg G. (2010) Modern biotechnological polymer synthesis: a review. *Food Technology and Biotechnology* **48**(3), 255–269.

Kothuis B., Schelleman F. (1998). Environmental economic comparison of biotechnology with traditional alternatives. In: Meesters KHP, editor. Production of poly-(3-hydroxyalkanoates) from waste streams. Delft: Tudelft Press; p. 4.

Lee I. Y., Kim M. K., Chang H. N., Park Y. H. (1994) Effects of propionate on accumulation of poly(beta-hydroxybutyrate-*co*-beta-hydroxyvalerate) and excretion of pyruvate in *Alcaligenes-eutrophus*. *Biotechnology Letters* **16**(6), 611–616.

Lee S. Y. (1996a) Bacterial polyhydroxyalkanoates. *Biotechnology and Bioengineering* **49**(1), 1–14.

Lee S. Y. (1996b) Plastic bacteria? Progress and prospects for polyhydroxyalkanoate production in bacteria. *Trends in Biotechnology* **14**(11), 431–438.

Lee S. Y. (1997) *E. coli* moves into the plastic age. *Nature Biotechnology* **15**(1), 17–18.

Lee S. Y., Choi J. I. (1998) Effect of fermentation performance on the economics of poly(3-hydroxybutyrate) production by *Alcaligenes latus*. *Polymer Degradation and Stability* **59**(1–3), 387–393.

Lee S. Y., Choi J-i. (1999) Production and degradation of polyhydroxyalkanoates in waste environment. *Waste Management* **19**(2), 133.

Lee S. Y., Choi J. I., Wong H. H. (1999) Recent advances in polyhydroxyalkanoate production by bacterial fermentation: mini-review. *International Journal of Biological Macromolecules* **25**(1–3), 31–36.

Lee Y., Lee S. Y. (1996) Enhanced production of poly(3-hydroxybutyrate) by filamentation-suppressed recombinant *Escherichia coli* in a defined medium. *Journal of Environmental Polymer Degradation* **4**(2), 131–134.

Lemos P. C., Serafim L. S., Reis M. A. M. (2006) Synthesis of polyhydroxyalkanoates from different short-chain fatty acids by mixed cultures submitted to aerobic dynamic feeding. *Journal of Biotechnology* **122**(2), 226–238.

Li R., Zhang H. X., Qi Q. S. (2007) The production of polyhydroxyalkanoates in recombinant *Escherichia coli*. *Bioresource Technology* **98**(12), 2313–2320.

Liu H. Y., Hall P. V., Darby J. L., Coats E. R., Green P. G., Thompson D. E., Loge F. J. (2008) Production of polyhydroxyalkanoate during treatment of tomato cannery wastewater. *Water Environment Research* **80**(4), 367–372.

Lopez-Vazquez C. M., Song Y. I., Hooijmans C. M., Brdjanovic D., Moussa M. S., Gijzen H. J., van Loosdrecht M. C. M. (2007) Short-term temperature effects on the anaerobic metabolism of glycogen accumulating organisms. *Biotechnology and Bioengineering* **97**(3), 483–495.

Majone M., Massanisso P., Carucci A., Lindrea K., Tandoi V. (1996) Influence of storage on kinetic selection to control aerobic filamentous bulking. *Water Science and Technology* **34**(5–6), 223–232.

Majone M., Dircks K., Beun J. J. (1999) Aerobic storage under dynamic conditions in activated sludge processes: the state of the art. *Water Science and Technology* **39**(1), 61–73.

Majone M., Beccari M., Dionisi D., Levantesi C., Renzi V. (2001) Role of storage phenomena on removal of different substrates during pre-denitrification. *Water Science and Technology* **43**(3), 151–158.

Mato T., Ben M., Kennes C., Veiga M. C. (2008) PHA production using brewery wastewater. 4th Sequencing Batch Reactor Conference Rome, April 7–10, pp. 59–66.

Mengmeng C., Hong C., Qingliang Z., Shirley S. N., Jie R. (2009) Optimal production of polyhydroxyalkanoates (PHA) in activated sludge fed by volatile fatty acids (VFAs) generated from alkaline excess sludge fermentation. *Bioresource Technology* **100**(3), 1399–1405.

Mino T., Van Loosdrecht M. C. M., Heijnen J. J. (1998) Microbiology and biochemistry of the enhanced biological phosphate removal process. *Water Research* **32**(11), 3193–3207.

Moo-Young M., Tamer L. M., Chisti Y. (1998) *A process for low-cost recovery of microbially produced poly(beta-hydroxybutyric acid) thermoplastic*. Abstracts of Papers of the American Chemical Society **216**, 185-BIOT.

Odegaard H., Gisvold B., Helness H., Sjovold F., Zuliang L. (2000) High rate biological/chemical treatment based on the moving bed biofilm process combined with coagulation. *Chemical Water and Wastewater Treatment* **6**, 245–255.

Oehmen A., Lemos P. C., Carvalho G., Yuan Z. G., Keller J., Blackall L. L., Reis M. A. M. (2007) Advances in enhanced biological phosphorus removal: from micro to macro scale. *Water Research* **41**(11), 2271–2300.

Page W. J., Knosp O. (1989) Hyperproduction of poly-beta-hydroxybutyrate during exponential-growth of *Azotobacter-vinelandiiuwd*. *Applied Environmental Microbiology* **55**(6), 1334–1339.

Paul E. (2010). PHB production under phosphorus limitation in fed batch culture inoculated directly with activated sludge. Unpublished report, INSA, Toulouse, France.

Paul E., Wolff D. B., Ochoa J. C., da Costa R. H. R. (2007) Recycled and virgin plastic carriers in hybrid reactors for wastewater treatment. *Water Environment Research* **79**(7), 765–774.

Pisco A. R., Bengtsson S., Werker A., Reis M. A. M., Lemos P. C. (2008) Use of industrial by-products for polyhydroxyalkanoates production by glycogen-accumulating organisms. Proceedings of the 5th IWA Leading-Edge Conference on Water and Wastewater Technologies, Zurich, Switzerland, June, 1–4.

Pisco A. R., Bengtsson S., Werker A., Reis M. A. M., Lemos P. C. (2009) Community structure evolution and enrichment of glycogen-accumulating organisms producing polyhydroxyalkanoates from fermented molasses. *Applied Environmental Microbiology* **75**(14), 4676–4686.

Reddy C. S. K., Ghai R., Kalia V. C. (2003) Polyhydroxyalkanoates: an overview. *Bioresource Technology* **87**(2), 137–146.

Reis M. A. M., Serafim L. S., Lemos P. C., Ramos A. M., Aguiar F. R., van Loosdrecht M. C. M. (2003) Production of polyhydroxyalkanoates by mixed microbial cultures. *Bioprocess and Biosystems Engineering* **25**(6), 377–385.

Rhu D. H., Lee W. H., Kim J. Y., Choi E. (2003) Polyhydroxyalkanoate (PHA) production from waste. *Water Science and Technology* **48**(8), 221–228.

Salehizadeh H., van Loosdrecht M. C. M. (2004) Production of polyhydroxyalkanoates by mixed culture: recent trends and biotechnological importance. *Biotechnology Advances* **22**(3), 261–279.

Satoh H., Mino T., Matsuo T. (1992) Uptake of organic substrates and accumulation of polyhydroxyalkanoates linked with glycolysis of intracellular carbohydrates under anaerobic conditions in the biological excess phosphate removal processes. *Water Science and Technology* **26**(5–6), 933–942.

Satoh H., Mino T., Matsuo T. (1994) Deterioration of enhanced biological phosphorus removal by the domination of microorganisms without polyphosphate accumulation. *Water Science and Technology* **30**(6), 203–211.

Satoh H., Iwamoto Y., Mino T., Matsuo T. (1998a) Activated sludge as a possible source of biodegradable plastic. *Water Science and Technology* **38**(2), 103–109.

Satoh H., Ramey W. D., Koch F. A., Oldham W. K., Mino T., Matsuo T. (1996) Anaerobic substrate uptake by the enhanced biological phosphorus removal activated sludge treating real sewage. *Water Science and Technology* **34**(1–2), 9–16.

Satoh H., Mino T., Matsuo T. (1998b) Anaerobic uptake of glutamate and aspartate by enhanced biological phosphorus removal activated sludge. *Water Science and Technology* **37**(4–5), 579–582.

Satoh H., Mino T., Matsuo T. (1999) PHA production by activated sludge. *International Journal of Biological Macromolecules* **25**(1–3), 105–109.

Senior P. J., Dawes E. A. (1971) Poly-beta-hydroxybutyrate biosynthesis and regulation of glucose metabolim in *Azotobacter-beijerinckii*. *Biochemical Journal* **125**(1), 55–66.

Serafim L. S., Lemos P. C., Oliveira R., Ramos A. M., Reis M. A. M. (2004a) High storage of PHB by mixed microbial cultures under aerobic dynamic feeding conditions. European Symposium on Environmental Biotechnology, pp. 479–482.

Serafim L. S., Lemos P. C., Oliveira R., Reis M. A. M. (2004b) Optimization of polyhydroxybutyrate production by mixed cultures submitted to aerobic dynamic feeding conditions. *Biotechnology and Bioengineering* **87**(2), 145–160.

Serafim L. S., Lemos P. C., Rossetti S., Levantesi C., Tandoi V., Reis M. A. M. (2006) Microbial community analysis with a high PHA storage capacity. *Water Science and Technology* **54**(1), 183–188.

Serafim L. S., Lemos P. C., Albuquerque M. G. E., Reis M. A. M. (2008) Strategies for PHA production by mixed cultures and renewable waste materials. *Applied Microbiology and Biotechnology* **81**(4), 615–628.

Takabatake H., Satoh H., Mino T., Matsuo T. (2000) Recovery of biodegradable plastics from activated sludge process. *Water Science and Technology* **42**(3–4), 351–356.

Tamer I. M., Moo-Young M., Chisti Y. (1998a) Disruption of *Alcaligenes latus* for recovery of poly(beta-hydroxybutyric acid): Comparison of high-pressure homogenization, bead milling, and chemically induced lysis. *Industrial and Engineering Chemistry Research* **37**(5), 1807–1814.

Tamer I. M., Moo-Young M., Chisti Y. (1998b) Optimization of poly(beta-hydroxybutyric acid) recovery from *Alcaligenes latus*: combined mechanical and chemical treatments. *Bioprocess Engineering* **19**(6), 459–468.

Tohyama M., Shimizu K. (1999) Control of a mixed culture of *Lactobacillus delbrueckii* and *Ralstonia eutropha* for the production of PHB from glucose via lactate. *Biochemical Engineering Journal* **4**(1), 45.

Tsuge T., Tanaka K., Ishizaki A. (2001) Development of a novel method for feeding a mixture of L-lactic acid and acetic acid in fed-batch culture of *Ralstonia eutropha* for poly-D-3-hydroxybutyrate production. *Journal of Bioscience and Bioengineering* **91**(6), 545–550.

vanAalastvanLeeuwen M. A., Pot M. A., van Loosdrecht M. C. M., Heijnen J. J. (1997) Kinetic modeling of poly(beta-hydroxybutyrate) production and consumption by *Paracoccus pantotrophus* under dynamic substrate supply. *Biotechnology and Bioengineering* **55**(5), 773–782.

van Loosdrecht M. C. M., Pot M. A., Heijnen J. J. (1997) Importance of bacterial storage polymers in bioprocess. *Water Science and Technology* **35**, 41–47.

Vollbrecht D., Schlegel H. G. (1979) Excretion of metabolites of hydrogen bacteria: 3. D(−)-3-hydroxybutanoate. *European Journal of Applied Microbiology and Biotechnology* **7**(3), 259–266.

Wallen L., Rohwedder W. (1974) Poly-β-hydroxyalkanoate from activated sludge. *Environment Science and Technology* **8**, 576–579.

Wang F., Lee S. Y. (1997) Poly(3-hydroxybutyrate) production with high productivity and high polymer content by a fed-batch culture of *Alcaligenes latus* under nitrogen limitation. *Applied Environmental Microbiology* **63**(9), 3703–3706.

Witholt B., Kessler B. (1999) Perspectives of medium chain length poly (hydroxyalkanoates), a versatile set of bacterial bioplastics. *Current Opinion in Biotechnology* **10**(3), 279–285.

Yu J. (2001) Production of PHA from starchy wastewater via organic acids. *Journal of Biotechnology* **86**, 105–112.

INDEX

Biological Sludge Minimization and Biomaterials/Bioenergy Recovery Technologies, First Edition.
Edited by Etienne Paul and Yu Liu.
© 2012 John Wiley & Sons, Inc. Published 2012 by John Wiley & Sons, Inc.

Printed and bound by CPI Group (UK) Ltd, Croydon, CR0 4YY

16/04/2025

14658589-0002